HEADLAND'S THERAPEUTICS.

The Action of Medicines; or, the mode in which Therapeutic Agents introduced into the Stomach produce their peculiar Effects on the Animal Economy. Being the Prize Essay to which the Medical Society of London awarded the Fothergillian Gold Medal for 1852. 8vo. cloth, $1 50.

"A text-book of the action of medicines. It is a well-timed publication."—*Association Journal.*

"We can speak of this work in unqualified terms of approbation. The author has brought to his task a sound, logical mind, extensive knowledge of the literature of his subject, perfect acquaintance with the principles of modern science, and a large number of original observations."—*Athenæum.*

"It is a full and clear exposition of the doctrines which have now begun to prevail in regard to the manner in which medicines produce their Physiological and Therapeutical effects. It is well and carefully written, and deserves to be carefully studied."—*Am. Journal of Pharmacy.*

"We recommend the work as replete with information; the practitioner cannot fail to obtain from it many valuable hints."—*Am. Med. Journal.*

"In our opinion, it is the ablest, the most philosophical and satisfactory treatise on the action of medicines, that has ever been issued."—*St. Louis M. and S. Journal.*

A REVIEW OF MATERIA MEDICA FOR THE USE OF STUDENTS.

By JOHN B. BIDDLE, M.D., late Professor of Materia Medica in the Franklin Medical College, Fellow of the College of Physicians, &c. In one volume, 12mo. Price $1 00.

"This is an admirable summary of Materia Medica, and to the student will prove a very useful handbook. Valuable as are the United States Dispensatory and Pereira's Materia Medica, they are far too voluminous to be used profitably as text-books. Dr. Biddle's Review is just such a manual as the student wants to recall the chief points to which he has attained."—*Western Journal of Med. & Surg.*

PEREIRA'S PRESCRIPTION BOOK.

Containing Lists of Terms, Phrases, Contractions, and Abbreviations used in Prescriptions, with Explanatory Notes.

Also, the Grammatical Constructions of Prescriptions, &c., to which is added a Key, containing the Prescriptions in an abbreviated form, with a literal translation, intended for the use of Medical and Pharmaceutical Students. By JONATHAN PEREIRA, M.D. Price 63 cts. in Cloth. 75 cts. in Tucks with pocket.

WYTHES' DOSE AND SYMPTOM BOOK.

Containing the Doses and Uses of all the Principal Articles of the Materia Medica and Chief Officinal Preparations, etc. By JOSEPH H. WYTHES, M.D. Author of "The Microscope," "Curiosities of the Microscope," &c. &c. Price 63 cts. in cloth. 75 cts. in Tucks with pocket.

BEASLEY'S PRESCRIPTION-BOOK.

THE BOOK OF PRESCRIPTIONS: containing Two Thousand, Nine Hundred Prescriptions, collected from the Practice of the most Eminent Physicians and Surgeons. By HENRY BEASLEY, Author of "The Medical Formulary," "The Druggists' Receipt-Book," &c. &c. In one volume, duodecimo. Price, $1 50.

The editor, carefully selecting from the mass of materials at his disposal, has compiled a volume, sufficiently comprehensive, and yet sufficiently portable, in which both physician and druggist, prescriber and compounder, may find, under the head of each remedy, the manner in which that remedy may be most effectively administered, or combined with other medicines in the treatment of various diseases. The alphabetical arrangement adopted renders this easy; and the value of the volume is still further enhanced by the short account given of each medicine, and the lists of doses of its several preparations. This is really a most useful and important publication, and, from the great aid which it is capable of affording in prescribing, it should be in the possession of every medical practitioner. Amongst other advantages is, that, by giving the prescriptions of some of the most able and successful practitioners of the day, it affords an insight into the methods of treatment pursued by them, and of the remedies which they chiefly employed in the treatment of different diseases. The volume is small, and its cost trifling.—*Lancet.*

BEASLEY'S FORMULARY.

(NEW EDITION.)

THE MEDICAL FORMULARY: comprising Standard and Approved Formulæ for the Preparations and Compounds employed in Medical practice. By HENRY BEASLEY. Second American, from the Sixth London, Edition. In one volume. Price, $1 50.

The fact that Mr. Beasley's Formulary has reached a sixth edition, is a sufficient proof of the estimation in which it is held by the medical and pharmaceutical public. It is, in fact, a very comprehensive work, containing a great mass of information in a very small compass. The arrangement is alphabetical, as being most convenient. It contains selections from the American, French, German, and other foreign Pharmacopœias, in addition to the Formulæ from the three British ones. The work, however, is so well known, that it is unnecessary to do more than announce the present edition, and to state that the doses of the various medicines have now been added.—*Medical Times and Gazette.*

BEASLEY'S DRUGGISTS' RECEIPT-BOOK.

(WITH UPWARDS OF 200 NEW FORMS, RECEIPTS, AND PROCESSES.)

Containing Numerous Recipes for Patent and Proprietary Medicines, Druggists' Nostrums, &c., &c., Factitious Mineral Waters, and Powders for Preparing them. Also, Numerous Recipes for Perfumery, Cosmetics, Beverages, Dietetic Articles, and Condiments, Trade Chemicals, Miscellaneous Compounds, used in the Arts, Domestic Economy, &c.; with many other Useful Tables and Memoranda. Also, a Copious Veterinary Formulæ and Materia Medica, &c. By HENRY BEASLEY. Second (Improved) Edition. In one volume. Price, $1 50.

The "General Receipt-Book" is an extensive appendix to the "Formulary." No Pharmaceutist who possesses the former should be without the latter, for the two form a complete counter-companion.—*Annual of Pharmacy.*

THE MEDICAL FORMULARY:

COMPRISING

STANDARD AND APPROVED

FORMULÆ

FOR THE

PREPARATIONS AND COMPOUNDS EMPLOYED IN MEDICAL PRACTICE.

BY

HENRY BEASLEY.

WITH ADDITIONS

FROM THE SIXTH LONDON EDITION.

PHILADELPHIA:
LINDSAY & BLAKISTON.
1856.

ADVERTISEMENT

TO THE SIXTH EDITION.

This little work was originally intended as a counter companion to the Dispensing Chemist; and it was the compiler's aim to furnish, in the compass of one small volume, and under an alphabetical arrangement—as most convenient for reference—a comprehensive collection of formulæ required in the compounding of prescriptions. In addition to the formulæ and processes of the last editions of the three British Pharmacopœias,—as well as many which have been successively rejected from previous ones, but which are still occasionally required,—it comprises a copious selection from the American, French, German, and other foreign pharmacopœias; from the well-known Formularies of Magendie, Dunglison, Foy, Bouchardat, Swediaur, and others; from the pharmacopœias of the principal hospitals of this and other countries; from the best systematic works on Medicine, Materia Medica, Surgery, and Pharmacy; from single treatises on particular remedies; and from the British and Foreign periodicals. Care has been taken to include the new remedies most recently introduced up to the date of publication.

At the suggestion of medical friends, the doses of the several preparations are now generally annexed; and other additions have been made to meet the wishes and requirements of the medical practitioner and student.

LIST OF THE PRINCIPAL WORKS

CONSULTED IN COMPILING THE POCKET FORMULARY AND SYNOPSIS OF THE PHARMACOPŒIAS.

British Pharmacopœias. LONDON: EDINBURGH: DUBLIN.

Dispensatories. Edinburgh Dispensatory, edited by Dr. Rotheram; by Dr. A. Duncan; Supplement to ditto; Dr. Christison's *Dispensatory; London Dispensatory*, by Dr. A. T. Thomson; *Conspectus*, by the same; *Complete English Dispensatory*, by Quincy; *General Dispensatory* by Dr. R. Brooks; and Gaubius' *Complete Extemporaneous Dispensatory.*

The Dispensatory of the United States of America, by Drs. Wood and Bache.

Pharmacopœia Bateana, edited by Salmon; Dr. Fuller's *Pharmacopœia Extemporanea;* Wilson's *Pharmacopœia Chirurgica; Pharmacopœia Medico-Chirurgica;* Swediaur's *Pharmacopœia Medici Practici Universalis;* Dr. Hugh Smith's *Formulæ Medicamentorum;* Dr. R. Pearson's *Thesaurus Medicaminum;* Dr. Ryan's *Formulary of Hospitals;* Fox's *Formulæ Medicamentorum Selectæ; Pharmacopœia Augustana*, by Zwelfer; Plenk's *Pharmacologia*, &c.

Pharmacopœia of the United States of America.

Materia Medica. Cullen's, Lewis's, Alston's, Boerhaave's, and other works on; Dr. W. Ainslie's *Materia Indica;* Dr. Fleming's *Catalogue of Indian Medicinal Plants and Drugs*, Calcutta.

Materia Medica and Pharmacy. Brande's *Dictionary of Materia Medica and Practical Pharmacy;* Gray's *Supplement to the Pharmacopœia;* Professor Redwood's improved edition of the same work; Rennie's *Supplement to the Pharmacopœia;* Kane's *Elements of Pharmacy;* Davies' *Manual of Materia Medica and Pharmacy*, from the French of Edwards and Vavassour.

Elements of Materia Medica and Therapeutics, by Dr. Pereira; Dr. Paris's *Pharmacologia* and *Appendix;* Dr. Royle's *Manual of Materia Medica*, &c.; Dr. Neligan's *Medicines and their Uses.*

Phillips' (Mr. R.) *Examination of the Pharmacopœia Londinensis;* and *Translation of the Ph. Londin.;* Dr. G. F. Collier's *Translation of the Pharmacopœia;* and *Companion to the same;* Drs. Barker and Montgomery's *Observations on the Dublin Pharmacopœia.*

Hospital Pharmacopœias, (British). Guy's; University College; Charing Cross; St. Bartholomew's; St. George's; Middlesex; Manchester; &c.

The Bengal Dispensatory. Edited by Dr. O'Shaughnessy.

Pharmacopœia Suecica; Pharmacopœia Borussica; Pharmacopœia Batava, &c.

Pharmacopée Universelle, ou Conspectus des Pharmacopées, &c. Par A. J. L. Jourdan. This work embraces the principal pharmacopœias, dispensatories, formularies, &c., of all countries.

Codex, Pharmacopée Française. [A considerable portion of this work has been incorporated in the present volume.]

Alibert's *Nouveaux Elémens de Matière Médicale,* 2 vols.; Virey's *Traité de Pharmacie,* &c., 2 vols.; Baume's *Eléments de Pharmacie;* Lemery's *Dictionnaire des Drogues.*

Dictionnaire Universel de Matière Médical et de Thérapeutique générale, by Merat and De Lens. 6 vols.; and *Supplement.*

Soubeiran's *Nouveau Traité de Pharmacie theorique et pratique.* 2 vols.

Henry and Guibourt's *Pharmacopée Raisonnée, ou Traité de Pharmacie,* &c.

Dorvault's *L'Officine ou Répertoire général de Pharmacie pratique.*

Magendie's *Formulaire pour le préparation et l'emploi de plusieurs Nouveaux Médicaments,* with an *Appendix* by Dr. Marinus. Brussels.

Richard's *Formulaire de Poche;* D'Etilly's *Formulaire Eclectique;* Foy's *Formulaire de practiciens;* Ratier's *Formulaire pratique des Hôpitaux;* Edward's and Vavassour's *Nouveau Formulaire pratique des Hôpitaux,* by Mialhe; Bouchardat's *Nouveau Formulaire Magistral.*

Bouchardat's *Annuaire de Thérapeutique,* &c.

Mr. Braithwaite's *Retrospect of Medicine.*

Dr. Ranking's *Half-Yearly Abstract of Medical Sciences.*

Transactions of the Medico-Botanical Society.

Besides the above works, the editor has had occasion to consult the well-known chemical works of Berzelius, Brande, Graham, Kane, Turner, Ure, &c. The Dictionary of Practical Medicine, by Dr. Copland; the Library of Practical Medicine; the works of Sydenham, and other medical writers: also several works on Systematic and Medical Botany. Many separate treatises on particular remedies have also been referred to, as Fleming on Aconite; Turnbull on the Ranunculaceæ; Manson on Iodine; Brandish on Caustic Alkali; Jongh de tribus Olei Jecoris Aselli Speciebus; Scudamore on Inhalation; Venables on Aerated Waters, &c., &c. Also the following periodicals:—The Pharmaceutical Journal; Lancet; Medical Gazette; Chemist; Pharmaceutical Times; Dublin Journal of Medical Sciences; Medico-Chirurgical Review; British and Foreign Medical Review; Chemical Gazette; Journal de Pharmacie; American Journal of Pharmacy. With respect to several of the above, both the recent numbers and the back volumes for several years have been carefully perused with a view to the present work. Many volumes of periodicals, now discontinued, in some cases the entire series, have also been looked through: Annals of Chemistry and Practical Pharmacy; London Medical Repository; Medical Review; Medical Essays; Duncan's Annals of Medicine; Medical Museum, &c., &c.

SIGNS, ABBREVIATIONS, ETC.,

USED IN THE FORMULÆ.

C or Cong. Congius. Imperial Gallon.

O Octarius. Pint, of 20 fluid ounces.

℔ Libra. Apothecaries', or Troy Pound.

℥ Uncia. Troy Ounce.

f℥ Fluiduncia. Fluid Ounce.

ʒ Drachma. Drachm, (60 grains.)

fʒ Fluidrachma. Fluid Drachm, (60 minims.)

℈ Scrupulus. Scruple, (20 grains.)

♏ Minimum. Minim, (1-60th of fʒj.)

gr. Granum, *or* grana. Grain or grains.

ss. Semis. A half.

Sesqui. One and a half.

q. p. Quantum placet. As much as you please.

q. s. Quantum sufficiat. As much as is sufficient.

p. æq. Partes equales. Equal parts.

Aa, Ana, and Sing. Of each ingredient.

M. Misce. Mix.

S. A. Secundum Artem. According to art.

O. M. Old wine measure.

Co. or Comp. Compound.

Av. Avoirdupois weight.

Imp. Imperial measure.

Pulv. *or* p. Pulvis. Powder.

Sp. Gr. Specific Gravity.

REFERENCES.

L. London Pharmacopœia or College.

E. Edinburgh Pharmacopœia or College.

D. Dublin Pharmacopœia or College,

U. S. Pharmacopœia of the United States.

P. The Paris Codex, or French Pharmacopœia.

Aust., Bat., Prus., Rus., Span., Ph., &c. The Austrian, Batavian, Prussian, Russian, Spanish Pharmacopœias, &c.

Ch. Pharmacopœia Chirurgica, and Ph. Medico Chirurgica.

M. Magendie's Formulary.

H. Hospital Formularies, as Guy's H., St. B. H., Char. H., Mid. H., U. C. H., St. Geo. H., &c. Those of Guy's, St. Bartholomew's, Charing Cross, Middlesex, University College, and St. George's Hospitals.

Fr. H., It. H., Germ. H. French, Italian, and German Hospitals. [These are chiefly taken from the latest edition of the "Nouveau Formulaire Pratique des Hôpitaux," edited by Mialhe.]

The Individual Names attached to the Formulæ are those of the Authors to whom they are commonly attributed, or from whose works they have been taken.

THE POCKET FORMULARY.

Acetas Calcis. See Calcis Acetas. [The Salts *generally* are placed under their respective bases; as *Potassæ* Acetas; *Plumbi* Acetas; *Sodæ* Acetas.]

Acetica. *Medicated Vinegars.* The solid ingredients, previously cut or bruised, are macerated with the vinegar, in glass vessels, for the time prescribed, shaking the mixture occasionally. The liquid should then be strained off, and the ingredients pressed, unless otherwise directed. If the liquor does not become clear by subsidence, filter it.

Acetone. See Naphtha.

Acetum. Vinegar is procured in this country from malt, by fermentation, &c. French vinegar (Acetum Gallicum, E., Acetum Vini, D.) is made from wine.

Acetum Allii. Fresh garlic ʒvj, distilled vinegar Oiij, proof spirit f ʒiv. Macerate 3 days.

Acetum Antihystericum. Castor ℥ij, galbanum 3iv, rue ʒj, vinegar ℔ij. Macerate and strain.

Acetum Antisepticum. *Four-Thieves' Vinegar.* See Acidum aceticum aromaticum. E.

Acetum Aromaticum. P. *Aromatic Spirit of Vinegar.* Strong acetic acid Oj, camphor ʒij, oil of lavender gr. ix, oil of cloves 3ss, oil of cinnamon gr. xx.

Acetum Cantharidis [Epispasticum]. L. Cantharides in powder ʒij, acetic acid f ℥xx. Macerate 8 days, and strain. E. Cantharides p. ʒiij, acetic acid f ℥v, pyroligneous acid f ℥xv, euphorbium ℥ss. 7 days. [To promote prompt vesication. See also Tinctura Canthar. Acetica.]

ACETUM CAPSICI. Capsicum ℥j, vinegar f℥xxiv. See Tinctura Capsici Acetici.

ACETUM COLCHICI. L. E. & D. Fresh colchicum ℥j, distilled vinegar f℥xvj. Macerate for 3 days, and add f℥j of proof spirit to the clear liquid. [℈viij of the dried cormus is considered equivalent to ℥j of the fresh. Dose fℨss to fℨjss.]

ACETUM DESTILLATUM. L. From Oviij of vinegar, in a glass retort, distil Ovij, by the heat of a sand-bath. D. rejects the first 10th. E. & D. direct French vinegar.

ACETUM LAVANDULÆ. P. Digest ℥j of dried lavender flowers, with ℥xij of vinegar for 8 days.

ACETUM LOBELIÆ. W. PROCTER. Lobelia seeds bruised ℥iv, distilled vinegar f℥xxiv. Macerate 24 hours, strain, and filter, adding more vinegar to make up f℥xxiv.

ACETUM OPII. E. & D. Opium, sliced ℥iv, distilled vinegar f℥xvj. Triturate the opium with a little of the vinegar, add the rest, macerate 7 days, strain, press, and filter. [Dose, 6 drops to 24. 20 drops equal to 30 of tinct. opii.]

ACETUM ROSÆ. P. From dried roses, as Acet. Lavandulæ.

ACETUM ROSMARINÆ. As Acet. Lavandulæ.

ACETUM RUBI IDÆI. P. *Raspberry Vinegar.* Macerate 3 parts of the fruit with 2 parts of wine vinegar for 15 days, and strain without pressure. The vinegars of other fruits are prepared in the same manner.

ACETUM RUTÆ. E. 1744. Rue ℔j, vinegar Cj. Digest and strain.

ACETUM SALVIÆ. P. Sage flowers ℥j, vinegar ℥xij.

ACETUM SAMBUCI. E. 1744. Dried elder flowers ℔j, vinegar Cj.

ACETUM SCILLÆ. L. Dried squill ℥xv, distilled vinegar Ovj. Digest with a gentle heat 24 hours, strain, and add Oss of proof spirit. E. and D. nearly the same. Dose fℨss to fℨjss.

ACETUM SINAPIS. BERAL. Mustard ℥j, vinegar f℥xij. Distil f℥viij. *For outward use.*

ACIDUM ACETICUM. L. Acidum aceticum fortius. L. 1824. *Strong Acetic Acid.* Put ℔ij of acetate of soda into a glass retort; add ℥ix of sulphuric acid previously mixed with f℥ix of water, and distil by the heat of a sand-bath. [A stronger acid may be obtained by carefully drying the acetate of soda, or by the following processes:—E. Take of acetate of lead, dried at 320° by an oil or metal bath (but Mr. Phillips says it may be sufficiently dried at 212°), ℥vj, sulphuric acid f ℨixss. Distil to dryness at 320°. The product to be shaken with a little red oxide of lead and redistilled. D. directs it to be distilled from 52 parts of sulphuric acid, and 100 of acetate of potash. Acidum Acetosum, L. 1788, was made by distilling, by the heat of a sand-bath, crystallized verdigris, bruised and thoroughly dried; and redistilling the product. These stronger acids are chiefly used in preparing Aromatic Vinegar.]

Acidum Aceticum Dilutum. L. 1824. (Acidum Aceticum. L. 1809.) *Distilled Vinegar.* See Acetum Destillatum. It is imitated by mixing 15 parts of strong acetic acid (Ac. Acet. L.) with 85 parts of distilled water; or so much that 100 grs. of the diluted acid may saturate 13 grs. of crys. subcarbonate of soda.

Acidum Aceticum Aromaticum. E. 1839. Dried rosemary ℥j, lavender flowers ℥ss, origanum ℥j, bruised cloves ℨss, acetic acid Oiss. Macerate 7 days, strain, express, and filter. This is substituted for the old Acetum Antisepticum, or *Four-Thieves' Vinegar*, which contained, in addition, rue, garlic, &c. E. 1817 directed distilled vinegar, for which the strong acid was substituted in 1839; in 1841 the preparation was omitted.

Acidum Aceticum Camphoratum. E. & D. Camphor (pulverized with spirit) ℥ss, strong acetic acid f℥viss. [f℥vi, D.]

Acidum Antimonicum. [Ac. Stibicum, P.] Antimonic acid is precipitated when diluted sulphuric acid is added to the washings of *Diaphoretic Antimony* (Antimonium Calcinatum).

Acidum Arseniosum. See Arsenicum Album.

Acidum Arsenicum. Brande. White arsenic 8 parts, nitric acid 24 parts, muriatic acid 4 parts. Distil to dryness, and heat the residue to dull redness.

Acidum Benzoicum. L. & E. *Flowers of Benzoin.* Gradually heat Benzoin, in a proper [glass E.] vessel placed in sand, till the acid sublimes. Press this between blotting paper, and resublime. [The Benzoin may be mixed with clean sand, and put into a shallow iron vessel, covered with porous paper tightly pasted to the rim, and over this a cone or hat of stiff cartridge paper. The acid, passing through the former, will be deposited on the latter sufficiently pure for use. The vessel should be heated on an iron plate on which sand has been spread. Dose, gr. v to xv.]

ACIDUM BORACICUM. M. WACKENRODER. Dissolve 40 parts of borax in 100 of boiling water, and add 25 of hydrochloric acid to the hot solution. Let the acid, which crystallizes on cooling, be collected on a filter, drained, washed with cold water, and lastly dried at 234° F. It may be rendered more pure by re-crystallizing. [It is usually precipitated by sulphuric acid, a portion of which it obstinately retains.]

ACIDUM CARBONICUM. Mix fragments of marble, or chalk, with water, and add sulphuric acid previously diluted with an equal quantity of water.

ACIDUM CITRICUM. L. To Oiv of lemon juice, made hot, add ℥ivss of prepared chalk. Let it settle, pour off the liquid, and wash the sediment repeatedly with warm water. Then add to it f℥xxvijss of diluted sulphuric acid, mixed with Oij of distilled water, and boil for a quarter of an hour. Strain through linen with strong pressure; evaporate the clear liquid, and set it aside that crystals may form. Purify them by resolution and recrystallization. E. and D. substantially the same. They direct 8 times as much dilute sulphuric acid as of chalk to be used.

ACIDUM GALLICUM. Mix powdered nut-galls into a thin paste with water, and expose it to the air 4 or 5 weeks, adding water to keep it moist. Squeeze it dry, boil it in water, and filter whilst hot. Let the acid which is deposited on cooling be boiled with 8 parts of water, and one-fifth of animal charcoal, and the hot solution filtered and cooled. [Dose, as an astringent, gr. iij, to gr. x. Larger doses have been given to expel the tapeworm. Externally as a styptic.]

ACIDUM HYDRIODICUM. Dr. BUCHANAN'S *Medicinal Hydriodic Acid* is made by dissolving separately 264 grs. of tartaric acid, and 330 grs. of iodide of potassium, each in f℥iss of distilled water. Mix the solutions, agitate; and when settled, decant the clear liquid, adding water to make up the measure f℥vj½. [fʒj contains gr. j of iodine. Dose fʒj, gradually increased to fʒiv, or more.]

ACIDUM HYDROCHLORICUM. L. *Muriatic or Hydrochloric Acid.* Put into a glass retort 24 parts of dried chloride of sodium (common salt), and add 20 parts of sulphuric acid, previously mixed with 12 of water. Put 12 parts of distilled water into the receiver, and distil with a gradually increased heat, by means of a sand-bath. D. By a similar process from 87 parts of sulphuric acid, 100 of dried salt, and 124 of water. Sp. gr. of each, 1·160.

ACIDUM HYDROCHLORICUM PURUM. [Ac. Muriaticum purum, E.] Take equal weights of pure muriate of soda (see Sodæ Murias Purum) well dried, sulphuric acid, and water. Put the salt into a glass retort, and add the sulphuric acid, previously mixed with a third of the water, and cooled. Fit on a receiver containing the rest of the water. Distil with a gentle heat as long as any acid passes over, keeping the receiver constantly cool. Density, 1·170. [Commercial hydrochloric acid sometimes contains *arsenic*, from which it may be freed by redistilling it with pieces of bright copper.]

ACIDUM HYDROCHLORICUM DILUTUM. L. Acidum muriaticum dilutum E. Hydrochloric acid f℥iv, distilled water f℥xij, mix. The D. acid is much stronger, f℥x of acid to f℥xj of water.

ACIDUM HYDROCYANICUM DILUTUM. L. *Diluted or medicinal Prussic acid.* Sulphuric acid ℥iss, water f℥iv; mix, and when cool, put them into a tubulated retort, and add ferro-cyanide of potassium ℥ij dissolved in f℥x of water. Pour f℥viij of distilled water into the receiver; and having connected the retort (and adopter), distil f℥vj with a gentle heat, keeping the receiver constantly cool. To the product add f℥vj of distilled water, or q. s. that 12·7 grains of nitrate of silver, dissolved in water, may be accurately saturated by 100 grains of the diluted acid; indicating 2 per cent. of real hydrocyanic acid. Or it may be more quickly made from 48½ grains of cyanide of silver, added to a mixture of 39½ grains of hydrochloric acid and f℥j of distilled water, and shaken together in a stopped phial; decanting the clear liquid when the sediment has subsided. [Dose, from 2 to 5 ♏.]

ACIDUM HYDROCYANICUM. E. Ferro-cyanide of potassium ℥iij, sulphuric acid f℥ij, water f℥xvj. Dissolve the salt in f℥xj of water, add the acid mixed with f℥v of water, and distil f℥xiv. Add distilled water to the product to make up the measure exactly f℥xvj. [Dose ♏ j to iij.]

ACIDUM PRUSSICUM. D. Cyanuret (bicyanide) of mercury ℥j, muriatic acid f℥vij, water f℥viij. From a glass retort, distil into a cooled receiver f℥viij; to be kept in a well-stopped bottle, in a cool, dark place. This last direction should be observed with all the varieties of this acid. The D. acid contains

1·5 or 1·6 per cent. of real acid. (Dr. KANE.) SCHEELE'S *Prussic acid* is frequently prescribed; but this name indicates no certain strength. (See Appendix 3.)

ACIDUM HYDROCYANICUM VEGETABILE. SCHRADER. Essential oil of bitter almonds ʒj, rectified spirit ʒix, distilled water ʒix. [Dose, 2 to 3 drops, in sugared water.]

ACIDUM HYDROSULPHURICUM AQUA SOLUTUM. P. Pass a current of sulphuretted hydrogen gas (procured by acting on sulphuret of iron by diluted sulphuric acid) through cold distilled water, till it ceases to be absorbed.

ACIDUM IODICUM. M. BOURSON. Treat one part of iodine with four parts of strong nitric acid (sp. gr. 1·5) by the aid of a gentle heat. Evaporate to dryness, and leave the mass exposed to the air till it deliquesces. Then place it in a warm, dry place, till crystals form.

ACIDUM LACTICUM. To Ovj of milk add ℥viij of bicarbonate of soda. Expose it to the air for some days, till it becomes sour, and saturate it with more soda. Repeat this as often as it becomes acid. Boil, filter, evaporate to the consistence of syrup, and digest with alcohol. Filter the solution, and add sulphuric acid as long as it occasions a precipitate. Again filter, and concentrate the clear solution by evaporation, till its density is about 1·215.

ACIDUM MECONICUM. *Meconic acid.* Mix ℥j meconate of lime (formed in making muriate of morphia by the E. process) with Oj of boiling water, and add ℥iij of muriatic acid; redissolve the crystals, which the liquor deposits in cooling, in the same quantity of water and acid, till they are freed from lime.

ACIDUM MURIATICUM. D. and E. See Acidum Hydrochloricum.

ACIDUM NITRICUM. L. Distilled from equal weights of dry nitre, and oil of vitriol. Sp. gr. 1·500. The commercial acid is usually from 1·38 to 1·40.

ACIDUM NITRICUM PURUM. E. As the last; but the nitre is purified by two or more crystallizations, till its solution is no longer disturbed by nitrate of silver. The acid may be rendered colourless by gently heating it in a retort. The commercial acid may be concentrated by distilling it with an equal measure of oil of vitriol, until two-thirds of the nitric acid are brought over. Mr. REDWOOD.

ACIDUM NITRICUM DILUTUM. L. Nitric acid f ℥j, distilled water f ℥ix. E. 1841. Pure nitric acid f ℥j (or commercial n. acid f ℥j ʒv), d. water f ℥ix. [The D. and former E. pharm. direct f ℥iij of acid to f ℥iv of water.]

ACIDUM NITROSUM. The red fuming nitric acid (nitric acid with nitrous acid gas) is so termed.

ACIDUM NITROSUM DILUTUM. L. 1788. Equal weights of nitrous acid and water. [*Aqua Fortis* is made of various strengths for different purposes in the arts. Dr. Pereira states, that the *aqua fortis duplex* of the shops has a sp. gr. of 1·36; *aqua fortis simplex*, of 1·22.]

ACIDUM NITRICUM ALCOHOLISATUM. P. Nitric acid, commercial, one part; rectified spirits, 3 parts. Mix. [Dose, ʒss.]

ACIDUM NITRO-MURIATICUM. D. Nitro-hydrochloric acid. *Aqua Regia.* Nitric acid f ℥j, muriatic acid f ℥ij. Mix, and keep it in a dark place. [Dose, ♏iij to iv.]

ACIDUM NITRO-MURIATICUM [NITRO-HYDROCHLORICUM] DILUTUM. Mid. H. Muriatic acid f ℥iij, nitric acid f ℥ij, water f ℥v. [Dose, ♏v to viij; but chiefly used for making the acid bath. See Balneum Acidum.]

ACIDUM OXALICUM. *Acid of Sugar.* Put into a glass or earthen retort equal weights of bruised sugar and nitric acid (sp. gr. 1·286). Connect with an adopter, and a receiver furnished with a tube to convey the vapours into a chimney. Heat moderately, till the vapours cease. The next day, remove and drain the crystals, and concentrate the residual liquor for more. Purify them by crystallization. Potato starch is economically substituted for sugar. *Poisonous.* Antidote; chalk, whiting, or magnesia.

ACIDUM PHOSPHORICUM DILUTUM. L. Mix nitric acid f ℥iv, with distilled water f ℥x; put them into a glass retort placed in a sand-bath, add ℥j of phosphorus, and apply heat till f ℥viij have distilled. Return these into the retort, and again distil f ℥viij, which are to be thrown away. Evaporate what remains in the retort in a platina capsule to f ℥ij f ʒvj; and add to the acid, when cooled, sufficient distilled water to make up f ℥xxviij. [It contains about 10 per cent. of real P. acid. Dose, from ♏x to f ʒss, properly diluted.]

ACIDUM PICIS. Crude Pyroligneous Acid.

ACIDUM PRUSSICUM, *vel* BORUSSICUM. See Acidum Hydrocyanicum.

ACIDUM PYROLIGNEUM. E. An impure acetic acid procured by the destructive distillation of wood. Sp. gr. 1·034. 100 grains neutralize 53 of carb. soda.

ACIDUM SACCHARICUM. Saccharic acid is obtained by accurately decomposing saccharate of barytes by sulphuric acid.

ACIDUM SUCCINICUM. D. *Acid*, or *Salt of Amber*. Mix amber with its weight of sand, and distil. Press the crystals in bibulous paper, and resublime. Dose, 4 to 12 or 15 grains.

ACIDUM SULPHURICUM PURUM. E. & D. The commercial acid purified by distillation in glass, rejecting the first 12th or 16th part. [No luting, or corks, should be used. A few strips of platinum in the retort will moderate the ebullition. "Sulphuric acid may be freed from *nitrous acid*, by heating f ℥viij with 10 or 15 grs. of sugar." E. A little sulphuret of barium, in solution, will remove the metallic impurities.]

ACIDUM SULPUHRICUM DILUTUM. L. *Spirit of Vitriol.* To f ℥xivss of distilled water, add gradually f ℥iss of sulphuric acid, and mix. E. directs f ℥j of acid to f ℥xiij of water. D. One part by weight of acid to 7 of water. Dose, ♏x to xxx, properly diluted.

ACIDUM SULPHURICUM ALCOHOLISATUM. P. *Eau de Rabel.* Add gradually 1 part of sulphuric acid to 3 parts of rectified spirit, by weight. [From ʒss to ʒj to Oij of water as an acidulous drink. Externally as an escharotic. It is sometimes coloured with cochineal.]

ACIDUM SULPHURICUM AROMATICUM. E. *Elixir of Vitriol.* Sulphuric acid f ℥iijss, rectified spirit Oiss, cinnamon bruised ℥iss, ginger bruised ℥j. Digest for 6 days and strain. L. 1746, directs ℥iv, by weight, of sulphuric acid, to be added to f ℥xvj of compound tincture of cinnamon. Dose, ♏v to xv.

ACIDUM SULPHYDRICUM (HYDROSULPHURICUM) AQUA SOLUTUM. P. Cold water fully saturated with sulphuretted hydrogen gas, procured from sulphuret of iron, and dil. sulphuric acid.

ACIDUM SULPHUROSUM AQUA SOLUTUM. P. Sulphurous acid gas (procured by gently heating 3 parts of sulphuric acid with 2 of quicksilver, in a glass matrass) is to be conveyed, first through a very little water to purify the gas, and then into the water to be charged, till the latter is fully saturated. A Woolfe's apparatus should be used, with a tube passing from the last bottle into a vessel of moistened chalk, to absorb the excess of gas.

ACIDUM TANNICUM. U. S. *Tannin* or *Tannic Acid.* Cause washed æther to percolate through powdered nut-galls, in a glass adopter, closed at the lower end with carded cotton. The liquor obtained divides into two portions; pour off the upper layer, and evaporate the denser liquid to obtain the acid. [*Astringent.* Dose, from 1 to 3 grains.]

ACIDUM TARTARICUM. L. Bitartrate of potash ℔iv, boiling distilled water Ciiss, prepared chalk ℥xxv¾, diluted sulphuric acid Ovij f℥xvij, hydrochloric acid f℥xxviss, or q. s. Boil the bitartrate with Cij of water, and add gradually half the chalk; afterwards add the rest of the chalk previously dissolved in the hydrochloric acid, and the remaining water. When settled, pour away the clear liquid, and wash the precipitate with distilled water till it is tasteless; then pour on it the diluted sulphuric acid, boil for a quarter of an hour, strain, and evaporate the clear liquor, that crystals may form. Redissolve the crystals, filter, concentrate the solution, and set it aside to crystallize. Repeat this till the crystals become colourless. E. Substantially the same. D. directs 10 parts of the bitartrate, 4 of chalk, 7 of sulphuric acid, 120 of water, and q. s. water of muriate of lime.

ACIDUM VALERIANICUM. PRINCE L. L. BONAPARTE. Distil not less than 40℔s. of valerian root, with 8 times its weight of distilled or rain water; collect the oil in a separatory, continuing the distillation as long as the water is decidedly acid. Agitate the oil with milk of lime, which takes up the acid which it contains; nearly saturate the acid water by milk of lime (first adding that already used, and then fresh); and lastly, add lime water in excess. Concentrate the solution till a pellicle appears, and when cold decompose it by nitric acid in a long narrow flask with a ground stopper; decant the valerianic acid which floats on the surface of the liquid, and distil it with a gentle heat till the distilled liquid ceases to be oily. [Several methods of increasing the product of acid have been proposed: as boiling the root with carbonate of soda, and distilling the decoction with an excess of sulphuric acid; also by exposing the distilled water to the air; or treating it with chromic acid. See Zinci Valerianas. The addition of acids to the root in the still contaminates the product with formic and acetic acids.]

ACONITINA. L. Take of monkshood root, dried and bruised ℔ij; boil it in three successive gallons of rectified spirit for an hour, in a retort connected with a cooled receiver, pouring off the liquor, and adding with the fresh spirit, that which distils over. Mix the strained tinctures, distil off the spirit, and evaporate what remains to an extract. Dissolve this in water, filter, and evaporate the solution to the consistence of syrup. Add sufficient diluted sulphuric acid, mixed with distilled water, to dissolve the aconitine, and throw down the latter by solution of ammonia. Redissolve the precipitate by more acid and water, agitate the solution with animal charcoal, filter, and again precipitate with ammonia. Wash the precipitate and dry it. [Other authorities direct the expressed juice of the plant to be boiled, filtered, neutralized by carbonate of potash; the mixture agitated with æther, and the ætherial solution evaporated. *It is an energetic poison, only used in outward applications.*]

Adeps Myristicæ. *Oil of Mace.* It is obtained from nutmegs by strong pressure.

Adeps Præparatus. L. 1824. Cut the raw hog's fat into pieces, melt it over a slow fire, and strain through linen. L. 1836, directs the lard of the shops to be well washed with water.

Adeps Oxygenatus. See Unguentum Acidi Nitrosi. [Another preparation of lard, intended to facilitate its combination with quicksilver, may here be described. The fat is melted and poured in a shower or fine stream into a large vessel filled with cold water; it is then placed on a hair or wicker sieve, in a cool dry cellar, for a few weeks or months.]

Adeps Ovillus Præparatus. Mutton suet is prepared in the same way as lard. Other fats are similarly treated.

Ærugo Præparata. Verdigris (diacetate of copper) prepared in the same manner as chalk. See Creta Præparata.

Æther Aceticus. P. Rectified spirit ℥xxx, strong acetic acid ℥xx, sulphuric acid ℥vj½. Distil ℥xl; agitate the product with dry carbonate of potash, and redistil, to obtain ℥xxx.

Æther Chloricus. The so-called medicinal chloric æther is an alcoholic solution of chloroform, of variable strength. Mr. Guthrie obtained it by putting into a large glass retort ℔iij of chloride of lime, and two wine-gallons of rectified spirit, and carefully distilling one gallon. Mr. Redwood states that what is sold in this country consists of one part of chloroform to six or eight of alcohol. Dose, ʒss in water, as an antispasmodic.

Æther Muriaticus. Into a retort connected with a Woolfe's apparatus, put equal weights of alcohol and muriatic acid, and distil with a gentle heat. The first bottle should contain a little warm water, and the others be surrounded with ice.

ÆTHER NITRICUS. *Nitrous*, or *Hyponitrous Æther*. E. Rectified spirit f℥xv, pure nitric acid f℥vij. Put the spirit, with a little clean sand, into a quart matrass fitted with a cork, through which pass a safety tube, and another tube connected with a refrigeratory. The safety tube being filled with pure nitric acid, add through it gradually, f℥iijss of the acid; and when the action has subsided, add the rest by half ounces, at intervals, keeping the refrigeratory very cool. Agitate the distilled æther first with milk of lime, and afterwards with half its volume of strong solution of muriate of lime, and decant. [LIEBIG has proposed a more productive process (by the use of starch), but the product is contaminated with prussic acid. PEDRONI says it may be safely and readily made by adding to 11 parts of crystallized nitrate of ammonia in a glass retort, 8 parts of sulphuric acid previously mixed with 9 of alcohol, and distilling by a naked fire, into a cooled receiver.]

ÆTHER SULPHURICUS. L. Æther Rectificatus. L. 1824. *Æther*, or *Rectified Æther*. Pour ℔ij of rectified spirit into a glass retort, add ℔ij of sulphuric acid, and mix; place it in sand, and heat quickly to boiling; let the liquor distil into a receiver, kept very cool, till a heavier portion passes over; to what remains in the retort, when sufficiently cooled, add ℔j more spirit, and let the æther distil as before. Mix the distilled liquors, pour off the supernatant part, and add to it ℥j of recently ignited carbonate of potash, and redistil. E. Rectified spirit Oijss, sulphuric acid f℥x. Pour f℥xij of the spirit gently over the acid, in an open vessel, and stir them well together. Transfer the mixture into a glass matrass connected by tubes with a refrigeratory, and with a raised reservoir containing the rest of the spirit. Raise the heat quickly to about 280°, and let the spirit flow into the matrass in a continuous stream in a quantity equal to that which distils over. When f℥xlij have passed over, and all the spirit has been added, the process may be stopped. Agitate the æther with f℥xvj of saturated solution of muriate of lime, to which ℥ss of slaked lime has been added; decant the æther, and redistil with a gentle heat, so long as the liquid which passes over has a density not above 735. D. directs liquor æthereus sulphuricus to be distilled from ℥xxxij each of sulphuric acid and rectified spirit, and f℥xx drawn over. From this, with ʒij dried subcarbonate of potash, f℥xij of æther sulphuricus are to be distilled.

ÆTHER LOTUS. Commercial æther generally contains a little alcohol, which may be removed by agitating it with twice its bulk of water, and decanting it. The æther retains a little water, which does not impair its fitness for *inhalation*, and which perhaps renders it more suitable for the preparation of *tannic acid*. If the æther is *acid*, lime-water may be substituted for water, when intended for inhaling.

ÆTHER SULPHURICUS CUM ALCOHOLE. See Spiritus Ætheris Sulphuricus.

ÆTHER SULPHURICUS IODURETUS. M. Iodine ℈ij, sulphuric æther f℥iss. Dose, 4 to 10 drops.

ÆTHER PHOSPHORATUS. P. Macerate 1 part of phosphorus with 50 of æther, for a month, in a dark place, shaking occasionally. Decant the clear solution and keep it in a dark place. Dr. COPLAND directs 2 grains of pure phosphorus, and ℈j of oil of peppermint, or oil of valerian, to be digested with ℥j of æther. Dose, 5 to 10 drops, with some mucilaginous liquid.

ÆTHER TEREBINTHINATUS. DURANDE. Æther 3 parts, rectified oil of turpentine 1 part. From 20 to 40 drops in whey, as a solvent for biliary calculi.

Other Æthereal preparations will be found among the Tinctures, Solutions, and Spirits.

ÆTHIOPS ABSORBENS. Hydrargyrus cum Cretâ.

ÆTHIOPS ANTIMONIALIS. PRUS. P. Quicksilver ℥j, sesquisulphuret of antimony ℥ij, sulphur ℥j. Triturate together till the quicksilver is no longer visible. *Alterative.* Dose, a few grains. Dr. PLUMMER'S Æthiops was prepared from equal parts of golden sulphur of antimony and calomel. PORT. PH. directs 3 parts of precipitated sulphuret of antimony, and 2 of purified mercury.

ÆTHIOPS GRAPHITICUS. Triturate 2 parts of plumbago with 1 of quicksilver. Dose, gr. viij.

ÆTHIOPS MARTIALIS. Black oxide of iron. See Ferri Oxydum Nigrum.

ÆTHIOPS MINERALIS. See Hydrargyri Sulphuretum cum Sulphure.

ÆTHIOPS SACCHARATUS. SPAN. P. Quicksilver 1 part, white sugar 2 parts. Triturate together with a few drops of water, till the quicksilver is extinct. BAUME (*sucre vermifuge mercuriel*), Æthiops mineral 2 parts, quicksilver 3, sugar 7.

ÆTHIOPS VEGETABILIS. Bladder-wrack (Fucus Vesiculosus) dried, and burnt in a covered crucible, with a perforated lid, till the vapours cease. Dose, gr. x. to ʒij.

ALCOHOL. Chloride of calcium (dried muriate of lime) ℔j, rectified spirit Cj, mix and distil Ovij f℥v. Sp. gr. 0·815. The E. process affords a stronger spirit. Rectified spirit Oj, fresh lime broken small, ℥xviij. Put them into a glass matrass, and heat gently till the lime begins to slake; withdraw the heat till the slaking is finished, keeping the upper part of the matrass cool with damp cloths. Then attach a proper refrigeratory, and with a gradually increasing heat, distil f℥xvij. [Sp. gr. 0·796.]

ALCOHOL AMMONIATUM. See Spiritus Ammoniæ.

ALCOHOL DILUTIUS, and ALCOHOL FORTIUS. E. The former names of *proof* and *rectified spirit.* See Spiritus.

ALCOHOL SULPHURICUM. P. See Acidum Sulphuricum Alcoholisatum.

ALLOXANUM. *Aloxane.* To nitric acid (sp. gr. 1·45 to 1·5) in a porcelain vessel, gradually add half its weight of dry uric acid, mixing each portion very carefully, and waiting till the effervescence is over, and the liquid cool, before adding more. Put the mass on porous paper, or brick, for 24 hours, to dry; then dissolve it by heat in its own weight of water, filter, and set it aside in a warm place, that crystals may form. [LIEBIG suggests its use in some diseases of the liver. Its dose is undetermined, but it does not appear to be poisonous. It is diuretic.]

ALOE COLATA. Aloes heated by steam in a tinned vessel, and strained, while warm, through a hair sieve.

ALUMEN EXSICCATUM. L. E. & D. *Dried* or *burnt alum.* Melt alum in an earthen (or iron, E.) vessel, and increase the heat till it ceases to boil. [Reduce to powder, E. & D.]

ALUMEN SACCHARINUM. Alum ℥vj, white lead ʒvj, sulphate of zinc ʒiij, white sugar ℥iss. Mix the powder into a paste with vinegar and white of egg. Used in eye-waters and cosmetic washes.

ALUMINA. *Earth of Alum.* Dissolve alum in water, and precipitate by carbonate of potash; wash the precipitate freely with distilled water; redissolve it in hydrochloric acid, precipitate by ammonia, and wash it as before.

ALUMINÆ ACETAS. Dissolve fresh precipitated alumina in strong acetic acid; filter the solution, and evaporate it to a gelatinous consistence.

AMMONIÆ AQUA. See Liquor Ammoniæ.

AMMONIÆ ACETATIS AQUA. See Liquor Ammoniæ Acetatis.

AMMONIÆ ARSENIAS. Saturate solution of arsenic acid with ammonia (which should be in slight excess), and evaporate by a gentle heat, that crystals may form on cooling. See Liquor Ammoniæ Arseniatis.

AMMONIÆ BENZOAS. Mix benzoic acid with 8 parts of water, and add a slight excess of ammonia. Digest the solution with purified animal charcoal, filter, concentrate by evaporation at a gentle heat, and crystallize by refrigeration.

AMMONIÆ BICARBONAS. D. Dissolve ℥iv of sesquicarbonate of ammonia in f ℥xv of water, and pass carbonic acid gas through it, till it is fully saturated. Set it aside, and let the crystals which form be dried without heat. Dose, gr. v to xx.

AMMONIÆ SESQUICARBONAS. L. Sesquicarbonate (formerly carbonate or subcarbonate) of ammonia. *Volatile Salts.* Mix ℔j of powdered sal ammoniac (ammoniæ hydrochloras) with ℔jss of prepared chalk, and sublime with a gradually increased heat. Dose, gr. v to xv.

AMMONIÆ HYDRIODAS. P. *Ammonii Iodidum.* Digest iodine with half its weight of clean iron-filings, in distilled water, till a colourless solution is obtained. Filter, and immediately add sesquicarbonate of ammonia in slight excess. Filter, concentrate by rapid evaporation, and crystallize by refrigeration. It it rather more active than iodide of potassium.

AMMONIÆ HYDROCHLORAS. Ammoniæ Murias. *Sal Ammoniac.* It is made by saturating ammoniacal gas liquor, or bone-spirit, with sulphuric acid; crystallizing the sulphate, mixing it with common salt, and subliming. The commercial sal ammoniac should be purified by crystallization for internal use. Dose, gr. v to xxv.

AMMONIÆ HYDROSULPHURETUM. E. Pass sulphuretted hydrogen gas (from muriatic acid ℥viij, water ℔ijss, and sulphuret of iron ℥iv) through f℥iv of solution of ammonia. D. directs 7 parts of sulphuric acid, 5 of sulphuret of iron, 32 of water, for 4 of water of ammonia. *Poisonous.* Dose, 4 to 8 drops, in water, diabetes.

AMMONIÆ NITRAS. Saturate diluted nitric acid, with sesquicarbonate of ammonia; filter, and concentrate by evaporation at a gentle heat, that crystals may form on cooling. Dose, ℈j, refrigerant and diuretic.

AMMONIÆ NITROSULPHAS. Pass nitric oxide gas through a solution of sulphite of ammonia in five or six volumes of water of ammonia; let the crystals which form be quickly washed with liquid ammonia, dried without heat, and preserved in closely-stopped bottles. Dose, gr. xij in typhoid fevers.

AMMONIÆ OXALAS. E. Dissolve ℥viij (probably ℥iv intended) of carbonate of ammonia in Oiv of water; add gradually ℥iv of oxalic acid, concentrate by boiling, and set aside to crystallize. As a test for lime.

AMMONIÆ PHOSPHAS. Saturate dilute phosphoric acid with carbonate of ammonia, and evaporate, that crystals may form.

AMMONIÆ PRÆPARATA. *Ammoniæ Sesquicarbonas.*

AMMONIÆ SUCCINAS IMPURUS. P. Spirit of hartshorn, neutralized with succinic acid (salt of amber), and filtered. Dose, a few drops, as an antispasmodic.

AMMONIÆ SULPHAS. Saturate diluted sulphuric acid with sesquicarbonate of ammonia, and evaporate the solution, that crystals may form as it cools.

AMYGDALINA. Boil well-pressed cake of bitter almonds twice in strong alcohol; strain through linen, and press the residue. Remove any oil that may appear, heat the liquid again, and filter. In a few days, part of the amygdaline crystallizes. Concentrate the residuary liquor to a sixth part, and add æther, which will throw down the amygdaline. Press it between blotting paper, wash it with æther, redissolve in boiling alcohol, and set aside to crystallize. [Seventeen grains with f℥jss of sweet almond emulsion form a substitute for (strong) Aqua Amygdàlæ Amaræ. This quantity is equivalent to one grain of real prussic acid, or 50 grains (55♏) of Ac. Hydroc. dil. P. L.]

AMYLI IODIDUM. Dr. BUCHANAN. Triturate 24 grains of iodine with a little water, and gradually add ℥j of powdered white starch. Continue the trituration till the compound assumes a deep and uniform colour. Dose, from ʒss, gradually increased to ʒiv or more.

AMYLUM CUM CERA. Melt wax, and stir into it four times its weight of starch or arrow-root. *Demulcent.*

ANTHRACOKALI. POYLA. Carbonate of potash, ℥vj, lime, ℥iijss, water Oiv. Proceed as in making liquor potassæ; and concentrate the clear solution, by boiling in an iron vessel, till an oily-looking liquid remains; then stir in ℥v of finely-powdered mineral coal; remove from the fire, and continue stirring till the whole is reduced to an uniform powder, which is to be immediately put into small dry bottles. Dose, 2 gr. twice or thrice a day, for skin diseases, scrofula, chronic rheumatism, &c.

ANTHRACOKALI SULPHURATUM. As the last, adding, with the coal, ʒiv of sulphur. Dose and uses the same.

ANTIMONIUM CALCINATUM. L. 1788. *Diaphoretic Antimony. Calx of Antimony.* Sesquisulphuret of antimony ℥viij, powdered nitre ℥xxiv. Mix and deflagrate by spoonfuls, in a crucible heated to redness. Burn for half an hour, and when cold, powder. [When washed with distilled water it forms *Calx Antimonii Lota.* The washings yield *Antimonic Acid* by the addition of sulphuric acid.]

ANTIMONII CALX SULPHURATA. HUFELAND. Mix 10 parts of burnt oyster shells, 4 of sulphur, and 3 of crude antimony; and calcine them in a luted crucible for an hour.

ANTIMONII CERUSSA. BATE. As Antimonium Calcinatum, substituting metallic antimony for the sulphuret. The *Ant. Cerussa Solaris* was made by igniting antimony by means of a lens.

ANTIMONII CHLORIDUM. *Sesquichloride, Muriate,* or *Butter of Antimony.* Distilled from a mixture of 1 part of sesquisulphuret of antimony, and 2 of corrosive sublimate, (L. 1745,) or from 1 part of crocus of antimony, 2 of common salt, and 1 of sulphuric acid, (L. 1788.) But the *liquid chloride* is more usually obtained by dissolving the crude or roasted sulphuret in muriatic acid. (See Antimonii Oxychloridum.) P. directs the muriatic solution to be evaporated to one-third, and the remainder heated in a retort, so long as what passes over does not precipitate with water. Then change the receiver for a dry one, and preserve what passes over in long narrow vials. The chloride of the shops contains iron and free acid.

ANTIMONII CINIS. *Antimony Ash.* The roasted sesquisulphuret.

ANTIMONII CROCUS. L. 1788. *Crocus,* or *Saffron of Antimony.* Powdered sesquisulphuret of antimony ℔j, nitre ℔j, common salt ℥j. Mix and deflagrate by portions in a heated crucible. Pour out the fused mass, and separate it from the scoriæ. When reduced to powder, boiled, and afterwards repeatedly washed with water, it forms *Crocus Antimonii Lotus.* This crocus is also formed in the first part of the L. process for Antim. p.-tartras.

ANTIMONIUM DIAPHORETICUM ABLUTUM. See Antimonium Calcinatum. The PRUS. Ph. directs 4 parts of nitre, to 1 of sesquisulphuret of antimony.

ANTIMONII OXYCHLORIDUM. Antimonii Oxydum Nitro-Muriaticum. D. *Algaroth's Powder.* Prepared sulphuret of antimony 20 parts, muriatic acid 100 parts, nitric acid 1 part. Digest the sulphuret with the mixed acids in a glass vessel, (avoiding the fumes,) with a gradually increased heat. Boil for an hour, and pour the cooled and filtered liquid into a gallon of water. Wash the precipitate with plenty of water till the latter no longer reddens litmus paper, and dry the oxide on bibulous paper.

ANTIMONII OXYDUM. E. *Sesquioxide of Antimony.* Powdered sesquisulphuret of antimony ℥iv, muriatic acid Oj. Dissolve as in the last; and having poured the solution into Ov of water, collect the precipitate in a calico bag, wash it well with cold water, then with a weak solution of carbonate of soda, and again with water. Dry over a vapour-bath. [L. 1809 directs subcarbonate of potash. P. Bicarbonate of potash with heat. M. TYSON recommends sesquicarbonate of ammonia.] Dose, gr. ¼ to 1.

ANTIMONII OXYDUM. L. 1815. Dissolve separately ℥j of tartarized antimony, and ʒij of sesquicarbonate of ammonia in water. Boil the mixed solutions, collect and wash the precipitate, and dry it. [These oxides are much more active than the calx of antimony. A crystallized oxide is obtained by heating metallic antimony, and condensing the vapours in a suitable apparatus.]

ANTIMONIUM OXYSULPHURETUM. L. *Oxysulphuret*, or *Precipitated Sulphuret of Antimony.* Take of sesquisulphuret of antimony, in powder, ℥vij, solution of potash Oiv, distilled water Cij. Mix, and boil them over a slow fire for two hours, stirring frequently, and adding more water as it wastes. Filter the solution through linen, and add gradually diluted sulphuric acid q. s. to throw down the oxysulphuret, avoiding the poisonous fumes. Wash the preceipitate with water, and dry it with a gentle heat. [If the solution be allowed to cool slowly, before adding the acid, *Kermes mineral* is deposited, and the acid afterwards added throws down *golden sulphur of antimony.* Each of them requires to be washed with distilled water, pressed, and dried. In the P. and other foreign Ph., soda is directed instead of potash, and is said to yield a finer Kermes. See Kermes Minerale.]

ANTIMONII POTASSIO-TARTRAS. L. *Emetic Tartar.* Take of powdered s. sulphuret of antimony ℔ij, nitre ℔ij, hydrochloric acid f℥iv. Mix accurately, ignite the mixture on an iron plate, reduce the residue when cold to a fine powder, and wash it with boiling water till tasteless. Mix with it ℥xiv of bitartrate of potash, and boil for half an hour in a gallon of distilled water. Filter the liquor whilst hot, and set it aside to crystallize. Let the remaining liquid be evaporated for more crystals. E. directs ℥iij of the oxide (Antim. oxydum, E.), ℥iv½ of bitartrate of potash, to be boiled for an hour with f℥xxvij of water. D. 4 parts of the oxychloride, 5 of bit. potash, and 34 of water. P. 200 parts of glass of antimony, 300 of bit. of potash, and 2000 of water.

ANTIMONII PULVIS COMPOSITUS. See Pulvis Antimonii Comp.

ANTIMONII REGULUS. *Metallic Antimony* is obtained by heating the susquisulphuret with half its weight of clean iron-filings, in a covered crucible; or by heating the oxide or oxychloride with twice its weight of cream of tartar, to dull redness.

ANTIMONII SULPHURETUM AUREUM. E. Nearly as Antim. Oxysulphuretum. L.

ANTIMONII SUBHYDROSULPHAS. See Kermes Minerale.

ANTIMONII SULPHURETUM PRECIPITATUM. L. 1824. As Antimonii Oxysulphuretum. L. 1836.

ANTIMONII SESQUISULPHURETUM. L. Black or crude antimony is obtained from the native ore by heating it in a proper furnace, and separating the fused sulphuret from the less fusible earthy matter with which it is combined.

ANTIMONIUM PRÆPARATUM. The sesquisulphuret prepared as *Creta Præparata.*

ANTIMONIUM VITRIFACTUM. *Glass of Antimony.* L. 1788. Burn powdered (sesquisulphuret of) antimony in a shallow earthen vessel till the sulphurous vapours cease. Put it into a crucible, of which it will occupy two-thirds, and, having fitted a cover, apply a gradually increased heat till the matter fuses; and pour it on to an iron plate.

ANTIMONII VITRUM CERATUM. L. 1746 and Dr. YOUNG. Melt ʒj of yellow wax in an iron ladle, and add ℥j of glass of antimony in fine powder. Keep it over a gentle fire, free from flame, for about half an hour, or till it becomes nearly the colour of snuff. Pour it out on white paper, and when cold reduce it to powder. Dose, from 4 to 9 or 10 grains in dysentery.

APOZEMA ANTISCORBUTICUM. P. Roots of burdock, patience, and horseradish, fresh leaves of scurvy-grass, buck-bean, and water-cress, each ℥ss, boiling water Oiijss. Infuse for 2 hours, strain, and press; let the sediment subside, and decant.

APOZEMA ANTICOLICUM. DEGLAND'S mixture for Lead Colic. Senna ℥ij, sulphate of soda ℥j, syrup of buckthorn ℥ij, water ℥xvj.

APOZEMA CONTRASTIMULANS. LAENNEC. See Mistura Antimonialis.

APOZEMA DIURETICUM. The 5 roots (species diureticæ) ℥j, boiling water ℥xvj. Infuse half an hour, strain, and add nitre ℈j, syrup of the 5 roots ℥j.

APOZEMA EMETO-CATHARTICUM. Emetic tartar gr. j, sulphate of soda ʒiv, veal broth f℥xvj. By glassfuls, and repeat till it operates. The Eau de Trévez (Fr. H.) consists of sulphate of magnesia ℥j, emetic tartar gr. ss, water Oij.

APOZEMA FEBRIFUGUM. *Decoctum Cinchonæ.*

APOZEMA DICTUM DE FELTZ. *Decoctum Sarzæ cum Ichthyocollâ.*

APOZEMA PURGANS. See Mistura Purgans. P.

APOZEMA DICTUM PTISANA REGALIS. P. Senna ʒiv, sulphate of soda ʒiv, aniseed ʒj, cinnamon ʒj, fresh chervil ʒiv, cold water Oj¾, one lemon, sliced. Macerate for 24 hours, stirring occasionally; strain, press, and filter.

APOZEMA SUDORIFICUM. Decoctum Guaiaci Compositum.

APOZEMA VERMIFUGUM. *Decoctum Granati Vermifugum.*

AQUÆ DESTILLATÆ. *Simple Distilled Waters.* The plants, &c., are put into the still with twice as much water as is intended to be drawn off. Some recommend a previous maceration, but this is not directed by the British Colleges. L. directs f℥vij of proof spirit, and E. f℥iij of rectified spirit, to be added in the still, for each gallon of product, but the utility of this addition is very questionable. The waters should be kept in a cool place. The L. & E. colleges allow to be substituted for most of the distilled waters, mixtures of the essential oils and water. L. directs fʒij of the essential oil to be rubbed with ʒij of carbonate of magnesia, and a gallon of distilled water gradually added. When the sediment has subsided, filter the liquid. [A better method is to rub the oil with ℥j of precipitated chalk (Calcis Carbonas Precipitatum) and f℥ij of rectified spirit, and afterwards by degrees, the water. In a few minutes it may be filtered. But Mr. Warrington objects both to magnesia and chalk, as being to some extent soluble; and prefers fine porcelain clay, or calcined flints; he finds the waters keep better without the addition of spirit.]

AQUÆ SPIRITUOSÆ. The distilled spirits were formerly so called. See Spiritus.

AQUÆ MEDICATÆ. Besides the distilled waters, the following list contains imitations of the principal mineral waters (Aquæ Minerales Factitiæ); and a few saline solutions, &c., to which the name *Aqua* is commonly applied, though the L. college now restricts the term to Distilled Waters.

AQUA ABSINTHII. Wormwood tops ℔ij, water q. s. Distil ℔iv.

AQUA FLORUM ACACIÆ. As Aq. Rosæ, from fresh flowers of Robinia pseudo-acacia. It contains prussic acid. ZELLER.

AQUA ACETATIS AMMONIÆ. E. See Liquor Ammoniæ Acetatis.

AQUA ACIDI CARBONICI. U. S. *Aqua Aerata.* Water charged by pressure with 5 times its volume of carbonic acid gas.

AQUA ACIDULA ALKALINA. See Liquor Potassæ Effervescens; and Liq. Sodæ Effervescens.

AQUA AERE ORBATA. Water deprived of air by boiling, and cooled in close vessels. It should always be used in preparing sulphuretted and chalybeate waters; and is preferable for those containing carbonic acid gas.

AQUA ÆTHEREA. *Eau Ethérée.* P. Mix 1 part of æther with 8 of water; agitate frequently in a bottle with a ground stopper; let it rest 24 hours, separate the supernatant æther, and keep the water for use.

AQUA ÆTHEREA CAMPHORATA. Camphor ʒij, æther ʒvj, distilled water f℥xv. Dissolve the camphor in the æther, and add the water. Shake the mixture occasionally, and in 24 hours decant, or draw off the water as required.

AQUA ALBUMINOSA. White of 2 eggs, water ℔ij. Beat up the whites with a little of the water, and add the rest. Strain through a sieve. As an antidote for corrosive sublimate.

Aqua Alexiteria Simplex. L. 1746. Fresh mint ℔j, tops of sea wormwood ℔j, angelica leaves ℔j, water q. s. Distil Cong. ijss.

Aqua Alexiteria Spirituosa. See Spiritus Alexiterius.

Aqua Aluminosa Bateana. *Liquor Aluminis Compositum.*

Aqua Ammoniæ. See Liquor Ammoniæ.

Aqua Amygdalæ Amaræ. P. Mix ℔ij of fresh cake of bitter almonds (from which the oil has been expressed) with enough water to form a thin pap. In 24 hours distil ℔iv, by means of steam conducted to the bottom of the still by a tube connected with a boiler. Filter the distilled water through wet paper. Another method is to add the above thin pap (after 24 hours' maceration) to water already boiling in the still, which is to be immediately luted. The Prus. and Hamb. pharmacopœias (Aqua Amygd. am. Concentrata) direct ℔ij of the water to be drawn from ℔ij of bruised bitter almonds, ℥ij of spirit, and ℔ij of water. It is estimated to contain, when fresh, about one grain of real Prussic acid (equivalent to 50 grains or 55♏ of Ac. Hydrocyan. dil. L.) in ℥j. There are many other formulæ for this water in the foreign pharmacopœias, differing widely in strength, but most of them very powerful. M. Hænle proposes to mix ʒss of essential oil of bitter almonds, and ʒx of diluted hydrocyanic acid (L.) with ℥xij of distilled water. The mixture to be well shaken, and then filtered. For another substitute see Emulsio Amygdalæ cum Amygdalinâ. Dose, from 10 to 40 drops. A concentrated water, obtained in distilling the essential oil, is sometimes used to flavour confectionary, and as an external application: but for internal use it is scarcely ever prescribed in this country, not often in France, but more frequently in Germany, in the above doses. An overdose proves rapidly fatal. A very dilute almond water is sometimes sold for Aqua Cerasi Nigri.

Aqua Anethi. L. & E. Bruised dill seed ℔jss, proof spirit f℥vij, [rect. spt. f℥iij, E.] water Cij, distil Cj. It may also be made with the oil without distillation. See Aquæ Destillatæ, above.

Aqua Angelicæ. P. Angelica seeds ℔iij, water q. s. Distil Cj. [Guibourt directs the root.]

Aqua Anthemidis. Dried chamomile flowers ℔viij, water ℔lxxij. Distil ℔xlviij.

Aqua Antimoniata. M. Lenthois' remedy for consumption, consists of one grain of emetic tartar in from 6 to 12 pints of water: to be taken as a common beverage.

Aqua Anisi. From aniseeds, as Aqua Anethi. P. As Aqua Angelicæ.

Aqua Anisi Stellati. From star-anise or badian seeds; as Aqua Anisi.

Aqua Armoraciæ. P. Horse-radish root ℔ij, water q. s. distil ℔iv.

Aqua Aromatica. Prus. Ph. Sage ℥viij, rosemary ℥iv, peppermint ℥iv, lavender flowers ℥iv, fennel seeds ℥ij, cinnamon ℥ij, rectified spirit ℔iv, water ℔xx. Macerate 24 hours, and draw off ℔xij.

Aqua Florum Aurantii. L. Orange flowers ℔x, proof spirit ℥vij, water Cij. Distil Cj.

Aqua Corticis Aurantii. L. 1746. Rind of oranges ℥v, water q. s. Distil Cj.

Aqua Barytæ Muriatis. See Liquor Barii Chloridi.

Aqua Benedicta. The old name of Liquor Calcis. But *Eau bénite* of H. de la Charité is a solution of gr. v. emetic tartar in Oj of water. *Eau bénite de Ruland* is Vinum Antimonii.

Aqua Benzoata Aerata. Benzoate of potash, borax, of each gr. xv; bicarbonate of potash ʒss, water f℥xvj. Charge with carbonic acid gas.

Aqua Bergamii. From bergamot peel; as Aqua Corticis Aurantii.

Aqua Binelli. A styptic nostrum, supposed to contain creasote.

Aqua Bonnensis. Aqua sodii sulphureti serves as a substitute for the waters of Bonnes, Cauterets, St. Sauveur, &c.

Aqua Brominii. See Solutio Brominii.

Aqua Boraginis. P. From fresh Borage; as Aqua Lactucæ.

Aqua Bryoniæ. See Spiritus Bryoniæ.

Aqua Calcis. E. & D. See Liquor Calcis.

Aqua Calcis Composita. D. 1807. (*Aqua Benedicta Composita.*) Rasped guiacum wood ℥vj, liquorice root ℥j, sassafras bark ℥ss, coriander seeds ʒiij, fresh lime-water Ov. Macerate 2 days in a close vessel, and strain.

Aqua Calcis Carbonatis. *Carara Water.* Contains carbonate of lime held in solution by carbonic acid gas. *Antilithic.*

Aqua Calcis Muriatis. See Liquor Calcii Chloridi.

Aqua Camphoræ. Camphor Mixture. See Mistura Camphoræ.

Aqua Camphorata Bateana. See Aqua Cupri Sulphatis Camphorata.

Aqua Carmelitana. See Spiritus Melissæ Compositus.

Aqua Carui. L. From caraway seeds, or the oil, as Aqua Anethi.

Aqua Caryophylli. P. Cloves ℔ij, water q. s. Macerate for 12 hours, and distil ℔viij.

Aqua Cascarillæ. P. Cascarilla bark ℔iij, water q. s. Distil Cj.

Aqua Cassiæ. E. Cassia bark ℔jss, rectified spirit f℥iij, water q. s. Distil Cj. [Guy's H. substitutes ℥xv of cassia buds.]

Aqua Castorei. L. 1746. Castor ℥j, water q. s. Distil ℔ij.

Aqua Cerasi Nigri. Prus. P. Black cherries (crushed in the hands, and the stones broken in a mortar) ℔x, water q. s. Distil ℔xx. [It contains prussic acid. A very dilute water of bitter almonds is often substituted for it. It should never be administered unless its exact strength is known.]

Aqua Chalybeata Aerata. Soubeiran. Water freed from air Oj, sulphate of iron gr. ss. Charge with 5 volumes of carbonic acid gas. Or, sulphate of iron, gr. j, carbonate of soda, gr. iv; water, freed from air and charged with 5 volumes of gas, Oj. [Bewley's *Aqua Chalybeata* is a solution of citrate of iron in aërated water flavoured with orange peel.]

Aqua Chenopodii Vulvariæ. Stinking goose-foot ℔j, water ℔vj. Distil ℔iij.

Aqua Chlorinii. D. *Aqua Oxymuriatica.* Pass chlorine gas (see Chlorinium) through cold water till it ceases to be absorbed. Aqua Chlorinei, E. is prepared by triturating ʒj of muriate of soda, and 350 grains of red oxide of lead; putting them into a stoppered bottle with f℥viij of water, and adding fʒij of sulphuric acid. After shaking the mixture, leave it to settle and decant. Dose fʒss to fʒij diluted.

Aqua Cinnamomi. L. Bruised cinnamon ℔jss (*or* oil of cinnamon ʒij), proof spirit f℥vij, water Cij. Distil Cj. It may also be made without distillation.

AQUA COCHLEARIÆ. P. Fresh scurvy-grass ℔ij, water q. s. Distil ℔ij.

AQUA COLONIENSIS. *Eau de Cologne.* P. Oil of bergamot ℥iij, oil of lemon ℥iij, oil of rosemary ℥jss, oil of neroli ℥jss, oil of lavender ℥jss, oil of cinnamon ʒvj, rectified spirit Oxxiv, compound spirit of balm Oiij, spirit of rosemary Oij. Mix, and after 8 days distil Oxxiv.

AQUA COPAIBÆ. Dr. CATTELL. Oil of copaiba ℥ij, water Cong. vss. Distil 3 or 4 gallons.

AQUA CORIANDRI. GUIBOURT. From coriander seeds, as Aqua Angelicæ.

AQUA CREASOTI. Creasote ʒj, distilled water ℥x. Shake together, and filter.

AQUA CUBEBÆ. From oil of cubebs, as Aqua Copaibæ. [Both are used as injections.]

AQUA CUPRI SULPHATIS CAMPHORATA. BATES' *Camphorated Lotion.* Sulphate of copper gr. xv, bole gr. xv, powdered camphor gr. iv, boiling water f℥iv. When cold, filter. [As a collyrium this requires dilution. Mr. Ware directs the above quantity to be diluted with Oiv of distilled water.]

AQUA DESTILLATA. L. From 10 gallons of water, distil 8, rejecting the first 2. E. directs the first 20th to be rejected and the next half preserved.

AQUA FABARUM. From bean-flowers: as Aqua Sambuci.

AQUA FŒNICULI. L. & E. From sweet fennel seeds: as Aqua Anethi.

AQUA FORMICARUM. BRUNS. P. Red ants q. v., water q. s. Distil three-fourths, express the residue, and distil the liquor nearly to dryness.

AQUA FORTIS. See Acidum Nitrosum Dilutum.

AQUA FRAGARIÆ. SAX. P. Strawberries ℔ij, water q. s. Distil ℔iij.

AQUA GOULARDI. See Liquor Plumbi Diacetatis Dilutus.

AQUA HORDEATA. See Decoctum Hordei.

AQUA HUNGARICA. *Queen of Hungary's Water.* See Spiritus Rosmarini.

AQUA HYDROCYANICA VEGETABILIS. SCHRADER. Essential

oil of bitter almonds, ʒj, rectified spirit ℥jss, distilled water ℥xvj. Mix well, and filter through wet filtering paper. [Intended as a substitute for Aqua Lauro-Cerasi.]

AQUA HYDROGENII. Water charged by pressure with hydrogen gas.

AQUA HYDROSULPHURATA. See Acidum Hydrosulphuricum Aqua Solutum.

AQUA HYSSOPI. P. From fresh hyssop: as Aqua Melissæ.

AQUA HYSTERICA. As Spiritus Bryoniæ Comp., omitting the Bryony.

AQUA IODURETÆ. LUGOL'S original ioduretted waters consisted respectively of ½, ¾, and 1 grain of iodine, dissolved in alcohol, ℥xvj of water, and ℥ij of sea salt. For the present form see Solutiones Iodinii.

AQUA JAVELLI. *Eau de Javelle.* See Liquor Potassæ Chlorinatæ.

AQUA JUNIPERI. P. Bruised juniper berries ℔iij, water q. s. Distil Cj.

AQUA LACTUCÆ. P. Fresh lettuces bruised ℔x, water ℔xx. Distil ℔x.

AQUA-LAURO CERASI. E. and D. Fresh leaves of cherry-laurel chopped small ℔j, water Oijss. Distil Oj, agitate the distilled liquor well, filter it through wet paper, and add compound spirit of lavender ℥j. [Dr. NELIGAN says the spirit of lavender is generally omitted. The dose is from ♏x to xx. It is more frequently prescribed in this kingdom than Aq. Amygd. Amaræ, but is liable to the objection that the quantity of prussic acid it contains is variable. M. HÆNLE proposes to substitute the following:—Mix ℥xij of distilled water with ʒss of essential oil of cherry-laurel, and ʒvj of diluted hydrocyanic acid, and filter.]

AQUA LAVANDULÆ. P. Flowering tops of lavender ℔ij, water q. s. Distil by steam ℔iv. [The simple and perfumed spirit of lavender are also termed *lavender water.* See Spiritus Lavandulæ.]

AQUA LILIORUM CONVALLIUM. BRUNS. Ph. Flowers of the lily of the valley ℔j, water ℔iv. Distil ℔ij.

AQUA LIMONIS. E. 1817. Fresh lemon-peel ℔ij, water q. s. Distil ℔x.

AQUA LITHARGYRI ACETATI. See Liquor Plumbi Diacetatis.

AQUA MAGNESIÆ CARBONATIS. See Liquor Magnesiæ Carbonatis.

AQUA MARINA FACTITIA. *Sea Water.* Common salt ℥xvj, sulphate of soda ℥vij, muriate of lime ℥jss, muriate of magnesia ℥vj, iodide of potassium ℈j, bromide of potassium ℈ss, water 4 gallons. The salts are to be in crystals. A simpler substitute is used as a bath; ℔j of salt to ℔xxx of water.

AQUA MATRICARIÆ. From feverfew: as Aqua Menthæ.

AQUA MELILOTI. P. Dried flowers of melilot ℔ij, water q. s. Distil ℔vij.

AQUA MELISSÆ. P. Fresh tops of balm ℔xij, water q. s. Distil Cj.

AQUA MENTHÆ PIPERITÆ. L. and E. Dried peppermint ℔ij (or ℔iv of the fresh herb; or ʒij of the essential oil), water Cij, proof spirit f℥vij, [rectified spirit f℥iij, E.,] distil Cj. It may also be made from the oil by trituration. See Aquæ Destillatæ.

AQUÆ MENTHÆ VIRIDIS (vulgaris, 1745; sativæ, 1788). L. and E. From common mint, as Aqua Menthæ Piperitæ.

AQUA MENTHÆ PULEGII. L. and E. From pennyroyal herb or oil, as Aqua Menthæ Piperitæ.

AQUA MYRTI. GRAY. Myrtle flowers ℔iij, water q. s. Draw a gallon.

AQUA NAPHÆ. Aqua Florum Aurantii.

AQUA NIGRA. GERM. H. See Lotio Hydr. Chloridi.

AQUA NITROGENII PROTOXIDI. See Aqua Oxygenii.

AQUA OPII. GUIBOURT. Opium in small pieces ℔j, water ℔vj. Macerate for 48 hours, and distil ℔j. Some authorities direct ℔iij to be distilled. Dose ʒij or more.

AQUÆ OPHTHALMICÆ. *Eye Waters.* See Collyria.

AQUA OXYGENII. Water charged by pressure with oxygen gas. But what is sold as oxygenous water, is stated by Dr. PEREIRA to be an aqueous solution of protoxide of nitrogen (laughing gas); each bottle containing about a quart of the gas.

AQUA OXYMURIATICA. See Aqua Chlorinii.

AQUA ORIGANI. P. As Aqua Meliloti, from wild marjoram flowers.

Aqua Persicæ. P. Fresh peach-leaves cut small ℔ij, water ℔iv. Distil gently ℔ij.

Aqua Petroselini. P. From parsley-seed: as Aqua Angelicæ.

Aqua Phagedænica. See Lotio Hydrargyri flava.

Aqua Picis. D. and Bp. Berkeley. Mix a quart of wood tar with Cj of cold water; stir together for a quarter of an hour, and filter. Keep it in a closed vessel. Taken, in various chronic disorders, to the amount of a pint or more daily.

Aqua Plantaginis. P. From fresh plantain-leaves: as Aqua Lactucæ.

Aqua Pimentæ. L. Bruised pimento ℔j (or ʒij of the oil), proof spirit f℥vij, water Cij. Distil Cj.

Aqua Pimentæ Diluta. Guy's H. Pimento water ℥vj, water ℥x. Other waters, similarly diluted, are directed in Hospital Formularies.

Aqua Potassæ. See Liquor Potassæ.

Aqua Potassæ Sulphureti. See Aq. Sulph. Potassæ.

Aqua Pulegii. From dried or fresh pennyroyal, or the oil: as Aqua Menthæ Piperitæ.

Aqua Pullna Artificialis. Sulphate of soda ℥iv, sulphate of magnesia ℥v; muriate of lime ʒj, muriate of magnesia ʒiv, muriate of soda ʒij; water Cj, carbonic acid gas Cv.

Aqua Rabelii. See Acidum Sulphuricum Alcoholisatum.

Aqua Raphani. See Aqua Armoraciæ.

Aqua Regia. The former name of nitro-muriatic acid.

Aqua Rhodii. Guibourt. Rhodium wood 1 part, water 8. Macerate, and distil 4 parts.

Aqua Rosæ. L. and E. Hundred-leaved roses ℔x, water Cij, proof spirit f℥vij, [rectified spirit ℥iij, E.] Distil a gallon. [Fresh petals should be preferred: but those which have been preserved by beating them with twice their weight of salt, are allowed by E.]

Aqua Rosmarini. Aqua Anthos. Rosemary in flower ℔j, water q. s. Infuse 24 hours, and distil a gallon.

Aqua Rubi Idæi. Fresh raspberries ℔vj, water q. s. Distil Cj. Pruss. P. directs ℔x of the cake left after expressing the juice, ℥ij of carbonate of potash, ℔xxx of water. Distil ℔xx.

AQUA RUTÆ. Fresh rue 1 part, water q. s. Macerate 24 hours, and distil 10 parts.

AQUA SALVIÆ. P. As Aqua Lavandulæ.

AQUA SAMBUCI. L. From fresh elder flowers: as Aqua Rosæ. [This water cannot be prepared from the oil. The flowers preserved by salt are sometimes used when the fresh flowers cannot be obtained.]

AQUA SANTALI. From yellow saunders: as Aqua Rhodii.

AQUA SAPPHIRINA. Liquor Cupri Ammoniati.

AQUA SASSAFRAS. P. Sliced sassafras ℔iij, water q. s. Distil Cj.

AQUA SEDLITZENSIS. P. Crys. sulphate of magnesia ℨij, water Oj, dissolve, and charge the solution with 3 volumes of carbonic acid gas.

AQUA SELTERANA. *Selters, or Seltzer Water.* P. Chloride of sodium ℈j, cr. carbonate of soda gr. xv, cr. phosphate of soda gr. jss, water ℥x. Dissolve also muriate of lime gr. v, muriate of magnesia, gr. iv, in water ℥x. Mix the solution, and aerate with 5 volumes of carbonic acid gas.

AQUA SERPYLLI. P. From mother of thyme: as Aqua Meliloti.

AQUA SINAPIS NIGRÆ. GUIBOURT. Mix one part of ground black mustard-seed with 8 of water; macerate for 12 hours, and distil 4 parts, by means of steam conducted by a tube from a boiler to the bottom of the still. Filter through moistened paper to separate the oil. Used externally as a rubefacient.

AQUA SODÆ EFFERVESCENS. See Liquor Sodæ Effervescens.

AQUA SODII SULPHURETI. *Eau Sulfurée. Bareges Waters.* Crys. sulphuret of sodium ℈j, cr. carbonate of soda ℈j, muriate of soda ℈j, water freed from air Cj. A stronger solution is prepared for baths; see Solutio ad Balneum Baretginense.

AQUA SPADANA. *Spa Water.* Carbonate of soda ℨss, carbonate of lime gr. ij, carbonate of magnesia gr. ijss, protochloride of iron gr. v, aerated water Cj.

AQUÆ SPIRITUOSÆ. Many of the distilled spirits were formerly termed waters. See Spiritus.

AQUA SULPHURATA. L. 1745. Water ℔ij, sulphur ℔ss. Burn the sulphur in successive portions, in an iron spoon, over the water in a closed vessel.

AQUA SULPHURETI AMMONIÆ. See Ammoniæ Hydrosulphuretum.

AQUA SULPHURETI POTASSÆ. D. Sulphur 1 part, solution of potash 11 parts. Boil for 10 minutes, and filter. Dose ℞ x to xl. P. directs a solution of the liver of sulphur in cold water, of the density of 1·261. It contains one-third its weight of the sulphuret.

AQUA TANACETI. P. Flowering tops of tansy ℔vj, water q. s. Distil Cj.

AQUA TILIÆ. P. From lime-tree flowers: as Aqua Meliloti.

AQUA ULMARIÆ. From the fresh flowers of Meadow sweet: as Aqua Sambuci. It is said to contain prussic acid.

AQUA VALERIANÆ. P. Valerian root ℔iij, water q. s. Distil Cj.

AQUA VANILLÆ. NIEMANN. Vanilla ℔j, water ℔xij. Maccrate 24 hours, and distil ℔vj.

AQUA VICENSIS. *Eau de Vichy.* Carbonate of soda ʒij, muriate of soda gr. ij, muriate of lime gr. viij, sulphate of soda gr. viij, sulphate of iron gr. $\frac{1}{3}$, sulphate of magnesia gr. iij, water Oj. Charge with $3\frac{1}{2}$ volumes of carbonic acid gas.

AQUA VIOLARUM. Violets 1 part, water 4. After 6 hours, distil 2 parts.

AQUA VITRIOLICA CAMPHORATA. L. 1788. Sulphate of zinc ℥ss, water f ℥xxxij, spirit of camphor ℥ss. Mix and filter.

AQUA VULNERARIA. From the same herbs as Spiritus Vulnerarius, but with water only.

ARGENTI AMMONIO-CHLORIDUM. SERRE. Saturate boiling liquor ammoniæ with fresh-precipitated and carefully-washed chloride of silver: filter whilst boiling hot and let the crystals, which form on cooling, be dried between blotting paper, and immediately put into well-stopped bottles. Dose from $\frac{1}{14}$th of a grain.

ARGENTI CHLORIDUM. Precipitate solution of nitrate of silver by an excess of muriate of soda; wash the precipitate thoroughly with distilled water, dry it quickly, and keep it from the light. Dose, $\frac{1}{2}$ gr. to 3 gr., or more, as a tonic and antispasmodic. It is the *Calx Lunæ* of BATE, &c., who extended the dose to gr. x.

ARGENTI CYANIDUM. L. Dissolve ʒxviij of nitrate of silver in

Oj of distilled water. Add Oj of diluted hydrocyanic acid, collect the precipitate, wash, and dry it. Dose, $\frac{1}{12}$th to $\frac{1}{8}$th of a grain.

ARGENTI IODIDUM. Dr. PATTERSON. Dissolve separately, in distilled water, equal weights of iodide of potassium and nitrate of silver. Mix the solutions, wash the precipitate with distilled water, and dry it with a gentle heat. Dose, $\frac{1}{8}$th to $\frac{1}{4}$th of a grain in stomach affections; gradually increased to $\frac{1}{2}$ or 1 gr. in epilepsy.

ARGENTI NITRAS. L. *Lunar Caustic.* Dissolve ℥jss of pure silver in f℥j of nitric acid mixed with f℥ij of distilled water. Evaporate the solution to dryness, fuse, and pour into greased moulds. E. the same. D. 37 parts of silver, and 60 nitrous acid. [It may be procured in *crystals* by concentrating the solution so that crystals may form in cooling. More may be obtained by evaporating the residual liquid. Let the crystals drain in a funnel, and wash them with a few drops of cold distilled water. If impure silver is used, the copper may be removed by washing the salt with pure nitric acid, or heating it in an iron spoon, and again dissolving and crystallizing.] Dose, gr. $\frac{1}{6}$th to gr. iij. Tonic.

ARGENTI OXYDUM. Mr. LANE. To a solution of ʒiv nitrate of silver, add solution of ʒij of hydrate of potash; wash the precipitate well, and dry it in the shade, with a moderate heat. Dose, $\frac{1}{2}$ gr. to gr. j, in cases of gastralgia, pyrosis, nervous affections, &c., twice or thrice a day.

ARGENTI PULVIS. Heat the oxide to dull redness in a porcelain crucible; when cold, triturate it in an agate mortar, and pass it through a sieve.

ARSENICI IODIDUM. M. BIETT. Mix 16 parts of metallic arsenic with 100 of iodine, and heat them in a glass retort till the iodide sublimes. Or digest them with water till combined, and evaporate the filtered solution to dryness at a very gentle heat. See Liquor Arsenici Periodidi.

ARSENICUM ALBUM SUBLIMATUM. *Arsenious Acid.* Commercial arsenic powdered and resublimed.

ARSENICUM ANTIMONIATUM. JUSTAMOND'S *Caustic.* Mix ℥ij of black sulphuret of antimony with ℥j of white arsenic, and melt together, avoiding the fumes.

ASPARAGINUM. *Asparagine,* or *Althein.* From asparagus juice;

but more conveniently from marsh-mallow root. Slice the root, macerate it twice in cold water, evaporate the mixed liquor to half, strain repeatedly through flannel, and evaporate to the consistence of syrup. Expose it to the air for some days; wash the crystals which form with a little water, and purify by re-crystallization. The juice of the climbing vetch is said to yield it abundantly.

AURI PULVIS. P. Triturate leaf-gold with 10 or 12 times its weight of sulphate of potash, and wash out the latter with boiling water. Dose, gr. $\frac{1}{5}$th to 1 grain; or applied in frictions to the tongue.

AURI [TER]-CHLORIDUM. P. Dissolve gold in 3 parts nitro-muriatic acid; evaporate till vapours of chlorine begin to appear, and set aside to crystallize. Dose, $\frac{1}{20}$th to $\frac{1}{16}$th of a grain.

AURO-CHLORIDUM SODII. P. *Soda-muriate of Gold.* Dissolve 85 parts chloride of gold, and 16 chloride of sodium, in a little water; concentrate by evaporation, that crystals may form as it cools. Dose, as the last. Both require to be very cautiously administered.

AURI CYANIDUM. DEFOSSES. Boil fresh precipitated oxide of gold (washed, but not dried) with diluted hydrocyanic acid, till the liquid assumes a beautiful yellow tint; and evaporate the clear solution to dryness at a gentle heat. Dose, $\frac{1}{16}$th to $\frac{1}{10}$th of a grain.

AURI IODIDUM. P. To a solution of chloride of gold add a solution of iodide of potassium as long as it occasions a precipitate. Wash this with alcohol, and dry it with a gentle heat. M. MEILLET substitutes hydriodate of ammonia for iodide of potassium. Dose, as the last.

AURI OXYDUM. P. *Teroxide of Gold*, or *Auric Acid.* To a solution of 1 part of chloride of gold in 40 of distilled water, add 4 parts of fresh calcined magnesia. Boil together, and wash the sediment with distilled water, then with pure nitric acid diluted with 20 parts of water, and again with water. Dry it in the shade. Dose, from $\frac{1}{10}$th to $\frac{3}{4}$ths of a grain.

AURUM MUSIVUM. See Stanni Persulphuretum.

AURUM STANNO-PARATUM. P. *Purple of Cassius.* Dissolve 1 part of chloride of gold in 200 parts of distilled water. Dissolve also 1 part of pure tin in 3 of nitro-muriatic acid, without heat, and dilute with 100 parts of distilled water. Add the solution of tin very gradually to the solution of gold so long as it causes a precipitate. Wash this by decantation, and dry it by a gentle heat.

BALNEÆ MEDICATÆ. Baths of cold or heated water, vapour, and heated air, are used medicinally. The following are the temperatures at which they are usually applied. WATER. *Cold*, 50° to 75° F. *Temperate*, 75 to 85. *Tepid*, 85 to 92. *Warm*, 92 to 98. *Hot*, 98 to 112. VAPOUR. If breathed—*Tepid*, 90 to 100. *Warm*, 100 to 110. *Hot*, 110 to 130. If not breathed—*Tepid*, 96 to 106. *Warm*, 106 to 120. *Hot*, 120 to 160. HOT AIR. As a *Sudorific*, 85 to 100. As a *Stimulant*, 100 to 130. Water (usually warm), vapour, and heated air, are often medicated by being charged with the active principles of various herbs and other drugs. The principal kinds in use are mentioned below. There are various contrivances for applying them either to particular parts, or to the whole surface, except that of the head. Dr. LYNCH has suggested one which combines a vapour and hot air bath. In the absence of suitable apparatus, Dr. SERRES suggests a simple plan of applying hot vapour,—a lump of quick lime, wrapped in a wet cloth, and covered with a dry one, is placed on each side of the patient in bed, and allowed to remain until perspiration is established. Probably the vapour might be *medicated* by placing the required ingredients between the two cloths.

BALNEUM ACIDUM. Dr. SCOTT'S *Nitro-muriatic Bath.* Muriatic acid f℥iij, nitric acid f℥ij, water f℥v. Mix. As a knee or foot bath, or for sponging, f℥iij of this diluted acid are mixed with each gallon of water. In winter it should be warmed. Time of application 20 or 30 minutes daily, for 2 or 3 weeks; afterwards every 2d or 3d day. As a *general* bath, it should be weaker. SOUBEIRAN prescribes from 4 to 16 ounces of nitro-muriatic acid to 60 gallons of water; the same quantity of muriatic acid is sometimes used.

BALNEUM ALKALINUM. F. H. Washing soda ℥viij to ℥xvj, warm water 60 gallons, or q. s. As a *foot-bath* ℥ij of subcarbonate of potash to q. s. of water.

BALNEUM AMMONIÆ HYDROCHLORATIS. ℔iv of sal ammoniac to a bath, for an adult.

BALNEUM ANTIMONIALE. SOUBEIRAN. Emetic tartar ℥j to ℥ij, water 64 gallons, or q. s. In lumbago, and some diseases of the skin.

BALNEUM AROMATICUM. F. H. Aromatic herbs (Species Aromaticæ) ℥xxxij, water q. s. Boil for a quarter of an hour, and add soap liniment ℥iv, sal ammoniac ℥ij. The aromatic *vapour* bath is made by causing steam to pass through the same herbs.

BALNEUM ASTRINGENS. MOST. Dissolve ℔iv of alum in cold water, and add 6 or 8 pailfuls of whey. In extensive burns.

BALNEUM BARETGINENSE. Add f℥x of concentrated Bareges water (solutio ad balneum baretginense) to a bath of 60 or 70 gallons.

BALNEUM BENZOICUM. Benzoin is sometimes used in the same way as camphor. See next article.

BALNEUM CAMPHORÆ. About ℥ss of camphor is placed upon a heated plate within, or communicating with, the chamber of the bath.

BALNEUM CARBONICUM. Carbonic acid gas (procured by the action of diluted sulphuric acid on chalk or marble) is applied to the body (except the head), or to particular parts, by means of a suitable apparatus.

BALNEUM CHLORINII. M. Chlorine gas (procured by gently heating in a glass retort ʒiv to ʒviij of black oxide of manganese, ℥jss of common salt, and ℥j of sulphuric acid previously mixed with ℥j of water) is applied in the same way as carbonic acid (see B. Carbonicum), at the temperature of 104° to 115° F. [Mr. WALLACE says 150°] for half an hour. The quantity of materials may be gradually increased to triple this quantity. Care must be taken to confine the gas securely, so that the patient shall not breathe it.

BALNEUM CONII. It. H. A decoction of fresh or dried hemlock is added to an ordinary bath. The quantity is not accurately indicated. [8 or 10 pinches of the herb. FANTONETTI.]

BALNEUM ELECTRICUM. The patient, insulated on a glass-legged seat, is put in contact with the prime conductor of an electrical machine.

BALNEUM FERRI IODIDI. PIERQUIN. Iodide of iron ℥j, water q. s. for a bath.

BALNEUM FURFURIS. Boil ℔iv of bran with Cj of water and add it to the bath, which should be used at 90°.

BALNEUM GELATINOSUM. F. H. Flanders glue ℔ijss, water Cij. Dissolve by heat, and add it to a warm bath.

BALNEUM HYDRARGYRI BICHLORIDI. F. H. *Bains antisyphilitiques.* From 5 to 10 grains of corrosive sublimate in water q. s. for a bath. Rarely used. Some authorities prescribe ʒij of sublimate.

BALNÆ IODURETÆ. LUGOL. For *Adults*, ʒij of iodine to ʒiv of iodide of potassium to be dissolved in Oj of water and added to a warm bath of 50 to 70 gallons. For *Children*, from f℥iij to f℥iv of the same solution may be used for a bath of 9 to 30 gallons. Wooden vessels must be used.

BALNEUM MARIS FACTITIUM. See Aqua Marina. Or dissolve 1 part of common salt in 30 of water. As a pediluvium, add a handful of salt to a pail of water; to which a little mustard is sometimes added.

BALNEÆ PNEUMATICÆ. Air of different temperatures, and variously impregnated with volatile remedies, is applied locally or generally to the body. Lately, compressed air has been applied locally; and M. TABARIE has caused patients to *breathe* compressed air for 2 or 3 hours daily, in some cases of *aphonia.* On the other hand, the removal of the pressure of the atmosphere, by dry cupping or an exhausting syringe, is employed as a revulsive.

BALNEUM RESOLVENS. F. H. Common salt ℥ij, sulphuret of potassium ℥j, subcarbonate of soda ℥ss, decoction of sage q. s. Dissolve, and add warm water for a bath.

BALNEUM SALINUM. See Balneum Maris.

BALNEUM SALINUM GELATINOSUM. Common salt ℔j, Flanders glue ℔ij. Dissolve separately in water by heat, and add water q. s. for a bath.

BALNEUM SAPONIS. F. H. Soap ℔ijss, dissolve in hot water q. s. and add to the bath.

BALNEUM SINAPIS. Flour of mustard ℥iv, mix it with a little water, and add it to the warm bath.

BALNEUM SODÆ CHLORINATÆ. F. H. Liquid chlorinated soda ℔jss, water q. s. for a bath. But the French solution is weaker than that of our pharmacopœia.

BALNEUM SULPHUROSUM. The fumes of burning sulphur, with hot air or vapour, are employed in the cure of itch, &c. About ℥ss of sulphur is used at once. Care must be taken to prevent the patient breathing the fumes.

BALNEUM SULPHURATUM. F. H. Liver of sulphur (sulphuret of potassium) ℥jss to ℥iv (or liquid sulphuret of potash ℥v) warm water C 25 to 50. Sulphuret of soda is sometimes used. G. H. employ sulphuret of lime ℥ij to a bath; adding at the time of using 30 or 40 drops of sulphuric acid. The Bareges water (see Balneum Baretginense) is less disagreeable.

BALNEUM SULPHURATUM GELATINOSUM. DUPUYTREN. Add to the Balneum Sulphuratum, ℔ij of Flanders glue, dissolved in hot water.

BALNEUM VAPORIS. See BALNEÆ.

BALSAMUM ACETICUM CAMPHORATUM. M. PELLETIER. Curd soap ʒv, camphor ʒv, oil of thyme ℈ij, acetic æther ℥v. Digest the soap in the æther till dissolved, and add the rest. [Dr. Sanchez' gout balsam is similar.]

BALSAMUM ACOUSTICUM. Dr. HUGH SMITH. Ox-gall ʒiij, balsam of Peru ʒj. Mix. In fœtid discharges from the ear.

BALSAMUM ACOUSTICUM CUM CREASOTO. BOUCHARDAT. Comp. spirit of balm ʒijss, almond oil ʒv, ox-gall ʒx, creasote 10 drops.

BALSAMUM ANODYNUM. BATE. See Linimentum Opii.

BALSAMUM AD APOPLECTICOS. E. 1744. Expressed oil of nutmeg ℥j; liquefy, and add oil of cloves, of lavender, and of rosemary, each ʒss, oil of amber, ♏x, balsam of Peru ʒj.

BALSAMUM FIORAVENTI. P. Venice turpentine ℥xvj, elemi, tacamahaca, amber, styrax, galbanum, and myrrh, each ℥iij, aloes ℥j, bayberries ℥iv, galangal, zedoary, ginger, cinnamon, cloves, and nutmegs, each ℥jss, dittany of Crete ℥j, rectified spirit ℔viij (Ovi½). Macerate six days, and distil ℔vij.

BALSAMUM GUAIACINUM. L. 1745. Guaiac ℔j, balsam of Peru ʒiij, rectified spirit Oij.

BALSAMUM HYDRIODATUM. See Linimentum Ioduretum Gelatinosum.

BALSAMUM LOCATELLI. E. 1744. Melt ℔j of yellow wax with f℥xxiv of olive oil, and add Venice turpentine ℔jss. Remove from the fire, and add balsam of Peru ℥ij, powdered dragon's blood ℥j, and stir till cold. L. 1746 directed olive oil ℥xvj, Venice turpentine ℔ss, yellow wax ℔ss, red saunders ʒvj.

BALSAMUM NERVINUM. *Baume Nerval.* P. Expressed oil of nutmegs (oil of mace) ℥iv, beef marrow ℥iv; melt, and add oil of rosemary ʒij, oil of cloves ʒj, balsam of Tolu ʒij, camphor ʒj, dissolved in alcohol ℥iv.

BALSAMUM ODONTALGICUM. Opium ℈j, rectified oil of turpentine ʒjss, oil of cloves ʒss, oil of cajeput ʒss, balsam of Peru ʒij.

BALSAMUM OPODELDOCH. P. Curd soap ℥j, camphor ʒvj, water of ammonia ʒij, oil of rosemary ʒjss, oil of thyme ʒss, rectified spirit ℥viij. In imitation of Steer's Opodeldoc.

BALSAMUM AD PERNIONES. LEJEUNE. Camphor ʒj, tincture of benzoin ʒv, iodide of potassium ʒv, diacetate of lead ʒx, rectified spirit, reduced to proof with rosewater, ʒxx. Mix, and add a warm solution of curd soap ʒx, in spirit (as above) ʒxx.

BALSAMUM PICEUM. E. H. Tar ℥iv, rectified spirit f℥xvj. Digest 3 days, and decant.

BALSAMUM POLYCHRESTUM. L. 1721. Rectified spirit ℔ijss (Oij), guaiacum ℥xvj, balsam of Peru ℥ss. Digest, and strain. See Elixir Polychrestum, E.

BALSAMUM SAPONACEUM. Linimentum Saponis.

BALSAMUM SATURNINUM. BATE. Acetate of lead ℥iv, oil of turpentine ℥xij. Digest for some days.

BALSAMUM SUCCINI. BATE. Digest powdered amber with twice its weight of turpentine. The residue in redistilling oil of amber is also so termed.

BALSAMUM SULPHURIS. See Oleum Sulphuratum.

BALSAMUM SULPHURIS ANISATUM. Originally made by digesting 1 part of sulphur with 4 of oil of aniseed. But a mixture of oil of aniseed with balsam of sulphur is usually sold for it.

BALSAMUM SULPHURIS TEREBINTHINATUM. Digest 1 part of sulphur with 4 of oil of turpentine till dissolved.

[Similar compounds were formerly made with sulphur and Barbadoes tar; and with the empyreumatic oils of amber, benzoin, &c.]

BALSAMUM TEREBINTHINATUM. Olive oil ℥vj, oil of turpentine ℥ij, yellow wax ℥j, balsam of Peru ʒij, camphor ʒjss.

BALSAMUM TRANQUILLANS. P. Fresh leaves of belladonna, henbane, black nightshade, tobacco, poppies, and stramonium, of each ℥iv; dried tops of wormword, hyssop, lavender, marjoram, round-leaved mint, costmary, St. John's wort, rue, and sage, of each ℥j; dried flowers of elder and rosemary, each ℥j; olive oil Ovj. Bruise the fresh plants, heat them with the oil until their moisture is dissipated, and leave them to digest for 2 hours: strain with pressure, pour the hot oil on the tops and dried flowers; macerate for a month, strain, press, and keep the oil in close bottles in a cool, dark place. *Baume Tranquille de Chomel* is made by boiling ℔j each of the henbane, houndstongue, and tobacco in 3 pints white wine to 2 pints; and boiling the strained liquor with as much olive oil.

BALSAMUM TRAUMATICUM. Tinctura Benzoes Composita.

BALSAMUM VIRIDE. E. 1744. Linseed oil ℔j, oil of turpentine ℔j, powdered verdigris ʒiij. Boil, and stir till cold.

BALSAMUM VITÆ. Several aloetic compounds, represented by Tinctura Rhei et Aloes, and Decoctum Aloes comp., are sometimes named *Baume*, or *Elixir de Vie*. But Hoffmann's Balsamum Vitæ is—oil of cinnamon, lemon, cloves, lavender, nutmegs, of each ℈j; ambergris, oil of rue and of amber, of each ℈ss; balsam of Peru ℈j; rectified spirit ℥x. That of Gaubius is similar. *Baume de Vie externe de Plenk* consists of soap ℥ij, oil of turpentine ℥iv, solution of carbonate of potash ʒiij. Or, according to Swediaur, soap ʒiij, oil of turpentine ʒiij, spirit of thyme ℥iij, liquid ammonia ʒj to ʒiv.

BARII BROMIDUM. M. Boil a solution of bromide of iron (see Solutio Ferri Bromidi. MOHR) with fresh precipitated carbonate of barytes; filter, and evaporate to dryness.

BARII CHLORIDUM. L. Barytæ Murias. E. Dissolve ℥x of carbonate of barytes in f℥x of muriatic acid diluted with Oij of water, and evaporate that crystals may form.

BARII IODIDUM. M. Heat a fresh solution of iodide of iron with excess of carbonate of barytes; filter, and evaporate to dryness. Redissolve, and crystallize.

BARII SULPHURETUM. Mix native sulphate of barytes, finely powdered, with an equal quantity of flour (or s. barytes ℔ij, charcoal ℥v, powdered black resin ℥j); and calcine the mixture in a covered crucible, at a white heat, for an hour or two. By treating the mass with hot water, the sulphuret is dissolved out, and may be obtained in crystals from the filtered solution.

BARYTÆ CARBONAS. Carbonate of barytes is found native; but is also procured, for pharmaceutical purposes, by precipitating the nitrate or muriate, by a carbonated alkali.

BARYTÆ MURIAS. See Barii Chloridum.

BARYTÆ NITRAS. Dissolve carbonate of barytes in nitric acid, and evaporate to dryness. Dissolve it in water, filter, and evaporate the solution that crystals may form.

BEBEERINA. From the fruit and bark of the Bebeeru, or Greenheart tree, similar in its uses and properties to quina. Dr. RODIE. The bark is exhausted with water acidulated with sulphuric acid, and ammonia added as long as it occasions a precipitate. To purify it, Dr. MACLAGAN directs the impure alkali to be washed and mixed with an equal weight of moist oxide of lead (Plumbi oxydum hydratum), the mass dried and exhausted with alcohol. The clear solution decanted and evaporated, leaves the alkaloid, which may be further purified by dissolving it in pure æther. Tonic and antiperiodic. Dose, from 2 to 12 grains.

BEBEERINÆ SULPHAS. By dissolving bebeerine in diluted sulphuric acid, till the acid is neutralized, and evaporating the solution.

BERBERINA. Treat a watery extract of barberry root with rectified spirit as long as the latter acquires a bitter taste. Distil off the spirit, and let the residue cool. Let the crystals which form be recrystallized, first from rectified spirit, and then from water. Dose, 8 to 10 grains. Tonic.

BISMUTHUM PURIFICATUM. P. Pulverize bismuth, and mix it with $\frac{1}{20}$th of its weight of nitre. Heat the mixture to redness in a crucible, and let it cool. Repeat the operation if required.

BISMUTHI TRISNITRAS. L. *Bismuthum Album.* E. *Trisnitrate, subnitrate,* or *magistery of bismuth.* Dissolve ℥j of pure bismuth in f ℥jss of nitric acid mixed with ℥j of water. Mix the solution with Oiij of water; collect and wash the precipitate, and dry it with a gentle heat, [in a dark place, E.] D. nearly the same. Dose, gr. v to xv, as a tonic and antispasmodic, particularly in pyrosis and gastrodynia.

BISMUTHI VALERIANAS. RIGHINI. Dissolve bismuth in nitric acid, as directed for the trisnitrate, and decompose it with a solution of valerianate of soda, to which a little valerianic acid has been added. Wash the precipitate, and dry it carefully.

BOLI. *Boluses,* are extemporaneous compounds, which may be regarded as single doses of electuaries, or as large pills. They may be conveniently taken wrapped in moistened wafer paper.

BOLUS ANTIPERIODICUS. See Bolus ad Quartanum.

Bolus Astringens. F. H. Cubebs ℥ss, balsam of copaiba ʒij, sulphate of iron ʒj, powdered resin ʒiij. In boluses of gr. viij each. Ger. H. Copaiva ʒij, p. gum Arabic ʒij, orange flower water ℈ij; triturate and add powdered cubebs ʒij. For 6 boluses, one 3 times a day.

Bolus Cambogiæ. Guy's H. Powdered gamboge gr. x, bitartrate of potash ℈j, ginger gr. ij, syrup q. s.

Bolus Camphoræ. Guy's H. Camphor (pulverized by spirit) gr. iij, conserve of roses gr. vj.

Bolus Camphoræ cum Nitro. Nitre gr. v, camphor gr. v, conserve of roses q. s.

Bolus Castorei. E. H. Castor ℈j, carbonate of ammonia gr. v, syrup q. s.

Bolus Catechu. U. C. H. Extract of catechu gr. x, aromatic confection gr. vj, syrup q. s.

Bolus Catechu Opiatus. Guy's H. Catechu ℈j, powder for confection of opium gr. vj, syrup q. s.

Bolus Catharticus. U. C. H. Jalap gr. xv, supertartrate of potash ℈j, syrup q. s.

Bolus Copaibæ. Mr. Evans. Mix pure copaiva with $\frac{1}{16}$th its weight of recently calcined magnesia, till thoroughly incorporated. Set it aside for a few days to become solid, form it into oval boluses of ʒss each, on a hot slab, and wrap each in wafer paper. Place them in water for a minute before taking them. Righini prescribes ʒv of copaiba, ʒjss of extract of rhatany, gr. xv oil of sassafras, with magnesia q. s. For 80 boluses, 4 or 5 daily. See also Bolus Astringens, and Bolus Cubebæ.

Bolus Cubebæ. Velpeau. Powdered cubebs ʒvj, balsam of copaiva ʒij, calcined magnesia q. s. For 36 boluses, to be taken in 2 days. See also Electuarium Cubebæ.

Bolus Febrifugus. F. H. Cinchona ʒv, rhubarb ʒss, muriate of ammonia ʒss, syrup of peach leaves q. s. For 10 doses. See also Bolus ad Quartanum.

Bolus Ferri et Myrrhæ. U. C. H. Carbonate of iron gr. xij, myrrh gr. vj, aromatic confection q. s.

Bolus Guaiaci. Home, *in Quinsy*. Guaiacum resin ʒss, elder rob q. s.

Bolus Guaiaci Compositus. Guy's H. Guaiacum ʒjss, ipecacuanha gr. vj, opium gr. vj, confection of hips q. s. Divide into 6 boluses. One, once or twice a day, in rheumatism, &c.

BOLUS KINO COMPOSITUM. GUY'S H. Kino gr. x, compound chalk powder with opium gr. xv, syrup of poppies q. s.

BOLUS AD QUARTANUM. F. H. Cinchona ℥j, carbonate of potash ʒj, tartarized antimony gr. xv, syrup q. s. To be divided into 60 boluses; to be taken in 24 hours, during the intermission.

BOLUS RHEI OPIATUS. GUY'S H. Rhubarb gr. xv, co. powder of chalk with opium, gr. x, syrup of ginger q. s.

BOLUS SCILLÆ ET HYDRARGYRI. Dr. GOWER, *in Chronic Hydrocephalus.* Quicksilver ʒj, manna ʒij, fresh squill ʒss. Triturate till the quicksilver disappears, and add liquorice powder q. s. For 6 doses; one 3 times a day.

BOLUS VERMIFUGUS. Dr. CAMPBELL. Basilic powder ℈j, conserve of wormwood q. s. In 1 bolus. FOY. Powdered pomegranate root ʒj, assafœtida ʒss, croton oil 3 or 4 drops, syrup q. s. Divide into 15 boluses; 5 daily for tape-worm. F. H. Wormseed ℈j, calomel gr. v, camphor gr. xv, syrup q. s. For 3 doses; 1, 2, or 3 in the day.

BRODIUM. See Jusculum.

BROMINIUM. From bittern; or from the mother-lye of certain brine springs. To a gallon of the mother-liquor, in a retort, add ℥j of binoxide of manganese, and ℥v or ℥vj of hydrochloric acid, and distil by the heat of a sand-bath into a cooled receiver. See Solutio Brominii.

CALAMINA PRÆPARATA. L. Burn the calamine, grind it, and prepare it in the same manner as chalk. See Creta Præparata. [A large proportion of what is sold as Lapis Calaminaris contains little or none of this mineral. It should dissolve in sulphuric acid.]

CALCII BROMIDUM. M. Precipitate a solution of bromide of iron with an excess of slaked lime; evaporate to dryness; redissolve in water, and evaporate the filtered liquid.

CALCII CHLORIDUM. L. Chloride of calcium. *Dried Muriate of Lime.* Chalk ℥v, muriatic acid f℥x, water f℥x. Dissolve, filter, evaporate to dryness, and fuse. Keep it from the air.

CALCII IODIDUM. From iodide of iron and slaked lime: as Calcii Bromidum.

Calcii Oxydum. *Quick Lime.* See Calx.

Calcis Acetas. Add prepared chalk to acetic (or purified pyroligneous) acid till fully saturated; filter and evaporate, that crystals may form.

Calcis Carbonas Præcipitatum. D. To 5 parts of solution of muriate of lime, (Aq. Calcis Muriatis. D.,) add a solution of 3 parts of carbonate of soda in 4 parts of water. Wash, collect, and dry the precipitate. The solutions should be cold.

Calcis Hydras. L. *Slaked Lime.* Fresh lime, sprinkled with water, till it falls into powder.

Calcis Hypochloris. See Calx Chlorinata.

Calcis Lactas. Henry. Evaporate sour whey to a syrup, treat the residue with alcohol, saturate the alcoholic solution with chalk or milk of lime; distil off the spirit, dissolve the residue in a little water, and crystallize.

Calcis Murias. See Calcii Chloridum. D. directs it to be made by evaporating to dryness the residual liquor left in preparing liquor ammoniæ.

Calcis Phosphas Precipitatum. D. Digest 1 part of calcined and powdered bones with 2 of diluted muriatic acid and 2 of water for 12 hours, and filter the liquor. Add q. s. of water of ammonia; wash the precipitate, and dry it. Dose ʒss in rickets, &c. An excellent basis for tooth-powders.

Calcis Sulphuretum. P. Sulphur ℥x, slaked lime ℥xxx, water Oijss. Boil together till a portion dropped on a cold surface becomes solid; pour it on a marble slab, and when solidified, break it up and keep it in well-closed vessels. Or by strongly calcining in a covered crucible, 100 parts of calcined gypsum with 15 of lampblack.

Calx Antimonii. See Antimonium Calcinatum.

Calx. L. Calx Viva. *Quick Lime.* Burn fragments of chalk for an hour in a very strong fire. E. orders pieces of marble to be burnt for three hours.

Calx e Testis. L. 1824. From oyster-shells, as from chalk.

Calx Chlorinata. L. Chloride (Hypochlorite) of lime. Pass chlorine gas (see Chlorinium) into a vessel, or chamber, in which slaked lime is thinly spread, till the latter is fully saturated with chlorine.

CALOMELAS. See Hydrargyri Chloridum.

CALOMELAS PRECIPITATUM. D. Purified mercury 17 parts, diluted nitric acid [D.] 15 parts; digest at a gentle heat in a glass vessel for 6 hours, shaking frequently; boil for a short time, [it is better to keep the heat below the boiling point, Mr. PHILLIPS,] decant the clear solution, and mix it with 7 parts of muriate of soda, dissolved in 400 parts of boiling water. Wash the precipitate with warm distilled water as long as the washings are affected by water of potash (Liquor Potassæ), and dry it.

CALUMBINA. Exhaust powdered columbo root with rectified æther, and leave the æthereal tincture to evaporate spontaneously.

CANNABINUM. See Resina Cannabis Indicæ.

CANTHARIDINA. P. Exhaust powdered cantharides with strong alcohol by percolation; distil off the spirit from the filtered tincture, and leave the residue to deposit crystals, which may be purified by dissolving them in boiling alcohol, digesting with animal charcoal, filtering the hot solution, and crystallizing by refrigeration.

CARBO ANIMALIS. Bone-black (called ivory-black) is obtained by burning bones [or flesh, L.] in close vessels.

CARBO ANIMALIS PURIFICATUS. L. and E. Hydrochloric acid ℥xij, water f℥xij; mix and pour it gradually on bone-black ℔j; digest for 2 days with a gentle heat, stirring frequently. Set aside, pour off the liquor, wash the charcoal frequently with water till no longer acid, [till the liquid scarcely precipitates with carbonate of soda, E.,] and dry it.

CARBONIS BISULPHURETUM. *Sulphuret*, or *Bisulphuret of Carbon.* Heat iron pyrites with one-fifth its weight of dry charcoal in a stone retort, furnished with a glass tube dipping in water. Separate the sulphuret which collects at the bottom of the water, and carefully re-distil it from muriate of lime. Or pass the vapour of sulphur over charcoal heated to redness in a porcelain tube. Dose, as a sudorific in rheumatism, 2 or 3 drops gradually increased to 5 or more. *Externally*, in liniments for rheumatic pains, &c. It is also dropped (40 or 50 drops) on the part to promote the reduction of strangulated hernia, (KRIMER.)

CARBONIS TER-CHLORIDUM. What is sold under the name of ter-chloride of carbon appears to be an alcoholic solution of chloroform, and to be identical with the so-called chloric æther.

See Æther Chloricus and Chloroformum. Mr. TUSON prescribes from 1 to 4 drops in water 2 or 3 times a day in cancer, &c. Externally ʒj to ʒij to Oj water. It is not chloroform which he employs, but the precise quantity contained in the solution he employs is not stated.

CARYOCOSTINUM. Confectio Scammonii. But the old preparation contained less scammony.

CASCARILLINA. M. DUVAL. Exhaust cascarilla by percolation with cold water; add acetate of lead to the liquid, and filter. Remove excess of lead from the filtrate by sulphuretted hydrogen gas, and evaporate the filtered liquid to two-thirds; add a little animal charcoal, and again filter. Evaporate at a low temperature till a pellicle appear, and allow it to cool. To purify the product, moisten the powder with a little cold, weak spirit, and after a few hours, wrap it in linen, express strongly, and dry the residue. It may be further purified by redissolving it in boiling alcohol, and leaving the clear solution to spontaneous evaporation.

CATAPLASMA SIMPLEX. *Simple Poultice.* D. Oatmeal 2 parts, linseed meal 1 part, mixed with boiling water q. s. GUY'S H. Linseed meal 1 part, ground bran 2. The simple linseed poultice and bread poultice are also so named. [In some hospitals, poultices are nearly exploded, simple water being preferred. A new material, called spongio-piline, has been introduced as a medium of applying water, or medicated liquids.]

CATAPLASMA ACETI. *Vinegar Poultice.* Oatmeal, or bread crumbs, with vinegar. Applied cold, for sprains, &c. [Verjuice is sometimes preferred.]

CATAPLASMA ACIDI PYROLIGNOSI. Dr. REECE. Bran ℔j, linseed meal ℥j, impure pyroligneous acid q. s. [To scrofulous ulcers, occasionally ♏xxx tinct. ferri muriatis, and ʒiij extract or powder of hemlock are added.]

CATAPLASMA ALUMINIS. D. Alum ʒj, white of 2 eggs. Agitate together till a coagulum is formed. Applied between fine linen, to inflamed eyes, and also to chilblains.

CATAPLASMA ANODYNUM. P. Poppy-heads ℥j, dried henbane ℥ij, water ℥xxiv. Boil, strain, and add to the liquor q. s. of emollient meals (see Farinæ Emollientes) to form a poultice. E. H. Simple poultice ℥xvj, wine of opium ʒj.

CATAPLASMA ANTISEPTICUM. F. H. Barley flour ℥vj, powdered

Peruvian bark ℥j, water q. s. Boil, and when cool enough, add camphor in powder ʒj. REUSS. Powdered bark ℥j, bruised rue ℥j, powdered camphor ʒss, simple poultice ℔j. Mr. ALLARD prescribed under this name—Two bottles of porter, half a pint of yeast, ℥j of treacle; mix and stir in linseed meal and oatmeal q. s., and set it near the fire to ferment. See also Cat. Tonicum.

CATAPLASMA AROMATICUM. Similar to Cataplasma Cumini.

CATAPLASMA ASTRINGENS. FOY. Catechu ℥j, powdered oak bark and *barley meal each ℥j, cold water q. s.*

CATAPLASMA BELLADONNÆ. Dr. REECE. Extract of belladonna made in vacuo ʒj, oatmeal ℔ss, boiling water q. s.

CATAPLASMA BYNES. GUY'S H. Ground malt, with yeast q. s. to form a poultice; to be applied warm.

CATAPLASMA CALCIS. Slaked lime ℥ij, oatmeal ℥ij, lard ℥iv. Formerly used at Bath Hospital.

CATAPLASMA CALCIS SULPHATIS. Sir W. BLIZARD. Paris plaster, mixed with water to a soft paste, and applied before it hardens. Formerly applied to ulcers to form an artificial scab; now occasionally used to afford mechanical support in some surgical cases.

CATAPLASMA CANTHARIDIS. IT. H. Powdered Cantharides ℥j, dough ℥jss, vinegar of squills to form a paste. See also Epithema Vesicatorium.

CATAPLASMA CARBONIS. D. Charcoal powder and simple poultice q. s.

CATAPLASMA CEREVISIÆ. GUY'S H. Ale-grounds, thickened with oatmeal; to be applied cold, twice or thrice in the day.

CATAPLASMA CONII. L. Extract of hemlock ℥ij, water Oj, ground linseed q. s. GUY'S H. directs a decoction of the leaves (℥jss of dried leaves in Ojss of water to Oj) to be thickened with the powder for cataplasms; others with bread-crumb. D. directs the same decoction to be thickened with powdered hemlock.

CATAPLASMA AD CONTUSIONES ET LIVOREM FACEI. ZWELFER. Solomon's seal ℥ss, orris, resin, olibanum, of each ʒjss, camphor ʒss, bread-crumb ℥jss, mucilage of tragacanth q. s.

CATAPLASMA CUMINI. L. 1788. Cumin seeds ℔j, bayberries,

scordium leaves, serpentaria root, of each ℥iij, cloves ʒj; to be powdered together and mixed with thrice their weight of honey. GUY'S H. Cumin seeds ℔j, bayberries ℥iij, wormwood ℥vj, pimento ℥j, treacle q. s.

CATAPLASMA DAUCI. D. Carrots, boiled till soft, and bruised.

CATAPLASMA DIGITALIS. Mr. ALLARD. A strong decoction of fox-glove, with bread-crumb, or linseed meal q. s.

CATAPLASMA DISCUTIENS. E. H. Barley meal ℥vj, fresh hemlock ℥ij, vinegar q. s. Boil, and add sal ammoniac ℥ss. F. H. the same, with acetate of lead ʒij.

CATAPLASMA EFFERVESCENS. Fresh wort, thickened with oatmeal, and a spoonful of yeast added.

CATAPLASMA EMETICUM. Bruised groundsel (Senecio vulgaris) applied over the stomach, produces vomiting.

CATAPLASMA EMOLLIENS. P. Emollient meals (Farinæ Emollientes) ℥iv, cold water q. s. Mix, and boil together to a due consistence, stirring constantly.

CATAPLASMA FARINÆ COMPOSITUM. Dr. H. SMITH. Rye flour ℔j, old yeast ℥iv, salt ℥ij, hot water q. s.

CATAPLASMA FÆCULÆ. P. Potato starch ℥ij; mix with a little cold water, add it to f℥xvj of boiling water, and boil for an instant.

CATAPLASMA FERMENTI. L. Flour ℔j, yeast Oss; mix, and apply a gentle heat till it begins to rise.

CATAPLASMI FÆCULÆ CEREVISIÆ. See C. Cerevisiæ.

CATAPLASMA FUCI. Dr. RUSSELL. Fresh bladder fucus (*sea wrack*) bruised. Applied to glandular tumours, &c.

CATAPLASMI FURFURIS. Fine bran with one-tenth of linseed meal, with boiling water q. s. Mr. PAYNE recommends, as a cheap hospital poultice, 3½ pecks of pollard, 14℔ linseed meal, and ¼℔ lard.

CATAPLASMA GALBANI. Lily roots ℥iv, figs ℥j; boil till soft, and bruise them with ʒjss of onions, and ℥ss of galbanum triturated with yolk of egg, and linseed meal q. s. See C. Maturans.

CATAPLASMA GOULARDI. See Cataplasma Plumbi.

CATAPLASMA HUMULI. Dr. TROTTER. Hops, softened with hot water. To foul ulcers.

CATAPLASMA IODURETUM. LUGOL. To a common poultice add rubefacient solution of iodine (See Solutiones Iodinii) q. p.

CATAPLASMA JUGLANDIS. Mr. PERFECT. The fresh leaves of walnut, bruised, and mixed with honey. Applied over the abdomen as a vermifuge.

CATAPLASMA LILII. The bulb of the white lily, boiled, and bruised.

CATAPLASMA LINI. L. Ground linseed, mixed with boiling water q. s. E. & D. direct the linseed meal to be made from the cake left after the oil has been expressed from the seeds.

CATAPLASMA MALI. The soft pulp of roasted apple. Applied to inflamed eyes: other ingredients are sometimes added.

CATAPLASMA MARCHANTIÆ. Two handfuls of the fresh plant (Marchantia Hæmispherica) to be boiled till soft, and beaten to a pulp, with linseed meal q. s. Applied over the abdomen in ascites.

CATAPLASMA MATURANS. L. 1745. Pulp of figs ℥iv, resin ointment ℥j, strained galbanum ℥ss. *Cataplasme Maturatif.* P. Resolvent meals (Farinæ Resolventes) ℥iv, decoction of mallows q. s. Mix, and while hot add resin ointment ℥j, softened with a little oil.

CATAPLASMA OXALIS. Mr. SANDFORD. Bruised sorrel leaves, mixed with oatmeal and beer.

CATAPLASMA PANIS. Pour boiling water on bread-crumb, cover it up till soaked, pour off the water, press gently, and beat it up with a spoon. A little oil may be added. Milk is frequently used, but is apt to become sour. Linseed meal renders it more adhesive.

CATAPLASMA PAPAVERIS. CH. Decoction of poppy-heads, thickened with bread-crumb.

CATAPLASMA PLUMBI. Goulard water ℔j, bread-crumb q. s.

CATAPLASMA PLUMBAGINIS. *Bengal Dispensatory.* The powdered bark of *Plumbago Rosea,* with flour and water q. s. Applied for half an hour it blisters.

CATAPLASMA POTASSÆ ACETATIS. *Cataplasma Neutrale.* Acetate of potash ℥j, water Oj, crumb of bread q. s. To ill-conditioned sores.

CATAPLASMA QUERCUS MARINÆ. See Cataplasma Fuci.

CATAPLASMA RAPI. GUY'S H. Peel turnips, boil them till soft, beat them to a pulp, and apply it warm.

CATAPLASMA RESOLVENS. F. H. Resolvent meals (Farinæ Resolventes. P.) ℥viij, emollient decoction q. s., liquid diacetate of lead ʒij. See also Cataplasma Saponis.

CATAPLASMA ROSÆ. CH. Powdered alum ʒss, confection of roses ℥ij. Mix.

CATAPLASMA RUBEFACIENS. P. Barley meal lightly roasted ℥iv, strong vinegar ℥j, whites of 3 eggs, water q. s. to form a cataplasm; spread it on linen, and sprinkle it over with ℥ss each of powdered fennel seed and black pepper.

CATAPLASMA SAPONIS. E. H. White soap ℥j, milk Oj, crumb of bread ℥viij. Boil slightly. F. H. Almond soap ℥iv, barley flour ℥viij, water q. s.

CATAPLASMA SIMPLEX. See above. Bread poultice is also so termed.

CATAPLASMA SINAPIS. L. Ground linseed ℔ss, flour of black mustard ℔ss, hot vinegar q. s. [P. directs warm water.]

CATAPLASMA SODÆ CARBONATIS. CH. Carbonate of soda ʒiv, muriate of soda ʒiv, linseed meal ℥j, oatmeal ℥v, hot water q. s. *In strumous enlargements.*

CATAPLASMA SODÆ CHLORINATÆ. St. B. H. Linseed meal, made into a poultice, with equal parts of water and liquor sodæ chlorinatæ.

CATAPLASMA SODÆ SULPHATIS. Dr. KIRKLAND. Sulphate of soda ℥j, boiling water ℔ss, crumb of bread q. s. *In Xerophthalmia.*

CATAPLASMA SOLANI TUBEROSI. Raw potatoes, scraped, grated, or pounded in a mortar. To be used cold. See also Cataplasma Fæculæ.

CATAPLASMA STIMULANS. Dr. HUGH SMITH. Rye flour ℔j, old yeast ℥iv, common salt ℥ij.

CATAPLASMA STOMACHICUM. E. H. Aromatic cataplasm ℥j, oil of mace (expressed oil of nutmegs) ʒij, anodyne balsam q. s.

CATAPLASMA SUPPURANS. E. 1774. To an emollient cataplasm add bruised onions ℥jss, basilicon ointment ℥j.

CATAPLASMA TEREBINTHINÆ. Dr. REECE. Oil of turpentine ʒij, olive oil ℥j, linseed meal ℥j, oatmeal ℥iv, boiling water q. s. To indolent ulcers; and, with more turpentine, to deep burns or scalds, and chilblains.

Cataplasma Tonicum. Germ. H. Powdered bark ℥j, charcoal ℥j, camphor ʒjss, oil of turpentine q. s.

Cataplasma Ulmi. The powdered bark of the slippery elm (Ulmus Fulva) mixed with hot water q. s.

Cathartina. Cathartine is obtained from senna, but is not suited for medicinal use.

Causticum Ammoniacale. Gondret. See Unguentum Ammoniacale.

Causticum Antimoniale. See Antimonii Chloridum.

Causticum Anticancrosum. Plunkett's *Caustic for Cancers.* Upright crow-foot, lesser spear-wort, of each ℥j, levigated white arsenic ʒj, sulphur ℈v; beat together to form a uniform paste, which is made into balls, and dried in the sun. The powdered paste is mixed, when required for use, with yolk of egg, and applied on bladder.

Causticum Aureum. Recamier. Chloride of gold gr. v, nitro-muriatic acid ℥j.

Causticum Commune Fortius. L. 1746. See Potassæ cum Calce.

Causticum Commune Mitius. L. 1746. Soft soap and quick-lime in equal parts; to be mixed at the time of using.

Causticum Hydrargyri Nitratis. See Hydrargyri Deutonitras Liquidus.

Causticum Lunare. *Argenti Nitras.*

Causticum Opiatum. Mr. Else. Potash with lime ʒiij, opium ʒss, soft soap q. s. Opium is occasionally added to other caustics.

Causticum Zinci. Dr. Canquoin's *Caustics,* Nos. 1, 2, and 3. Mix 1 part of chloride of zinc with two, three, and four parts of wheat flour, and sufficient water to form a paste. The powdered chloride and flour being quickly and carefully mixed, add the water to half the quantity, to form a soft paste, and mix with this as much of the remaining powder as will render it stiff. Form it into cakes, or wafers, of from half a line to 4 lines in thickness, according to circumstances. It is to remain on 24 hours or more, then to be gently removed, and the part covered with a poultice. Dr. Rankin says it should not be thicker than 1 or 2 lines, nor left on longer than from 6 to 10 hours.

This will produce an eschar of quarter inch depth. *In Cancers, Lupus, Nævi, &c.* Dr. URE substitutes Paris plaster for flour.

CAUSTICUM ZINCI ANTIMONIALE. Dr. CANQUOIN'S *Caustic*, No. 4. Chloride of zinc 1 part, chloride of antimony ½ part, flour 2½ parts. To be mixed as before, but formed into crayon-shaped rolls, of a consistence to be moulded to any required form. *In nodulated Cancerous Tumours.*

CAUSTICUM ZINCI OPIATUM. Powdered opium may be mixed with either of the preceding, to mitigate the pain.

CERA PURIFICATA. D. Melt bees-wax with a gentle heat; and after allowing it to settle, carefully decant the wax from the sediment.

CERATUM. L. *Ceratum Simplex.* L. 1824. Yellow wax ℥iv, olive oil f℥iv. Melt the wax with a gentle heat, add the oil, and mix.

CERATUM ÆRUGINIS. DEN. Ph. Wax 12 parts, resin 6, Venice turpentine 5, verdigris 1.

CERATUM ALBUM. L. 1745. See Ceratum Cetacei.

CERATUM AMMONIACALE. RECHOUX. Carbonate of ammonia ʒj, simple cerate ℥j.

CERATUM ARSENICI. U. S. White arsenic ℈j, cerate ℥j. Mix.

CERATUM BELLADONNÆ. Extract of belladonna 1 part, soap cerate 2 or 3 parts.

CERATUM CALAMINÆ. L. Ceratum Epuloticum. *Turner's Cerate.* Yellow wax ℔ss: melt, add olive oil f℥xvj, and stir in prepared calamine ℔ss.

CERATUM CALAMINÆ CUM HYDRARGYRO. CH. Calamine cerate ℔ss, nitric oxide of mercury ℥ss. Mix.

CERATUM CALMANS. ROUX. Cerate ℥j, cherry-laurel water ℥ss. Mix. Or, oil of almonds 4, white wax 1, cherry-laurel water 3.

CERATUM CALOMELANOS. Calomel ʒj, spermaceti cerate ʒiv.

CERATUM CALOMELANOS COMPOSITUM. Calomel ʒj, calamine cerate ʒiv.

CERATUM CAMPHORATUM. *Pommade du frère Cosme.* Olive oil ℥xvj, yellow wax ℥viij; melt together, and add camphor ʒj;

stir till it begins to thicken. F. M. H. one part of camphor to 10 of Ceratum Galeni.

CERATUM CANTHARIDIS. L. Spermaceti cerate ℥vj, powdered cantharides ℥j. Mix. F. H. Cantharides ℥j, water ℥xij; boil for half an hour, filter, evaporate to ℥v: add lard ℥vj, olive oil ℥iv, white wax ℥iv. Evaporate the water, and when cool, add powdered camphor ʒij.

CERATUM CETACEI. L. Spermaceti ℥ij, white wax ℥viij, olive oil Oj; melt together, and stir till cool.

CERATUM CINCHONÆ. Extract of bark ʒj, simple cerate ℥ss. Mix.

CERATUM CINNABARIS. ALIBERT'S *Antiherpetic Cerate.* Vermilion ʒj, camphor ℈j, cerate ℥j.

CERATUM CITRINUM. L. 1746. *Ceratum Resinæ.*

CERATUM CONII. St. B. H. Ointment of hemlock ℔j, spermaceti ℥ij, white wax ℥iij.

CERATUM COPAIBÆ. Dr. HOULTON. White wax ℥j, balsam of copaiva ℥ij. Add the balsam to the wax, previously melted, and stir till cool.

CERATUM COSMETICUM. *Pommade en Crème.* Oil of almonds ℥iv, white wax ʒiij, spermaceti ʒiij, rose water ℥iij, tincture of balsam of Mecca ʒij. Mix. VAN MONS. White wax 1 part, oil of almonds 4, butter of cacao 1.

CERATUM CRETÆ ACETATIS. See Ceratum Neutrale, and Unguentum Plumbi Compositum.

CERATUM CROTONIS. M. CAVENTOU. Melt 2½ parts of lard with half a part of wax, and when nearly cold, mix with it one part of croton oil. [One part of croton oil with 4 of soap cerate may be advantageously substituted. These applications are more convenient than liniments for producing counter-irritation.]

CERATUM CUPRI. SWEDIAUR. Solution of ammoniated copper ʒj, cerate ℥j. Mix.

CERATUM DIAPIPEROS GALENI. ZWELFER. Litharge ℔j, white lead ℔j, olive oil ℔ij, wax ℥vj, turpentine ℥iij, frankincense ℥ss, alum ʒvj, pepper ʒiij. *A stimulant application to indolent ulcers.*

CERATUM FUSCUM. See Emplastrum Fuscum.

CERATUM GALENI. P. *Cold Cream.* White wax ℥iv, oil of

almonds ℥xvj : melt, and gradually add in ℥xij of rose water, stirring till cold.

Ceratum de Gratiæ Dei Nicolai. Resin ℔j, wax ℥iv, mastic ℥j : melt together, and boil with a decoction of one handful of vervain, bettony, and pimpernel in wine, till incorporated; then remove from the fire, and add ℔ss of common turpentine.

Ceratum Goulardi. See Ceratum Plumbi Compositum.

Ceratum Hydrargyri Compositum. L. Mercurial ointment (strong) ℥iv, soap cerate ℥iv, camphor ℥j. Mix.

Ceratum Hydrargyri Nitratis. St. B. H. Ointment of nitrate of quicksilver ℥j, spermaceti cerate ℥j. Mix.

Ceratum Limacum. White wax 3 parts, spermaceti 3, oil of almonds 32, mucilage of snails 24, otto of roses q. s.

Ceratum Lithargyri. Ch. Lead plaster ℔ss, lard ℔ss, wax ʒj; melt them together, and gradually add Goulard's extract (liquor plumbi diac.) ʒiv. Stir till cold.

Ceratum Lithargyri Acetatis. See Ceratum Plumbi Compositum.

Ceratum Mellis. Ch. Olive oil ℔ss, wax ʒiv, lead plaster ʒiv; melt together, and add ℔ss of honey. Galbanum plaster is sometimes substituted for simple lead plaster.

Ceratum Mellis cum Terebinthina. Paracelsus. Common turpentine ℔j, the yolks of 20 eggs, honey ℔j. Beat together the honey and yolks, and add the turpentine, softened by heat.

Ceratum Mercuriale. L. 1746. Strong mercurial ointment ʒvj, lard ʒiij, yellow wax ʒvj. Mix.

Ceratum Metopii. Dr. Barham. Hog-gum (gum of Rhus Metopium) ʒiv, lard ʒiv, white wax ʒij, powdered root of sweet aristolochia (a. odoratissima) ʒij, yellow resin ʒj. *In rheumatic pains.*

Ceratum Mezerei. Exhaust fresh mezereon bark, by repeated digestion with rectified spirit. Mix the liquors, add milk of lime, (1 part of lime and 3 of water for 3 parts of mezereon,) and digest till the colour becomes of a yellowish green. Distil off most of the spirit, add water to the residue, and collect the soft green substance which separates. Mix 1 part of this with 4 of yellow wax, and 8 of olive oil.

CERATUM NEUTRALE. KIRKLAND. *Cer. Cretæ Acetatis.* Lead plaster ℥viij, olive oil ℥iv, chalk ℥iv, distilled vinegar ℥iv, Goulard's extract of lead ℥ss. Melt together the plaster and oil, add the chalk, and lastly, the diacetate of lead, mixed with the vinegar.

CERATUM OPIATUM. GIBERT. Cerate ℥j, wine of opium ʒj. LAGNEAU. Opium ʒss, yolk of 1 egg; mix, and add cerate ℥j.

CERATUM PLUMBI ACETATIS. L. Acetate of lead finely powdered ʒij, white wax ℥ij, olive oil f℥viij. Melt the wax with f℥vij of the oil, and add the acetate of lead, previously triturated with f℥j of the oil.

CERATUM PLUMBI COMPOSITUM. L. Yellow wax ℥iv, olive oil f℥viij; melt together, remove from the fire, and when it begins to thicken, gradually add liquor of diacetate of lead f℥iij; stir till cool, and lastly, add camphor ʒss, dissolved in olive oil f℥ij.

CERATUM QUINÆ. Sulphate of quinine gr. vj, cerate ʒj. *Used endermically.*

CERATUM RESINÆ. L. Yellow resin ℔j, wax ℔j; melt together, add olive oil f℥xvj, and strain while warm through linen.

CERATUM ROSATUM. P. *Lip Salve.* Oil of almonds ℥ij, white wax ℥j, alkanet root ʒj; melt, and digest till coloured sufficiently, then strain, and add 6 drops of otto of roses.

CERATUM RUBRUM. CH. Yellow wax, and lard, of each ℔ss, resin ℥ss, red sulphuret of mercury gr. xvj. Mix. *As a common dressing.*

CERATUM SABINÆ. L. Fresh savine ℔j, wax ℔ss, lard ℔ij. Melt together the lard and wax, add the bruised savine, and strain by pressure through linen. D. and E. direct the savine to be *boiled* in the lard, (and wax, E.;) but a heat below boiling is sufficient.

CERATUM SAPONIS. L. Common vinegar Cj, powdered litharge ℥xv; boil till they combine, add Castile soap ℥x; boil till the moisture is evaporated, and mix with it yellow wax ℥xijss, previously melted with olive oil Oj. [The Ceratum Saponis of U. S. is *white.* Solution of diacetate of lead f℥xxxij, soap ℥vj, white wax ℥x, olive oil f℥xvj. Boil gently the diacetate with the soap to the consistence of honey, heat in a water-bath until the moisture is dissipated, then add the wax melted with the oil, and mix.]

CERATUM SAPONIS DURUM. The soap cerate may be rendered harder and more adhesive than it usually is by thoroughly evaporating the moisture. Some add diachylon plaster. See Emplastrum Cerati Saponis.

CERATUM SIMPLEX. E. Spermaceti 1 part, white wax 3, olive oil 6 parts.

CERATUM SULPHURATUM. P. Washed sulphur ʒj, cold cream (Ceratum Galeni) ℥iijss, oil of almonds ʒss.

CERATUM TABACI. GER. H. Tobacco juice ℥iij, wax ℥iij, resin ʒss, olive oil q. s.

CERATUM ZINCI COMPOSITUM. MID. H. Equal parts of zinc ointment, and compound lead ointment.

CERATUM ZINCI CUM LYCOPODIO. HUFELAND. Cerate ʒss, oxide of zinc gr. xv, lycopodium gr. xv. Mix.

CEREI *vel* CEREOLI. *Bougies* are made by dipping strips of soft linen cloth, rather wider at one end than the other, into certain emplastic or elastic compositions, folding them up firmly, and rolling them on a smooth slab. For elastic bougies, pieces of catgut, bundles of thread or cotton, or strips of fine open silk, are sometimes used. The following are some of the compositions which have been held in most repute :—

1. BELL'S. Lead plaster ℥iv, yellow wax ʒjss, olive oil ʒiij.

2. HUNTER'S. Olive oil ℔iij, yellow wax ℔j, red lead ℔jss. Boil together over a slow fire till combined.

3. SWEDIAUR'S *white*. White wax ℔j, spermaceti ʒiij, sugar of lead from ʒij to ʒj. Boil together slowly.

4. ST. B. H. *Red.* Wax ℔j, Chio turpentine ℥iv; melt together and add vermilion ʒj. It must be well stirred.

5. PIDERIT'S *Wax.* Yellow wax 6 parts, olive oil 1 part.

6. GOULARD'S. Yellow wax, melted and mixed by stirring with from one 24th to one 3d of extract of lead. PRUS. PH. ʒij Goulard's extract to ℥vj yellow wax.

7. FALK'S *Mercurial.* Mercurial plaster ʒj, turpentine ʒss, powdered shell-lac gr. xv, calomel ʒj, red oxide of mercury ℈j.

8. DARAN'S. Olive oil (in which hemlock, tobacco, flowers of sweet trefoil, and St. John's wort, have been infused) 50 parts, lard 15, wax 10, litharge 20. DARAN'S *Emollient.* White wax ℥iv, spermaceti ℥jss, rose ointment ʒj, ceruss plaster P. ʒj.

9. SHARP'S. Lead plaster ʒij, Burgundy pitch ℈ij, prepared antimony ʒss; mix, and add quicksilver ʒj triturated with oil of sulphur q. s.

10. *Elastic.* Boiled linseed oil (drying oil) ℥xij, amber ℥iv, oil of turpentine ℥iv, caoutchouc ℥v. This varnish is repeatedly applied to the web.

11. Dr. REECE. Lead plaster, tar, and powdered belladonna, on linen.

CEREVISIA ABIETINA. *Spruce Beer.* Dr. WOOD. Essence of spruce Oss, pimento and ginger, bruised, each ℥v, hops ℥v, water Ciij. Boil for 5 or 10 minutes, strain, add Cxj of warm water, yeast Oj, molasses Ovj. Let it ferment for 24 hours.

CEREVISIA ANTISCORBUTICA. P. *Sapinette.* Fresh scurvy-grass ℥j, horseradish root ℥ij, buds of spruce fir ℥j, new beer Oiijss. Macerate for 4 days, strain, press, and filter for use.

CEREVISIA ARMORACIÆ. HUFELAND. Scraped horseradish ℥v, new beer Oij: digest in a close vessel for 24 hours; strain, and add ℥j of syrup. A cupful twice a day.

CEREVISIA CANNABIS. BUCHAN, *in Jaundice.* Boil ℥ij of hemp seed in Oiv of ale; sweeten with sugar.

CEREVISIA CATHARTICA. Senna ℥ij, centaury ℥jss, wormwood ℥jss, aloes ʒij, ale 3 or 4 gallons.

CEREVISIA CINCHONÆ. Bruised bark ℥j, rectified spirit ℥j; mix, macerate for 2 days in Ojss of new beer, and filter. MUTIS directs 1 part of bark, 8 of sugar, and 80 of water, to be mixed, and allowed to ferment for 4 or 5 days.

CEREVISIA DIURETICA. E. H. Whole mustard seed ℥viij, juniper berries ℥viij, wild carrot seed ℥iij, wormwood ℥ij, new small ale Cx.

CEREVISIA PICIS. DUHAMEL. *Tar Beer.* Bran Oij, tar Oj, honey Oss, water Ovj. Mix them in an earthen pipkin, and let the mixture simmer over a slow fire for 3 hours. When cool, add Oss of yeast, and let it work for 36 hours, then strain. Dose, a wineglassful before every meal. *In bronchial diseases, incipient consumption, &c.*

CEREVISIA ZINGIBERIS. DONOVAN. Infuse ℥ijss bruised ginger in Civ of boiling water. When cold, strain, and add ℔iv of loaf sugar, Oss of solid yeast, and ℥ij of cream of tartar. Ferment in a warm situation. When the fermentation subsides, rack off the clear liquor, and return it into the cooler, previously cleaned. In a day or two, bottle it.

CEREVISIA STOMACHICA. QUINCY. Centaury tops, Roman wormwood, of each 4 handfuls; gentian root ℥ij, thin peels of 6 Seville oranges, Spanish angelica root, and Winter's bark, bruised, of each ℥j, new ale Cvj.

CETRARINA. Digest bruised Iceland moss in rectified spirit, express, distil off most of the spirit, and filter the solution whilst hot. Purify the cetrarin which is deposited, by again dissolving it in spirit. *Febrifuge;* dose, gr. ij to v, every 3 hours.

CHARTA ANTIRHEUMATICA. M. BERG. Euphorbium 30, cantharides 15, alcohol 150 parts. Digest 8 days, filter, and add black resin 60, turpentine 50 parts. Thin paper to be brushed over 2 or 3 times with this varnish. The following is said to resemble Poor-man's plaster. Black resin 3 parts, tar 2, yellow wax 1.

CHARTA EPISPASTICA CUM CANTHARIDIBUS. *For keeping blisters open.* White wax ℥j, spermaceti ʒiij, olive oil ʒiv, turpentine ʒj, cantharides (for No. 1) ʒj, (for No. 2) ℈iv, water ʒx. Boil slowly in a tinned vessel for 2 hours, constantly stirring, and filter through flannel. Dip slips of paper into the melted mixture, and draw them between two wooden rules. Or the paper may be spread on one side only by the usual method. [WISLIN'S plan of spreading paper with emplastic compositions is this:—Cut white printing paper in strips; melt the composition in a plate over boiling water; take one extremity of the paper in the left hand, and raise the other end with the right, so as to form the arc of a circle; draw the under side of the paper over the surface of the composition, gradually lowering the right hand.]

CHARTA EPISPASTICA CUM MEZEREO. GUIBOURT. The ingredients are the same as the last, substituting for the cantharides ʒss or ℈ij of ethereal extract of mezereon dissolved in a little alcohol. The whole should be melted by a gentle heat, and stirred constantly till the alcohol is evaporated, and then strain through linen, and spread as above.

CHARTA PRO FONTICULIS. SOUBEIRAN. *Issue Paper.* White wax 10 parts, spermaceti 5, elemi 5, turpentine 6. Melt over a slow fire, and strain. To be spread on paper by a proper machine.

CHARTA VESICATORIA. See Tela Vesicatoria, and Sparadrapum Vesicans.

CHLORINIUM. Chlorine gas may be procured by gently heating muriatic acid with half its weight of black oxide of manganese, in a flask or retort.

CHLORINEI AQUA. E. See Aqua Chlorinii.

CHLOROFORMUM. Chloroform is obtained from 1 part of chloride of lime, 3 of water, and 3 of alcohol. These are put into a capacious retort, and distilled by a gentle heat into a receiver kept very cool. The heavy oily fluid (chloroform) is separated from the water, and may be rectified by redistilling it with oil of vitriol.

CHOCOLATA. The nuts are picked, slightly roasted to loosen the envelopes, broken, winnowed, and cleansed from the skins, &c., again heated, and ground in a mill. The powder is then beaten to a paste in a warm iron mortar, and mixed with sugar.

CHOCOLATA SIMPLEX VEL SALUTIS. Chocolat de Santé. P. 96 pounds each of the richer and inferior kind of cacao (Cacao Caraque and Maraignan), treated as above, with 160 pounds of sugar, and 1 ounce of cinnamon.

CHOCOLATA LICHENIS. P. Chocolate (as above) 32 parts, powdered sugar 29 parts, dried jelly of Iceland moss 11 parts. [Another form directs—sugar ℔vij, cacao ℔vij, cinnamon ℥j, dry extract of lichen (freed from bitter) ʒxiij, jelly of lichen ℔j; to be finely ground with a muller on a warm slab.]

CHOCOLATA MARTIS. TROUSSEAU. Spanish chocolate ʒxvj, subcarbonate of iron ʒss. Triturate, on a warm slab, and divide into cakes of ʒj each. Others direct levigated filings of iron.

CHOCOLATA IODIDI FERRI. PIERQUIN. Iodide of iron ℈ij, chocolate ʒxvj.

CHOCOLATA PAULLINIÆ. Guarana ʒj, simple chocolate ʒxvj.

CHOCOLATA PURGANS. Calomel ℈ij, jalap ℈iij, chocolate ℈xxxj. Divide into ℈j cakes.

CHOCOLATA CUM SALEP. P. To ʒxvj of prepared chocolate add ʒss of powdered salep. Arrow-root, and tapioca, are mixed with chocolate in the same proportion.

CHOCOLATA CUM VANILLA. P. To ʒxvj of chocolate add ℈ss of vanilla powdered with a portion of the sugar.

CIGARRÆ ARSENICALES. TROUSSEAU. Dip white paper in a solution of 1 part arseniate of soda in 30 of water; make it into cigars the length of the finger. 4 or 5 inspirations twice or thrice daily, in phthisis.

CIGARRÆ BELLADONNÆ OPIATÆ. Extract of opium gr. j, belladonna leaves ℈j. Dissolve the extract in water, and moisten the leaves with the solution. Dry them, and form into cigars.

CIGARRÆ CAMPHORÆ. M. RASPAIL. These are used cold.

Pieces of camphor may be included in a quill, straw, or other tube, confined by blotting paper, and the air drawn through it.

CIGARRÆ MERCURIALES. M. BERNARD proposes to steep tobacco leaves (previously deprived of narcotine by repeated washing) in a weak solution of corrosive sublimate and opium (½ gr. of the former and ¼ gr. of the latter to ℨss of tobacco), and to smoke it in paper, as a mercurial inhalation.

CIGARRÆ STRAMONII. Stramonium leaves, rolled into the form of cigars. *Smoked for the relief of asthma*, but often *without benefit.* Henbane and belladonna are also used in this form.

CIGARRÆ TABACI. Tobacco leaves are formed into cigars for smoking. Dr. APJOHN attributes to this practice "the pallid, emaciated visages, debilitated frames, and deranged digestion of the young men of the present day."

CINCHONIA. Cinchonine is prepared from the disulphate, in the same manner as quina. The acetate, arseniate, hydrochlorate, nitrate, and other salts of cinchonia are obtained in the same way as those of quina.

CINCHONIÆ DISULPHAS. Boil coarsely powdered pale (gray) bark with 8 or 10 parts of water acidulated with 2 parts of muriatic acid. Let the decoction cool, filter; add powdered lime till the liquor is alkaline, wash the precipitate with a little water and dry it. Boil it in alcohol, mix the solution with water, distil off the spirit, neutralize the residue with diluted sulphuric acid, evaporate, and crystallize. Uses and doses as disulphate of quina.

CINGULUM ANTIRHEUMATICUM. MARJORLIN. Camphor ℨss, benzoin ℨj, euphorbium ℨj, muriate of ammonia ℨij. Powder them finely and sprinkle on wadding, which is to be slightly quilted between two folds of flannel, to form a belt, to be applied over the seat of rheumatic pains.

CINGULUM MERCURIALE. Agitate ℨiij of quicksilver with ℥ij of lemon juice: pour off the liquid, and mix the quicksilver with the white of an egg and ℈j of tragacanth. Spread on the belt of flannel. *A popular remedy for the Itch.*

CODEIA. This is left in solution when ammonia is added to ordinary muriate of morphia, and is obtained by evaporating the residual liquor, crystallizing, treating the salt by liquor potassæ, dissolving the precipitate in æther, and evaporating. MAGENDIE says it is half the strength of morphia.

COLCHICINA. Digest colchicum seeds in boiling alcohol, precipitate by magnesia, treat the precipitate with boiling alcohol, and evaporate the filtered solution. Very poisonous; dose, undetermined.

COLLUTORIA. *Mouth washes;* usually of a thicker consistence than gargles. They are altogether extemporaneous.

COLLUTORIUM ACIDUM. Muriatic acid ʒj, honey of roses ℥iij.

COLLUTORIUM ACIDI OXALICI. M. NARDO. Oxalic acid ʒj, barley water ℥xv.

COLLUTORIUM ANTISEPTICUM. WENDT. Extract of bark ʒj, rue water ℥ij, muriatic æther ʒij, honey of roses ℥j.

COLLUTORIUM ASTRINGENS. NEUHOF. Alum ʒj, honey of roses ℥ij, tincture of myrrh ʒss. KOEKER prescribes tincture of catechu ʒij, clarified honey ʒij, infusion of sage ℥vss.

COLLUTORIUM BORACIS. SWEDIAUR. Borax ʒij, water ℥j, tincture of myrrh ℥j, honey of roses ℥ij. BAHI. Mucilage of quince seeds f℥viij, borax ʒiij, honey of roses ℥ij.

COLLUTORIUM DETERGENS. PRINGLE. Infusion of roses ℥jss, borax ʒiij, honey of roses ℥ij.

COLLUTORIUM HYDRIODATUM. RIGHINI. Dissolve ℈j of iodide of potassium in ℥iv of water, and ℥ij of rose water, and add 10 drops of tincture of iodine, and fʒiv of simple syrup. *In mercurial salivation.*

COLLUTORIUM MYRRHÆ. CH. Lime water ℥jss, tincture of myrrh ʒij, honey of roses ʒij.

COLLUTORIUM PYRETHRI. U. S. D. Pellitory root ʒiv, vinegar ʒvj, extract of opium gr. iij. Infuse for an hour. See also Gargarisma.

COLLYRIA. *Eye Waters.* Aquæ Ophthalmicæ.

COLLYRIUM ACETI. SCARPA. Vinegar f℥j, brandy f℥j, rose water f℥viij. WARE. Vinegar fʒiv, spirit of rosemary fʒiij, elder water f℥vij.

COLLYRIUM ACIDUM. KRIMER. Muriatic acid ♏xx, mucilage ʒj, rose water ℥ij. For removing particles of iron from the eye.

COLLYRIUM ALOETICUM. *Collyre de Brun.* Aloes ʒj, rose water ℥jss.

COLLYRIUM ALUMINIS. GUY'S H. Alum ℈j, distilled (or rose) water ℥vj. MID. H. Burnt alum gr. iv, water f℥j.

COLLYRIUM AMMONIÆ ACETATIS. CH. Liquid acetate of ammonia f ℥j, rose water f ℥vij. WARE. Liquid acetate of ammonia f ʒvj, elder water f ℥vij. WARDROP. Liquid acetate of ammonia f ℥ij, camphor mixture ℥vj. BEER adds gr. x of soft extract of opium.

COLLYRIUM ANODYNUM. F. H. Saffron ʒj, decoction of linseed ℥iv, wine of opium ʒj.

COLLYRIUM ANTIMONIALE. PEREIRA. Potash-tartrate of antimony gr. j, distilled water f ℥ij. *In chronic ophthalmia, and spots on the cornea.*

COLLYRIUM ARGENTI NITRATIS. MACKENZIE. Nitrate of silver gr. ij to iv, distilled water f ℥j. A stronger solution is used in some cases.

COLLYRIUM BATEANUM. BATE'S camphorated water (Aqua cupri sulphatis camphorata) f ʒij, distilled water f ℥iv. GUTHRIE. Sulphate of copper gr. viij, bole gr. viij, camphor gr. ij, hot water f ℥viij. Mix and filter.

COLLYRIUM BORACIS. RICHARD. Borax ʒss, white sugar ʒj, rose water f ℥ij.

COLLYRIUM CADMII. ROSENBAUM. Sulphate of cadmium gr. j to ij, rose water f ℥j.

COLLYRIUM CALCIS CHLORIDI. VARLEZ. Chloride of lime ℈j, water ℥j; dissolve and filter.

COLLYRIUM CAPSICI. CH. Capsicum gr. viij, distilled water ℥viij. Infuse without heat for 3 hours, and filter. *In Amaurosis,* 2 or 3 drops to be used daily.

COLLYRIUM CUPRI ACETATIS. Verdigris gr. viij, rose water f ℥viij, sedative solution of opium ʒij.

COLLYRIUM CUPRI AMMONIATI. CH. Verdigris gr. iv, lime water f ℥viij, muriate of ammonia ʒss. Digest 24 hours, and decant.

COLLYRIUM CUPRI SULPHATIS. See Col. Bateanum.

COLLYRIUM DIVINUM. Dissolve ʒj of the compound called Lapis Divinus (P.) in f ℥xxxvj of water, and filter.

COLLYRIUM EMOLLIENS. F. H. Marsh-mallow root ʒj, boil in water q. s. to obtain ℥iv of decoction. CRUVEILHIER. White of egg ℥jss, emulsion of the cold seeds ℥iij, sugar-candy ʒj.

COLLYRIUM HYDRARGYRO IODO-CYANIDI POTASSII. Cyanhydrargyrate of iodide of potassium gr. iv, water f ℥iv.

Collyrium Hydrargyri Submuriatis. Mr. Ware. Calomel ʒss, water ℥ss. Agitate the bottle when used, and drop 3 drops into the eye, in scrofulous ophthalmia.

Collyrium Hydrargyri Bichloridi. Travers. Sublimate gr. ij to iv, distilled water f℥viij. Germ. H. Sublimate gr. ss, rose water ℥iij, mucilage of quince seeds ʒj, cherry-laurel water ʒss. Mackenzie. Sublimate gr. j, water f℥viij.

Collyrium Hydrargyri et Plumbi Acetatis. Dr. Reece. Acetate of mercury gr. ij, acetate of lead gr. v, distilled vinegar fʒss, distilled water f℥vj. Mix. [ʒss of opium is occasionally added.]

Collyrium Iodinii. M. Iodine gr. i to ij, iodide of potassium ℈j, rose water ℥vj. Dr. Lohsse prescribes a stronger solution for dropping into the eye in opacity of the cornea. Iodine gr. j, iodide of potassium gr. ij, water fʒvj. A similar solution has been proposed for removing particles of iron from the eye.

Collyrium Juglandis. M. Negrier. Decoction of walnut leaves f℥viij, extract of belladonna ℈j, wine of opium ♏xiv. *In Scrofulous Ophthalmia.*

Collyrium Lithargyri Acetatis. See Col. Plumbi.

Collyrium Morphiæ. Dr. C. Lee. Sulphate of morphia gr. ij, distilled water f℥j.

Collyrium Opiatum. P. Extract of opium gr. iv, rose water ℥iv. Lawrence. Soft extract of opium gr. x, camphor gr. vj, hot water f℥xij. See Col. Anodynum.

Collyrium Opii Compositum. Guy's H. Liquor of acetate of ammonia f℥iij, wine of opium f℥j.

Collyrium Papaveris. Beer. Decoction of poppy-heads f℥iv, rose water f℥ij, camphor mixture f℥ij.

Collyrium Plumbi. Ch. Solution of diacetate of lead 10 drops, distilled water (or rose, or elder-flower water) f℥iv. [♏xx of wine of opium, or of spirit of camphor, are occasionally added.]

Collyrium Plumbi Acetatis. Mid. H. Acetate of lead gr. ij, d. water ℥j.

Collyrium Plumbi Carbonatis. Mr. Cam. Compound ceruss powder ʒj, rose water f℥viij.

Collyrium Resolvens. Alibert. Melilot flowers ℈j, boiling water f℥xij. Infuse, strain, add acetate of lead ʒss. U. C. H. Distilled water f℥x, muriate of ammonia gr. xij, liquor of diacetate of lead fʒss.

Collyrium Sedativum. U. C. H. Distilled water f℥viij, opium ℈j, ferro-prussiate of potash ℈j. Mix, and filter.

Collyrium Siccum. Dupuytren. White sugar ʒj, red oxide of mercury ℈ss, oxide of zinc ℈j. Or, sugar-candy, calomel, and oxide of zinc, equal parts. Recamier prescribes equal parts of oxide of zinc and sugar-candy. Lagneau, sugar-candy and nitre. Velpeau, trisnitrate of bismuth and candy, e. p. These powders should be triturated till perfectly impalpable, and a small pinch blown into the eye through a quill. [For Collyrium Siccum Ammoniacale, P., see Pulvis Ammoniatus Aromaticus.]

Collyrium Sodæ Muriatis. Dr. J. Hays, *in Granular Ophthalmia.* A saturated solution of common salt. Tavignot prescribes from ʒiv to ʒx of salt to ℥iv of water.

Collyrium Sodæ Chlorinatæ. Dr. Herzberg. Labarraque's solution gr. xv, distilled water ℥iv.

Collyrium Strychniæ. Henderson. Strychnia gr. ij, distilled vinegar fʒj, water f℥j. Mix, and filter. *In Amaurosis.*

Collyrium Tabaci. Dr. Vetch. Tobacco ʒj, boiling water f℥viij. Infuse, and strain.

Collyrium Tannini. M. Cavarra. Tannin gr. ij to iij, water f℥j.

Collyrium Zinci Acetatis. Ware. Acetate of zinc gr. xv to ʒss, distilled water f℥xij.

Collyrium Zinci Cyanidi. Koch. Cyanide of zinc gr. viij, wine of opium ♏xxiv, powdered gum acacia ʒij, cherry-laurel water ʒvj, black cherry water ℥iij.

Collyrium Zinci Iodidi. Mannoir. Iodide of zinc gr. iv, distilled water ℥vj.

Collyrium Zinci Oxydi. De Haen. Oxide of zinc ℈j, elder flower water f℥ij. H. des Enfans. Gr. j of oxide, to ℥j of plantain water.

Collyrium Zinci Sulphatis. Various authorities direct from

gr. ss to iv of the sulphate to each f℥j of distilled water, rose water, or elder water. Extract or wine of opium is frequently added.

COLLYRIUM ZINCI CAMPHORATUM. GUY'S H. Sulphate of zinc ℈j, tincture of camphor f℥j, distilled water f℥viij; mix, and filter.

COLLYRIUM ZINCI COMPOSITUM. GUY'S H. Sulphate of zinc gr. xij, water f℥vj, wine of opium f℥ij.

COLOCYNTHINUM. *Colocynthin* is obtained by digesting watery extract of colocynth in alcohol, evaporating the clear tincture to dryness, washing the residue with cold water, and again drying it.

CONFECTIO AMYGDALÆ. L. [Conserva Amygdalæ. E.] Sweet almonds, blanched by maceration and peeling ℥viij, powdered gum acacia ℥j, white sugar ℥iv. Beat them together to a uniform mass. The confection keeps longer if the ingredients, powdered separately, are merely mixed, and only beaten into a mass at the time of using.

CONFECTIO ALKERMES. L. 1745. Strained juice of kermes ℔iij, rose water f℥vj, white sugar ℔j, oil of cinnamon ℈ss.

CONFECTIO ALUMINIS. ST. B. H. Powdered alum ℥ss, confection of roses ℥iij. Dose, ʒj three times a day. FOY directs ʒj alum to ℥j of confection.

CONFECTIO AROMATICA. L. Cinnamon ℥ij, nutmegs ℥ij, cloves ℥j, cardamom-seeds ℥ss, saffron ℥ij, prepared chalk ℥xvj, white sugar ℔ij. The ingredients, finely powdered and uniformly mixed, are to be kept in a close vessel; and a portion of the powder mixed with water q. s. when required for use. E. Aromatic powder [E.] 1 part, syrup of orange-peel 2 parts. Mix.

CONFECTIO AURANTII. L. Fresh bitter orange-peel rasped ℔j, white sugar ℔iij; beat together in a marble mortar with a wooden pestle.

CONFECTIO CASSIÆ. L. Cassia pulp ℔ss, manna ℥ij, tamarind pulp ℥j, syrup of roses f℥viij. Dissolve the bruised manna in the syrup, add the pulps, and evaporate to a due consistence.

CONFECTIO CINCHONÆ. St. B. H. Powdered bark (yellow) ʒvj, ginger ʒss, treacle ℥iijss. Dose, ʒj—ij.

CONFECTIO CONII. Dr. OSBORNE. Fresh hemlock-leaves, beaten

up with an equal weight of treacle. Dr. O. proposes to preserve other narcotic plants in the same manner. Dr. M. Hall had previously recommended the use of *sugar* for the same purpose.

Confectio Cynosbati. See Confectio Rosæ Caninæ.

Confectio Damocratis. *Mithridate.* L. 1745. It consisted of 45 ingredients, and contained 1 grain of opium in ℥ss.

Confectio Ferri Subcarbonatis. St. B. H. Subcarbonate (sesquioxide) of iron ℥ss, treacle q. s. Dose ʒss. See *Electuarium* Ferri Subcarb.

Confectio Ferri Tartarizati. St. B. H. Bitartrate of potash ℥jss, tartarized iron ʒij, powdered ginger ℈j, treacle ℥ijss. Dose ʒij, 3 times a day.

Confectio Hamech (purgative), and Confectio de Hyacintho (astringent), are obsolete.

Confectio Hydrargyri. Dr. D. Davies. Quicksilver rubbed to extinction, with an equal weight of treacle or manna.

Confectio Jalapæ Composita. St. B. H. Powdered jalap ʒij, cream of tartar ℥jss, ginger ℈j, treacle ℥ijss. Dose ʒij.

Confectio Opii. L. Opium ʒvj, long pepper ℥j, ginger ℥ij, caraway seeds ℥iij, tragacanth ʒij. Mix the ingredients, finely powdered, with f℥xvj of hot syrup. The powder should be kept in a close vessel, and the syrup added when it is required for use. The proportion will be f℥j of syrup to ʒiijss of the powder.

Confectio Paulina. L. 1745. Zedoary, cinnamon, long pepper, black pepper, styrax, galbanum, castor, opium, of each ℥ij; thick syrup ℔iv. Mix.

Confectio Piperis Nigri. L. *Ward's Paste.* Black pepper ℔j, elecampane ℔j, fennel seed ℔iij, white sugar ℔ij. Reduce them to a very fine powder, and keep it in a close vessel. When required for use, mix it with ℔ij of honey, [or ℥vij of the powder with ℥ij of honey.]

Confectio Potassæ Nitratis. St. B. H. Nitrate of potash ʒiv, confection of roses ℥iij. Mix. Dose ʒj, 3 times a day.

Confectio Potassæ Bitartratis. St. B. H. Bitartrate of potash ℥iij, ginger ʒss, syrup ℥iij.

Confectio Resinæ. Dr. Watson. Pulverized resin ℥j, clarified honey ℥v. Mix. Dose ʒij to ʒiij. If the stomach will bear it, ℥ss balsam copaiva may be added. *In hemorrhoids with constipation.*

Confectio Rosæ Caninæ. L. *Confection* (or *Conserve*) *of Hips.* Pulp of fruit of dog-rose ℔j, white sugar ℥xx. Heat the pulp gently in an earthen vessel, gradually add the sugar, and rub together till they are incorporated. E. To 1 part of hips, deprived of carpels, and beaten to a pulp, gradually add 3 parts of sugar.

Confectio [Conserva, E. and D.] Rosæ Gallicæ. L. Red roses (the unblown flowers deprived of their heels) ℔j, pure sugar ℔iij. Beat the roses in a marble mortar, add the sugar, and beat them together. [D. the same. E. ℔ij sugar.]

Confectio Rutæ. L. Rue dried, caraway seed, bay berries, of each ℥jss, sagapænum ℥ss, black pepper ʒij. Powder them finely, and mix with honey ℥xvj.

Confectio Scammonii. L. [*Electuarium Caryocostinum.* L. 1720.] Scammony ℥jss, cloves ʒvj, ginger ʒvj; powder finely, and add syrup of roses q. s.; rub together with oil of caraway f ʒss. The powders are directed to be kept mixed, and the syrup and oil added when required for use.

Confectio Sennæ. L. Electuarium Sennæ, E. *Lenitive Electuary.* Figs ℔j, liquorice root ℥iij, water Oiij; boil to half, press, and strain. Reduce by evaporation by water-bath to f ℥xxiv, and add white sugar ℔ijss to form a syrup; to which add pulp of tamarinds, cassia, and prunes, of each ℔ss, powdered senna ℥viij, and powdered coriander seeds ℥iv. E. directs ℔j pulp of prunes, and omits the tamarind and cassia, adding ¼ pint more water. Mix. [See Electuarium Sennæ, D.]

Confectio Sennæ Composita. St. B. H. Confection of senna ℥ij, jalap powder ʒj, supertartrate of potash ʒij, ginger ʒjss, syrup q. s. Dose ʒj.

Confectio Spongii. St. B. H. Burnt sponge ℥j, syrup of orange-peel q. s. Dose ʒj, 3 times a day.

Confectio Stanni. St. B. H. Powdered tin ℥j, confection of dog-rose ℥ij. Mix. Dose ℥ss every morning.

Confectio Sulphuris Composita. St. B. H. Precipitated sulphur ℥ss, supertartrate of potash ʒj, clarified honey ℥j. Mix. For other Confections, see *Conserva* and *Electuarium*.

CONIA. GEIGER. *Concine* is obtained by distilling soft alcoholic extract of hemlock-seeds (fruit) with its weight of water and a little caustic potash. The salts of conia are obtained by neutralizing it with the diluted acids.

CONSERVA ABSINTHII MARITIMI. L. 1788. Beat the fresh leaves of sea-wormwood in a marble mortar, with a wooden pestle, first alone, and then with thrice their weight of refined sugar, till they are incorporated. [The other conserves are prepared in the same way unless otherwise directed. Dr. BLEY preserves the *narcotic plants* by beating one part of the fresh plant with two of sugar.]

CONSERVA ARI. Fresh root of spotted arum ℔ss, sugar ℔jss. Beat together.

CONSERVA AURANTII. See Confectio Aurantii.

CONSERVA COCHLEARIÆ. L. 1788. From fresh scurvy-grass; as Cons. Absinthii.

CONSERVA LAVANDULÆ. From 1 part of fresh flowers, and 3 of sugar.

CONSERVA LUJULÆ. Leaves of wood-sorrel 1 part, sugar 3 parts.

CONSERVA MALVÆ. Mallow flowers 1 part, sugar 3 parts.

CONSERVA MENTHÆ. L. 1745. As Conserva Absinthii. [Many other conserves are directed in Foreign Pharmacopœias from the leaves and flowers of plants, with twice or thrice their weight of sugar.]

CONSERVA PRUNI SYLVESTRIS. L. 1788. Put sloes into water over the fire, taking care they do not break; then press them through a hair sieve, and form the pulp into a conserve, with thrice its weight of sugar. *Astringent.*

CONSERVÆ ROSÆ. E. & D. See Confectio Rosæ.

CONSERVA ROSÆ ACIDA. G. H. Confection of red rose ℔j, sulphuric acid ʒj. Mix.

CONSERVA RUTÆ. D. See Confectio Rutæ.

CONSERVA SCILLÆ. Fresh squill ℥j, sugar ℥v. Beat together.

CONSERVA TAMARINDI. P. Pulp of tamarinds ℥iv, powdered sugar ℥vj. Evaporate in a water-bath to the consistence of honey.

CORALLIA PRÆPARATA. Corals are prepared as chalk. See Creta Præparata.

CORNU USTUM. L. Burn pieces of stag's horn in an open vessel till they are perfectly white; then powder and prepare them as chalk.

CORTEX AURANTIORUM CONDITUS. L. 1746. Steep fresh peels of Seville oranges in repeated waters till they lose their bitterness; then boil them in syrup till tender and transparent. Lemon and citron peels are candied in the same manner.

CREASOTON. P. Distil wood-tar in a wrought-iron retort till white vapours appear; collect the heavy oily matter which forms the lower layer of the product, and wash it with water slightly acidulated with sulphuric acid. Then distil it in a glass retort (rejecting the first portions, which are chiefly *eupione*), and treat the product with solution of potassa at 1·12 sp. gr., shaking the mixed liquids strongly. When it is settled, pour off the layer of eupione from the surface, and expose the combined potash and creasote to the air till it becomes black. Then saturate with diluted sulphuric acid, pour away the watery liquid, and distil the product in glass. Repeat the treatment by exposure, potash, sulphuric acid, and distillation three times or oftener, until the combination of creasote and potash ceases to become coloured by the action of the air; then saturate it with concentrated phosphoric acid, and distil the creasote, rejecting the first portions.

CREMOR LITHARGYRI ACETATI. Dr. KIRKLAND. Solution of diacetate of lead ʒj, cream ℥j. Mix.

CREMOR TARAXACI. Dr. COLLIER. Wash fresh dandelion roots, cut them in slices, and sprinkle them with spirit of juniper; then express the juice by means of an iron press. The creamy juice will keep for a considerable time. Dose, a tablespoonful twice or thrice a day.

CRETA PRÆPARATA. L. Rub chalk very fine with a little water, stir this into a large quantity of water, and when the coarser particles have subsided pour off the supernatant milky water into another vessel, and let it settle. Pour off the water and dry the sediment.

CRETA PRECIPITATA. See Calcis Carbonas Precipitatum.

CRYSTALLI FERRI IODIDI SACCHARATI. See Saccharum Ferri Iodidi.

CUPRUM ALUMINATUM. See *Lapis Divinus.* P.

CUPRUM AMMONIATUM. E. & D. *Cupri Ammonio-sulphas.* L. Sulphate of copper ℥j, sesquicarbonate of ammonia ℥jss; rub together till no more carbonic acid gas escapes, wrap the mass in blotting paper, and dry in the air. Keep it in well-closed bottles.

CUPRI ACETAS ET DIACETAS. The *diacetate* of copper (C. Subacetas, D.) or common verdigris, is prepared by the action of fermenting *marc* of grapes, or of vinegar, on copper plates. The *acetate,* by dissolving the diacetate in acetic acid, and crystallizing. Cupri subacetas *præparatum* (D.) is prepared in the same way as chalk.

CUPRI DINIODIDUM. To a solution of 1 proto-sulphate of copper, and 2¼ proto-sulp. of iron, add solution of iodide of potassium; wash the white precipitate, and dry it.

CUPRI SULPHAS. It may be made by evaporating a solution of copper in diluted sulphuric acid, and crystallizing; but is generally obtained from copper pyrites, by the action of air, heat, and moisture; and also as a product in the refining of silver.

DECOCTA. *Decoctions.* The roots, barks, woods, and other solid ingredients require to be sliced or bruised. *Distilled* water is generally ordered by the L. college, and is always preferable when it can be obtained; otherwise the purest and softest water should be selected for the purpose. When sufficiently boiled, the liquid should be immediately strained; and again decanted before it is cold, from any sediment which may have subsided.

DECOCTUM ACANTHI. Bear's-breech ℥j, water Oj; boil for a quarter of an hour and strain.

DECOCTUM ADSTRINGENS. SWEDIAUR. Oak bark, pomegranate peel, tormentil root, of each ʒij, water ℔j, milk ℔j; boil for a quarter of an hour; adding towards the end ʒij of cinnamon, and strain.

DECOCTUM ALOES COMPOSITUM. L. Extract of liquorice ʒvij, carbonate (subc.) of potash ʒj, aloes, myrrh, saffron, of each ʒjss, water Ojss; boil to Oj, strain, and add compound tincture of cardamom f℥vij. E. and D. Aloes, myrrh, saffron, of each ʒj, extract of liquorice ℥ss, carbonate of potash ℈ij, water f℥xvj. Boil to f℥xij, filter, and add comp. tincture of cardamom f ℥iv. [The foreign extract of liquorice is not suitable for this purpose, as it deposits much sediment. A purified extract obtained from it by the action of cold water is sometimes substituted for the extract of the Pharmacopœia; but the latter is preferable, especially that of the Ed. Ph.]

Decoctum Album Sydenhami. See Mistura Cornu Cervi.

Decoctum Alconorco. Niemann. American Alconorque bark ℥ss, water ℥xvj; boil to ℥viij, and strain. Dose f ℥j. *In Phthisis.*

Decoctum Alni. Bark of common alder ℥j, water Oj; boil to f ℥xvj.

Decoctum Althææ. See Mistura Althææ. E.

Decoctum Amarum. Bitter herbs (species Aromaticæ, P.) ℥j, water Ojss; boil to Oj.

Decoctum Amyli. L. [Mucilago Amyli, E. and D.] Pure starch ʒiv, (ʒiij, D.,) water Oj. Triturate the starch with a little of the water, add the rest, and boil slightly.

Decoctum Anthemidis. See Decoctum Chamæmeli Compositum. D.

Decoctum Anticolicum Deglandi. See Apozema Anticolicum.

Decoctum Apocyni. Dr. Griscom. Root of Apocynum Cannabinum ℥j, juniper berries ℥j, water Oiij; boil to Oij. [The Apocynum Cannabinum is sometimes called *Indian hemp*, but is altogether different from the *Cannabis Indica*. It is chiefly used in dropsies.]

Decoctum Artemisiæ Vulgaris. Dunglison. Mugwort-root ℥j, water f ℥xxiv; boil for half an hour. Dose f ℥jss or f ʒij every 2 hours. *In Epilepsy.*

Decoctum Asclepiadis Tuberosæ. Pleurisy-root ℥j, water Oij; boil to Oj. Dose, a teacupful every 3 or 4 hours, warm. For children, in dentition, ʒij of the root in f ℥xviij of milk, boiled to f ℥xij. Dose f ℥j. *Diaphoretic.*

Decoctum Asparagi. Roots of asparagus ℥j, water ℔ij; boil for 10 or 15 minutes.

Decoctum Astragali. Crichton. Root of astragalus exscapus (hairy-podded milk vetch) ʒx, water Oiij; boil to Oij. A wine-glassful 3 or 4 times a day. *In syphilis.*

DECOCTUM ASTRINGENS. SWEDIAUR. Oak bark, pomegranate peel, and tormentil root, of each ℥ij, water ℔j, milk ℔j. Boil for ¼ of an hour, adding towards the end ʒij of cinnamon, and strain.

DECOCTUM AVENÆ. *Gruel.* GUY'S H. Oatmeal ℥j, cold water f℥iv; mix them, and add it to Oiij of boiling water; boil for an hour, and strain through a hair sieve. Dr. CULLEN directs it to boil 4 hours. Dr. A. T. THOMSON recommends ℥iv of washed groats to be boiled with Oiv of water till reduced to Oij.

DECOCTUM AZEDERACH. Fresh root-bark of poison-berry tree (Melia Azederach) ℥iv, water Oij; boil to Oj. *Anthelmintic.* Dose, f℥ss every 2 or 3 hours until it produces sickness or purging.

DECOCTUM BALLOTÆ LANATÆ. BRERA. Siberian or woolly ballota ℥j, water Oj; boil to f℥xij. Dose, from f℥vj to f℥xij in the day. *In rheumatic, gouty, and dropsical affections.*

DECOCTUM BARDANÆ. LEWIS. Dried roots of burdock ℥ijss, water Oiij; boil to Oij, and strain. A pint daily.

DECOCTUM BECCABUNGÆ. COPLAND. Fresh brooklime ℥iij, water Oj; boil for 15 minutes, and strain.

DECOCTUM BIGNONIÆ CATALPÆ. Dr. GRANVILLE. Pods of catalpa ℥ss; boil in water q. s. to strain f℥viij. AUTOMARCHI directs the seeds and diaphragms of 3 or 4 pods to be boiled with ℥xv of water till reduced to ℥vj, and this quantity to be taken daily, in asthmatic affections, &c.

DECOCTUM BISTORTÆ. Bistort root ℥ij, water Ojss. Boil 15 or 20 minutes, and strain. *Astringent.* Dose, f℥j to f℥ij.

DECOCTUM BORAGINIS. F. H. A handful of borage to Oj of water.

DECOCTUM CAINCÆ. F. H. Cahinca root (*chiococca racemosa*) ʒij, water Ojss. Boil slightly. *Purgative, emetic, and diaphoretic.*

DECOCTUM CHINÆ. SWEDIAUR. China root ℥j, grocer's currants ℥j, water Oiv; boil to Ojss.

DECOCTUM COLUMBÆ COMPOSITUM. U. S. Calumba, quassia, of each ʒij, orange peel ʒj, rhubarb ℈j, subcarbonate of potash ʒss, water ℥xx. Boil to ℥xvj, strain, and add compound tincture of lavender ℥ss.

DECOCTUM CEDRELÆ. Bark of *Cedrela febrifuga* (deprived of its epidermis) ℥ss, water Oj; boil to Oss. To be taken in 24 hours. *In intermittents.*

DECOCTUM CENTAURII. F. H. Lesser centaury ℥ij, water Oij, boil for a few minutes, and strain.

DECOCTUM CETRARIÆ. L. *Decoctum Lichenis.* Iceland moss ʒv, water Ojss; boil to Oj and strain. Dose, f℥ij frequently. *In phthisis*, &c.

DECOCTUM CETRARIÆ [cum Lacte]. GUY'S H. Decoction of Iceland moss Oj, new milk Oj, sugar ℥jss. Boil a little, and strain. The bitterness is sometimes removed by first infusing the moss in Oj of boiling water for a quarter of an hour, rejecting the water. *Taken as the last.*

DECOCTUM CHAMÆMELI COMPOSITUM. D. Chamomile flowers ℥ss, fennel seed ʒij, water Oj; boil and strain. *In fomentations and clysters.*

DECOCTUM CHENOPODII. Dr. WOOD. Fresh leaves of American wormseed (*Chenopodium anthelminticum*) ℥j, milk Oj; boil. Dose, a wineglassful, with some aromatic.

DECOCTUM CHIMAPHILÆ. L. Dried pyrola (*winter green*) ℥j, water Ojss; boil to Oj and strain. D. (*Dec. Pyrolæ*) Pyrola umbellata ℥j, water f℥xxxij; macerate 6 hours, bruise the root, and boil to f℥xvj. Dose, f℥j–ij. *In dropsies.*

DECOCTUM CHIRAYTÆ. Dried chiretta ʒiv, water Oj; boil for 15 minutes. There is no authorized form; but this is sometimes used.

DECOCTUM CHONDRI. Macerate ℥ss of carrageen (Irish moss) for 10 minutes in cold water, take out the moss, and having shaken off the water, boil it in Oiij of milk, or water, for 15 minutes, and strain. It may be flavoured and sweetened to the taste. *Ad libitum.*

DECOCTUM CIMICIFUGÆ. Black snake root (*Cimicifuga racemosa*) ℥j, water f℥xvj; boil for 10 minutes. Dose, ℥j to ℥ij. *In rheumatic and dropsical affections.*

DECOCTUM CINCHONÆ. Peruvian bark bruised ʒx, water Oj; boil for 10 minutes and strain. L. directs the pale, yellow, or red cinchona to be used; E. the crown, gray, yellow, or red; D. the pale. *Tonic and antiperiodic.* Dose, ℥ij.

DECOCTUM CINCHONÆ ACIDULATUM. SIR J. WYLIE. Cinchona

bark ℥j, water f℥xvj, diluted sulphuric acid ʒj; boil for 10 minutes, and strain while hot.

Decoctum Cinchonæ cum Serpentaria. Sir J. Pringle. Peruvian bark ʒiij, water Oj; boil to Oss, and infuse in the hot decoction ʒiij of serpentaria root.

Decoctum Colocynthidis. Bat. Ph. Colocynth pulp ʒj, water ℥viij; boil for 10 minutes, strain, and when cool, add syrup of orange peel ℥j, æther ʒj. Dose, ℥ss, 3 times a day. *In dropsies*, &c.

Decoctum Commune. Decoctum Malvæ Compositum.

Decoctum Cornu Cervi. See Mistura Cornu Cervi.

Decoctum Cornus Floridæ. U. S. Bark of Jamaica dogwood ℥j, water f℥xvj; boil 10 minutes, and strain. As a substitute for Cinchona, but is more astringent. Other species of Cornel are also employed.

Decoctum Cydoniæ. L. Quince seeds ʒij, water Oj; boil for 10 minutes, and strain.

Decoctum Digitalis. D. 1807. Dried fox-glove ʒj, water q. s. to produce f℥viij of strained decoction. Set it on a slow fire, and when it begins to boil, remove it, let it digest 15 minutes, and strain.

Decoctum Dulcamaræ. L., E., & D. Bitter-sweet stalks ʒx, water Ojss; boil to Oj, and strain.

Decoctum Dulcamaræ Compositum. Augustin. Dulcamara ʒiv, burdock root, liquorice root, sassafras, guaiacum wood, of each ʒij, water ℔ij. Boil to ℥xvj. Foy directs ℥ij dulcamara. A wineglassful frequently.

Decoctum pro Enemate. L. 1788. Decoctum Malvæ Compositum.

Decoctum Ergotæ. Pereira. Ergot of rye ʒj; water f℥vj; boil for 10 minutes, and strain. For 3 doses.

Decoctum Eupatorii Cannabini. Hemp-agrimony ℥j, water Oj; boil, and strain.

Decoctum Euphorbiæ [pilosæ, or palustris]. Krebel. Boil ʒj of the root in Oj of water to f℥xvj. To prevent hydrophobia, let the wound be washed with it, and a wineglassful taken daily for 3 or 4 days. [These species of spurge are not found in England.]

DECOCTUM FILICIS. Dried fern root ʒv, water Ojss; boil to Oj, and strain.

DECOCTUM FŒNUGRECI. TADDEI. Fœnugrec seeds ℥j, water Oj; boil and strain. *Mucilaginous, chiefly used in fomentations.*

DECOCTUM PRO FOMENTO. L. 1788. Dried southernwood, wormwood tops, and chamomile flowers, of each ℥j, dried bay leaves, ℥ss, water Ov; boil slightly, and strain.

DECOCTUM FUCI AMYLACEI. Ceylon moss ʒv, water Oij; boil for 20 minutes, and strain.

DECOCTUM FULIGINIS. M. BLAUD. Wood-soot two handfuls, water ℥xvj; boil for half an hour, and strain. Dr. NELIGAN. Wood-soot ℥iv, water Ojss; boil to Oj. As a lotion to chronic skin diseases, ulcers, &c., and as an enema in ascarides. Dr. HEWSON.

DECOCTUM FULIGINIS CUM CAFFÆA. M. TROUSSEAU. Wood-soot ʒij, roasted coffee ʒj; boil in water q. s., strain, and sweeten. *As a vermifuge for children.*

DECOCTUM FURFURIS. Bran ℥iv, water Oj; boil, and strain.

DECOCTUM GALLÆ. Galls ℥ss, water Ojss; boil to Oj.

DECOCTUM GEI. Dr. A. T. THOMSON. Avens root ℥j, water Oj; boil for 15 minutes, and strain. *Astringent and febrifuge.* Dose ℥ss to ℥j.

DECOCTUM GEOFFRÆÆ. E. 1817. Powdered cabbage-tree bark ℥j, water ℔ij; boil to ℔j, and strain. D. Bruised bark ℥j, water f℥xxxij; boil to f℥xvj, strain, and add syrup of orange peel ℥ij. *Vermifuge,* but requires caution. Dose for an adult ℥ss to ℥j; for children, from fʒss to fʒjss, promoting its operation with warm water and a dose of castor oil.

DECOCTUM GERANII. Dried root of spotted crane's bill ℥j, water f℥xxiv; boil to f℥xvj. Dose f℥j to ℥ij. *Astringent.* Dr. CHAPMAN says the root boiled in milk is an excellent remedy for the cholera of infants.

DECOCTUM GLYCYRRHIZÆ. D. Liquorice root ℥jss, water f℥xvj; boil for 10 minutes, and strain.

DECOCTUM GOSSYPII. Dr. BOUCHELLE. Inner bark of the root of the cotton plant ℥iv, water Oij; boil to Oj. Dose, f℥ij, every 20 or 30 minutes. *As a parturifacient.*

DECOCTUM GRAMINIS. *Tisane de Chiendent.* Dog-grass root ℥j, water Oij; boil for half an hour, and infuse in it ʒij of liquorice root for an hour.

DECOCTUM GRAMINIS IODURETUM. M. Decoction of dog-grass ℥xxxij, iodide of potassium ʒss, syrup of peppermint ℥ij.

DECOCTUM GRANATI. L. Pomegranate peel ℥ij, water Ojss; boil to Oj.

DECOCTUM GRANATI VERMIFUGUM. *Apozême Vermifuge.* P. Dried bark of the pomegranate root ℥ij, water ℥xxiv; boil slowly to ℥xvj, and strain. [The form used in India is ℥viij of the fresh root bark, boiled with Oiij of water to Oij. Dose, a wine-glassful, repeated every half-hour, or as the patient can bear it. Dr. FLEMING. Dr. ROYLE says, ℥ij fresh bark to be macerated 12 hours in Ojss water, then boiled to Oj; dose ℥ij—iv, in the morning fasting, and repeated every 2 hours for 3 times.]

DECOCTUM GUAIACI [Compositum. D.] E. *Decoctum Lignorum.* Guaiac turnings ℥iij, raisins ℥ij, water Oviij; boil to Ov, adding towards the end, liquorice root ℥j, sassafras ℥j; strain.

DECOCTUM HÆMATOXYLI. E. Logwood ℥j, cinnamon ʒj, water Oj; boil to Oss. D. Logwood ℥jss, cinnamon ʒj, water f℥xxxij; boil to f℥xvj. Dose ℥j—ij.

DECOCTUM HELENII. ROYLE. Elecampane root ℥ss, water Oj; boil. NIEMANN directs f℥vj of decoction to be made from ℥ss of the root. The former is given by wine-glassfuls, the latter by spoonfuls.

DECOCTUM HELENII COMPOSITUM. F. H. Elecampane root ℥j, hyssop ʒij, ground ivy ʒij, water ℥xxxij; boil, strain, and add syrup of honey, ℥ij.

DECOCTUM HELLEBORI NIGRI. Dr. A. T. THOMSON. Black hellebore root ʒij, water Oj; boil a quarter of an hour. Dose f℥j, every 4 hours.

DECOCTUM HELMINTHOCORTI. Corsican moss ʒv, water Ojss; boil to Oj, and strain. Dose, a wine-glassful. *Vermifuge.*

DECOCTUM HEMEDESMI. PEREIRA. Root of Indian sarsaparilla (*Hemedesmus Indicus*) ℥ij, water Ojss; boil to Oj. By wine-glassfuls.

DECOCTUM HIPPOCASTANEI. NIEMANN. Horse-chestnut bark

℥jss, water Ojss; boil to ℥x, adding towards the end ʒj of liquorice root, and strain.

DECOCTUM HORDEI. L. *Barley Water.* Pearl barley ℥ijss, wash it with cold water, boil it a few minutes with Oss of water, throw this away, and boil the barley with Oiv of water to Oij, and strain. [D. nearly the same.]

DECOCTUM HORDEI COMPOSITUM. L. Decoction of barley Oij, figs ℥ijss, raisins ℥ijss, liquorice root ʒv, water Oj; boil to Oij.

DECOCTUM HORDEI ACIDULATUM. Decoction of barley ℔iij, lemons sliced No. 2; boil to ℔j, strain, and add sugar ℥iij. GUY'S H. Decoction of barley Oj, syrup of lemon f℥j; or dilute sulphuric acid fʒj, syrup ℥j. Other usual additions to barley water are gum arabic ℥ss, nitre ʒj; or cream of tartar ʒj, to each Oj.

DECOCTUM HYDRARGYRI. Quicksilver boiled with twice its weight of water for half an hour. Dose, f℥ss to f℥ij. *As a vermifuge.* A portion of the metal is said to be taken up by the water.

DECOCTUM ILLICIS. FOY. Holly leaves ʒiv, water ℥xvj; boil to ℥xij. For 3 doses. *In Intermittents.*

DECOCTUM INULÆ. See Dec. Helenii.

DECOCTUM JUGLANDIS. GENEVA PH. Peels of green walnuts ℥j, water Oss; boil for a quarter of an hour.

DECOCTUM JUGLANDIS [*foliorum.*] M. NEGRIER. Fresh walnut leaves one handful, water Oij; boil for 15 minutes.

DECOCTUM JUJUBARUM. Boil ℥ij of jujubes (stoned) for an hour, in water q. s. to produce Oij of decoction.

DECOCTUM JUNIPERI COMPOSITUM. St. B. H. Juniper berries ℥ij, cream of tartar ʒiij, water Oiv; boil to Oij, strain, and add compound spirit of juniper f℥ij.

DECOCTUM LAPPÆ. See Decoctum Bardanæ.

DECOCTUM LAURO-CERASI CORTICIS. Dr. KASTNER. Cherry-laurel bark ℥ij, water Oj; boil. To be taken in 24 hours. *In Amenorrhœa.*

DECOCTUM LEPIDII. Narrow-leaved pepperwort ℥ss, water f℥xvj; boil to f℥viij, and strain. *In Intermittents;* ℥j every 2 hours.

DECOCTUM LICHENIS. See Decoctum Cetrariæ.

Decoctum Lignorum. Decoctum Guaiaci Comp.

Decoctum Limacum. M. Monchou. Flesh of vine or garden snails (cleansed from shell and intestines) ℥v, water Oij, simmer gently for 2 hours, adding towards the end maiden hair ℥ij, and strain.

Decoctum Limonum. M. Minsycht. Lemons sliced No. 5, water Oiijss; boil to Oij, and add sugar ʒiv.

Decoctum Lini. Guy's H. Linseed slightly bruised ℥jss, water Oiij; boil gently for 10 minutes, and strain.

Decoctum Lobeliæ Syphiliticæ. Swediaur. Boil ℥v of the dried root of blue cardinal flower with ℔xij of water to ℔viij. *Alterative and diuretic.* Dose, f℥viij to Ojss daily. This plant must not be confounded with lobelia inflata.

Decoctum Lusitanicum. *Lisbon Diet Drink.* The Dec. Sarzæ Comp. is now substituted for it. The original form is said to be—sarsaparilla ℥j, china root ℥j, dried peels of walnuts No. 20, black antimony ℥ij, pumice-stone powder ℥j, water Oviij: boil to Oiv. M. Pearson used sarsaparilla ʒiv, walnut peels ℥iv, guaiacum shavings ℥jss, black antimony ℥ss, water Oiv; boil to Oiij. The antimony and pumice to be tied up in rag. The black sulphuret of antimony sometimes contains sulphuret of arsenic, which in boiling becomes white arsenic. Its use therefore requires caution.

Decoctum Malti. Swediaur. Ground malt ℥vj, water ℔v; boil to ℔iv, and strain. ℥ij of syrup of lemons may be added. Others direct ʒj or ʒij of liquorice root to be added towards the end of the boiling.

Decoctum Malvæ Compositum. L. Dried mallows ℥j, chamomiles ℥ss, water Oj; boil for 15 minutes.

Decoctum Marchantiæ. Marchantia conica ℥j, water Ojss; boil to Oj. By glassfuls, in dropsies and gravel.

Decoctum Maticonis. Dr. Jeffreys. Matico leaves ℥j, water Oj; boil for 10 or 15 minutes, and strain. Dose, f℥j, 3 times a day. *Astringent.*

Decoctum Menyanthis. Buckbean ℥j, water Ojss; boil to Oj.

Decoctum Mezerei. E. Root-bark of mezereon ʒij, liquorice root ℥ss, water Oij; boil gently to Ojss, and strain. St. B. H. Mezereon bark ℥j, water Oxij; boil to Cj, adding towards the end liquorice root ℥j.

Decoctum Narcoticum. F. H. Dried black nightshade ℥j, poppy-heads 2, water ℥xvj; boil and strain. *As a fomentation.*

Decoctum Nitrosum. E. 1745. Nitre ℥ss, white sugar ℥ij, cochineal ℈j, water Oij; boil to Ojss, and when cold, decant. U. C. H. (*Decoctum Nitratum.*) Barley water Oj, nitre ʒiv.

Decoctum Oryzæ. See Ptisana Oryzæ.

Decoctum Papaveris. L. Poppy-heads (without the seeds) ℥iv, water Oiv; boil 15 minutes, and strain. [E. Oiij of water; D. f℥xxxij.]

Decoctum Pareiræ. Guy's H. Pareira brava root ℥j, water Ojss; boil to Oj, and strain. Brodie prescribes ʒiv of the root; Geoffroy ʒiij. Dose f℥j to f℥ij, 3 times a day. Brodie's from f℥viij—xij in the day.

Decoctum Parietariæ. Ratier. Wall pellitory ʒj, water Ojss; boil to Oj, and strain.

Decoctum Patientiæ. See Decoctum Rumicis.

Decoctum Pruni Padi. M. Broerland. Fresh bark of bird-cherry ℥viij, (or dried bark ℥vj,) water ℔viij; boil to ℔iv. Dose f℥iv, 4 times a day.

Decoctum Pyrolæ. D. See Decoctum Chimaphilæ.

Decoctum Pyrethri. Guy's H. Pellitory root ℥j, water Ojss; boil to Oj, and strain. Dose f℥j to f℥ij.

Decoctum Quercus. L. Oak bark ʒx, water Oij; boil to Oj, and strain.

Decoctum Rhamni Frangulæ. Black alder bark ℥j, water Ojss; boil to Oj, and strain. Dose, a wine-glassful twice a day as a purgative and alterative. The *fresh* bark is said to vomit; the *dry* to purge.

Decoctum Rhododendri. Leaves of rhododendron chrysanthemum ʒiv, water Oss; boil, and strain.

Decoctum Ribis Nigri. M. Colombat. Boil a handful of black currant root in Oij of water, and strain. A cupful occasionally as an astringent.

Decoctum Rosæ Vinosum. F. H. Red roses ℥ij, red wine ℔ij. Heated in a covered vessel to near boiling, and let it stand near the fire for half an hour. *For outward use.*

Decoctum Rubi. Dr. Wood. Smaller roots (or bark of larger

roots) of American blackberry ℥j, water f℥xxiv; boil to f℥xvj. *Astringent.* Dose f℥ij, 3 or 4 times in 24 hours. Our common bramble also possesses astringent properties.

Decoctum Rumicis Aquatici. Dr. A. T. Thomson. Water-dock root ℥j dried, or ℥ij fresh, water Oj; boil for 15 minutes, and strain. R. obtusifolius and other species of dock are also used. *In chronic skin-diseases,* &c.

Decoctum Salicariæ. Dr. A. T. Thomson. Spiked loosestrife (fresh) ʒx, water Oj; boil 15 minutes, and strain.

Decoctum Salicis. Wilkinson. Broad-leaved willow bark ℥jss, bruise, and macerate in water ℔ij for 6 hours, boil for 15 minutes, and strain. Or, it may be made as Dec. Cinchonæ.

Decoctum Sambuci. Sydenham. Inner bark of elder ℥j, water Oj, milk Oj; boil to Oj.

Decoctum Santonici. Worm seed (*semen-contra*) ℥ss, water Ojss; boil, and strain.

Decoctum Saponariæ. Swediaur. Soap wort ℥ij, water ℔iv; boil to ℔ij, and strain. Taken as Dec. Sarzæ.

Decoctum Sarzæ. L. and E. Sarsaparilla ℥v, boiling water Oiv; macerate for 4 [E. 2] hours near the fire, take out and bruise the root, return it to the liquor, and again macerate for 2 hours; boil down to Oij, and strain.

Decoctum Sarzæ Compositum. L. and E. Boiling decoction of sarsaparilla Oiv, sassafras, guaiacum wood, liquorice root, each ʒx, mezereon root-bark ʒiij [E. ʒiv]; boil for a quarter of an hour, and strain.

Decoctum Sarzæ cum Icthyocolla. *Tisane de Feltz.* Sarsaparilla ℥iij, isinglass ℥ss, sulphuret of antimony (tied up in rag) ʒiij, water Ov; boil to Oijss and strain.

Decoctum Sarzæ cum Senna. *Tisane de Vinache.* Cadet. Sarsaparilla ℥jss, china root ℥jss, guaiacum wood ℥jss, sulphuret of antimony (in rag) ℥ij, water Ov; boil to Oiij, and add sassafras ʒiv, senna ʒiv, infuse for an hour, and strain.

Decoctum Scillæ Compositum. Dried squill ʒiij, juniper berries ℥iv, senega ℥iij, water Oiv; boil to Oij, strain, and add spirit of nitric æther ℥iv.

Decoctum Scoparii Compositum. L. Broom-tops, juniper berries, dandelion root, of each ʒiv, water Ojss; boil to Oj, and

8*

strain. E. omits the dandelion, and adds bitartrate of potash ʒiij. Dose, a wine-glassful 3 times a day.

Decoctum Secalis Cornuti. See Decoctum Ergotæ.

Decoctum Senegæ. L. Senega root ʒx, water Oij; boil to Oj, and strain. Guy's H. adds liquorice root ℥ss. The *infusion* is a better preparation. Dose f℥j—iij.

Decoctum Sevi. *Artificial Goat's Milk.* Tie a piece of mutton suet in muslin, and let it boil gently in new milk.

Decoctum Simaroubæ. Dr. Wright. Simaruba bark ʒij, water f℥xxiv; boil to f℥xij, and strain.

Decoctum Spigeliæ. India pink ʒv, water Oj; boil for a few minutes and strain. Senna ʒv, may be infused in the boiling decoction.

Decoctum Spongiæ. Hufeland. Burnt sponge ℥j, water ℔j; boil, digest for 12 hours, strain, and add cinnamon water f℥ij. Dose, f℥j.

Decoctum Staphisagriæ. Stavesacre seeds ℥j, water Oij; boil for a few minutes, and strain. *For external use.*

Decoctum Suberis. Pierquin. Rasped cork ℈ij, water Oiij; boil to Ojss. *Astringent.*

Decoctum Sudorificum. The Dec. Guaiaci Compositum, and Dec. Sarzæ Comp. are so termed.

Decoctum Symphyti. Niemann. Comfrey root ℥ss, water ℥xvj; boil to ℥viij.

Decoctum Taraxaci. D. & E. Fresh dandelion ℥v, [E. ℥viij,] water Oij; boil to Oj, and strain.

Decoctum Tormentillæ. L. Tormentil root ℥ij, water Ojss; boil to Oj, and strain. *Astringent.*

Decoctum Tussilaginis. Fresh coltsfoot leaves ℥ij, (or flowers ℥j,) water Oij; boil to Oj and strain.

Decoctum Ulmi. L. Fresh elm bark ℥ijss, water Oij; boil to Oj, and strain. *In scaly skin diseases.*

Decoctum Ulmi Compositum. Jeffreys. Decoction of elm Oviij, sassafras ℥j, guaiacum wood ℥j, mezereon ʒiij, liquorice root ℥j; boil for an hour, and strain.

Decoctum Uvæ Ursi. L. Bearberry leaves ℥j, water Ojss; boil to Oj, and strain.

DECOCTUM VERATRI. L. White hellebore root ʒx, water Oij; boil to Oj, and strain, and add rectified spirit f ℥iij, [f ℥ijss, D.] *For external use.*

DECOCTUM VERBASCI. Dr. HOME. Leaves of great mullein ℥ij, water Oij; boil for 20 minutes, and strain. Dose, f℥iv. *In diarrhœas.* Also as a fomentation.

DECOCTUM VISCI. NIEMANN. Misletoe ℥j, water Oij; boil to Oj. *In epilepsy;* by wine-glassfuls, frequently.

DECOCTUM XANTHOXYLI. Dr. WOOD. Bark of prickly ash ℥j, water f℥xlviij; boil to f℥xxxij, and strain. *Stimulant and diaphoretic,* from f℥xij to f℥xvj, in 24 hours.

DELPHINIA. *Delphine.* Treat alcoholic extract of stavesacre seeds with water acidulated with sulphuric acid as long as anything is dissolved; add ammonia to the filtered solution, collect and dry the precipitate, and redissolve it in rectified spirit; filter through charcoal, and evaporate it carefully to dryness. Its salts are made by saturating the diluted acids with delphine, and evaporating to dryness. Dose, gr. ss; also used outwardly as veratria.

DIASCORDIUM. This is replaced by the Electuarium Catechu. E.

DIGITALINA. *Digitaline.* HENRY. Exhaust powdered digitalis by percolation or digestion, with spirit of ·860 sp. gr. Filter, distil off the spirit, dissolve the residue in water acidulated with acetic acid, precipitate with infusion of nutgall, collect the precipitate, mix it with powdered litharge and a little spirit, dry the paste, digest it at a very gentle heat with rectified spirit, distil off the spirit, and agitate the residue with ether. What remains is digitaline. It is said to be 100 times as strong as powdered foxglove.

ELÆOSACCHARUM ANISI. P. Essential oil of aniseed, 1 drop, refined sugar ʒj; triturate in a mortar till perfectly mixed. [Other authorities direct 2 drops of the oil.] Elæosacchara of the other essential oils are prepared in the same manner, except the following:—

ELÆOSACCHARUM LIMONIS. Rub the outer rind of a lemon with ʒij of refined sugar, in lumps, and triturate the product in a mortar. In the same manner prepare the elæosacchara of citrons, oranges, and bergamots.

ELATERINUM. Dr. MORRIES. Elaterine is obtained by evaporating tincture of elaterium, made with rectified spirit, to the consistence of thin oil, and throwing it into boiling distilled water. When cold, collect the crystalline precipitate, and dry it with a gentle heat. Dose, to commence, one-sixteenth of a grain.

Electuaria. Electuaries consist of powders mixed up to a soft paste, with syrup, honey, or other thick article. They are included by the L. college, together with Conserves, under the term *Confections*. For other Electuaries see Confectio and Linctus.

Electuarium Anticachecticum. *Bath Electuary*. Select the heaviest and bluest clinkers from a blacksmith's forge, powder them finely, and mix with enough treacle to form a stiff paste. To ℥viij of this add carbonate of magnesia, and powdered ginger, each ℥ss. Give a teaspoonful twice a day for 3 days, then omit it for 3 days, and repeat this as long as is considered necessary. [This is sometimes termed Elect. Ferri Compositum.]

Electuarium Aromaticum. E. Aromatic powder [E.] one part, syrup of orange peel two parts. Mix. For L. & D., see Confectio Aromatica.

Electuarium Antimonii. Ch. Electuary of senna ℥j, guaiacum resin, æthiops mineral, prepared sulphuret of antimony, each ℥ss, syrup q. s. Dose, ʒj to ʒij, twice a day.

Electuarium Antiepilepticum. Dr. Mead. Peruvian bark ʒj, valerian ℥ss, tin ʒss; mix the powders with syrup q. s. to form an electuary.

Electuarium Antidysentericum. E. 1745. Electuary of catechu ℥ij, balsam of Locatellus ℥j. Mix.

Electuarium Anticholericum. A compound of equal parts of lard, charcoal, and maple sugar, is said to have been used with success in the treatment of cholera.

Electuarium Antirheumaticum. *Chelsea Pensioner*. Guaiacum resin ʒj, rhubarb ʒj, bitartrate of potash ℥j, sulphur ℥ij, one nutmeg; mix the powders with sufficient honey, or treacle.

Electuarium Arabicum. Sarsaparilla ℥v, parched nutshells ʒj, China root ʒj; cloves No. iv. Reduce to a fine powder, and form an electuary with honey, q. s. [This forms part of the *traitment Arabique*, for the cure of obstinate skin diseases. A pill (see Pil. Arabicæ) is given every night and morning, followed by a glass of decoction of sarsaparilla, and an hour after a dose of this electuary.] The diet for 25 to 40 days to be purely vegetable (as dried fruits, &c.), and the only drink allowed decoction of sarsaparilla. [There is a want of agreement in the published formulæ and doses.]

Electuarium e Baccis Lauri. See Confectio Rutæ.

Electuarium Carbonis. Prepared charcoal ʒij, carbonate of soda, ʒij, confection of senna ℥ij.

Electuarium Catechu. E. [Comp. D.] *Confectio Japonica.* Catechu ℥iv, kino ℥iv, cinnamon ℥j, nutmeg ℥j [℥ij, D.] opium ʒjss; diffuse the opium in a little sherry, powder the rest finely, and mix the whole with syrup of red roses, [of ginger, D.] (boiled to the consistence of honey) Ojss, [℔ijss D.]

Electuarium Cephalicum. E. H. Valerian ℥j, misletoe of the oak ℥j, syrup q. s.

Electuarium Cinchonæ Compositum. Copland. Yellow bark ℥j, confection of roses ℥ss, diluted sulphuric acid ʒj, syrup of ginger ℥jss. Dose, ʒj or ʒij, 3 or 4 times a day. Quarin's Electuary consists of powdered red bark ℥j, gentian ʒj, ammoniated iron ʒj, oxymel of squills, and syrup of five roots (species diureticæ) q. s. P. Gray bark ʒxviij, muriate of ammonia ʒj, honey ℥ij, syrup of wormwood ℥ij.

Electuarium Copaibæ. Caspar. Blanched almonds ʒvj, marsh-mallow powder ʒj, catechu ʒss, balsam of copaiva, ʒiij.

Electuarium Cubebæ et Copaibæ. Bouchardat. Copaiva ℥j, cubebs in fine powder ℥jss, oil of peppermint 8 drops, spirit of nitric æther 15 drops, powdered sugar q. s.; to form a paste. To be taken in 4 days, wrapped in wafer paper.

Electuarium Dentifricium. P. Prepared coral ℥iv, sepia-bone ℥j, bitartrate of potash ℥ij, cochineal ℥j, alum ʒss, Narbonne honey ℥x. Mix, and add any suitable essential oil.

Electuarium Deobstruens. Copland. Bitartrate of potash ℥j, borax ʒiij, precipitated sulphur ʒvj, confection of senna ℥jss, syrup of ginger ʒvj, syrup of poppies ʒij. Mix. Dose, ʒj every night.

Electuarium Dolichos. See Elect. Mucunæ.

Electuarium Febrifugum. E. H. Peruvian bark ℥j, muriate of ammonia ʒj, syrup of lemons q. s. See also Elect. Cinchonæ Comp. P.

Electuarium Ferri Subcarbonatis. Copland. Subcarbonate of iron ℥ss, syrup of ginger ℥ss, conserve of orange peel ℥ij; mix. Dose, the size of a nutmeg, twice or thrice a day. Mid. H. Sesquioxide of iron ℥j, treacle ℥j, boiling water f ʒij. See also Confectio Ferri.

Electuarium Guaiaci Compositum. Mid. H. Guaiacum resin ʒij, rhubarb ʒj, sulphur ʒij, nitre ʒij, syrup of poppies q. s. Mix. Dose, ʒss to ʒj.

Electuarium Kermetis Mineralis. *Marmelade de Zanetti.* Manna ℥ij, syrup of marsh-mallow ℥jss, pulp of cassia ℥j, oil of almonds ℥j, butter of cacao ʒij, orange-flower water f ʒiv, Kermes mineral gr. iv. Mix.

Electuarium Hæmorrhoidale. U. C. H. Manna ℥ij, sulphate of potash, nitre, precipitated sulphur, each ʒij, syrup q. s. E. H. Confection of senna ℥ij, sulphur ℥ss. Dr. Copland. Nitrate of potash ʒij, confection of senna ℥jss, syrup of ginger ℥jss, elder rob ℥j. Mix. Dr. Graves. Confection of senna ℥j, sulphur ℥j, jalap ʒj, balsam of copaiva ℥ss, ginger ʒss, bitartrate of potash ℥ss, syrup q. s.

Electuarium Lenitivum. See Confectio Sennæ.

Electuarium Mucunæ. Chamberlain's. Dip the dolichos pods in treacle, and scrape off the hairs, repeating fresh pods till it becomes sufficiently thick. Guy's H. Dolichos hairs ℥ss, treacle q. s. to form a soft electuary. Dose, a dessert-spoonful every morning.

Electuarium Nigrum. Trousseau's *Black Tonic.* Perchloride of iron ʒiv, tannin ʒj, confection of roses ℥ij, syrup of orange peel ℥j. Mix.

Electuarium Olibani. Ch. Olibanum ℥ss, balsam copaiva ℥ss, conserve of hips ℥j, syrup q. s. Dose, ʒij twice a day, for gleets, &c.

Electuarium Opii. E. Aromatic powder ℥vj, senega ℥iij, opium diffused in a little sherry ℥ss, syrup of ginger ℔j. Mix. See Confectio Opii.

Electuarium Phyllanthi. Dr. Roxburgh states that the leaves, fruit and flowers of phy. simplex, with their weight of sugar, form an electuary used by the natives of India for the cure of gonorrhœa. Dose, ʒj.

Electuarium Pigmenti Indici. Indigo ℥ss, water q. s. Rub together to form a smooth paste, and add aromatic powder ʒss, syrup ℥j.

Electuarium Pectorale. E. 1744. Conserve of roses ℥ij, compound powder of tragacanth ℥ss, flowers of benzoin ʒj, syrup of balsam of Tolu q. s.

Electuarium Potassæ Nitratis. Guy's H. Nitre ʒjss, confection of roses ℥j.

Electuarium Prunorum. Zwelfer. Pulp of prunes, boiled to a due consistence, ℔ij; pure sugar ℔j.

Electuarium Scillæ Compositum. Guy's H. Oxymel of squills f℥ij, bitartrate of potash ℥iij. Dose, fʒij.

Electuarium e Scordio. *Diascordium.* Replaced by Electuarium Catechu.

Electuarium Sennæ. D. Senna ℥iv, pulp of prunes ℔j, pulp of tamarinds ℥ij, molasses f℥xxiv, oil of caraway ʒij. Mix, s. a. See Confectio Sennæ for L. & E. A cheaper form for hospital use is thus prepared. Mid. H. Powdered senna, coriander, jalap, bitartrate of potash, ginger, liquorice root, of each ℥ij; treacle ℥xlviij. Dose, ʒj to ʒij.

Electuarium Sennæ Compositum. U. C. H. Senna ʒiv, supertartrate of potash ℈iv, jalap ʒij, syrup of ginger f℥jss.

Electuarium Sinapis. Guy's H. Mustard seed lightly bruised ℥j, sulphur ʒij, syrup of orange peel f℥j. Dose, ʒj 3 or 4 times a day.

Electuarium Stanni et Ferri. Dr. Cheston. Pure tin filings or powder ℥iv, carbonate of iron ℥j, conserve of wormwood ℥iij.

Electuarium Sulphuris Compositum. Guy's H. Sulphur ℥j, bitartrate of potash ℥ss, treacle ℥iij. Mix. Mid H. Sulphur ℥ss, cream of tartar ℥ss, electuary of senna ℥ij, treacle q. s.

Electuarium Terebinthinæ. St. B. H. Common turpentine ℥j, honey ℥ij. Mix.

Electuarium Olei Terebinthinæ. Dr. Copland. Oil of turpentine ℥j, clarified honey ℥ij, liquorice powder q. s. to form an electuary.

Electuarium Vermifugum. Bresmer. Worm-seed ℥ss, tansy seed ℥ss, valerian ʒij, jalap ʒjss, sulphate of potash with sulphur ʒjss, oxymel of squills q. s. See also Electuarium Stanni. For other Electuaries see Confectio, Conserva, and Linctus.

Elixir. This name is applied to certain compound tinctures, and other solutions of the active principles of drugs.

Elixir Acidum Halleri. Equal weights of sulphuric acid and rectified spirit, very gradually mixed. It is stronger than *Eau de Rabel.* See Acidum Sulphuricum Alcoholisatum. Dippel's Acid Elixir consists of 1 part of sulphuric acid, 5 of spirit, and 2 of kermes and saffron. Vogler's, of equal weights of sulphuric acid and nitrous æther.

Elixir Aloes Compositum. Copland. Acetate of potash, aloes, inspissated ox-gall, myrrh, each 2 parts, saffron 1 part, brandy 24 parts. Macerate, and strain.

Elixir Anticatarrhale. Hufeland. Extract of blessed thistle ʒj, extract of dulcamara ʒj, fennel water ℥j, cherry-laurel water ʒj. Mix. Dose, ʒj 4 times a day.

Elixir Antiscrofulosum. P. *Tinctura Gentianæ Ammoniata.*

Elixir Antivenereum. Quincy. *Jesuit's Drops.* Copaivi ℥j, guaiacum ʒij, oil of sassafras ʒj, subcarbonate of potash ʒss, rectified spirit f℥v. Digest 3 days.

Elixir Dictum *de Garus.* P. Aloes ℥j, myrrh ℥ss, saffron ℥j, cinnamon ℥ss, cloves ℥ss, nutmeg ℥ss, proof spirit Oxij, orange-flower water f℥xvj. Macerate for 2 days, and distil Ovj; add syrup of capillaire Ovijss, and colour with a little saffron.

Elixir Longæ Vitæ. *Tinctura Rhei et Aloes.*

Elixir Myrrhæ. *Tinctura Sabinæ Composita.*

Elixir Paregoricum. *Tinctura Camphoræ Compcsita.*

Elixir Paregoricum Scoticum. *T. Opii Ammoniata.*

Elixir Pectorale. E. 1745. Balsam of Tolu ℥ij, benzoin ℥jss, saffron ℥ss, rectified spirit f℥xxxij. Digest in a sand heat for 4 days, and strain.

Elixir Polychreston. E. 1745. Guaiacum ℥vj, balsam of Peru ℥ss, rectified spirit f℥xxxij. Digest in a sand heat for 4 days, strain, and add oil of sassafras ʒij.

Elixir Proprietatis. *Tinctura Aloes Composita.*

Elixir Sacrum. *Tinctura Rhei et Aloes.*

Elixir Salutis. *Tinctura Sennæ Composita.*

Elixir Stomachicum. *Tinctura Gentianæ Composita.*

Elixir Viscerale Hoffmanni. *Vinum Centaurii.*

ELIXIR VITRIOLI ACIDUM. *Acidum Sulphuricum Aromaticum.*

ELIXIR VITRIOLI DULCE. *Spiritus Ætheris Aromaticus.* For other Elixirs, see Tincturæ.

EMBROCATIONES. *Embrocations* do not differ materially from *Lotions.* See Lotio.

EMBROCATIO ACONITINÆ. Dr. TURNBULL. Aconitina gr. viij, rectified spirit f ℥ij.

EMBROCATIO ALUMINIS. CH. Alum ʒij, vinegar f ℥viij, weak spirit f ℥viij. *For chilblains,* &c.

EMBROCATIO AMMONIÆ ACETATIS. Embrocatio Communis. GUY'S H. Sesquicarbonate of ammonia ℥iv, vinegar Ov, or q. s. to saturate. Mix, and add proof spirit Oijss.

EMBROCATIO AMMONIÆ ACETATIS CUM SAPONE. Equal parts of solution of acetate of ammonia, and soap liniment.

EMBROCATIO CONTRA ALOPECIAM. E. WILSON. Eau de Cologne f ℥ij, tincture of cantharides f ʒij, oil of rosemary ♏x, oil of lavender ♏x. *To promote the growth of the hair.*

EMBROCATIO CANTHARIDIS. Dr. STRUVE, *in Pertussis.* Tartarized antimony ℈j, water f ℥ij, tincture of cantharides f ℥ss. To be rubbed over the region of the stomach, covering the part afterwards with flannel.

EMBROCATIO CANTHARIDIS CUM CAMPHORA. CH. Equal parts of tincture of cantharides and spirit of camphor.

EMBROCATIO DELPHINIÆ. Dr. TURNBULL. Delphinia ℈j, rectified spirit f ℥ij.

EMBROCATIO QUINÆ. Dr. GUSTAMACCHIA. Disulphate of quinine gr. viij to xij, rectified spirit ℥j. Rubbed over the spine, in intermittents.

EMBROCATIO VERATRIÆ. Dr. TURNBULL. Veratria ℈j to ʒj, rectified spirit ℥ij. For other Embrocations see Lotio and Linimentum.

EMETINA MEDICINALIS. P. Prepare an extract of ipecacuanha with spirit at 0·824; dissolve it in 4 parts of cold water, filter, evaporate to the consistence of syrup, spread it thinly with a brush on plates, and let it dry in a stove.

EMETINA PURA. P. Dissolve one part of alcoholic extract of ipecacuanha in 10 of cold water, filter, add 1 part of calcined magnesia, evaporate to dryness with a gentle heat; wash the product on a filter with 4 or 5 parts of very cold water, dry it again and treat it with boiling alcohol. Evaporate the filtered tincture, redissolve the residue in a little water acidulated with sulphuric acid, decolorize with animal charcoal, filter, precipitate with ammonia, and dry the precipitate with a gentle heat. For the mode of administering Emetine, see Mistura Emetinæ, and Syrupus Emetinæ.

EMPLASTRA. *Plasters* should be of such a consistence as to retain their form at the temperature of the body; merely becoming soft and adhesive without melting. The resins, gum-resins, &c., should be previously strained; and in melting them, no greater heat should be employed than is necessary.

EMPLASTRUM ADHÆRENS. See *Emp. Saponis Compositum.*

EMPLASTRUM ADHÆSIVUM. See *Emp. Resinæ*, and *Emp. Saponis Comp.* D. Mr. BAYNTON'S adhesive plaster, for bad legs, consisted of ʒvj of resin, with ℔j of lead plaster, spread on calico.

EMPLASTRUM ADHÆSIVUM CALCAREUM. Soap of lime, 200 parts, boiled turpentine 100 parts, suet 25 parts.

EMPLASTRUM ÆRUGINIS. P. *Corn Plaster.* Yellow wax ℥iv, Burgundy pitch ℥ij, Venice turpentine ℥j; melt together, add prepared verdigris ℥j, and stir till nearly cold.

EMPLASTRUM AMMONIÆ. Dr. KIRKLAND'S *Volatile Plaster.* Scraped soap ʒij, lead plaster ℥ss; melt together, and when nearly cold, add finely powdered sal ammoniac ʒss. *It should be renewed every* 24 *hours.*

EMPLASTRUM AMMONIACI. L. Strained ammoniacum ℥v, distilled vinegar f℥viij [ix E.]; dissolve and evaporate to a due consistence, stirring constantly. D. Ammoniacum ℥v, vinegar of squills f℥viij.

EMPLASTRUM AMMONIACI CUM CICUTA. E. 1744. Ammoniacum ℥viij, vinegar of squills q. s., juice of hemlock ℥iv. Boil to a plaster. CH. Strained ammoniacum ℥iij, extract of hemlock ʒij; melt, and add liquid diacetate of lead ʒj.

EMPLASTRUM AMMONIACI CUM HYDRARGYRO. L. Triturate quicksilver ℥iij with sulphurated oil fʒj, till the globules of quicksilver are no longer visible, and mix them with strained ammoniacum, melted with a gentle heat, ℔j.

EMPLASTRUM AMMONIACI CUM SCILLA. Guy's H. Strained ammoniacum ʒvij, vinegar of squills fʒij. Mix, and spread immediately on leather.

EMPLASTRUM SANCTI ANDREÆ A CRUCE. P. *Emp. Glutinans.* P. White pitch ℥viij, elemi ℥ij, Venice turpentine ℥j, oil of bays, ℥j. Melt, and strain through linen.

EMPLASTRUM ANODYNUM. Emplastrum Opii.

EMPLASTRUM ANTIMONII TARTARIZATI. U. C. H. Sprinkle finely powdered tartar emetic lightly on the surface of a compound pitch plaster.

EMPLASTRUM ANTICANCROSUM. RICHTER. Extract of hemlock ℥j, extract of henbane ʒiv, powdered belladonna ʒj, acetate of ammonia q. s.

EMPLASTRUM ANTIHYSTERICUM. See Emplastrum Assafœtidæ.

EMPLASTRUM AROMATICUM. D. Strained resin of spruce fir, (Thus) ℥iij, yellow wax ℥ss; melt together, and when nearly cool, add powdered cinnamon ʒvj, oil of pimento ʒij, oil of lemon ʒij.

EMPLASTRUM ASSAFŒTIDÆ. E. Lead plaster ℥ij, assafœtida ℥ij, galbanum ℥j, yellow wax ℥j. Melt and mix.

EMPLASTRUM ATTRAHENS. See Emplastrum Ceræ.

EMPLASTRUM BELLADONNÆ. L. & E. Resin plaster ℥iij, extract of belladonna ℥jss; add the extract to the plaster, previously melted with a gentle heat, and agitate briskly. D. directs *Emp. Saponis* ℥ij, ext. of belladonna ℥j.

EMPLASTRUM BRYONIÆ. BOERHAAVE. Strained galbanum ℥iv, wax plaster ℥ix, olive oil ℥j; melt together, and add powdered briony root ℥ij, flowers of sulphur ℥j, Æthiop's mineral ʒij; stir till cold.

EMPLASTRUM CALEFACIENS. D. Blistering plaster 1 part, Burgundy pitch 7 parts. Melt together with a moderate heat, and mix. [Dr. Thomson truly observes that the quantity of blistering plaster is too great.]

EMPLASTRUM CAMPHORATUM. Camphor is best applied by sprinkling the powder on the warm surface of a spread adhesive, or other plaster. Blisters are treated in this way to prevent strangury.

EMPLASTRUM CANTHARIDIS. L. *Blistering Plaster.* Wax plaster ℔jss, lard ℔ss; melt together, and when they begin to cool, sprinkle in powdered cantharides ℔j, and mix. [Or, lard 6½, yellow wax 7½, prepared suet 7½, resin 2½. Melt together, strain if necessary, and stir in powdered flies 12 parts. Keep the ointment melted by a water-bath for some hours; then stir till cool.] E. directs equal weights of cantharides (in fine powder), resin, beeswax, and suet. D. Cantharides in fine powder, ℔j, wax ℔j, resin ℥iv, suet ℔ss, lard ℔ss.

Emplastrum Olei Cantharidis. Mr. J. Smith. Digest the powdered flies for 14 days with twice their weight of olive oil, and to ℥iv of the strained oil add wax ℥iijss, resin ℥ss.

Emplastrum Cantharidis Dilutum. Dr. Pereira. Blistering plaster 1 part, soap cerate 3 parts. *For Children.*

Emplastrum Cantharidis Compositum. E. Venice turpentine 18 parts, Burgundy pitch 12, powdered cantharides 12, wax 4, verdigris 2, flour of mustard 1, black pepper 1. Melt the pitch and wax, add the turpentine, sprinkle into the mixture the powders, and stir till cool.

Emplastrum Cephalicum. See Emp. Ladani Compositum.

Emplastrum Ceræ. L. *Emp. Attrahens.* Yellow wax ℔iij, suet ℔iij, resin ℔j; melt together and strain.

Emplastrum Cerati Saponis. Soap cerate rendered hard by boiling, till the whole of the vinegar is expelled; or by the addition of a portion of lead plaster; or by varying the proportion of the ingredients.

Emplastrum Ceroneum. P. Burgundy pitch ℥xij, black pitch ℥iij, yellow wax ℥iij ʒvj, suet ʒx, bole ℥iij ʒij, myrrh ʒv, olibanum ʒv, finely powdered red lead ʒv.

Emplastrum Cerussæ. P. Carbonate of lead ℥xvj, olive oil ℥xxxij; mix them thoroughly in a large basin, add Ojss of water, and boil till they combine. Make it into rolls as Emp. Plumbi. Remelt it and add ℥iij of white wax.

Emplastrum Cicutæ. See Empl. Ammoniaci cum Cicutâ, and Emp. Conii.

Emplastrum Commune. *Diachylon.* See Emplastrum Plumbi.

Emplastrum Conii. Swed. Ph. Wax ℔ss, olive oil ℥iv, ammoniacum ℥ss; melt, and add powdered hemlock ℔ss. Bat. P. Lead plaster ℔j, yellow wax ℔j, olive oil ℥vj, powdered hemlock ℔j. See also Emp. Ammoniaci cum Cicutâ.

EMPLASTRUM CROTONIS. M. BOUCHARDAT. Melt 4 parts of lead plaster, and when nearly cold, mix with it 1 part of croton oil.

EMPLASTRUM CUMINI. L. 1788. Cumin seed, caraway, bayberries, of each ℥iij, Burgundy pitch ℔iij, yellow wax ℥iij; melt the pitch with the wax, and add the powdered seeds.

EMPLASTRUM DIACHYLON. See Emplastrum Plumbi.

EMPLASTRUM DIAPALMA. P. Lead plaster 32 parts, yellow wax 2; melt together, and add sulphate of zinc 1, dissolved in a little water, and keep the mixture over a slow fire, constantly stirring, till the water is evaporated. E. 1744. Litharge ℔iij, olive oil ℔iij, lard ℔ij.

EMPLASTRUM DIASULPHURIS RULANDI. Balsam of sulphur ℥iij, yellow wax ℥ss, resin ʒiij; melt together.

EMPLASTRUM EUPHORBII. GUY'S H. Burgundy pitch plaster ℥iv, powdered euphorbium ʒss; melt together, and mix.

EMPLASTRUM FERRI. E. Litharge plaster ℥iij, resin ʒvj, olive oil ʒiijss, bees-wax ʒiij, red oxide of iron ℥j. Rub the oxide with the oil, and add to the rest, melted together.

EMPLASTRUM "FLOS UNGUENTORUM" DICTUM. L. 1720. Resin ℔ss, frankincense ℔ss, wax ℔ss, suet ℔ss, olibanum ℥iv, common turpentine ℥ijss, myrrh ℥j, camphor ʒij, white wine f℥viij. Boil together to form a plaster.

EMPLASTRUM FUSCUM. P. Olive oil ℔ij, lard ℔j, butter ℔j, suet ℔j, wax ℔j; heat together in a copper pan till they begin to smoke; add gradually finely powdered litharge ℔j, stir constantly till the mixture assumes a deep brown colour, and add black pitch melted and strained ℔¼.

EMPLASTRUM GALBANI. L. *Diachylon with the Gums.* Galbanum ℥viij, common turpentine ʒx; melt together, and add powdered resin of spruce fir ℥iij, and lastly, add plaster (melted with a gentle heat) ℔iij. D. Litharge plaster ℔ij, galbanum ℔ss, wax ℥iv.

EMPLASTRUM GLUTINANS. *Emplâtre d'André de la Croix.* P. White pitch ℥viij, elemi ℥ij, Venice turpentine ℥j, oil of bays ℥j. Melt and strain.

EMPLASTRUM GUMMOSUM. E. Litharge plaster ℥iv, ammoniacum, galbanum, bees-wax, of each ℥ss. Melt and mix.

EMPLASTRUM HYDRARGYRI. L. Quicksilver ℥iij, sulphurated

oil f℥j; triturate till the globules disappear, add gradually ℔j of melted lead plaster, and mix. E. Mercury ℥iij, olive oil f℥ix, resin ℥j, litharge plaster ℥vj.

EMPLASTRUM HYOSCIAMI. SWED. PH. As Emplastrum Conii.

EMPLASTRUM ICTHYOCOLLÆ. *Court Plaster* is made by repeatedly brushing over stretched sarcenet with a solution of 1 part of isinglass in 8 of water mixed with 8 parts of proof spirit, and finishing with a coat of tincture of benzoin, or of balsam of Peru. The *transparent* isinglass plaster is made by brushing over oiled silk with a similar solution. An improved method of making Mr. Liston's plaster is by brushing over one surface of the peritoneal membrane of the cæcum of the ox, (prepared in the same manner as gold-beater's skin,) with solution of isinglass, and the other with drying oil.

EMPLASTRUM IODINII. Lead plaster ʒvj, resin plaster ʒij; melt together, and add iodine ℈j rubbed with olive oil ʒss. RODERBURG prescribes ʒss of iodine (or ʒj of iodide of potassium), rubbed with a few drops of spirit and olive oil, and incorporated with ℥j of simple plaster previously melted.

EMPLASTRUM IODINII COMPOSITUM. St. GEO. H. Iodine ʒij, iodide of potassium ʒiij, lead plaster ℔j, opium plaster ℥ij. Melt the plasters, and add the iodine and iodide in a fine powder, and mix.

EMPLASTRUM IODINII CUM BELLADONNA. Iodine ℥ss to ℥ij, Venice turpentine ʒij, olive oil ʒj, belladonna plaster ℔j; mix, and spread with a cool iron. In these plasters an iodide of lead is formed.

EMPLASTRUM LADANI COMPOSITUM. L. 1788. Ladanum ℥iij, frankincense ℥j; melt, and add powdered cinnamon ℥ss, expressed oil of mace (nutmegs) ℥ss, oil of mint ʒj. Mix.

EMPLASTRUM LITHARGYRI. *Litharge*, or *Lead Plaster*. The D. and E. name for Emplastrum Plumbi.

EMPLASTRUM LITHARGYRI BURGUNDICUM. CHESELDEN'S *Sticking plaster*. Lead plaster ℔j, Burgundy pitch ℥ss. Melt and mix.

EMPLASTRUM LITHARGYRI CUM GUMMI. Empl. Galbani.

EMPLASTRUM LITHARGYRI CUM HYDRARGYRO. See Empl. Hydrargyri.

EMPLASTRUM LITHARGYRI CUM RESINA. D. Empl. Resinæ.

EMPLASTRUM LYTTÆ. *Empl. Cantharidis.*

EMPLASTRUM MELILOTI. E. 1744. Fresh melilot bruised ℔vj, suet ℔iij; boil till the herb is almost crisp, strain with pressure, and add white resin ℔viij, yellow wax ℔iv. Boil to make a plaster.

EMPLASTRUM E MINIO. L. 1746. Olive oil ℔iv, finely powdered red lead ℔ijss. As Empl. Plumbi; but requires more water and greater care to preserve the colour. When discoloured by heat, it forms *Emp. de minio fuscum.* With a fifth part of soap, it forms Emp. e Minio cum Sapone, E. 1744.

EMPLASTRUM E MUCILAGINIBUS. L. 1746. Yellow wax 40 parts, oil of mucilages 8, ammoniacum 6, common turpentine 2. To the ammoniacum melted with the turpentine, add the wax melted with the oil, and mix.

EMPLASTRUM NIGRUM. Mr. SHARP'S black plaster was formed by boiling together olive oil ℥xiij, wax ℥ijss, carbonate of lead ℥x.

EMPLASTRUM OPII. L. Lead plaster ℔j, melt, and add powdered opium ℥ss, powdered resin of spruce fir ℥iij, water f℥viij; boil to a proper consistence. E. & D. Burgundy pitch ℥iij, litharge plaster ℥xij; melt, and add powder of opium ℥ss. GUY'S H. Spread wax plaster, and cover the surface with extract of opium, softened with water.

EMPLASTRUM OPII ET CAMPHORÆ. Dr. PARIS. Opium and camphor, each ʒss, lead plaster, q. s. Mix.

EMPLASTRUM OXYCROCEUM. E. 1744. Wax ℔j, black pitch ℔ss, galbanum ℔ss; melt, and add Venice turpentine, myrrh, olibanum, of each ℥iij, powdered saffron ℥ij; mix. *The saffron is often omitted.*

EMPLASTRUM PARACELSI. Olive oil ℥vj, wax ℥jss, litharge ℥ivss, ammoniacum ℥ss, bdellium ℥ss, galbanum ℥vj, opoponax, oil of bays, calamine, both the birthworts, myrrh, frankincense, of each ʒij, turpentine ℥j. Mix into a plaster s. a.

EMPLASTRUM PICIS. [Compositum, 1824.] L. Burgundy pitch ℔ij, resin of spruce fir ℔j, resin ℥iv, wax ℥iv, expressed oil of nutmegs ℥j, olive oil f℥ij, water f℥ij. Melt together the pitch, resin, and wax, add the rest, and boil to a proper consistence.

EMPLASTRUM PICIS [ABIETINÆ ET NIGRÆ.] GUY'S H. Burgundy pitch [or black pitch] ℥vj, wax ℥ss, common turpentine ʒj. Melt, and mix.

EMPLASTRUM PLUMBI. L. (Empl. Lithargyri D. and E.) *Lead* or *Litharge plaster; common plaster*, or *Diachylon*. Powdered litharge ℔vj, olive oil Cj, water Oij. Boil together over a slow fire, constantly stirring, till they unite; adding a little boiling water, if the water first used should be nearly evaporated. When sufficiently cooled, the plaster must be worked in the hands, to separate any uncombined water, and formed into rolls. E. and D. nearly the same.

EMPLASTRUM QUINÆ. VOISIN. Sulphate of quinine ʒij, mercurial plaster ℥iv. In enlargement of the spleen, after intermittent fevers.

EMPLASTRUM RESINÆ. L. Resin ℔ss, lead plaster ℔iij; to the melted plaster, add the powdered resin, and mix. E. ℥j of resin to ℥v of lead plaster; D. ℔ss to ℔iijss. See Empl. Adhæsivum.

EMPLASTRUM RESINÆ CUM CANTHARIDE. GUY'S H. Resin plaster ℥vj, cantharides plaster ℥j; liquefy, and mix.

EMPLASTRUM RESOLVENS. *Empl. ex mixtis quatuor*. P. Equal parts of hemlock plaster, galbanum plaster, mercurial plaster, and soap plaster. Melt, and mix by stirring.

EMPLASTRUM ROBORANS. See Empl. Thuris, and Empl. Ferri.

EMPLASTRUM SAPONIS. L. and D. Soap cut small ℔ss, lead plaster ℔iij; melt the plaster, add the soap, and boil to a proper consistence. E. Lead plaster ℥iv, galbanum plaster ℥ij, Castile soap in shavings ℥j.

EMPLASTRUM SAPONIS COMPOSITUM. D. *Empl. Adhærens*. Soap plaster ℥ij, resin plaster ℥iij. Melt, and mix. [St. B. H. Soap cerate ℥j, lead plaster ℥v. Melt, and mix.]

EMPLASTRUM SCILLÆ COMPOSITUM. CH. Galbanum ℥ss, soap ℥ss, litharge plaster ℥ij; melt together, and add opium ʒj, ammoniacum ℥ss, vinegar of squills ℥iij, mixed together; keep them over the fire, constantly stirred, till they are incorporated.

EMPLASTRUM SIMPLEX. E. *Wax Plaster*. (Wax ℥iij, suet ℥ij, resin ℥ij.) But Empl. Simplex, P. is simple Lead Plaster.

EMPLASTRUM STOMACHICUM. *Emplastrum Ladani*, or *Empl. Aromaticum*. D.

EMPLASTRUM THURIS. L. 1788. Frankincense ℔ss, dragon's blood ℥iij, lead plaster ℔ij; melt the plaster, add the rest finely powdered, and mix.

EMPLASTRUM VERMIFUGUM. RYAN. Aloes ʒj, essential oil of chamomile ♏viij, common turpentine q. s. Applied over the belly.

EMPLASTRUM VESICATORIUM. Emp. Meloes Vesicatorii. E. Former names of *Empl. Cantharidis.*

EMPLASTRUM VIGONIS. P. Lead plaster ℥xl, wax ℥ij, resin ℥ij, ammoniacum, bdellium, olibanum, myrrh, each ʒv, saffron ʒiij, quicksilver ℥xij, common turpentine ℥ij, liquid styrax ℥vj, oil of lavender ʒij. Make a plaster.

EMPLASTRUM VISCI QUERCINI. HARDY. To two parts of melted bees-wax, add gradually one part of juice of true oak misletoe, and form a plaster. *In neuralgic pains.*

EMULSIONES. The *Emulsions* of the British Pharmacopœias are now termed *Mixtures* (see Misturæ). But the old names of Mistura Acaciæ, and Mistura Camphoræ, of the new E. Pharmacopœia, are here retained, to distinguish them from the very different preparations to which these names are applied by the London College.

EMULSIO ACACIÆ. *Mistura Acaciæ.* E. 1839. Blanched almonds ʒx, sugar ʒv; beat them together with mucilage f℥iij; gradually add Oij of water, constantly stirring, and strain through linen or calico.

EMULSIO ARABICA. D. Powdered gum acacia ʒij, blanched almonds ℥ss, sugar ℥ss, water f℥xvj.

EMULSIO AMYGDALÆ. See Mistura Amygdalæ.

EMULSIO AMYGDALÆ CUM AMYGDALINA. WOEHLER. Form ℥j of emulsion with ʒij of sweet almonds, and dissolve in it gr. xvij of amygdaline. It is intended as a substitute for *Aqua Amygdalæ Amaræ.* Dose, 10 to 40 drops.

EMULSIO BALSAMI PERUVIANI. Balsam of Peru ʒiv, oil of almonds ʒvj, powdered gum arabic ℥j; triturate, and add rose water ℥iv. Dose, ℥ss.

EMULSIO CAMPHORÆ. *Mistura Camphoræ.* E. 1839. Camphor ℈j, pure sugar ℥ss; rub together, and add blanched almonds ℥ss; beat the whole into a smooth pulp, and gradually add water Oj, constantly stirring; then strain.

EMULSIO CANNABIS. P. Hemp-seed ℥j, sugar ℥j, water ℔ij. Form, an Emulsion.

EMULSIO CANNABIS INDICÆ. Mr. BROMFIELD. Rub ℈j of extract of Indian hemp in a warm mortar, with f ʒj of olive oil; then add gradually, still triturating the mixture, f ʒiv mucilage of acacia, and f ℥vijss of distilled water.

Emulsio Ceræ. Guibourt. White wax ℥j, powdered gum acacia ℥jss, water ℥xxiv, syrup ℥iv. Mix the syrup and water, put ℥iij with the wax in a mortar, heat to melt the wax, add the gum, and triturate briskly with a warm pestle, gradually adding the rest of the liquid, and stirring constantly while it cools.

Emulsio Cetacei. Spermaceti ʒij, yolk of one egg, or q. s.; beat together, and gradually add water f ℥vijss, syrup of Tolu f ℥ss, spirit of nutmeg ʒij.

Emulsio Copaibæ. Copaiva ℥ij, syrup ℥j, mucilage ℥j, water ℥xij. Triturate the balsam with the mucilage and syrup, and gradually add the water.

Emulsio Cubebæ. Dublanc. Essence of cubebs ℥iv, mucilage ℥iv. Mix. Dose, ʒj, three or four times a day. [Mr. Procter (of America) directs ʒij of his oleo-resinous extract of cubebs to be formed into an emulsion with ℥ss of p. acacia, ʒj of sugar, and f ℥iijss of water. Dose, a tablespoonful.]

Emulsio Oleosa. Brande. Powdered gum ℥ss, water f ℥ss; mix, and add, gradually, oil of almonds f ʒiij, rose water f ℥jss, distilled water f ℥iij, syrup f ʒiij.

Emulsio Papaveris. Poppy seeds ʒij, water ℥viij. Make an emulsion, and strain.

Emulsio Purgans cum Resina Jalapæ. P. Jalap-resin gr. x, white sugar ℥j, orange-flower water ʒij, water ℥iv. Triturate the resin with a little of the sugar, add gradually half the yolk of an egg, triturate for a long time, then add gradually the rest of the sugar and the water.

Emulsio Purgans cum Oleo Ricini. P. Castor oil ℥j, yolk of an egg, peppermint water ℥ss, water ℥ij, syrup ℥j. Mix the yolk with a little of the water, and add the oil, gradually rubbing them briskly in the mortar, then add very gradually the rest of the water and the syrup.

Emulsio Purgans cum Scammonio. P. Aleppo scammony ℈ss, milk ℥iv, sugar ℥ss, cherry-laurel water ʒij. The large proportion of cherry-laurel water in this mixture renders it unsafe to give a full dose. Planche directs, scammony gr. vij, sugar ʒij; triturate, and add gradually, new milk ℥iij, cherry-laurel water 3 or 4 drops, for one dose. See also Mistura Scammonii. E.

Emulsio Seminum Frigidorum. The 4 cold seeds ℥j, sugar ℥j, cold water ℥xxxij.

Emulsio Simplex. P. Blanched almonds ℥j, sugar ℥j, cold water ℥xxxij.

Emulsio Vermifuga. Saunders. Peach kernels ʒij, bitter almonds ʒij, scammony ℈ss, wormwood water ℥iij. Other emulsions will be found among the Mixtures [Misturæ].

Enema Aceti. Brande. Vinegar f℥ij, infusion of chamomile f℥v.

Enema Aloes. L. Aloes ℈ij, carbonate of potash gr. xv, decoction of barley Oss. Mix.

Enema Amyli. F. H. Decoction of starch ℥v, linseed oil ℥j.

Enema Anodynum. See Enema Opii, and En. Papaveris.

Enema Argenti Nitratis. Boudin. Nitrate of silver, gr. j to iij, distilled water f℥v.

Enema Assafœtidæ. St. B. H. Assafœtida ʒij, yolk of egg q. s., decoction of barley Oss.

Enema Astringens. F. H. Extract of rhatany, softened with spirit, ʒjss, water ℥iv. The decoction of galls, bistort, pomegranate, &c., are also used.

Enema Belladonnæ. Ratier. Belladonna ℈ss, boiling water f℥vj. Infuse.

Enema Carminativum. Buchan. Chamomiles ℥j, aniseeds ℥ss, water Ojss; boil to Oj.

Enema Catharticum. E. Senna ℥ss, boiling water f℥xvj. Infuse, strain, add sulphate of magnesia ℥ss, sugar ℥j, olive oil ℥j. D. Manna ℥j, comp. decoction of chamomile f℥x, olive oil ℥j, sulphate of magnesia ℥ss.

Enema Cevadillæ. Soubeiran. Cevadilla ʒij, water ℥x; boil to ℥vij, strain, and add milk ℥viij. *To destroy Ascarides.*

Enema Chloridi Calcis. Dr. Reid. Add gr. x of chloride of lime to a common enema.

Enema Cinchonæ. As Decoctum Cinchonæ.

Enema Colocynthidis. L. Compound extract of colocynth ℈ij, soft soap ℥j, water Oj. Mix.

ENEMA COLOCYNTHIDIS COMPOSITUM. GUY'S H. Colocynth pulp ʒj, water f ℥xij. Boil and strain, then add common salt ℥ss, syrup of buckthorn f ℥ss. MID. H. Comp. extract of colocynth ʒjss, boiling water Oj.

ENEMA COMMUNE. GUY'S H. Warm gruel f ℥xij, salt ℥j. Mix. U. C. H. Gruel ℥viij, salt ℥j, linseed oil f ℥ij. Mix.

ENEMA COPAIBA. Copaiva ℥iij, yolk of 2 eggs, gruel or warm water Ojss. For 4 or 6 injections.

ENEMA CREASOTI. Dr. WILMOT. Creasote ʒj, decoction of starch ℥xij. *In epidemic dysentery.*

ENEMA CROTONIS. SUNDELIN. Croton oil 2 to 4 drops, linseed oil ℥ij, gruel ℥iv.

ENEMA CUBEBÆ. F. H. Decoction of mallow ℥vj, powdered cubebs ʒvj.

ENEMA DOMESTICUM. E. H. Milk Oss, sugar ℥j, olive oil ℥j. See also Enema Commune.

ENEMA EMOLLIENS. Decoction of linseed, starch, or oatmeal, Oj, linseed or olive oil ℥j. Or Decoction of Emollient herbs, (species *Emollientes,*) P.

ENEMA ERGOTÆ. BOUDIN. Infuse ʒj of ergot in ℥viij of hot water, and strain.

ENEMA FELLIS. Dr. CLAY. *To soften indurated fæces.* Fresh ox-gall f ℥ij, warm water f ℥iv. Dr. ALLNATT prescribes ox-gall ℥ij, thin gruel f ℥viij.

ENEMA FERRI TARTARIZATI. GER. H. Infusion of yarrow ℥xij, potassio-tartrate of iron ʒjss, honey of roses ℥j.

ENEMA FILICIS. FR. H. Male fern root ʒj, water ℔j; boil, and strain.

ENEMA FŒTIDUM. E. To Enema Catharticum add tincture of assafœtida f ʒij. See also Enema Assafœtidæ.

ENEMA FULIGINIS. As Decoctum Fuliginis.

ENEMA GALLÆ ET OPII. Dr. RYAN. Decoction of galls ℥viij, tincture of opium ʒss.

ENEMA IPECACUANHÆ. U. C. H. Ipecac root bruised ʒj, boiling water f ℥viij. Macerate for an hour and strain.

ENEMA LAXATIVUM *vel* PURGATIVUM. FR. H. Senna ʒij to

ʒiv, decoction of linseed (or of emollient herbs) Oj. Infuse, strain, and add sulphate of soda ʒij to ʒiv.

ENEMA MORPHIÆ. BRERA. Morphia gr. jss, oil of almonds ℥j; triturate, and add infusion or decoction of linseed q. s.

ENEMA NUTRIENS. Strong beef tea, thickened with arrowroot.

ENEMA OLEI RICINI. GUY'S H. Castor oil f℥j, honey ℥j; mix, and gradually add boiling gruel Oss. Use it tepid.

ENEMA OLEOSA. MID. H. Olive oil f℥iv, decoction of barley f℥xvj.

ENEMA OPII. L. Decoction of starch f℥iv, tincture of opium fʒss. Mix. E. Starch ʒss, water f℥ij, tincture of opium fʒss to fʒj. D. Opium gr. j, tepid water f℥vj.

ENEMA PAPAVERIS. Poppy-heads without seeds ʒv (for children from ʒj to ʒiij), boiling water ℥xvj; infuse, and add starch ℥ss.

ENEMA QUINÆ. Sulphate of quinine gr. v to xv, decoction of starch f℥vj.

ENEMA RHATANIÆ. TROUSSEAU. See Enema Astringens. *For fissures of the anus.*

ENEMA RUTÆ. Confection of rue ℈j to ʒj, thin gruel f℥vj to f℥viij.

ENEMA SAPONIS. St. B. H. Soft soap ʒvj, hot water Oj.

ENEMA SODÆ CHLORINATÆ. Labarraque's solution 24 drops, decoction of mallows f℥xvj.

ENEMA SODII CHLORIDI. MID. H. Common salt ℥j, barley water Oss, olive oil ℥j.

ENEMA TABACI. L. Tobacco leaves ʒj, boiling water Oj. Macerate for an hour and strain. [Not more than a half or a third of this should be thrown up at once. Dr. PEREIRA.] E. Tobacco gr. xv to xxx, boiling water f℥viij.

ENEMA TABACI ET CROTONIS. MOLL. Tobacco ʒj, boiling water ℥vj, croton oil 3 drops, gum acacia ʒij. *In desperate cases of ileus.*

ENEMA TEREBINTHINÆ. L. and E. Oil of turpentine f℥j, yolk of egg q. s., decoction of barley f℥xix. GUY'S H. half the quantity. D. orders common turpentine ℥ss, 1 yolk of egg, tepid water f℥x.

ENEMA VERMIFUGUM. Several of the above are useful in dislodging ascarides; particularly Enema Aloes, Cevadillæ, Terebinthinæ, Fuliginis, and those containing salt. Decoctions of wormwood, tansy, and wormseed are also used, and tincture of muriate of iron. Dr. NELIGAN recommends oil of turpentine f ℥ss, syrup of garlic f ℥j, barley water f ℥vij. To be followed by a cathartic enema. For children, use half, or a fourth of the above.

ENEMA VINOSUM. *In suspended animation.* Warm water f ℥vj, brandy ℥ss to ℥iv, white wine ℥vj.

EPITHEMA ASTRINGENS. BRERA. Bole ℥j, p. rhatany ℥j, rose vinegar q. s. to form a paste; to be placed on the forehead to stop bleeding at the nose.

EPITHEMA LITHARGYRI. See Cremor Lithargyri.

EPITHEMA ROSÆ. CH. Conserve of roses ℥ij, alum ℥ss.

EPITHEMA TEREBINTHINÆ. Common turpentine ℥j, honey and flour q. s.

EPITHEMA VERMIFUGUM. HOFFMANN. Wormwood and centaury, beaten up with aloes and colocynth, and applied over the belly.

EPITHEMA VESICATORIUM. L. 1746. Cantharides in fine powder, and wheat flour, of each equal weights; make them into a paste with vinegar. ALIBERT directs rye and barley meal to be made into a paste with vinegar, and ʒss or ℈ij of finely powdered cantharides sprinkled over the surface. [Lately revived under the name of the magistral blister of M. Valleix.]

EPITHEMA VOLATILE. L. 1746. Common turpentine ℥j, water of ammonia ℥j. Mix. Epithem is a general name for local applications. See Cataplasma, Embrocatio, &c.

ERGOTINA. This name has been applied to different principles, or mixed products, obtained from ergot of rye. For BONJEAN'S Ergotine, see Extractum Ergotæ Aquosum.

ESSENTIÆ. *Essences.* This name is applied to certain strong alcoholic tinctures, to some essential oils, to solutions of these in alcohol, and, with less propriety, to fluid extracts, or concentrated infusions and decoctions; some of which will be noticed elsewhere. [See Liquor.]

ESSENTIA ABSINTHII. VAN MONS. Tincture of wormwood Oj, salt of wormwood ʒv, extract of wormwood ʒj.

ESSENTIA AMARA. Tinctura Absinthii Composita.

ESSENTIA AMYGDALÆ AMARÆ. Dr. PEREIRA. Essential oil of

bitter almonds f ℥j, rectified spirit f ℥vij. A stronger preparation (f ℥j to f ℥iij, Professor Redwood) is also employed.

ESSENTIA ANODYNA. GERM. H. Extract of opium ʒj, spirit of cinnamon ℥ix.

ESSENTIA ANTIHYSTERICA. P. Similar to Spiritus Ammoniæ Fœtidus.

ESSENTIA CAPSICI. See Tinctura Capsici Concentrata.

ESSENTIA CEPHALICA. Dr. WARD'S *Essence for the Headache.* Spirit of camphor ℔ij, strong water of ammonia ℥iv, essence of lemon ℥ss.

ESSENTIA CUBEBÆ. DUBLANC. Oleo-resinous extract of cubebs ℥j, brandy ℥iij. Dose, ʒj. A concentrated tincture of cubebs is sold under this name. See Tinct. Cubebæ.

ESSENTIA ERGOTÆ. See Ess. Secalis Cornuti.

ESSENTIA LEVISTICI. WURT. PH. Lovage root ℥ij, lovage seeds ℥j, rectified spirit ℥x. Digest, express, and filter. Dose, 60 to 80 drops, in dropsical affections.

ESSENTIA MENTHÆ PIPERITÆ. *Tinctura Menthæ, p.* U. S. Oil of peppermint f ℥ij, rectified spirit f ℥xvj. Dose, from 10 to 20 drops. Mr. Redwood directs 1 part of oil to 3 of spirit. A common form is 1 part to 7. It is sometimes coloured with spinage leaves.

ESSENTIA MENTHÆ VIRIDIS, and Ess. Menthæ Pulegii, may be made in the same way as the last.

ESSENTIA REGALIS. SOUBEIRAN. Ambergris ℈ij, musk ℈j, civet ℈ss, oil of cinnamon gr. vj, oil of rhodium gr. iv, attar of rose gr. iv, subcarbonate of potash ℈ss, rectified spirit ℥iij. Digest and filter.

ESSENTIA SAPONIS. P. White soap ℥iij, subcarbonate of potash ʒj, proof spirit ℥xij. Macerate till dissolved, and filter.

ESSENTIA SARSAPARILLÆ. GUIBOURT. Alcoholic extract of sarsaparilla ℥j, good white wine ℥iij. Dissolve, and filter. One part of the essence represents 2 parts of the root, or 16 of the decoction.

ESSENTIA SARSAPARILLÆ COMPOSITA. Compound extract of sarsaparilla ℥ij, white wine ℥xiv, oil of sassafras 2 or 3 drops.

ESSENTIA SECALIS CORNUTI. Bruised ergot ℥j, boiling water

f ℥ij. Infuse 24 hours, and add rectified spirit f ℥jss. Digest 10 days, and filter. [Lancet, 1827–8, p. 435.]

Essentia Secalis Cornuti Ætherea. Mr. Lever. Powdered ergot ℥iv, sulphuric æther f ℥iv. Digest 7 days, strain, and let the tincture evaporate spontaneously. Dissolve the residue in f ℥ij of æther. Dose ♏xv to xxx, on sugar. M. Bonjean states that *water* is the proper solvent for the hæmostatic principle of ergot, and that æther takes up chiefly the poisonous narcotic principle. See Extractum Ergotæ.

Essentia Zingiberis. Unbleached Jamaica ginger in coarse powder ℥iv, rectified spirit f ℥xvj. Prepare by digestion or percolation. There is no standard formula, but this is of about the usual strength.

Ether. See Æther.

Extracta. *Extracts* are made by evaporating the expressed juices of plants, or their decoctions, infusions, or tinctures, by a gentle heat. They are usually of a pilular consistence; but are sometimes prepared in a semi-fluid state (*fluid extracts*), and others in a dry state. In some instances, æther, wine, and vinegar are used as solvents of the vegetable principles. A few extracts are procured from animal substances. The juices or solutions are to be evaporated by the heat of a warm bath (L.) or vapour bath, (E. and D.,) and constantly stirred towards the end of the process. But "most of them may be obtained of a greatly superior quality by the process of evaporation *in vacuo*. And the extracts of expressed juices cannot, perhaps, be better prepared than by spontaneous evaporation in shallow vessels exposed to a current of air." E. "The softer extracts should be sprinkled with a little rectified spirit." L.

Extracts of expressed juices (*Succi Spissati*) are made by bruising the fresh plants, after they have begun to flower, sprinkled with water, in a marble mortar, and expressing the juice. L. & D. direct the expressed juices to be evaporated as directed above, without being filtered or otherwise clarified. E. directs them to be filtered cold. P. directs them to be heated till the albumen coagulates, and the coagulum to be removed by straining; some of the extracts to be also made from the unclarified juice (*Extracta cum Fæculâ*) evaporated in shallow dishes in a stove heated to 95° or 104° F. Righini recommends a tincture of the green coagulum to be added to the defæcated juice.

Watery Extracts (*Extracta Aquosa*. Ext. *Simpliciora*. D.)

are made by boiling the drug (after 12 hours' infusion, D.) with 8 (D.) or 10 times its weight of water, till reduced to one-half; the decoction is then strained, allowed to settle, decanted, and evaporated as above. Some watery extracts are preferably made by maceration in hot or cold water; or by percolation, as directed under Extractum Krameriæ, E.

Spirituous Extracts (*Extracta Alcoholica*) are made from tinctures prepared with rectified or diluted spirit. They are usually more active than the corresponding watery extracts, and should therefore not be used except when specially directed. The spirit distilled from the tinctures should be reserved for future operations. MOHR describes another mode of preparing alcoholic extracts of great activity, which is noticed under Ext. Belladonnæ Alcoholicum.

EXTRACTUM ABSINTHII. D. From a decoction of wormwood tops, as directed above for watery extracts. [A better extract is obtained by spirit.]

EXTRACTUM ACONITI. By evaporating the expressed juice of monkshood, without previous clarification (L. & D.), or after being clarified by heat (P.) E. directs the expressed juice to be mixed with a tincture prepared from the pressed residuum by percolation with rectified spirit; the mixture filtered, the spirit distilled off, and the residuum evaporated in a vapour-bath. P. (*Ext. Aconiti cum Fæcula*) directs the juice to be strained through linen, and exposed in shallow dishes to the heat of a stove, at a temperature of 95° to 104° F. until it becomes dry. Dose, gr. ss–ij, gradually increased, if necessary.

EXTRACTUM ACONITI ALCOHOLICUM. U. S. & P. Coarsely powdered aconite ℔j, proof spirit Oiij, (℔iijss, P.) Moisten the powder with half its weight of the spirit, and in 24 hours lixiviate it, packed in an apparatus of displacement (between two diaphragms in a tin cylinder, P.) with the rest of the spirit. When all the spirit has penetrated the powder, keep this covered with distilled water till the liquid begins to cause a precipitate on falling into that which had previously passed. Distil off the spirit from the tinctures, and evaporate the extract to a proper consistence. [Dr. FLEMING directs it to be made by evaporating a tincture of the root. (See Tinctura Radicis Aconiti.) The dose is from one-sixth to one-third of a grain. Dr. TURNBULL'S is made in the same way. The addition of 10 drops of liquor ammoniæ to each ʒj of the extract, forms his Ext. Aconiti Ammoniatum.]

Extractum Agarici. P. Macerate white agaric with 4 parts of cold water 24 hours, express lightly, and macerate again with 3 parts of water, express strongly; mix, filter the liquor, and evaporate by a water-bath.

Extractum Agrimonii. As Ext. Absinthii.

Extractum Alkakengi. As Extractum Bac. Sambuci.

Extractum Aloes Purificatum. L. Digest bruised aloes in 10 parts of water for 3 days, with a gentle heat; strain, let it settle, decant and evaporate the clear liquid. [D. directs it to be made from hepatic aloes, according to the general directions for watery extracts.]

Extractum Anemonis. P. From the juice of the pasque flower, or from the powder, by percolation with water or proof spirit.

Extractum Anthemidis. L. 1824. From a decoction of chamomile flowers, as Ext. Gentianæ.

Extractum Angelicæ. Prus. Ph. Angelica root, 2 parts, rectified spirit 2 parts, water 9 parts; digest, strain; and evaporate.

Extractum Arnicæ. From the flowers, (P.) or the root, (Baden Ph.) as Ext. Aconiti Alcoholicum.

Extractum Asparagi. The juice inspissated, as Ext. Aconiti cum Fæcula.

Extractum Balsaminæ. The inspissated juice of the balsam apple. Dose gr. v to xv. *In dropsy.*

Extractum Bardanæ. From the expressed juice, or decoction, or infusion, or by percolation, as Ext. Krameriæ. (P.)

Extractum Belladonnæ. L. and D. By inspissating, by the heat of water-bath, the expressed juice of deadly nightshade, [after filtration, E.] P. directs it to be prepared both with and without fæcula; and also by percolation of the powdered leaves with water. Dose from ¼ gr., cautiously increased as required. Its strength is variable. [Debreyne makes it by boiling the flowering herb for half an hour in water q. s., and evaporating the strained decoction.]

Extractum Belladonnæ Alcoholicum. U. S. and P. As Ext. Aconiti Alcoholicum. Dose from ¼ grain to 2 grains. [Another method is that of Mohr, or Pelletan. The juice of the plant is coagulated by heat, strained, and rapidly evaporated by water bath to the consistence of syrup; an equal measure of absolute alcohol is added, and the clear portion of the liquid evaporated. This forms a *quadruple* extract, chiefly employed in outward applications.]

EXTRACTUM BACCARUM BELLADONNÆ. P. Evaporate the expressed juice of the berries (without previous fermentation) to the consistence of thick honey. Dose, gr. ij to v.

EXTRACTUM BISTORTÆ. P. From the dried root, as Ext. Krameriæ. [It is also made by decoction. SPAN. PH.] Dose ℈j to ℈ij. *Astringent.*

EXTRACTUM BORAGINIS. P. From dried borage (P.), and also from the clarified juice of the fresh plant (PORT. PH.), or by decoction, (SP. PH.) Dose ℈j to ʒj.

EXTRACTUM BUXI. P. From the bark of the root of box, with proof spirit, as Ext. Ipecacuanhæ.

EXTRACTUM CAINCÆ. From dried cahinca root, as Ext. Ipecacuanhæ. Dose, gr. x to xx, in dropsies; repeated so as to keep up its diuretic and cathartic effect.

EXTRACTUM CALUMBÆ. P. As Ext. Ipecacuanhæ. Dose, gr. v to xv.

EXTRACTUM CANNABIS INDICÆ. BENGAL DISPENSATORY. Boil the dried tops of Indian hemp (*Gunjah*) in rectified spirit (about ℔j to Cj); distil off the spirit, and evaporate the extract by a gentle heat. In India and Persia it is also collected by mechanical means from the surface of the plant. Dose, in India, from gr. ss to gr. j, in painful and spasmodic affections; but in this country it is generally necessary to increase the dose. [For Messrs. Smith's *Cannabine,* see Resina Cannabis.]

EXTRACTUM CANTHARIDIS. P. From the powdered flies, as Ext. Ipecac. A stronger extract (Extractum Oleosum) is obtained by evaporating a tincture made by percolation or digestion, with sulphuric æther.

EXTRACTUM CANTHARIDIS ACETICUM. Cantharides in coarse powder 4 parts, pyroligneous acid 1 part, rectified spirit 16 parts. Digest by the heat of a water-bath, press, filter, and evaporate to a buttery consistence. See Tela Vesicatoria.

EXTRACTUM CARDUI BENEDICTI. As Ext. Absinthii.

EXTRACTUM CASCARILLÆ. L. 1788. As Ext. Jalapæ, L. BOUL-

DUC says, "Cascarilla yields to spirit all its active parts, the extract amounting to five-eighths of the bark."

EXTRACTUM CASSIÆ. L. The pulp, washed out of the pods by boiling water, strained through a hair sieve, and evaporated. P. directs cold water, and the solution to be strained through flannel.

EXTRACTUM CATECHU. P. Bruised catechu ℔j, boiling water ℔vj. Infuse for 24 hours, stirring the mixture occasionally; decant, and evaporate by water-bath.

EXTRACTUM CATHARTICUM. Ext. Colocynthidis Comp.

EXTRACTUM CENTAURII. From common, lesser, and American centaury, as Ext. Absinthii; or by percolation.

EXTRACTUM CERATONIÆ. SPAN. P. By evaporating an infusion of Carob bean pods.

EXTRACTUM CHELIDONII. The inspissated juice of greater celandine, (Chelidonium Majus.) Some Pharm. direct it to be made with rectified spirit; others, by decoction. Dose, gr. iij to x, in scrofula, visceral obstructions, &c.

EXTRACTUM CHENOPODII. The inspissated juice of stinking goose-foot, (*Ch. olidum.*) Mr. HOULTON prefers it prepared by spontaneous evaporation. Dose, gr. v to xv, as an emmenagogue. [The officinal chenopodium of the U. S. is a different species, *C. anthelminticum.*]

EXTRACTUM CHIMAPHILÆ. From the decoction. Dose, gr. x to xv. [PEREIRA.] Dr. Wood says ℈j to ʒss.

EXTRACTUM CHICOREÆ. P. From the clarified juice.

EXTRACTUM CINCHONÆ. L. Bruised yellow bark (or pale, or red, as prescribed) ℥xv, water Cj. Boil to Ovj, strain while warm. Boil the bark again with the same quantity of water 4 times; mix the strained liquids, and evaporate to a proper consistence. D. nearly the same, from *pale* bark. E. and U. S., and P. direct an alcoholic extract. "Coarsely powdered cinchona (the red or yellow varieties in preference) ℥iv, proof spirit f℥xxiv. Percolate, distil off the spirit, and evaporate what remains to an extract." (E.) P. as Ext. Ipecac.

EXTRACTUM CINCHONÆ SICCUM. P. *Lagaraye's Essential Salt of Bark.* Moisten crown bark, ground to a moderately fine powder, with half its weight of cold distilled water, and after 12 or 15 hours, pack it closely between two pierced diaphragms in a tin cylinder, and lixiviate it with distilled water, below 77° F., as long as the liquid is strongly charged with the bark. Evaporate the liquors to the consistence of thick syrup, and spread it thinly and uniformly on earthen dishes, dry it in a stove, chip it off with a blunt-pointed knife, and preserve it in close bottles. PRUS. PH. directs 3 ℔s of powdered yellow bark to be macerated in 36 ℔s of cold water for 48 hours; the strained liquor evaporated to 2 ℔s, then filtered, and evaporated to dryness.

EXTRACTUM CINCHONÆ CUM RESINA. L. 1788. As Ext. Jalapæ.

EXTRACTUM CINCHONÆ RESINOSUM. L. 1809. Bark ℔j, rectified spirit Oiij; macerate, strain, and evaporate.

EXTRACTUM CINCHONÆ FLUIDUM. Dr. NELIGAN directs it to be made by exhausting yellow bark by percolation with proof spirit, and afterwards with water, and concentrating the mixed liquors by cautious evaporation. See Liquor Cinchonæ.

EXTRACTUM COCCULI. VAN MONS. By evaporating the clarified decoction.

EXTRACTUM COCHLEARIÆ. P. From the clarified juice of scurvy-grass.

EXTRACTUM COLCHICI. L. Bruise the fresh bulbs, (*cormi*,) sprinkled with water, in a marble mortar, express the juice, and evaporate to an extract. Dose, gr. j, or from gr. ss to gr. ij. The bulbs should be gathered in July or August.

EXTRACTUM COLCHICI ACETICUM. L. Bruise ℔j of the fresh cormi, sprinkled with f ℥iij of acetic acid, express, and evaporate the juice. But Sir C. SCUDAMORE prefers an extract made by digesting the dried colchicum in distilled vinegar, and evaporating the liquid. Dose, as the last.

EXTRACTUM COLOCYNTHIDIS. L. Colocynth pulp ℔j, distilled water Cij. Boil slowly for six hours, supplying the waste of water; strain whilst hot, and evaporate to a proper consistence. E. & D. nearly the same. The latter directs the decoction to be reduced to half, and filtered. P. directs it to be made as Ext. Scillæ. The dose is from gr. iv to xx, generally in combination. Of the alcoholic extract, gr. ij to viij.

EXTRACTUM COLOCYNTHIDIS COMPOSITUM. L. & D. Pulp of colocynth ℥vj, proof spirit Cj. Macerate with a gentle heat for 4 days; strain the tincture, and add to it purified aloes [hepatic aloes, D.] ℥xij, scammony ℥iv, soap ℥iij, (both in powder.) Evaporate to an extract, adding towards the end finely-powdered cardamom seed ℥j. [L. 1809, directed water instead of spirit; the spirit was restored in 1815. Soap was introduced into the formula in 1809, omitted in 1815, and restored in 1824.] Dose, from 5 to 20 grains.

EXTRACTUM CONII. L. By evaporating the expressed juice of fresh hemlock by means of a water-bath. E. directs the juice to be filtered, and evaporated to a very firm extract either by the aid of heat *in vacuo*, or spontaneously, in shallow dishes, placed in a current of dry air, and protected by gauze screens. D. (*Succus Spissatus Conii.*) From the juice, defæcated by six hours' repose, and evaporated by a gentle heat. P. From the juice, both with and without the fæcula.

EXTRACTUM CONII ALCOHOLICUM. P. & U. S. By percolation with proof spirit.

EXTRACTUM COPAIBÆ. Mr. THORN. By carefully distilling balsam copaiba, the resin (amounting to 5-16ths of the whole) remains behind. Dose, gr. x to xv.

EXTRACTUM CORNUS. From the bark of Cornus florida, and also of Cornus sericea, and Cornus circinatus, and other species of *dog-wood.* As Extr. Ipecacuanhæ.

EXTRACTUM CROCI. P. As Extractum Scillæ.

EXTRACTUM CUBEBÆ. Mr. TOLLER. Exhaust cubebs by rectified spirit, distil off most of the spirit, and evaporate the residue over a water-bath at a low temperature to a pilular consistence, adding a little powdered soap. Dose, gr. xv twice a day. [Mr. Judd.]

EXTRACTUM CUBEBÆ FLUIDUM. By evaporating, with a very gentle heat, a tincture prepared by digestion or percolation with rectified spirit. PUCHE directs the cubebs to be treated by percolation with proof spirit, so as to obtain a liquid equal in weight with the cubebs.

EXTRACTUM CUBEBÆ OLEO-RESINOSUM. M. DUBLANC. Put ℔vj of fresh-ground cubebs into a still with Oxij of water, and let Ovj distil. Separate the oil, and return the distilled water into the still with ℔vj more cubebs, and again distil and separate the oil. Express the marc strongly, and exhaust it by rectified spirit. Distil the filtered tincture, evaporate the extract to the consistence of honey, and incorporate with it the essential oil. One part of this extract is equal to eight of the powder. Mr. PROCTER exhausts the powdered cubebs with *æther*, in a displacement apparatus, and distils the tincture in a water-bath. The oleo-resinous extract which remains, represents (according to Mr. P.) eight times its weight of cubebs; but, according to Mr. BELL, about six times its weight.

EXTRACTUM CUSPARIÆ. As Extractum Ipecacuanhæ.

EXTRACTUM CYNARÆ. Mr. COPEMAN. The inspissated juice of the fresh leaves of artichoke. Dose, gr. ij or iij three times a day, in rheumatism. Dr. BADELEY gives gr. v, with f℥j of the tincture.

EXTRACTUM DIGITALIS. L. From the unfiltered juice. E. As Ext. Conii. P. From the dried leaves, by percolation with proof spirit, and also with water.

EXTRACTUM DULCAMARÆ. From the stalks, by decoction; or percolation, U. S.

EXTRACTUM ELATERII. L. E. & D. Slice the fruit of the wild cucumber, (ripe, L. & D.; before it is quite ripe, E.,) and press very lightly, and strain the juice through a fine hair sieve. Set it aside, and when the thicker part has subsided, reject the supernatant liquid, and dry the fæculence (laid upon a linen cloth, and covered with another, D.) with a gentle heat. Dose, if of the best quality, from $\frac{1}{16}$th to $\frac{1}{4}$th of a grain; otherwise, from $\frac{1}{8}$th to 1 grain. Dr. THOMSON gives gr. $\frac{1}{10}$th with gr. j calomel, every six hours, until it begins to operate.

EXTRACTUM ERGOTÆ AQUOSUM. The *Ergotine* of M. BONJEAN. Exhaust powdered ergot by displacement with cold water; heat the solution in a water-bath, and filter; evaporate the filtered liquor to the consistence of syrup, and add rectified spirit to throw down the gummy matter; when settled, decant the clear liquid, and evaporate by water-bath. One ounce of ergot yields about 70 grains. M. BONJEAN says it possesses the hæmostatic without the toxic properties of ergot. The liquid must be evaporated without delay, as it rapidly decomposes.

EXTRACTUM ERGOTÆ ÆTHEREUM. WRIGHT. Exhaust the powdered ergot by percolation with æther, and let the solution evaporate spontaneously. M. BONJEAN states that the *undissolved residue*, after all the oil and resin have been removed by æther, is more efficient as an obstetric remedy.

EXTRACTUM FELLIS BOVINI. P. Strain fresh ox-gall through flannel, and evaporate it by means of a water-bath to a proper consistence. Dose, gr. iv to x. Dr. H. LANE recommends the evaporation to be continued until the extract is sufficiently dry to be reduced to powder, and to be kept, in close bottles, in that state.

EXTRACTUM FILICIS. See Oleum Filicis.

EXTRACTUM FULIGINIS. Boil wood soot in 8 parts of water for half an hour, strain, and evaporate to an extract. Dose, gr. iv to xvj daily.

EXTRACTUM FULIGINIS ACETICUM. As the last, using equal parts of vinegar and water.

EXTRACTUM FUMARIÆ. From the clarified juice of fumitory, or from a decoction of the dried plant.

EXTRACTUM GALLARUM. As Extractum Krameriæ; or by decoction, as Ext. Gentianæ.

EXTRACTUM GENISTÆ. L. 1788. From decoction of broom tops, (Spartium scoparium,) as Ext. Gentianæ. Dose, gr. x to ʒss.

EXTRACTUM GENTIANÆ. L. Gentian sliced ℔ijss, boiling distilled water Cij. Macerate for 24 hours, then boil to Cj; strain while hot, and evaporate to a proper consistence. D. directs 8 parts of water to 1 of gentian.

EXTRACTUM GENTIANÆ [per aquam frigidum.] E., U. S. & P. As Extractum Krameriæ.

EXTRACTUM GLYCYRRHIZÆ. L. As Ext. Gentianæ. But a finer extract is prepared (E. & U. S.) by percolation with cold water, as Ext. Krameriæ. [The foreign commercial extract, or *juice*, may be purified by the following process:—cut it into small pieces, and place it on a diaphragm in a tin vessel. Add enough cold distilled water to cover it, and when sufficiently divided, withdraw the liquid, strain it through flannel, and evaporate it to a firm extract. P.]

EXTRACTUM GRAMINIS. P. From the dried roots of dog's-grass, as Ext. Krameriæ. Also by decoction as Ext. Gentianæ, (HAMB. PH.) Others direct the inspissated juice. The fluid extract (*Mellago Graminis*) is prepared by evaporating the liquid to the consistence of syrup.

EXTRACTUM GRANATI CORTICIS. P. From the root-bark of pomegranate, as Ext. Ipecacuanhæ.

EXTRACTUM GRATIOLÆ. BADEN PH. directs a spirituous extract. GEOFFROY a vinous extract. Others direct it to be made by infusion, decoction, or the inspissation of the depurated juice. Dose, gr. ij to iv.

EXTRACTUM GUAIACI. P. & L. 1746. Boil rasped guaiacum wood repeatedly in water, concentrate the clear decoction, and when it becomes thick add a little rectified spirit, and evaporate to dryness.

EXTRACTUM GUARANÆ. See Ext. Paulliniæ.

EXTRACTUM HÆMATOXYLI. L. As Ext. Gentianæ.

EXTRACTUM HÆMOSTATICUM. See Ext. Ergotæ Aquosum.

EXTRACTUM HELLEBORI NIGRI. L. 1788. As Ext. Gentianæ. U. S. & P. With proof spirit, as Ext. Ipecacuanhæ. Dose, gr. iv. to viij.

EXTRACTUM HELLEBORI ALKALINUM BACHERI. Black hellebore root bruised ℔j, subcarbonate of potash ℥iij, proof spirit Oiij. Digest for 12 hours, and strain. Digest the root with white wine Oiij for 24 hours, make it boil, and strain. Evaporate the mixed liquids to a firm extract. Dose, gr. ij to vj.

EXTRACTUM HUMULI. See Ext. Lupuli.

EXTRACTUM HYOSCYAMI. L. E. D. U. S. & P. By the same processes as respectively directed for Ext. Conii, and Ext. Conii Alcoholicum. Dose of the inspissated juice, gr. ij to viij: of the alcoholic extract gr. ¼ to gr. ij. [In India the juice is evaporated by exposure to the heat of the sun, yielding an extract which produces decided effects in doses of 3 grains.]

EXTRACTUM SEMINUM HYOSCYAMI. P. Digest ℔j of the ground seeds with ℔iij of proof spirit with a gentle heat, strain; digest them with ℔iij more spirit, and again strain and press. Evaporate the filtered liquors to an extract, dissolve this in cold water, filter, and again evaporate. Dose, ½ gr. to 2 grains.

EXTRACTUM INULÆ. L. 1746. From the decoction of elecampane root. P. by percolation.

EXTRACTUM IPECACUANHÆ. P. Ipecacuanha root in moderately fine powder ℔ij, proof spirit ℔vij. Moisten the powder with ℔j of the spirit, and pack it between two diaphragms in a tin cylinder; after 12 hours lixiviate it with the rest of the spirit. When the last portions of spirit have been absorbed by the powder, keep the latter covered with distilled water till the liquid produces a precipitate on falling into that which had previously passed. Distil off the spirit and evaporate the residue to an extract.

EXTRACTUM JACOBÆÆ. Inspissated juice of ragwort (Senecio Jacobæa). Dose, gr. x or xv, in *Gonorrhœa.*

EXTRACTUM JALAPÆ. L. & D. Powdered jalap ℔ijss, rectified spirit Cj. Macerate 4 days, decant, boil the residue in 2 gallons of water to half a gallon. Strain the tincture and decoction separately, and boil the latter, and distil the former, till they each become thick. Mix them, and evaporate [by means of steam, D.] to a proper consistence. This extract should be kept both in a soft and dry state. Dose, gr. viij to xx.

EXTRACTUM JALAPÆ ALKALINUM. E. 1744. As the last, adding to the water ℥j, or q. s. of subcarbonate of potash.

EXTRACTUM *sive* RESINA JALAPÆ. E. Moisten powdered jalap with rectified spirit, and after 12 hours exhaust it with rectified spirit, in a percolator. Distil off the greater part of the spirit, and concentrate the residuum over a vapour bath to a due consistence. Dose, gr. iij to vj.

EXTRACTUM JUGLANDIS IMMATURÆ. The inspissated juice of the green walnut. An extract is also made by boiling the green shells with water, as Ext. Gentianæ. Dose, ℈ss to ʒss.

EXTRACTUM JUGLANDIS FOLIORUM. M. NEGRIER. From the dried leaves by decoction; or preferably by percolation. Dose, gr. iij, 2 or 3 times a day, in *Scrofula.*

EXTRACTUM JUGLANDIS CINEREÆ. U. S. From the inner bark of the root of the butternut, as Ext. Krameriæ. Dose ℈j to ʒss, as a purgative, or less as a laxative.

EXTRACTUM JUNIPERI. P. Juniper berries lightly bruised ℔j, distilled water ℔iij. Macerate at 77° to 86° F. for 24 hours, strain with gentle pressure, add more water to the berries, and let it stand 12 hours. Filter, and evaporate the mixed liquid to a soft extract.

EXTRACTUM KALDANÆ. BENGAL DISPENSATORY. An alcoholic extract of the berries of the Pharbitis Cerulea. Purgative, dose gr. x.

EXTRACTUM KRAMERIÆ. E. Reduce dried rhatany root to a moderately fine powder; mix it with half its weight of distilled water; in 12 hours put it into a percolator, and exhaust it by percolation with temperate distilled water; concentrate the liquid, filter before it becomes too thick, and evaporate it in a vapour-bath to a due consistence.

EXTRACTUM LACTUCÆ. L. By inspissating the unfiltered juice of garden lettuce. See also Lactucarium. *Thridace* is directed (P.) to be made by inspissating the juice of the *stalks* of the flowering plant, as *Ext. Aconiti cum fæcula.*

EXTRACTUM LACTUCÆ CONCENTRATUM. PROBART. From the external parts only of the stalks, and the old leaves, after the plants have flowered; by maceration and decoction; evaporating first by heat, and then drying in shallow dishes. About half the strength of *Lactucarium.*

EXTRACTUM LACTUCÆ VIROSÆ. P. The inspissated juice of wild lettuce.

EXTRACTUM LOBELIÆ INFLATÆ. Dried lobelia ℥iv, proof spirit Oiv, strong acetic acid f℥j. Macerate for 48 hours, filter, and evaporate by water-bath.

EXTRACTUM LUPULI. L. From dried hops, as Ext. Gentianæ, L.

EXTRACTUM MARRUBII. From the expressed juice, or the decoction; or thus (PORT. PH.): White horehound 1 part, rectified spirit 1 part, water 8 parts. Digest for 3 days, express, and evaporate.

EXTRACTUM MARTIS POMATUM *sive* CYDONIATUM. Digest ℔j of iron filings in ℔ij of sour apple or quince juice for some days; strain through cloth, and evaporate with a gentle heat.

EXTRACTUM MARTIS. P. By evaporating Tinctura Martis Tartarizata.

EXTRACTUM MENYANTHIS. P. Inspissated juice of buck-bean.

EXTRACTUM MEZEREI. The *alcoholic* extract is made by digesting mezereon bark in a water-bath with rectified spirit, and evaporating the tincture. The *æthereal* extract is best made from the alcoholic, evaporated only to the consistence of syrup. Let this be digested with æther in a stoppered bottle, the æthereal tincture decanted, and carefully evaporated.

EXTRACTUM MONESIÆ. From the Burhanem bark as Ext. Krameriæ. The imported extract may be purified as Ext. Catechu. Dose, gr. iv to viij.

EXTRACTUM MYRRHÆ AQUOSUM. Digest bruised myrrh in hot

water, set it aside, and when cool, strain, and evaporate to an extract. Some authorities direct it to be boiled.

EXTRACTUM MYRRHÆ [Alcoholicum]. P. As Extractum Scillæ.

EXTRACTUM NARCISSI. From dried flowers of daffodil, by percolation with proof spirit; or with water. Dose, gr. ss to gr. jss, in hooping cough.

EXTRACTUM NICOTIANÆ. See Ext. Tabaci.

EXTRACTUM NUCIS VOMICÆ. E. Exhaust nux vomica (which has been softened by steam, sliced, dried, and ground in a coffee-mill) by percolation, or boiling, with rectified spirit. Distil off the greater part of the spirit, and evaporate what remains to a proper consistence in a vapour-bath. D. directs proof spirit. P. a medium spirit, ·863. Dose, ½ a grain, cautiously increased to 2 or 3 grains.

EXTRACTUM OPII PURIFICATUM. L. Opium sliced ℥xx, distilled water Cj; soften the opium by maceration with a little of the water for 12 hours; then, the rest of the water being gradually added, triturate them together till perfectly mixed, and set aside till the dregs have subsided. Then filter the liquor, and evaporate to a proper consistence. E. directs repeated maceration and strong expression: and the extract to be again taken up by maceration with successive portions of cold water, and the filtered liquor evaporated.

EXTRACTUM OPII ABSQUE NARCOTINA. P. The extract, softened with cold water, is agitated and macerated with successive portions of æther as long as anything is taken up. The æther being poured off, the extract is evaporated to a pilular consistence. [Another process has been devised by M. Limouzin-Lamothe. Four parts of extract of opium are beaten in a mortar with one of resin, and triturated with enough water to form a liquid mass. This is boiled with 16 parts of water till reduced to half, then removed from the fire, and as much cold water added as has been boiled away. The resin is then removed, and the extract evaporated.]

EXTRACTUM OPII PER FERMENTATIONEM. DEYEUX. To an unstrained mixture of 1 part of opium in 8 of water, add yeast q. s., and leave it for a week at a temperature between 68° and 70° F. Then filter the liquor and evaporate it. M. LANGELOT dissolves the opium in juice of quinces, and ferments for a month. GUIBOURT prefers digesting opium and water at the above temperature without the yeast.

EXTRACTUM OPII TORREFACTI. GUIBOURT. Heat powdered

opium in a flat dish over a moderate fire, with constant stirring, till vapours cease to be disengaged. Treat it twice with six times its weight of cold water, and evaporate the filtered solution. [These last three extracts are supposed to contain the full proportion of morphine, without the irritating and virous principles of opium.]

EXTRACTUM OPII VINO PARATUM. P. Macerate ℔j of choice opium in ℔iv of white wine for 24 hours, stirring occasionally; strain and press, diffuse the residuum through ℔ij more wine, and after some hours express the liquid. Evaporate the strained liquors to an extract. [Other extracts are obtained from opium by digesting it with vinegar, lemon-juice, quince-juice, alcohol, &c.]

EXTRACTUM PAPAVERIS. L. Poppy-heads without the seeds ℥xv, boiling water Cj; macerate for 24 hours, boil to Oiv, filter whilst hot, and evaporate by water-bath to a proper consistence.

EXTRACTUM PAREIRÆ. L. By decoction, as Extr. Gentianæ; or by percolation (P.), as Extr. Krameriæ.

EXTRACTUM PATIENTIÆ. P. From the root of patience dock, as Extractum Krameriæ.

EXTRACTUM PAULLINIÆ. Dr. GAVRELLE. From the ground seeds of Paullinia sorbilis (Guarana), by boiling with proof spirit. *Tonic.* Dose, gr. viij to x in the day.

EXTRACTUM PETROSELINI. P. From parsley root, as Extractum Krameriæ. M. PERAIRE prescribes the inspissated juice of the *leaves* as a substitute for quinine. Dose, gr. viij to xv in 24 hours.

EXTRACTUM PHARBITIS. See Ext. Kaldanæ.

EXTRACTUM PIMPINELLA. Root of burnet saxifrage 2 parts, rectified spirit 3 parts, water 9 parts. Digest, strain, and evaporate. It is also made by boiling the root with six times its weight of water, and evaporating the decoction. Dose, ℈j.

EXTRACTUM PODOPHYLLI. U. S. From the root (rhizome) of May-apple, as Ext. Jalapæ. *Purgative.* Dose, gr. v. to xv.

EXTRACTUM PYROLÆ. See Extractum Chimaphilæ.

EXTRACTUM QUASSIÆ. E. From rasped quassia, by percolation, as Ext. Krameriæ.

EXTRACTUM QUERCUS. D. As Extractum Hæmatoxyli.

EXTRACTUM RHAMNI BACCARUM. By inspissating the juice of buckthorn berries, after it has undergone a slight fermentation. Dose, ℈j to ʒjss.

EXTRACTUM RHATANIÆ. See Extractum Krameriæ.

EXTRACTUM RHEI. L. & D. Rhubarb in powder ℥xv, proof spirit Oj, distilled water Ovij. Macerate for 4 days in a gentle heat; then strain, and set the solution aside to settle. Decant, and evaporate the clear liquid to a proper consistence. E. directs it to be prepared by maceration in successive portions of cold water, and the expressed and filtered liquids evaporated in a vapour-bath, or preferably *in vacuo*, to a proper consistence.

EXTRACTUM RHEI COMPOSITUM. PRUS. PH. *Extractum Panchymagogum.* Extract of rhubarb ʒiij, purified aloes ʒj, soap of jalap ʒj. Dissolve them in a little spirit, and evaporate to a proper consistence.

EXTRACTUM RHOIS TOXICODENDRI ET RADICANTIS. P. The inspissated juice of the leaves of the poison oak. An alcoholic extract of the dried leaves is probably more active.

EXTRACTUM RUBIÆ. HAMB. PH. By evaporating a tincture made with two parts of ground madder, three of rectified spirit, and nine of water.

EXTRACTUM RUDII. See Pilulæ Rudii.

EXTRACTUM RUTÆ. L. 1788 as Extr. Absinthii. P. as Extr. Aconiti Alcoholicum.

EXTRACTUM SABADILLÆ. Dr. TURNBULL. By evaporating the concentrated tincture of cevadilla seeds. Dose, ⅛th of a grain; as a substitute for veratria.

EXTRACTUM SABINÆ. L. 1788. By evaporating a decoction of dry savine. P. by percolation with proof spirit.

EXTRACTUM SALICIS. P. From powdered willow-bark, as Ext. Krameriæ.

EXTRACTUM SAMBUCI. *Elder Rob.* 1788. Evaporate the expressed and defæcated juice of elder-berries in a salt-water bath. E. directs the addition of ℔ss of sugar to Oiv of juice.

EXTRACTUM SAPONARIÆ. P. From the dried roots of soapwort, as Ext. Krameriæ. Other Pharm. direct the expressed juice of the plant to be inspissated. Dose, ℈j to ʒij.

EXTRACTUM SARZÆ. L. Ext. Sarsaparillæ, D. Sliced sarsaparilla ℔ijss, boiling distilled water Cij. Macerate for 24 hours, boil to Cj, strain while hot, and evaporate to a proper consistence.

EXTRACTUM SARZÆ FLUIDUM. E. Digest ℔j of sarza in chips, with Ovj of boiling water for 2 hours, take out the root, bruise, and replace it; boil for 2 hours, filter, and squeeze out the liquid. Boil the sarza in Oij of water, filter, and squeeze; evaporate the mixed liquors to the consistence of thin syrup, add when cool, rectified spirit q. s. to make up f℥xvj, and filter. It may be aromatized at will with various volatile oils or warm aromatics. D. directs ℔j of sarsaparilla to be twice boiled with cong. j of water, the decanted decoctions reduced to f℥xxx, and f℥ij of rectified spirit added. [f℥j of the fluid extract E., or f℥ij D. represent f℥vj of the decoction. A better preparation is made by macerating the root in temperate or tepid water. See Liquor Sarzæ.]

EXTRACTUM CORTICIS SARZÆ. By macerating or percolating the root-bark with temperate water, and evaporating the liquid to a solid or fluid extract.

EXTRACTUM SARZÆ ALCOHOLICUM. P. & U. S. As Extr. Ipecac. It yields one-eighth of its weight of extract, which is superior to the watery.

EXTRACTUM SARZÆ COMPOSITUM. PEREIRA. By mixing with extract of sarsaparilla an extract prepared by evaporating a decoction of a corresponding proportion of the other ingredients of the compound decoction, adding a small quantity of oil of sassafras. As commonly sold, it contains too much liquorice. GUIBOURT recommends it to be made by percolation with proof spirit. Mr. Hodgson (America) gives the following form.—Sarza ℥xvj, liquorice root, guaiacum wood, sassafras bark, each ℥ij, mezereon ʒvj, proof spirit Oviij o. m. (Ovjss, *Impl.*) Digest 14 days, express, filter, evaporate to f℥xij, then add ℥viij of white sugar, and remove from the fire as soon as it is dissolved.

EXTRACTUM SATURNI. See Liquor Plumbi Diacetatis.

EXTRACTUM *sive* RESINA SCAMMONII. E. Boil scammony in fine powder, in successive portions of proof spirit, till the spirit ceases to dissolve anything; filter, distil the liquid till little but water passes over. Then pour away the watery solution from the resin, wash the latter with boiling water, and dry it at a temperature not exceeding 240°.

EXTRACTUM SCILLÆ. P. Dried squill ℔j, proof spirit ℔iv. Macerate for some days, strain, press, and filter; digest the squill with ℔ij more spirit, and after 2 or 3 days, strain and press again. Distil off the spirit from the mixed tincture, and evaporate the residuum to an extract. Dose, gr. j to iij.

EXTRACTUM SCOPARII. See Ext. Genistæ.

EXTRACTUM SENEGÆ. P. As Ext. Ipecacuanhæ.

EXTRACTUM SENEGÆ ET SCILLÆ. Mr. ECKY. Macerate ℔ij each of senega and squills in proof spirit q. s. to cover them: transfer the whole to a displacement funnel, and pass proof spirit through it till it passes nearly tasteless. Strain, distil off most of the spirit, and reduce to ℔iv.

EXTRACTUM SENNÆ. P. By percolation with temperate water, as Ext. Krameriæ. Mr. HUSBAND says proof spirit yields a more active extract.

EXTRACTUM SENNÆ FLUIDUM. Mr. DUNCAN. Senna 15℔s, av. (℔xviij¼), boiling water 4 times its weight, or q. s. Exhaust the senna by displacement, concentrate the liquor to 10℔s. av. (℔xij); dissolve in it 6℔s av. (℔vij ℥iijss.) of treacle, previously concentrated over a vapour-bath, till it becomes nearly dry on cooling. Add f℥xxiv rectified spirit, and water q. s. to make up 15 pints, o. m. (Oxij imp.) Dose ʒij. Each f℥j corresponds with 1 oz. av. of senna.

EXTRACTUM SOLANI TUBEROSI. Dr. LATHAM. From the stalks and leaves of potato, as Ext. Conii. Dose, gr. iij.

EXTRACTUM STRAMONII [SEMINUM]. L. & D. Stramonium seeds ℥xv, boiling water Cj. Macerate near the fire for 4 hours, bruise and return the seeds, boil down to Ov, strain while hot, and evaporate to a proper consistence. E. directs the seeds to be ground, mixed with proof spirit into a thick pulp, placed in a percolator, and exhausted by proof spirit. The spirit is to be distilled off, and what remains evaporated in a vapour-bath.

EXTRACTUM STRAMONII [FOLIORUM]. P. directs the inspissated juice of the leaves, both with and without the fæcula, also a watery extract from the powdered leaves by percolation; and an alcoholic extract by percolation with proof spirit, as Ext. Aconiti.

EXTRACTUM STYRACIS. E. Boil powdered storax in successive portions of rectified spirit till exhausted, filter the spirituous solution, distil off the spirit, and evaporate to an extract.

EXTRACTUM TABACI. Mr. CHIPPENDALE. Shag tobacco ℥iv, distilled water Oij; boil, and let them simmer for 2 or 3 hours;

then strain, wash the tobacco with more boiling water, and evaporate the strained liquors to the consistence of an extract. *For external use in neuralgia.* See Unguentum Tabaci.

Extractum Taraxaci. L. & E. From a decoction of the fresh roots (herbs and roots D.) as Extractum Gentianæ. P. From the expressed juice clarified by heat. Mr. Houlton allows the expressed juice of the roots (taken up in August or September) to evaporate spontaneously in shallow vessels. The evaporation may be facilitated by various contrivances for increasing the current of dry air, and promoting the absorption of the moisture.

Extractum Taraxaci Fluidum. Usually made by evaporating the expressed juice or the decoction to the consistence of syrup, and adding a little spirit. For a better method, see Liquor Taraxaci.

Extractum Taxi. Loder. The inspissated juice of yew-leaves. Dose, from gr. j to viij, *in Epilepsy*, &c.

Extractum Tormentillæ. As Ext. Gentianæ.

Extractum Urticæ. P. The juice of nettles inspissated without clarification.

Extractum Uvæ Ursi. L. From the dried leaves, by decoction, as Ext. Gentianæ.

Extractum Valerianæ. D. As Ext. Gentianæ. P. by percolation with proof spirit, as Ext. Ipecac.

Extracta Narcotica cum Saccharo. Gauger. Dissolve ℥vj of alcoholic extract of the plant in ʒxiv or ℥ij of strong alcohol by trituration in a porcelain mortar, and mix with it ℥xxx of powdered white sugar gradually added with constant stirring. Set the mixture in a warm situation till dry. Add sugar q. s. to make up ℥xxxvj. These preparations are less liable to lose their efficacy than the simple extracts. Six grains represent one of the extract.

Fæcula. The fæcula of Arum, Briony, Chestnuts, &c., is obtained by rasping them, pressing the pulp, mixed with an equal weight of water, in a hair bag, straining the liquid, and after allowing it to settle, collecting, washing, and drying the sediment which subsides. Potatoes are rasped, the pulp diffused in water, and the fæcula obtained from the strained liquor as above. The *green* fæcula of narcotic and other plants, obtained by filtering or heating the expressed juice, is of a different nature, and retains a small and uncertain portion of the active principles of the plants.

FARINÆ EMOLLIENTES. See Species Emollientes.

FEL BOVINUM SPISSATUM, ET DESICCATUM. See Ext. Fellis.

FERRI ACETAS. D. *Peracetate of Iron.* Carbonate (sesquioxide) of iron 1 part, acetic acid 6 parts; digest for 3 days, and filter. [The acetic acid of the Dub. Ph. is much stronger than that of L.] Dose ♏vj to xxiv.

FERRI ACETATIS TINCTURA. See Tinctura Ferri Ac.

FERRI AMMONIO-CHLORIDUM. L. Sesquioxide of iron ℥iij, hydrochloric acid f℥x; digest in a proper vessel in a sand-bath for 12 hours. Add hydrochlorate of ammonia ℔ijss, previously dissolved in Oiij of distilled water; filter, evaporate to dryness, and reduce to powder.

FERRI AMMONIO-CITRAS. BERAL. Citric acid ℥xxiv, distilled water Oiij, water of ammonia (*Liquor ammoniæ,* L.) f℥xiss; heat to boiling, and gradually add moist hydrated oxide of iron (see *Ferrugo*) till a portion remains undissolved. About ℥liv or lv will be required. [Mr. PROCTER states that the temperature should be kept *below* boiling.] The filtered solution is evaporated to the consistence of treacle, and then spread thinly on dishes, or plates of glass, and gradually dried in a drying closet (not by heat applied to the bottom of the dishes) till it can be chipped off in scales. Mr. HEMINGWAY directs a known quantity of citric acid to be neutralized with ammonia, and a similar quantity of the acid added to the solution. To this, add the hydrated oxide gradually, till a portion remains undissolved. Evaporate the filtered solution as directed above. Soda-citrate and potash-citrate of iron are made in a similar way. Dose gr. iv to viij.

FERRI AMMONIO-TARTRAS. AIKIN. Dissolve 1 part of tartaric acid in q. s. of boiling water, add 2 or 3 parts of iron wire, or turnings, and digest in a warm place for 2 or 3 days. Add caustic ammonia in slight excess, mix by trituration, and pour off the solution, set it aside, decant the clear liquid, and evaporate it to dryness. Redissolve in distilled water, add a little more ammonia, filter, and evaporate the solution in shallow, porcelain dishes, by a gentle heat till it becomes brittle. Then chip it off with a blunt-pointed knife. [Mr. PROCTER, jun., of Philadelphia, gives a different process. Dissolve 50 drachms of tartaric acid in a gallon (o. m.) of water, saturate with carbonate of ammonia, and add 50 drachms more of acid. Heat the solution in a water-bath, and add moist hydrated oxide of iron, (derived from 53½ drachms of sesquioxide dissolved in muriatic acid q. s., and precipitated by ammonia.) Digest till the oxide is dissolved, filter, and finish as directed above.] Dose, gr. iv to vj.

Ferri Arsenias. Obtained by mixing solutions of arseniate of soda, and proto-sulphate of iron, and collecting, washing, and drying the precipitate. Dose, $\frac{1}{16}$th of a grain, *in herpetic and cancerous affections.* (Biett.) Also used *externally*, with 4 times its weight of phosphate of iron, by Carmichael; and in the form of ointment.

Ferri Bromidum. Mohr. Mix 1 part of iron filings with 3 parts of water in a stopped vial; add 1 part of bromine; close the bottle, and set it aside, shaking it occasionally. When the solution has assumed a greenish colour, filter, and evaporate to dryness. Dose, gr. ij to vj.

Ferri Carbonas. *F. Sub-carbonas.* When a solution of carbonate of soda is added to one of sulphate of iron, carbonate of iron is precipitated; but in drying, most of it becomes a sesquioxide. (See Ferri Sesqui-oxydum.) This, however, is in a great measure prevented by adding sugar to the washed and moist precipitate, as in

Ferri Carbonas Saccharatum. E. Sulphate of iron ℥iv, carbonate (subc.) of soda ℥v; dissolve each in Oij of water, and mix the solutions; collect the precipitate on a cloth filter, wash it with cold water, squeeze out as much water as possible, and without delay triturate the pulp with ℥ij of pure sugar in fine powder. Dry it at a heat not much above 120°. [The water used for washing should have been recently boiled, to expel the air, and cooled in a close vessel. Mr. R. Phillips, jun., advises to add the sugar, previously made into a thick syrup, to the washed precipitate without its being squeezed, and evaporating to dryness.] Dose, gr. v to viij.

Ferri Chloridum. P. The *proto-chloride* is made by adding clean iron turnings to muriatic acid, as long as any is dissolved, boiling the solution on excess of iron, decanting the solution as soon as it has settled, and evaporating quickly to dryness. The *perchloride* is made by evaporating to dryness a solution of red-oxide of iron in muriatic acid.

Ferri Citras. Beral. Citric acid ℥iv, water ℥iv; heat together in a platinum capsule, and gradually add moist peroxide of iron (see Ferrugo) as long as any is dissolved. Proceed as directed for Ferri Ammonio-citras. About ℥x of pure sulphate of iron will be required to furnish sufficient oxide. The more gradually the citrate is dried, the larger the scales. Dose, gr. iv to viij.

FERRI ET QUINÆ CITRAS. BERAL. Dissolve 4 parts of citrate of iron, and 1 of citrate of quinine, in distilled water, and evaporate the solution to dryness, as directed for Ferri Ammonio-citras.

FERRI FERRO-CYANURETUM [per cyanidum, L.] U. S. *Pure Prussian Blue.* Make a solution of persulphate of iron, as directed for Ferrugo; and gradually add to it ℥ivss of ferrocyanide of potassium, stirring after each addition; then pour the whole on a filter, wash till tasteless, dry, and pulverize. Dose, gr. iij to vj, *in Intermittents, Epilepsy,* &c.

FERRI IODIDUM. L. Iodine ℥vj, distilled water Oiv; mix, and add iron filings ℥ij; heat in a sand-bath, and when the solution assumes a greenish colour, pour it off, and wash what remains with Oss of hot water. Evaporate the filtered liquors to dryness, at a heat not above 212°, in an iron vessel. Keep it from the air and light. E. directs to proceed as in making Solutio Ferri Iodidi, but to evaporate to $\frac{1}{6}$th in contact with iron before filtering; and to evaporate the solution in a close vessel, in a basin surrounded with quick-lime. [It is difficult to prepare this in a perfect state, and almost impossible to preserve it so. It is therefore more frequently prescribed in the form of solution, syrup, or pills; which see.]

FERRI IODIDUM SACCHARATUM. See Saccharum Ferri Iodidi.

FERRI LACTAS. Dissolve ℥j of lactate of lime in ℥iv of boiling water; precipitate the lime by oxalic acid, avoiding excess, and filter. Heat the liquid with excess of iron filings for 6 or 8 hours, filter, set aside, wash the crystalline powder which is deposited with a little alcohol, and dry it. M. LEPAGE dissolves 100 parts of lactate of lime in 500 of boiling water; and 68 of crys. sulphate of iron in 500 parts of cold water. Mix the filtered solutions, add a little lactic acid, and heat the mixture with constant stirring, until decomposition is complete. Filter, and set aside to crystallize. On further evaporation, more crystals are obtained; wash them with a little alcohol, and dry on blotting paper. Dose, gr. j or ij.

FERRI LIMATURA PRÆPARATA. Care should be taken to procure

iron filings free from other metals, as these cannot be effectually removed by the method formerly used for their purification,—drawing them through a hair sieve with a magnet. P. directs them to be beaten in an iron mortar, the oxide and dust to be removed by a fine sieve, and the grosser parts by a coarse hair sieve.

FERRI LIMATURA LÆVIGATA. P. Ferrum Pulveratum. Prepared iron filings ground by means of a slab and muller of porphyry to a fine powder, without moisture. See Ferrum Reductum.

FERRI MALAS IMPURUM. See Extractum Martis Pomatum.

FERRI MURIATIS TINCTURA. See Tinctura F. M.

FERRI OXYDUM NIGRUM. Black Oxide of Iron, or Martial Ethiops. D. directs the scales from the smith's anvil to be prepared as chalk. See Creta Præp. P. by exposing moistened iron filings to the air for 2 or 3 days, stirring occasionally. But it is more elegantly prepared by precipitation. E. Dissolve ℥iij of sulphate of iron in Ojss of boiling water; add sulphuric acid f ʒij ♏ xl; boil and add by degrees pure nitric acid f ʒivss, boiling the liquid after each addition briskly for a few minutes. Dissolve ℥iij more of the sulphate in another Ojss of boiling water, mix thoroughly the two solutions, and immediately add f ℥ivss of strong liquid ammonia in a full stream, stirring briskly. Collect the powder on a calico filter, wash it with water till the water is no longer precipitated by nitrate of barytes, and dry it at a temperature not exceeding 180°. Dose, gr. v to xx.

FERRI OXYDUM MAGNETICUM. Dr. JEPHSON'S formula being much in use, is here inserted. It does not appear to differ essentially from the last. Crystallized sulphate of iron bruised ℥xxjss, water Oij, strong nitric acid f ℥iv, or q. s. Heat in an earthen vessel at 180°, stirring frequently, and adding the nitric acid gradually, till the solution no longer yields a blue precipitate with the red or *per*-prussiate of iron. When quite cool, add *suddenly* to this a solution of ℥x¾ of sulphate of iron in Oiij of water. Dissolve by heat, in a large iron pan, ℥xl of cryst. subcarbonate of soda in Oiij of water; add to this, gradually, the mixed solution of iron, stirring them well together. Boil briskly for half an hour; remove, settle, pour off the liquid, add Ovj of water, boil for half an hour, decant the liquid, wash the precipitate repeatedly, drain in muslin, and dry carefully at a moderate temperature.

12

FERRI SESQUIOXYDUM. L. (Formerly Ferri Carbonas, and Subcarbonas.) Dissolve separately sulphate of iron ℔iv, carbonate of soda (cryst. subc.) ℔iv ℥ij, each in cong. iij of boiling water. Mix the liquors, set them aside, and when the powder has subsided, pour off the liquid, wash the precipitate with water, and dry it.

FERRI OXYDUM RUBRUM. D. *Colcothar.* Roast dried sulphate of iron with a strong fire as long as it gives off acid vapours. Wash the product thoroughly, and dry it. E. nearly as Ferri Sesquioxydum, L. The latter is not a perfect peroxide. Mr. R. PHILLIPS, jun., proposes to form a definite peroxide by adding to a boiling mixture of solutions of 1168 parts of sulphate of iron, and 1728 of cr. carbonate of soda, 124 (rather 130) parts of chlorate of potash. The washed precipitate to be dried at 212°. Whether this can be substituted for the FERRUGO, E. as an antidote for arsenic remains to be ascertained.

FERRI PERCYANIDUM. See Ferri Ferro-cyanuretum.

FERRI PERNITRAS *vel* SESQUI-NITRAS. Mr. KERR. To iron wire ℥jss add nitric acid f℥iij diluted with f℥xv of water, set them aside till the action has ceased, decant, add muriatic acid ʒj, and water to make up f℥xxx. Dose, 6 or 8 drops, sometimes increased to 15.

FERRI PHOSPHAS. U. S. Dissolve separately pure sulphate of iron ℥v, and phosphate of soda ℥vj, in Oiv of water: mix, and when the phosphate has subsided, pour off the supernatant liquid, wash the precipitate with hot water, and dry it with a gentle heat. Dose, gr. v to x.

FERRI OXYPHOSPHAS. CARMICHAEL. To a solution of perchloride of iron add one of phosphate of soda, as long as a precipitate falls. Wash this, and dry it. Dose, ℈j.

FERRI POTASSIO-TARTRAS. L. (*Ferrum Tartarizatum.* E. *Tartarum Ferri,* D.) Digest ℥iij of sesquioxide of iron in f℥x of muriatic acid for 2 hours in a sand-bath; add Cij of distilled water, set it aside for an hour, then pour off the supernatant liquid. Add Oivss of solution of potash (*liquor potassæ*), wash the precipitate frequently with water, and boil it while still moist with ℥xjss of bitartrate of potash, previously mixed with Cj of water. If acid, neutralize with sesquicarbonate of ammonia. Lastly filter, and evaporate to dryness by a gentle heat. E. directs the moist oxide (prepared as directed under Ferrugo) from ℥v of sulphate of iron to be mixed with Oiv of water, and ℥v ʒj of bitartrate of potash, and boiled till the oxide is dissolved. When the solution is cold, pour off the clear liquid, add carbonate of ammonia so long as it occasions effervescence, and evaporate so that the residuum may be solid when cold. U. S. directs the moist oxide and supertartrate of potash to be digested for 30 hours at 140°, and the solution evaporated.

Ferri Proto-murias. *Hydrated proto-chloride of iron.* Digest sulphuret of iron in excess, with diluted muriatic acid; filter, and evaporate, that crystals may form. Keep them from the air.

Ferri Proto-sulphas. See Ferri Sulphas.

Ferri Proto-tartras. Dr. Ure. Digest ℥j of iron turnings, ℥ss of tartaric acid, and hot water q. s. till the action has ceased; diffuse the tartrate through the liquid, pour it off from the iron, collect the powder, wash, and dry it. Or dissolve separately in water 132 parts of crys. tartrate of potash, and 139 of pure sulphate of iron; wash the precipitate with boiling water, squeeze it strongly in a cloth, and dry it on a salt-water bath. Soubeiran.

Ferri Proto-sulphuretum Hydratum. Add a solution of bi-hydrosulphuret of soda to one of proto-sulphate of iron; wash the precipitate quickly on a cloth filter, squeeze out most of the water, and keep the paste from the air. In this state, it is used as an antidote for poisoning by corrosive sublimate. It may be safely taken in considerable doses. [For the anhydrous proto-sulphuret, see Ferri Sulphuretum, below.]

Ferri Per-sulphuretum Hydratum. Into a dilute solution of liver of sulphur, drop *very gradually* a neutral solution of per-sulphate of iron, prepared as directed under Ferrugo. Collect and preserve the precipitate as the last. M. Bouchardat prefers it to the proto-sulphuret as an antidote for sublimate, white arsenic, and the salts of lead and copper.

Ferri Rubigo. See Ferrugo.

Ferri Sulphas. L. Sulphuric acid ℥xiv, water Oiv; mix, add iron filings ℥viij, apply heat, and when the action has ceased, filter, and set aside, that crystals may form. More may be obtained by evaporating the remaining liquid. Let them all be dried. E. directs the commercial sulphate to be dissolved in its weight of boiling water with a little sulphuric acid, and the filtered solution set aside to crystallize.

Ferri Proto-sulphas Præcipitatum. Berthemot. To ℥xvijss of water, kept boiling, gradually add ℥xvj of pure sulphate of iron, and ℥ss of clean iron turnings; filter the boiling solution into a vessel containing ℥xij of rectified spirit, mixed with ʒij of sulphuric acid. Drain the crystalline powder, and dry it between blotting paper.

Ferri Sulphas Exsiccatum. E. Dry sulphate of iron with a moderate heat, in a porcelain or earthenware vessel not glazed with lead, till it becomes a grayish-white mass, and reduce it to powder.

Ferri Persulphas. This is formed in the process for Ferrugo (below). By evaporating the filtered solution to dryness at a moderate temperature, the salt is obtained.

Ferri et Ammoniæ Sulpho-tartras. Aikin. Dissolve sulphate of iron with half its weight of tartaric acid in a little cold water; add ammonia to saturation, filter, and evaporate to dryness. Redissolve, add a little more ammonia, filter, and again evaporate to dryness. Twelve grains equal to 10 of the sulphate. It is not precipitated by alkalies.

Ferri Sulphuretum. D. & E. Rub a rod of iron heated to full whiteness, on a roll of sulphur; let the melted sulphuret fall into a vessel of water. Separate it from portions of melted sulphur, and dry it. An inferior kind is made by heating in a crucible a mixture of 1 part of sulphur with 3 of iron filings, removing the crucible as soon as the mixture begins to glow, and covering it till the action has ceased.

Ferri Sulphocyanidum. Sulphocyanide of iron is formed by mixing a solution of sulphocyanide of potassium with a neutral solution of a persalt of iron.

Ferri Tannas. Benedetti. To a boiling solution of 90 parts of pure tannic acid add gradually 440 parts of subcarbonate (sesquioxide) of iron which has been prepared from pure sulphate of iron and carbonate of soda, and dried at a moderate heat. Agitate the solution till the effervescence ceases. Evaporate the mixture at 176° F. in a porcelain vessel, until it becomes thick; then spread it on glass or porcelain to dry, in a stove at 95°. In *Chlorosis* 2 or 3 grains three times a day, increasing the dose as required.

Ferri Valerianas. Ruspini. To clean iron filings, in a Wedgwood mortar, add by little and little an equal weight of valerianic acid, and stir continually. In an hour add distilled water, gently warm the whole in a flask, and filter. The surface in contact with the air becomes covered with a crystalline layer of valerianate of peroxide of iron. Collect this in a filter, and again expose the liquid to the air; pass it through the filter, and repeat this as long as it yields crystals. Dose, gr. j to ij.

FERRUGO. E. Rubigo Ferri. *Hydrated Sesquioxide of Iron.* Dissolve ℥iv of sulphate of iron in Oij of water, add f ʒiijss of oil of vitriol, and boil the solution; add f ʒix or q. s. of nitric acid (1·380) in small portions, boiling the liquid for a minute or two after each addition, until it acquires a yellowish-brown colour, and yields a precipitate of the same colour with ammonia. Filter and allow the liquid to cool; then add in a full stream f ℥iijss of strong ammonia, stirring briskly. Collect the precipitate on a calico filter, wash it thoroughly with water till the washings cease to precipitate with nitrate of barytes, then squeeze it strongly, and dry it at a heat not above 180°.

When it is intended as an antidote for poisoning with arsenic, it is preferable to preserve it in a moist state, after being simply squeezed. [It is used in the same state for making the citrate, ammonio-citrate, potash-tartrate, and some other salts of iron.]

[As its efficacy is impaired by long keeping, even in the moist state, it would perhaps be better to keep the solution, prepared as in the first part of the process, in readiness; and add the ammonia when required for use.]

FERRUM REDUCTUM. *Iron reduced by hydrogen.* Spread oxide of iron in a tube, heat the tube, and cause a stream of hydrogen gas to pass through it till the iron is reduced.

FLORES SAMBUCI SALITI. Fresh elder-flowers are strewed in a cask or jar with alternate layers of dry salt. *For distilling the water at any period of the year.*

FOLIA BELLADONNÆ OPIATA. M. CRUVEILHIER. Steep ℥ij of belladonna leaves in a solution of ℈j of opium in ℥ij of water, and dry them in the shade. *For smoking in phthisis.*

FOMENTUM (*vel* Fotus) ACETI. P. White vinegar ℥viij, cold water ℥xxxij.

FOMENTUM AMMONIÆ MURIATIS. CH. Decoction of mallow Ojss, muriate of ammonia ℥j; dissolve, and add spirit of camphor ℥ij. U. C. H. muriate of ammonia ℥j, water f ℥xij, proof spirit f ℥ij, liquid subacetate of lead f ʒij. Mix.

FOMENTUM ANTHEMIDIS. Chamomile flowers ℨij, water ℔iv; boil, and strain. 2 or 3 poppy-heads are sometimes added.

FOMENTUM ARNICÆ. GRAEFE. Flowers of Arnica ℨij, rue ℥j; infuse in sufficient boiling water to strain off f ℥xij. For black eyes, and other extravasations. See Lotio Arnicæ.

FOMENTUM CONII COMPOSITUM. GUY'S H. Dried hemlock ℨij, dried chamomiles ℥ss, boiling water Ojss; macerate for 2 hours, strain, and press.

FOMENTUM DIGITALIS. Dried foxglove ℨj, boiling water Ojss; infuse and strain.

FOTUS ANODYNUM. E. H. Poppies ℥j, elder flowers ℨss, water Oijss; boil to Ojss.

FOTUS ANTINEURALGICUM. MIALHE. Acetate of morphia gr. ij, acetic acid gutt. ij, eau de cologne ℥ij. *In facial neuralgia.*

FOTUS AROMATICUS. E. H. Cloves ℥j, mace ℥j, red wine ℔j; boil a little and strain. F. H. wormwood, bay-leaves, rosemary, each ℥j; water Oiv; boil and strain.

FOTUS ASTRINGENS. Decoction of oak bark, or of pomegranate Ojss, alum ℥iij.

FOTUS CALMANS. F. H. Mallows ℨj, henbane ℥j, poppy heads ℥j, water ℔iv; boil to ℔iij.

FOTUS COMMUNE. L. 1744. Dried southernwood, sea wormwood, chamomiles, of each ℨj, dried bay-leaves ℥ss, water Ov; boil slightly, and strain.

FOTUS EMOLLIENS. P. Emollient herbs (*species emollientes*) ℥j, boiling water Ojss. Infuse for an hour, and strain.

FOTUS NARCOTICUS. P. Narcotic herbs (*species narcoticæ*) ℥j, boiling water Ojss. Infuse for an hour, and strain.

FOTUS GALLÆ. CH. Bruised galls ℨss, boiling water ℔ij; macerate for an hour, and strain. In *prolapsus* and *hæmorrhoids.*

FOTUS PAPAVERIS. As *Decoctum Papaveris.*

FOTUS RESOLVENS. Infusion of elder flowers ℨviij, Goulard's extract ℥ss.

FOTUS SAMBUCI. P. Infusion of elder flowers.

FOTUS TANNINI. RICORD. Tannin ℈ij, aromatic wine ℨviij.

FOTUS VINOSUS. P. Red wine Oij, honey ℥ivss. See Lotio and Embrocatio.

FULIGOKALI. DESCHAMPS. Caustic potash 20 parts, powdered wood soot 100 parts, distilled water q. s.; dissolve the potash in a little water, and add the soot; boil for an hour, then add more water, and filter. Evaporate the clear solution to dryness, constantly stirring; and put the powder into dry bottles.

FULIGOKALI SULPHURATUM. Caustic potash 14 parts, sulphur 4 parts; heat them together with a little water till dissolved, add fuligokali 60 parts, and evaporate to dryness.

FUMIGATIO AROMATICA. Olibanum, amber, mastic, of each ʒiij; styrax ʒij, benzoin, and labdanum, each ʒj; throw the mixed powders on red-hot cinders. See the next.

FUMIGATIO BALSAMICA. Benzoin is burnt alone, or with styrax as a remedy for *Hooping Cough*, ℈j or ʒss of each being thrown on hot cinders or a heated iron in the patient's room. Dr. DOHRN prescribes olibanum ℔ij, benzoin ℔ss, styrax ℔ss, dried roses ℥vj, lavender flowers ℥vj.

FUMIGATIO BELLADONNA. M. SCHROEDER. About ʒij of the dried leaves are thrown on a pan of coals; to relieve hæmoptysis, and allay cough.

FUMIGATIO CHLORINII. *Suffumigatio Guytoniana*. P. Put into an earthen vessel 3 parts of common salt, 1 of oxide of manganese, and 2 of water; add 2 parts of sulphuric acid. Stir it with a glass rod, or tobacco pipe. *This is for unoccupied rooms only*.

FUMIGATIO IODINI ET SULPHURIS. SELLERS. Sulphur ℥iij, cinnabar ℈ij, iodine gr. x; in six powders. One to be thrown on to a heated iron at the bottom of a large jar, of sufficient size to receive the limb. In lepra, psoriasis, and tubercular eruptions; 20 minutes, 3 times a day.

FUMIGATIO MERCURIALIS. ABERNETHY directs the patient to be placed in a vapour-bath, in his under garments, and his neck secured by a towel; and exposed for 15 or 20 minutes to the vapour from ℥ij of black oxide of quicksilver put on to a heated iron. F. H. use ʒss to ʒiij of red sulphuret of mercury, either alone or mixed with ℥ij of olibanum. The sulphuret is also used by placing ʒss on a hot shovel covered with a funnel (or in an apparatus sold for the purpose) and the fumes inhaled to produce salivation. Mr. COLLES recommends the oxide or sulphuret to be mixed with melted wax, and formed into tapers; which are to be burned on a plate, covered with a curved funnel raised about an inch above the plate; and the vapour inhaled, or directed to any part.

FUMIGATIO ACIDI NITRICI. *Suffumigatio cum Acido Nitrico.* P. Put into a porcelain cup equal measures of sulphuric acid and water, and add to it from time to time powdered nitre.

FUMIGATIO NITROSA. Soak porous paper in a solution of nitre; roll it up, place it in a candlestick, and set it on fire. *In Asthma.* (American Journal.)

FUMIGATIO PICEA. Sir A. CRICHTON. Mix Norway tar with a little carbonate of potash (℥ss to ℔j) to neutralize the acid, and keep it heated by means of a spirit lamp.

GARGARISMA. St. B. H. [G. Simplex, GUY'S H.; Commune U. C. H.] Vinegar f℥ijss, decoction of barley Oj, honey, or honey of roses f℥jss. Mix.

GARGARISMA ACIDI MURIATICI. CH. Muriatic acid gutt. xxx, honey of roses f℥ij, decoction of barley f℥vj. St. B. H. Red roses ʒij, boiling water Oj, muriatic acid ʒjss. Macerate for an hour, and strain. F. H. Infusion of bark ℥iv, syrup of honey ℥j, muriatic acid 18 drops.

GARGARISMA ÆRUGINIS. GUY'S H. Liniment of verdigris (*oxymel Æruginis*) f℥ss, honey of roses f℥ij, decoction of linseed f℥iijss. MID. H. Liniment of verdigris f℥j, mucilage f℥ij, water f℥ix. Mix.

GARGARISMA ALUMINIS. SAUNDERS. Alum ℈j, infusion of roses ℥vij, honey of roses ℥j. U. C. H. Alum ʒj, decoction of bark f℥x, honey q. s. MID. H. Alum ʒij, water f℥xij. ZOBEL'S *Specific* consisted of alum ℥iij, nitre ℥iij, cream tartar ℥iv, vinegar ℔iv, evaporated to dryness. ʒiv of this to be dissolved in ℥viij of plantain water. In Quinsy.

GARGARISMA ANTISCORBUTICUM. P. Bitter species (*species amaræ*) ʒj, boiling water ℥viij; infuse for an hour, strain, and add syrup of honey ℥ij, antiscorbutic tincture ℥j.

GARGARISMA ANTISEPTICUM. F. H. Muriate of ammonia ℈ss, camphor ℈j, decoction of bark ℥vj.

GARGARISMA ASTRINGENS. A. T. THOMSON. Infusion of roses f℥vij, diluted sulphuric acid fʒj, tincture of catechu fʒvj, tincture of opium fʒjss. JANNART. Tannin ʒss, honey of roses ʒij, water ℥viij, rose water ʒij. Dr. NELIGAN. Decoction of pomegranate f℥vij, honey of borax ʒj. *In Aphthous Ulcerations.*

GARGARISMA BORACIS. U. C. H. Borax ʒij, water fʒvj, honey ʒj. MID. H. Borax ʒij, oxymel f℥ss, water f℥xj.

GARGARISMA CAPSICI. U. C. H. Tincture of capsicum fʒj, water fʒvj, vinegar f℥j. MID. H. Tincture of capsicum fʒij, water f℥xij.

GARGARISMA CINCHONÆ. BRANDE. Decoction of bark f℥iijss, infusion of roses f℥iijss, tincture of myrrh fʒij, muriatic acid ♏x.

GARGARISMA CHLORINII. MID. H. Chlorine water f℥ij, water f℥x. F. H. Chlorine water ℥ss, water ℥iv, syrup ℥ss, gum tragacanth gr. x.

GARGARISMA CALCIS CHLORINATÆ. Chloride of lime ʒij, water Oj; triturate, filter, and add clarified honey ℥j.

GARGARISMA DETERGENS. P. Honey of roses ℥ij, alcoholized sulphuric acid ℈ss, decoction of barley ℥viij.

GARGARISMA EMOLLIENS. BUCHAN. Althæa root ℥j, figs ʒij, water Oij; boil to Oj, and strain. F. H. Decoction of althæa ʒvij, syrup of honey ℥j.

GARGARISMA HYDRARGYRI BICHLORIDI. CH. Corrosive sublimate gr. ij, decoction of barley Oj, honey of roses ℥ij.

GARGARISMA HYDRARGYRI CYANURETI. PARENT. Cyanide of mercury gr. x, decoction of althæa, or of linseed Oj.

GARGARISMA IODINII. Dr. ROSS. Tincture of iodine ℈j to ℈ij, tincture of opium ʒj, water f℥vj. *In ulceration of the tonsils.*

GARGARISMA MANGANESII OXYDI. PEREIRA. Black oxide of manganese ʒij to ʒiij, decoction of barley f℥vj.

GARGARISMA MYRRHÆ. CH. Tincture of myrrh ʒss, honey of roses ℥jss, lime water ℥vj.

GARGARISMA NITRI. BRANDE. Nitre ℈ij, simple oxymel f℥j, barley water f℥vij.

GARGARISMA PLUMBI. RATIER. Liquid diacetate of lead ʒss, barley water ℔j, syrup ℥j.

GARGARISMA POTASSÆ CHLORATIS. Chlorate of potash ʒj, water ʒvij, honey of roses ℥j.

Gargarisma Pyrethri. Swediaur. Infusion of pellitory Oj, muriate of ammonia ʒij, vinegar ℥iij.

Gargarisma Rhois Glabri. An infusion of the inner bark of the root of smooth Sumach is used as a gargle in mercurial salivation.

Gargarisma Rosæ. Kenrick. Conserve of roses ℥iij, boiling water fʒxvj; infuse for an hour, add diluted sulphuric acid fʒij, and strain.

Gargarisma Sodæ Chlorinatæ. Guy's H. Solution of chloride of soda fʒxij, water fʒxij. Dr. Copland. Solution fʒxij, honey ℥ss, water f℥vj. St. B. H. fʒij of the solution to f℥iv of water.

Gargarisma Spiritus Vini. Dr. Watson. Brandy 1 part, water 5 parts. *In Salivation.*

Gargarisma Stimulans. Dr. Copland. Infusion of roses f℥vjss, diluted muriatic acid ♏xl, tincture of capsicum fʒjss, honey ʒiij.

Gargarisma Sulphuris Composita. Mid. H. Sulphur ʒj, acetate of lead ℈j, distilled water fʒxij.

Gargarisma Tannini. Jannart. Tannin (*acidum tannicum*) ʒss, honey of roses ℥ij, water ℥viij, rose water ℥ij.

Gargarisma Terebinthinatum. Geddings. Oil of turpentine ʒij, mucilage ʒviij. *In Salivation.*

Gargarisma Zinci. Dr. Copland. Sulphate of zinc ℈j, rose water f℥vij, simple oxymel f℥j.

Gelatina. *Patent Gelatine* is made by macerating cuttings of calves' skins with caustic soda, washing, exposing to fumes of sulphur, dissolving, drying the jelly, cutting it, washing it thoroughly, and again dissolving and drying it. [The process, which is secured by a patent, need not be more particularly described. In France, pure gelatine is termed *grenetine.*]

Gelatina Berberorum. E. 1744. Picked barberries ℔j, white Sugar ℔j; boil gently to a due consistence, and strain through flannel.

Gelatina Cornu Cervi. P. Hartshorn shavings ℥viij, water Oiij, white sugar ℥iv, and 1 lemon. Wash the hartshorn, boil it in the water gently till reduced to half; strain and press, add the sugar and lemon juice, and the white of an egg beaten up with water; clarify by heat, and reduce to a gelatinizing consistence. Add the lemon-peel, strain, and set it in a cool place.

GELATINA CHONDRI. Soak ℥j of Irish moss in cold water, drain, boil in Oij of water to a proper consistence, adding lemon &c. to the taste. MOUCHON directs ʒj of carragheen to be boiled for half an hour with f℥xvj of water, and ℥ijss of sugar, in lumps, to be added to the strained liquor, which is evaporated to ℥viij, and aromatized with a few drops of tincture of orange or lemon-peel. It is also made with milk. BERAL directs moss ℈iv, milk ℥xxiv, sugar ℥ss, cinnamon ℈j. DAN. PH. Soak ʒij of the moss in cold water, and boil it with ℥xij of milk.

GELATINA COPAIBÆ. M. CAILLOT. Isinglass 4, water 26; dissolve in water-bath, pour the clear liquid jelly into a warm mortar, and add copaiba 30; triturate, and pour in a vessel to jelly. In the same way prepare jelly of cod-liver oil, castor oil, &c.

GELATINA CYDONIORUM. E. 1744. Juice of quinces ℔iij, sugar ℔j; boil to a jelly.

GELATINA FUCI. Dr. RUSSEL. Bladder-wrack (*Fucus vesiculosus*) ℔ij, sea-water ℔ij; macerate for 15 days. *Applied to glandular tumours.*

GELATINA FUCI AMYLACEI. Dr. SIGMOND. Boil ℥ss of prepared Ceylon moss in Oij of water for 25 minutes, (or till a spoonful taken out jellies in two or three minutes.) Flavour with wine, lemon, &c., and strain.

GELATINA HELMINTHOCORTI. P. Boil ℥j of Corsican moss for an hour in water q. s., to yield ℥viij. Add ʒj of isinglass, first soaked in a little water, ℥ij refined sugar, and ℥ij white wine. Boil and strain.

GELATINA ICTHYOCOLLÆ. Soak the isinglass in cold water, then boil in water to a gelatinizing consistence. ℥jss makes Oj of strong jelly; to which may be added wine, sugar, &c. SOUBEIRAN directs, isinglass ʒvj, water ℥xxiv, sugar ℥xij, citric acid ʒss, tincture of fresh lemon or orange-peel ʒiij.

GELATINA IODURETA. *Gelée pour le Goître.* See Linimentum Ioduretum Gelatinosum.

GELATINA LICHENIS. P. Iceland moss ℥ij, white sugar ℥iv, isinglass ʒj. Wash the moss, and boil it for an hour in enough water to yield a strong solution. Strain, leave it to settle, decant; heat again with the isinglass (first steeped in water) and the sugar, and stir continually *till it boils.* Keep it gently boiling till sufficiently concentrated; remove the skin from the surface, put it into pots, and set it to cool. The moss is sometimes deprived of its bitterness, by macerating it in cold water (changed every six hours) for 3 days.

GELATINA LICHENIS CUM CINCHONA. P. Add to the last, while warm, ℥vj of syrup of bark. [Sulphate of quinine is sometimes substituted for syrup of bark in the proportion of ½ grain to each ℥j.]

GELATINA LICHENIS SICCATA. P. Iceland moss deprived of its bitterness ℔j; boil it in sufficient water for an hour, strain, and press; add sugar ℔j, and evaporate in a flat vessel to a firm consistence, stirring it constantly. Then spread it on plates, dry it in a stove, and reduce it to powder.

GELATINA MARANTÆ. Boil ℥xvj of water with a little sugar, and add to it ℥j of arrow-root previously rubbed to a smooth paste with a little cold water; let it boil for an instant, and pour it out. Jelly of potato arrow-root and of *tous les mois* is prepared in the same way. Sago and Tapioca require to be first soaked in cold water, then boiled with fresh water to a proper consistence; adding sugar, &c. to the taste. One ounce will be sufficient for a pint of jelly.

GELATINA SALEP. Ground salep ʒiv, sugar ℥iv, water q. s. Boil to f ℥xvj, and flavour to the taste.

GENTIANINA. M. *Gentianine.* Macerate powdered gentian in cold æther, concentrate the filtered tincture, and treat the crystalline residue with alcohol. Evaporate the solution, and set it aside to crystallize. Many subsequent steps are necessary to obtain the principle quite pure; but perhaps without any advantage to its medicinal efficacy. It appears to consist of two distinct principles, *Gentisic Acid*, and *Gentianite.* Dose, gr. ss to gr. 1.

GLOBULI CONTRAYERVÆ. These only differ from Pulvis Contrayervæ Comp. in form.

GLOBULI GASCOIGNII. *Gascoign's Balls.* The compound powder of crab's claws formed into balls with mucilage. The original balls contained pearls, and oriental bezoar; and were imitated by the following: crab's claw's ℥vij, calcined hartshorn and amber, each ℥j, powdered seeds of the amomum Plinii ʒij, mucilage q. s.

Globuli Martiales. P. They consist of tartarized iron with aromatics. They are not used in this country.

Glycerinum. *Glycerine*, or *the sweet principle of oil*, is obtained in making Emplastrum plumbi, from the water employed. Pass a current of sulphuretted hydrogen through the water until all the lead is thrown down; filter, and evaporate, *in vacuo* or over sulphuric acid, till the sp. gr. is 1·27. Used externally in skin diseases, diluted with water, or added to poultices.

Gummi Resinæ. See Vegetabilium Preparatio.

Guttæ Aconiti cum Antimonio. Richter. Extract of aconite ʒj, antimonial wine ℥j.

Guttæ Acousticæ. Oil of almonds ʒiv, oil of turpentine ℈ss, tincture of opium ℈ss. See also Balsamum Acousticum.

Guttæ Æthereæ Terebinthinatæ. M. Durande. Sulphuric æther ℈vj, rectified oil of turpentine ℈ij. *In Gallstones*. Dose, ♏xl to f ℈j.

Guttæ Anodynæ. See Liquor Morphiæ Acetatis.

Guttæ Antacidæ. U. C. H. Solution of potash f ℥iij, solution of ammonia f ℥j, myrrh ℥j. Triturate together, and filter.

Guttæ Anthelminticæ. Schwartz. Petroleum ℈iv, tincture of assafœtida ℈vj; dose, 40 drops. See also Oleum Anthelminticum.

Guttæ Antipertussicæ. Dr. Graves, or Dr. Beatty. Tincture of cantharides, and comp. tincture of camphor, of each f ℥ss; comp. tincture of bark f ℥v. A teaspoonful 3 times a day, in Hooping Cough.

Guttæ Antiscrofulosæ. Augustin. Muriate of iron ℈ss, muriate of barytes ℈ss, distilled water ℥j. Dose, from 20 drops.

Guttæ Emmenagogæ. Brande. Compound tincture of aloes f ʒj, tincture of valerian f ʒj, tincture of sesquichloride of iron f ℥ss. Dose, a teaspoonful in chamomile tea.

Guttæ Goddardianæ. This once famous remedy, for which King Charles II. gave 1500 pounds, was merely *oleum animale*, procured from human bones.

GUTTÆ HYDRARGYRI BICHLORIDI. Sir A. COOPER. Bichloride of quicksilver gr. j, tincture of cinchona bark f ℥ij. Dose, f ʒj.

GUTTÆ NIGRÆ. Dr. ARMSTRONG. *Lancaster Black Drop.* Opium ℔ss, verjuice Oiij, bruised nutmegs ℥jss, saffron ℥ss. Boil to a proper thickness, then add 2 spoonfuls of yeast, and let it stand in a warm place for 6 or 8 weeks, then in the open air till it is of the consistence of syrup. Then decant, filter, and bottle, adding a little sugar to each bottle. U. S. (Acetum Opii.) Take of opium in coarse powder ℥viij, nutmeg ℥ss, saffron ℥ss, distilled vinegar, or diluted acetic acid, f ℥xxiv: digest on a sand-bath for 48 hours. Digest the residue in the same quantity of vinegar. Then put the whole into a displacement apparatus, pouring distilled vinegar on the materials so as to obtain f ℥48. Dose, 7 to 10 drops. Similar to Rousseau's Drops. See Vinum Opii Fermentatione Paratum.

GUTTÆ ODONTALGICÆ. *Tooth-ache Drops.* Dr. COPLAND. Opium gr. x, camphor gr. x, rectified spirit q. s., oil of cloves ʒj, oil of cajeput ʒj. Dr. RIGHINI. Rectified spirit ʒiv, creasote ʒvj, tincture of cochineal ℈ij, oil of peppermint 12 drops. Dr. BLAKE. Alum finely powdered ʒj, spirit of nitric æther ℈vij. M. COTTEREAU. Saturate ether (cold) with camphor, and add a few drops of ammonia.

HAUSTUS. *Draughts* are single doses of liquid medicines, and are almost exclusively extemporaneous. A selection of useful formulæ is here given. See also Misturæ.

HAUSTUS ACIDI NITRICI CUM OPIO. Dr. COPLAND. Dilute nitric acid f ʒj, tincture of opium f ʒss, infusion of calumba f ʒxss.

HAUSTUS ACIDI HYDROCYANICI. MID. H. Dilute hydrocyanic acid ♏iv, sesquicarb. soda gr. x, water f ℥jss.

HAUSTUS ÆTHEREUS. Dr. NELIGAN. Sulphuric æther f ʒj, spermaceti gr. ij: rub together, and add peppermint water f ℈x.

HAUSTUS AMMONIÆ. BRANDE. Solution of ammonia ♏xv to xx, comp. tincture of cardamoms f ℈ss, tincture of gentian f ℈ss, camphor mixture f ℥jss.

HAUSTUS AMMONIÆ ACETATIS. Dr. PARIS. Camphor mixture f ℥jss, solution of acetate of ammonia f ʒiv, antimonial wine ♏xx. To this may sometimes be added, tincture of opium ♏x.

HAUSTUS AMMONIÆ CITRATIS. BRANDE. Carbonate of ammonia ℈j, water f ℥jss, citric acid gr. xxiv, syrup of Tolu f ʒss, spirit of nutmeg f ʒss. GUY'S H. (Effervescing.) Sesquicarbonate of ammonia ℈j, water f ℥j; mix, and add lemon-juice f ℥ss.

HAUSTUS AMMONIÆ TARTRATIS. MID. H. Sesquicar. of ammonia gr. xv, tartaric acid ℈j, water f ℥jss.

HAUSTUS ANODYNUS. Dr. COPLAND. Camphor mixture ʒix, nitrate of potash gr. vj, compound spirit of æther f ʒj, tincture of opium ♏x to xij, syrup of poppies f ʒij. To be taken at bedtime.

HAUSTUS ANTACIDUS. Carbonate of soda gr. xv, infusion of gentian (or calumba) f ʒvj, water f ʒvj, tincture of hops f ʒj. See Haustus Calcis Comp.

HAUSTUS ANTI-ARTHRITICUS. Sir H. HALFORD'S *Gout Preventive.* Infusion of gentian f ℥jss, bicarbonate of potash gr. xv, tincture of rhubarb f ʒj.

HAUSTUS ANTI-EMETICUS RIVERII. P. Bicarbonate of potash ʒss, lemon-juice ʒiv, syrup of lemon ℥j, water ℥iij.

HAUSTUS ANTILITHICUS. Dr. VENABLES. Borax gr. viij, bicarbonate of soda gr. x, aërated water f ℥viij. *In Red Gravel.* [Dr. PARIS. Subcarbonate of soda gr. x, infusion of quassia f ℥j, tincture of calumba ʒj.]

HAUSTUS ANTISPASMODICUS. Dr. GREGORY. Fœtid spirit of ammonia f ʒj, camphor mixture f ʒx, syrup of saffron f ʒj.

HAUSTUS APERIENS. Dr. PARIS. Infusion of senna f ℥j, tincture of senna f ʒj, tincture of jalap f ʒj, tartrate of potash ʒj, syrup of senna f ʒj. Mix. Dr. RYAN. Sulphate of magnesia f ʒiv, infusion of senna f ℥jss, tincture of senna f ʒjss, syrup of ginger f ʒj, aromatic spirit of ammonia ♏xx. See also Haustus Sennæ Comp.; H. Jalapæ; H. Scammonii; and Mistura Aperiens.

HAUSTUS APERIENS EFFERVESCENS. Dr. YOUNG. Subcarbonate of soda ʒijss, water f ℥viij, supertartrate of potash ʒiij. Cork securely in a strong bottle. Dr. BARKER. Bisulphate of potash gr. 73, or carbonate of soda 72; water q. s. Dissolve separately, and mix.

HAUSTUS APERIENS SEDLITZENSIS. Bicarbonate of soda ℈ijss, potash-tartrate of soda ʒij, water f ℥vj, or q. s. Dissolve, and add tartaric acid ℈ij. Dr. PARIS prescribes, tartarized soda ʒij, bicarbonate of soda ℈j; to be dissolved in water, and a table spoonful of lemon-juice added.

HAUSTUS AROMATICUS CUM RHEO. ST. B. H. Aromatic confection ʒj, infusion of rhubarb f ʒvj, cinnamon water f ℥vj.

HAUSTUS ASSAFŒTIDÆ CUM AMMONIA. Dr. PARIS. Carbonate of ammonia gr. v, assafœtida gr. iv, compound spirit of lavender f ℥ij, decoction of aloes f ℥x.

HAUSTUS ASTRINGENS. Dr. PARIS. Chalk mixture ℥jss, tincture of opium ♏xv, tincture of catechu f ℥j.

HAUSTUS BALSAMI PERUVIANI. St. B. H. Balsam of Peru f ℥ss, mucilage of acacia f ℥iv, water f ℥v, pimento water f ℥iij.

HASUTUS BALSAMI TOLUTANI. As the last.

HAUSTUS BISMUTHI. Dr. PARIS. Tris-nitrate of bismuth gr. viij, mucilage ℥ij, almond mixture f ℥j. Twenty drops of tincture of henbane, or of solution of muriate of morphia; or ♏xv of aromatic spirit of ammonia, are occasionally added.

HAUSTUS CAJAPUTI. Dr. PARIS. Oil of cajeput ♏iij, white sugar gr. x, infusion of calumba f ʒix, tincture of calumba f ʒj.

HAUSTUS CALCIS COMPOSITA. MID. H. Carb. magnesia gr. v, aromatic sp. of ammonia f ℥ss, lime water f ℥jss.

HAUSTUS CAMPHORÆ. GUY'S H. Camphor gr. vj, spirit q. s., white sugar ʒj, mucilage f ʒiij, water f ℥jss.

HAUSTUS CHLORINII. Dr. COPLAND. Chlorine water f ʒss, water f ℥jss, syrup of poppies f ʒss. *Every* 6 *hours.*

HAUSTUS CINCHONÆ. Dr. JOY. Decoction of bark f ℥jss, extract of bark gr. xv, tincture of bark f ℥j, aromatic spirit of ammonia ♏xxx. BRANDE. Infusion of bark f ʒxj, disulphate of quinine gr. j, comp. tincture of bark f ℥ss, syrup of poppies f ʒss. MID. H. Decoction of yellow bark f ℥vj, infusion of roses f ʒvj, diluted sulphuric acid ♏v.

HAUSTUS COLCHICI. Sir C. SCUDAMORE. Magnesia gr. xv to xx, sulphate of magnesia ℥j to ij, vinegar of colchicum f ℥j to f ʒij, cinnamon or other water f ℥ix, syrup ʒj. BRANDE. Wine of colchicum f ʒss, carbonate of magnesia gr. xv, cinnamon water f ʒiv, water f ℥j. WESTM. H. Colchicum wine f ʒss, solution of sulphate of magnesia ʒiij, carb. of magnesia ℈j, peppermint water f ℥j.

HAUSTUS CONII ET HYOSCYAMI. Dr. PARIS. Extract of hemlock gr. v, extract of henbane gr. v, mucilage f ʒij, solution of acetate of ammonia f ʒiv, water f ℥j, syrup of red poppies f ʒj.

HAUSTUS COPAIBÆ. St. B. H. As H. Balsami Peruviani.

HAUSTUS CRETÆ ET FERRI. Dr. PARIS. Chalk mixture f ℥vij, compound mixture of iron f ʒiij, sesquicarbonate of ammonia gr. v. *In Diarrhœa.*

HAUSTUS CRETÆ CUM RHEO. MID. H. Comp. powder of chalk with opium gr. x, rhubarb gr. xv, comp. tincture of cardamom f ʒss, caraway water f ℥jss.

HAUSTUS DIURETICUS. COPLAND. Acetate of potash ʒss, infusion of quassia f ℥vj, cinnamon water f ʒvj, vinegar of squills f ℥ss, spirit of nitric æther f ℥ss.

HAUSTUS EFFERVESCENS. Sesquicarbonate of soda ʒss, water q. s., dissolve and add f ℥ij of any syrup; then gr. xxv of citric or tartaric acid. See also Haustus Potassæ Citratis.

HAUSTUS EMETICUS. MID. H. Tartar emetic gr. j, ipecacuanha ℈j, water f ℥jss. GUY'S H. Antimonial wine f ℥ij, ipecacuanha wine f ʒvj.

HAUSTUS EMETICUS STIMULANS. SPRAGUE. Carbonate of ammonia ℈j, ipecacuanha ℥ss, peppermint water f ℥iij, tincture of capsicum f ℥ij. Dr. COPLAND prescribes only ♏xx of tinct. of capsicum, and adds oil of chamomile 10 drops. *In Poisoning by Narcotics.*

HAUSTUS EMETICO-CATHARTICUS. Dr. PICKFORD. Sulphate of zinc ℈j, sulphate of magnesia ʒiv, water q. s.

HAUSTUS FERRI EFFERVESCENS. Dr. MACMICHAEL. Bicarbonate of soda ℥j, water f ℥iv; dissolve, and add tinct. of chloride of iron f ℥j.

HAUSTUS FERRI AERATUS. Dr. VENABLES. Sulphate of iron gr. v, bicarbonate of potash gr. xij, aërated water f ℥viij.

HAUSTUS FERRI CUM MAGNESIA. Sir J. MURRAY. Fluid carbonate of magnesia f ℥jss, tincture of muriate of iron ♏x to xxx.

HAUSTUS FERRI IODIDI. A. T. THOMSON. Iodide of iron gr. ij to iv, water f ʒxj, tincture of orange-peel f ℥j. Twice or 3 times a day. [Dr. THOMSON has recently recommended the following form:—Syrup of iodide of iron (Thomson's) f ℥j, nitric acid ♏iij, tincture of roses (Squire's) f ʒj, infusion of orange-peel f ℥jss.]

HAUSTUS FERRI PROTOXYDI. DONOVAN. Calcined magnesia ℈ij, distilled water f ℥vj; triturate together, and add pure sulphate of iron in fine powder ʒiv, and tincture of quassia f ʒij. Put it immediately into ℥j bottles, and secure them from the air. Each draught contains about ℈ss of protoxide of iron.

HAUSTUS GENTIANÆ ET FERRI. GUY'S H. Comp. infusion of gentian f ʒx, tincture of sesquichloride of iron ♏x.

HAUSTUS GUAIACI COMPOSITUS. MID. H. Comp. tincture of guaiacum f ʒj, mucilage f ʒij, camphor mixture f ʒix.

HAUSTUS HYDRIODATIS ARSENICI ET HYDRARGYRI. DONOVAN. Solution of hydriodate of arsenic and mercury (*Liquor Hydriodatis Arsenici et Hydrargyri*) f ʒij, distilled water f ℥iijss, syrup of ginger f ℥ss. Mix, and divide into 4 draughts. One night and morning.

HAUSTUS HYDROCYANICUS. DONOVAN. Cyanide of potassium gr. j, distilled water f ℥iijss, syrup of lemons f ℥ss. Mix, and divide into 8 equal draughts; 1 for a dose.

HAUSTUS HYOSCYAMI CUM SCILLA. Dr. BREE. Extract of henbane gr. iij, tincture of squill ♏x, dilute nitric acid ♏vj, water f ℥jss.

HAUSTUS IPECACUANHÆ CUM SCILLA. St. B. H. Ipecac. wine, oxymel of squills, and weak pimento water, each f ℥ss. Mix.

HAUSTUS IPECACUANHÆ OPIATUS. St. B. H. Ipecacuanha gr. ij, confection of opium ℈j, water f ℥j, pimento water f ℥ss.

HAUSTUS JALAPÆ ET SCILLÆ. COPLAND. Tincture of jalap f ʒij, vinegar of squill f ʒj, mint water f ℥jss.

HAUSTUS LAXANS TONICUS. BRANDE. Sulphate of magnesia ʒss, infusion of roses f ʒvj, infusion of gentian f ʒvj, diluted sulphuric acid ♏x, syrup of ginger, f ʒj. *Daily.*

HAUSTUS LAXANS CUM TARAXACO. COPLAND. Infusion of senna f ʒvj, infusion of gentian (or calumbo) f ʒvj, sulphate of potash ʒss, extract of dandelion ʒss, comp. tincture of cardamoms f ʒjss.

HAUSTUS MAGNESIÆ EFFERVESCENS. Solution of bicarbonate of magnesia f ℥jss, syrup of orange-peel f ʒj, lemon-juice f ʒiij.

HAUSTUS MAGNESIÆ CITRATIS. BRANDE. Carbonate of magnesiæ ʒj, water f ʒix, syrup of balsam of Tolu f ʒj, spirit of nutmeg f ʒss, lemon-juice f ʒiij.

Haustus Magnesiæ Sulphatis. St. B. H. Sulphate of magnesia ʒvj, manna ʒiv, mint water f ℥ij.

Haustus Magnesiæ Sulphatis Acidus. Sulphate of magnesia ʒiij, peppermint water f ℥ij, tincture of jalap f ʒj, diluted nitric acid ♏xx.

Haustus Narcotinæ. Mr. Jeston. Narcotine gr. ij, diluted sulphuric acid ♏xx, infusion of roses f ℥jss. *Every 2 hours in the intermissions of Neuralgia.*

Haustus Niger. *Black Draught.* See Haustus Aperiens, Haustus Sennæ, Mistura Sennæ, and Mistura Aperiens.

Haustus Nitratis Potassæ. Nitre gr. xv, gum arabic gr. x, almond mixture f ℥jss.

Haustus Nucis Vomicæ. Dr. Joy. Powdered nux vomica gr. iij, powdered gum acacia ʒij, cinnamon water f ℥jss, comp. tincture of cardamoms f ʒj.

Haustus Olei Ricini. Guy's H. Castor oil ʒiv, yolk of egg q. s., syrup f ʒj, cassia or other distilled water f ℥j.

Haustus Opiatus. St. B. H. Tincture of opium ♏xij, water f ℥j, pimento water ʒiij, syrup of red poppies f ʒj.

Haustus Opii cum Antimonio. Add to the last, antimonial wine ♏xx.

Haustus Potassæ Acetatis. Mid. H. Acetate of potash ℥ss, bicarbonate of potash ℈j, peppermint water f ʒjss.

Haustus Potassæ Citratis. St. B. H. Carbonate of potash ℈j, water f ʒjss; dissolve, and add at the time of taking, citric acid gr. xvij. Guy's H. Carbonate of potash ℈j, mint water ʒjss, lemon juice f ʒiv.

Haustus Potassæ Tartratis. Mid. H. Bicarbonate of potash ℈j, tartaric acid gr. xv, sugar gr. vj, water f ʒj.

Haustus Quassiæ et Ferri. Dr. Paris. Infusion of quassia f ʒx, tincture of muriate of iron ♏x, tincture of calumbo f ʒj.

Haustus Quinæ. St. Geo. H. Disulphate of quinine gr. ij, dil. sulphuric acid ♏iv, water f ʒxj, tincture of orange-peel f ʒj.

Haustus Quinæ Acidus. Sulphate of quinine gr. ij. dilute sulphuric acid f ʒss, water f ʒixss, comp. tincture of cardamoms f ʒj, syrup f ʒj.

HAUSTUS QUINÆ ET ZINCI. COPLAND. Sulphate of zinc gr. ¼ to j, sulphate of quinine gr. ij, infusion of roses f ℥x, tincture and syrup of orange-peel each f ℥j.

HAUSTUS SCAMMONII. Dr. PARIS. Pure scammony gr. ij, sulphate of potash gr. x, mucilage f ℥ij, almond mixture f ℥j, spirit of nutmegs f ʒss. See also Mistura Scammonii, E., and Emulsio Purgans cum Scammonio, P.

HAUSTUS SCOPARII COMPOSITUS. St. B. H. Decoction of broom-tops f ℥xj, spirit of juniper f ℥j, tartrate of potash ℥j.

HAUSTUS SENNÆ. St. B. H. Infusion of senna ʒxj, sulphate of magnesia ʒjss, oil of peppermint ¼ of a drop.

HAUSTUS SENNÆ COMPOSITUS. GUY'S H. *Black Draught.* Senna ℥x, mint ℥x, boiling water Oij. Macerate for an hour, strain, and add sulphate of magnesia ℥viij. Dose, f ʒij to f ℥iv.

HAUSTUS TEREBINTHINÆ. As Haustus Balsami Tolutani.

HAUSTUS TONICUS. Disulphate of quinine gr. ij, diluted sulphuric acid ♏ v, infusion of cascarilla, or of gentian f ℥x, compound tincture of cardamoms f ℥jss, syrup of orange-peel f ʒj.

HEDERINUM. *Hederine.* By boiling the seeds of ivy (Hedera helix) in water with a little slaked lime, treating the dried precipitate with alcohol, and evaporating the filtered solution. *Febrifuge.*

HYDRARGYRI ACETAS. P. Dissolve protonitrate of mercury in 3 or 4 times its weight of water, slightly acidulated with nitric acid; and add to it gradually a solution of acetate of soda in slight excess. Wash the precipitate with cold water, and dry it in the shade. D. directs the acetate of potash. Dose, ⅙th of a gr. to 1 gr.

HYDRARGYRI AMMONIO-CHLORIDUM. L. and E. *White Precipitate.* Bichloride of mercury ʒvj, distilled water Ovj; dissolve by heat, and when cold add solution of ammonia f ℥viij, stirring occasionally. Wash the precipitate with cold water till tasteless, and dry it. [D. directs water of ammonia to be added to the liquor poured off from precipitated calomel. See Calomelas Precipitatum.]

HYDRARGYRI ET AMMONIÆ MURIAS. P. *Sal Alembroth.* Equal parts of bichloride of quicksilver and muriate of ammonia levigated together.

HYDRARGYRI BICYANIDUM. L. (Hydrargyri Cyanuretum, D.) Boil ʒviij of Prussian blue with ʒx binoxide of mercury in Oiv of distilled water for half an hour, and filter; evaporate and crystallize, wash what remains frequently with boiling distilled water, and evaporate the mixed liquors for more crystals. [It may also be made by adding red oxide of mercury to hydrocyanic acid. D. directs 6 parts of Prussian blue, 5 of nitric oxide of mercury, and 40 of distilled water.]

HYDRARGYRI BICHLORIDUM. L. (Sublimatus Corrosivus, E. Hydrargyri Murias Corrosivum, D.) *Corrosive Sublimate.* Quicksilver ℔ij, sulphuric acid ℔iij, boil to dryness, and when cooled, rub the mass with chloride of sodium ℔jss in an earthenware mortar; then sublime by a gradually increased heat. E. by a similar process from mercury ℥iv, sulphuric acid f℥ij fʒiij, pure nitric acid f℥ss, muriate of soda ʒiij. D. from 5 parts of persulphate of mercury, and 2 of dried muriate of soda. Dr. A. T. THOMSON's patent method of making this salt is by burning quicksilver in chlorine gas.

HYDRARGYRI CHLORIDUM. L. (Calomelas, E.; C. Sublimatum, D. Hydrargyri Chloridum Mite, U. S.) *Calomel.* Quicksilver ℔ij, sulphuric acid ℔iij; boil to dryness, and when cooled, rub the bipersulphate of mercury with ℔ij of quicksilver so as to mix them perfectly, and add chloride of sodium ℔jss, and rub them together till the globules disappear; then sublime. Rub the sublimate into a very fine powder, and wash it thoroughly with boiling distilled water, and dry it. E. by a similar process from ℥viij of mercury, f℥ij fʒiij of sulphuric acid, f℥ss pure nitric acid, fʒiij of muriate of soda. D. from 25 parts of persulphate of mercury, 17 parts of pure quicksilver, and 10 of dried muriate of soda. U. S. as L., but directs the washings to be tested with ammonia. [When sublimed into a vessel containing steam, it forms the *hydro-sublimed calomel.*]

HYDRARGYRI CHLORO-IODIDUM. M. CAVENTOU. Dissolve bichloride of mercury in alcohol, and add an equal weight of biniodide of mercury; then carefully evaporate the mixed solutions to dryness. It is said to be more active than either of its constituents.

HYDRARGYRI IODIDUM. L. Quicksilver ʒj, iodine ʒv; rub together, with a few drops of alcohol, till they combine; dry in the dark by a gentle heat, and keep it in a well-stopped bottle. [MIALHE states that protoiodide of mercury, prepared by trituration, always contains a portion of biniodide, which should be removed by alcohol.]

Hydrargyri Biniodidum. L. Mercury ℥j, iodine ʒx, alcohol q. s., proceed as in the last. E. directs it to be dissolved by boiling in Oiv of strong solution of salt, from which it is deposited in crystals. [A brighter product is obtained by precipitation. P. dissolve separately 100 parts of iodide of potassium, and 80 parts of bichloride of mercury in a large quantity of distilled water; add the latter solution to the former so long as a precipitate is produced, avoiding excess, (or rather leaving a slight excess of iodide of potassium, which is essential to obtaining a very bright-coloured product.) Wash with distilled water, and dry in the shade, by a very gentle heat.]

Hydrargyri Nitras. See Hydr. Proto-nitras, and Deuto-nitras, below.

Hydrargyri Proto-nitras. P. Put into a large flat-bottomed glass matrass equal parts of pure quicksilver, and nitric acid at 1·321 density; leave them in a cool place for 24 hours, remove the crystals, place them in a glass funnel, wash them with a little nitric acid, drain them, and keep them in closely-stopped bottles.

Hydrargyri Deuto-nitras Liquidus. P. (Acid nitrate of mercury.) Dissolve 1 part of quicksilver in 2 parts of nitric acid at 1·321 density; and evaporate the solution to three-fourths of its original weight. [Used as a caustic applied with a camel-hair brush.]

Hydrargyri Subnitras. Dr. Duncan. Dissolve mercury in excess of nitric acid by heat; pour the solution into water, collect the precipitate, and dry it. A darker coloured precipitate is obtained by boiling this in water. [Both are used for making extemporaneous Unguentum Hydrargyri Nitratis; ℈ij of the powder being mixed with ℥j of simple or spermaceti cerate. But the ointment so made is not identical with that of the Pharmacopœia.]

Hydrargyri et Potassii Iodo-cyanidum. Hydrargyro-iodo-cyanide of potassium. To a concentrated solution of bicyanide of mercury, add a solution of iodide of potassium, collect the crystalline precipitate, and dry it by a gentle heat. *As a test for foreign acids in prussic acid.*

Hydrargyri et Potassii Iodidum. Iodohydrargyrate of iodide of potassium. M. Boullay. Iodide of potassium 10 parts, biniodide of mercury 25 parts, distilled water 10 parts. Boil together in a glass matrass till the biniodide of mercury is dissolved; let the solution cool, pour off the clear liquid, and crystallize by evaporation and refrigeration. See Solutio Iodo-hydrargyratis Potassii.

HYDRARGYRI OXYDUM. L. Calomel ℥j, lime water Cj; mix, agitate together, set it aside, decant, wash the powder with distilled water, and dry it in the air wrapped in bibulous paper. D. (Hyd. ox. nigrum.) Calomel 1 part, warm solution of caustic potash 4 parts. Wash the precipitate, and dry it with a medium heat. [Mr. TYSON says the oxide is most effectually obtained by treating calomel first with solution of potash, and then with ammonia.]

HYDRARGYRI BINOXYDUM. L. Formerly made by keeping mercury in a tall glass heated to 600° till converted into red scales. Now precipitated from a solution of ℥iv of bichloride of mercury in Ovj of distilled water, by f℥xxviij of solution of potash. The precipitate to be carefully washed, and dried.

HYDRARGYRI OXYDUM RUBRUM. E. Mercury ℥viij, dilute nitric acid (sp. gr. 1280,) f℥v; dissolve half the mercury in the acid with heat, and evaporate to dryness, triturate the rest of the mercury with the dry salt, and heat the powder in porcelain, with constant stirring, until acid fumes cease to be discharged. D. Expose purified mercury in an open glass vessel, with a narrow mouth and broader bottom, to a heat of 600° until converted into red scales.

HYDRARGYRI NITRICO-OXYDUM. L. Quicksilver ℔iij, nitric acid ℔jss, water Oij; heat gently till the quicksilver is dissolved; boil to dryness, powder the residue, and heat it in a shallow vessel till the red vapours cease. D. (Hydr. oxydum nitricum) nearly the same.

HYDRARGYRI OXYDUM SULPHURICUM. D. See Hydrargyri Subsulphas Flavus.

HYDRARGYRI PRECIPITATUM ALBUM. E. As Hydr. Ammonio-chloridum, L.

HYDRARGYRI PRECIPITATUM NIGRUM. HAHNEMANN'S *Soluble Mercury.* Dissolve proto-nitrate of mercury by triturating it with distilled water slightly acidulated with nitric acid; and add to the filtered solution, by small quantities, solution of ammonia diluted with 15 or 20 times its weight of water, so long as the precipitate formed is nearly black, stirring with a glass rod. Wash the powder, and dry it in the shade. Dose ½ to 1 grain.

HYDRARGYRI PHOSPHAS. PRUS. PH. To a solution of nitrate of mercury, add solution of phosphate of soda acidulated with a little nitric acid. Wash and dry the precipitate.

HYDRARGYRI ET QUINÆ CHLORIDUM. *Double Chloride of Mercury and Quinine.* M'DERMOTT. Dissolve 1 part of bichloride of mercury, and 3 parts of hydrochlorate of quina, separately, in the smallest quantity of water, and mix the solutions. Collect the salt which separates, and dry it with a gentle heat. See Pil. Hydr. et Quinæ Chloridi.

HYDRARGYRI SUBMURIAS. See Hydrargyri Chloridum.

HYDRARGYRI SUBMURIAS AMMONIATUM. D. See Hydr. Ammonio-chloridum.

HYDRARGYRI PER-SULPHAS. *Bipersulphate of Mercury.* D. Quicksilver 6 parts, sulphuric acid 6 parts, nitric acid 1 part. Heat them in a glass vessel, till a dry white mass be obtained. [It is also formed in the L. process for making calomel.]

HYDRARGYRI SUB-SULPHAS FLAVUS. Hydr. Oxydum Sulphuricum. D. *Turpeth Mineral.* Triturate 1 part of persulphate of mercury with 20 parts of warm water, and pour off the supernatant liquor; wash the yellow powder with warm distilled water till the decanted fluid yields no precipitate with solution of potash, and dry it.

HYDRARGYRI SULPHURETUM CUM SULPHURE. L. (Hydrargyri Sulphuretum nigrum. D.) *Æthiops Mineral.* Rub together equal parts of quicksilver and sulphur till the globules are no longer visible. Dose from 5 to 30 grains *as an alterative.*

HYDRARGYRI BISULPHURETUM. L. *Vermilion,* or *factitious Cinnabar.* Quicksilver ℔ij, sulphur ℥v; mix the quicksilver with the sulphur liquefied over the fire, and as soon as the mass swells up, remove the vessel from the fire, and cover it firmly lest it inflame; then rub it into powder and sublime. Dose, as the last. Also used in mercurial fumigation, D. (*Hydr. Sulphuretum rubrum*) by the same process, from 19 parts of purified mercury, and 3 of sublimed sulphur.

HYDRARGYRI TARTRAS. P. *Proto-tartrate of Mercury* is made by adding a solution of proto nitrate of mercury in water slightly acidulated with nitric acid, to a solution of tartrate of potash as long as a precipitate forms. Wash it with distilled water, dry it in the shade, and keep it in bottles covered with black paper. Dose, 1 to 2 grains.

HYDRARGYRI POTASSIO-TARTRAS. A double salt (or a variable mixture of tartrate of mercury, tartrate of potash, and cream of tartar, SOUBEIRAN) was formerly used. Its solution formed *Liqueur de Pressavin;* but its effects were found uncertain.

HYDRARGYRI ET AMMONIÆ NITRAS. WARD. Nitric acid ℥xvj, add gradually sesquicarbonate of ammonia ℥viij; afterwards digest in a sand-bath with ℥iv of quicksilver, and when that quantity is dissolved, add more quicksilver by small quantities till the fluid ceases to act on it. Then evaporate the solution, and crystallize by refrigeration.

HYDRARGYRUM PURIFICATUM. P. Distil quicksilver from an iron or earthen retort, to which is fixed a flexible tube formed of folded linen, moistened, and dipping into water. Dry the distilled metal, and pass it through chamois leather. [Quicksilver may also be purified by heating it to 104° F., agitating it with a little strong solution of nitrate of mercury, and straining.]

HYDRARGYRUM CUM CRETA. L. & E. Quicksilver ℥iij, prepared chalk ℥v, rub together till the globules are no longer visible. D., as Hyd. cum Magnesia, substituting precipitated carbonate of lime for carb. magnesia. Dose, from 5 to 20 grains. A little water is said to aid the extinction of the mercury. [Mr. TYSON substitutes a mixture of one part of his black protoxide of mercury with 2 of prepared chalk, but this should not be used except when expressly ordered.]

HYDRARGYRUM CUM MAGNESIA. D. Quicksilver 2 parts, manna 2 parts, carbonate of magnesia 1 part. Rub the quicksilver and manna together, with enough water to give them the consistence of syrup, till the globules disappear; then add, still triturating, ⅛ part of the magnesia, and after the whole is well mixed, add 16 parts of hot water, and agitate the mixture. When it has settled, decant the fluid, and repeat the washing a second and third time. Then add the rest of the magnesia, and dry the powder on bibulous paper. [This contains nearly twice as much quicksilver as Hyd. cum Creta.]

HYDROLATA. Distilled waters. See Aquæ Destillatæ.

HYDROGENIUM. *Hydrogen* is readily procured by adding dilute sulphuric acid to fragments of zinc. *Carburetted* Hydrogen, in the form of coal gas, is sometimes employed as a palliative in consumption. Dr. R. CLANNY recommends it to be passed through water, then agitated with fresh precipitated carbonate of lead, and mixed in the gasometer with an equal quantity of common air. 12 cubic inches of the mixed gas to be inspired 3 or 4 times a day, and the quantity gradually increased to 20 C. I. For *Sulphuretted* Hydrogen, see Acidum Hydrosulphuricum.

HYDROMEL. P. Fine honey ℥ij, boiling water ℥xxxij. Dissolve, and filter.

INFUSA. *Infusions.* The ingredients, divided by bruising or cutting, being put into a warm vessel, boiling distilled water is to be poured on them, and the vessel covered. Having macerated the time prescribed, the liquor is to be strained off, through linen or calico. For infusions containing *acids*, vessels of glass, or of earthenware not glazed with lead, should be used. In a few instances, *cold* water is used, but unless so directed, boiling water is to be understood. Many substances might be advantageously treated by displacement to obtain infusions of any desired strength. The usual dose of infusions is from f℥j to f℥ij, or a wineglassful. The principal exceptions will be noticed.

INFUSUM ABSINTHII. BRANDE. Fresh wormwood ℥ij, boiling water Oj; macerate for 4 hours, and strain. Others direct from ℥ss to ℥j of the dry herb to Oj of water.

INFUSUM ABROTANI. TADDEI. Southernwood ℥j, boiling water Oj. Infuse 2 hours, and strain.

INFUSUM ACORI CALAMI. Dr. PARIS. Calamus root ʒvj, boiling water f℥xij. Macerate 2 hours. Dr. COPLAND, ʒiij to Oss.

INFUSUM ALLII. Mr. WHITE. Garlic ℔ss, water ℔j; let them digest in an oven for some hours, and strain. Two spoonfuls before and after every meal, *in epilepsy*.

INFUSUM ALKALINUM. Hickory ash Oj, wood soot O¼, boiling water cong. ½. Let them stand 24 hours, and decant. A wineglassful 3 or 4 times a day. A popular remedy in America for dyspepsia.

INFUSUM ALOES COMPOSITUM. Dr. FOTHERGILL. Aloes ʒj, rhubarb ʒiv, calumbo ʒiv, lime water f℥viij, spirit of horseradish fʒiv. Infuse 12 hours in a close vessel, and strain.

INFUSUM AMARUM PURGANS. L. 1746. Similar to Mist. Gentianæ Co.

INFUSUM ANGELICÆ. Angelica root from ʒiv to ℥j, boiling water Oj.

INFUSUM ANISI. Dr. PROUT. Aniseed ʒiv, warm water (at 120° F.) Oss. Infuse till cold.

INFUSUM ANTHEMIDIS. L. & E. Chamomile flowers ʒv, boiling water Oj. Macerate for 10 minutes, (20 minutes, E.) and strain. D., ʒij in f ℥viij, 24 hours.

INFUSUM ANTISCORBUTICUM. E. H. Marsh-trefoil ℥ij, orange-peel ℥ss, boiling water Oiij; infuse for a night, and add compound spirit of horse-radish ℥iv.

INFUSUM ARMORACIÆ COMP. L. & D. Horse-radish root ℥j, black mustard-seed ℥j, boiling water Oj (f ℥xvj, D.); macerate for 2 hours, (6 hours, D.) strain, and add comp. spirit of horse-radish f ℥j. [This infusion is more pungent if made in a *cold* jug, or with water below the boiling point. Mr. GREENISH.]

INFUSUM ARNICÆ MONTANÆ. PEREIRA. Arnica flowers ℥ss, boiling water Oj, macerate 2 hours, and strain. A. T. THOMSON. Leaves or flowers ʒjss, or ℈ij of the root, to f ℥xij of water.

INFUSUM AURANTII COMPOSITUM. L. & D. (Inf. Aurantii, E.) Dried bitter orange-peel ℥ss, fresh lemon-peel ʒij, cloves ʒj, boiling water Oj; macerate for 15 minutes, and strain.

INFUSUM AYÆ-PANÆ COMPOSITUM. Dr. CAMERA'S Sudorific Infusion. Leaves of Brazilian ayapana ʒij, aniseed ʒj, boiling water ℔ij.

INFUSUM BERBERIS. COPLAND. Barberry bark ℥j, boiling water Oj; macerate for 2 hours. *In jaundice*, &c.

INFUSUM BELLADONNÆ. Dr. PARIS. Dried belladonna gr. iv, boiling water f ℥ij. Infuse, for one dose. Dr. SAUNDERS prescribes ʒss of dried leaves to f ℥xij of water, adding to f ℥vij of the strained infusion f ℥j of comp. tincture of cardamoms.

INFUSUM BUCHU. E. & D. See Inf. Diosmæ.

INFUSUM CAFFEI. Dr. MACBRIDE. Macerate 30 unroasted coffee berries in Oij of cold water. Dose, Oss every morning *in calculous disorders*. M. HONORE gives daily an infusion of ʒvj roasted coffee in Oss of water, in *albuminuria*. BOUCHARDAT prescribes a strong infusion, by percolation, with the addition of a little brandy, in poisoning by opium, after emetics and ioduretted water.

INFUSUM CALUMBÆ. L. & D. Calumba root ʒv, boiling water Oj; infuse for 2 hours.

INFUSUM CALUMBÆ [cum Aqua Frigida]. E. Calumba in coarse powder ʒiv, triturate it with a little cold water so as to moisten it thoroughly, put it into a percolator, and transmit cold water through it till f ℥xvj of infusion be obtained.

INFUSUM CAPSICI. PEREIRA. Powdered capsicum ʒiv, boiling water Oj; macerate for 2 hours, and strain. Dose, f ʒiv. [A weaker infusion, gr. viij to f ℥viij of water, has been dropped in the eye in *Amaurosis.*]

INFUSUM CAPSICI COMPOSITUM. STEPHEN'S Pepper Medicine. Two table-spoonfuls of red pepper, 2 teaspoonsful of salt, boiling water Oss; when cold, strain, and add Oss of vinegar.

INFUSUM CARDUI BENEDICTI. NIEMANN. Blessed thistle (Cnicus benedictus) ʒvj, boiling water ℔j. A. T. THOMSON directs ʒvj of the herb to f ℥xvj of cold water. The warm infusion promotes vomiting and perspiration; the cold is tonic and stomachic.

INFUSUM CARYOPHYLLI. L. & E. Cloves ʒiij, boiling water Oj; macerate for 2 hours and strain. D., ʒj of cloves to f ℥viij of water.

INFUSUM CASCARILLÆ. L. & E. Cascarilla ℥jss, boiling water Oj; macerate 2 hours. D. nearly the same.

INFUSUM CASSIÆ. *Eau de Casse.* SOUBEIRAN. Cassia pods, bruised, ℥iv, boiling water Ojss. Infuse 6 hours, and strain. See Mistura Cassiæ.

INFUSUM CATECHU. E. Catechu ʒvj, cinnamon ʒj, boiling water f ℥xvij; infuse for 2 hours, strain, and add syrup f ℥iij.

INFUSUM CATECHU COMPOSITUM. L. & D. Catechu ʒvj, cinnamon ʒj, boiling water Oj; macerate an hour.

INFUSUM CENTAUREÆ. See Inf. Cardui Benedicti.

INFUSUM CENTAURII. Common centaury (Erythrea centaurium) ʒiv, boiling water Oj.

INFUSUM CEPHALICUM. E. H. Valerian root ℥ij, rosemary ʒiv, boiling water Oiij; infuse for 12 hours, strain, and add aromatic water ℥iv.

INFUSUM CHIRETTÆ. E. Chiretta ʒiv, boiling water Oj; macerate 2 hours, and strain. [Dr. ROYLE states that water of not more than 180° is preferable.]

INFUSUM CIMICIFUGÆ RACEMOSÆ. Black snake root ℥j, boiling water Oj, macerate for 2 hours. In *Rheumatism, Dropsies, affections of the Lungs, &c.*

INFUSUM CINCHONÆ. L. & E. Peruvian bark (pale, L., of any species prescribed, E.) ℥j, boiling water Oj; macerate 6 (4, E.) hours, and strain.

INFUSUM CINCHONÆ [sine calore]. D. powdered bark (pale) ℥j, cold water f℥xij; rub the bark with a little of the water, add the rest, macerate 24 hours, and filter. GUY'S H. directs fʒxij of tincture of bark to be added after straining; and the yellow bark to be used.

INFUSUM CINCHONÆ CUM AQUA CALCIS. U. S. Powdered bark ℥j, lime water f℥xvj; macerate 12 hours in a covered vessel.

INFUSUM CINCHONÆ CUM MAGNESIA. U. S. Powdered bark ℥j, calcined magnesia ʒj, water f℥xij; boil, digest for an hour, and strain. [The last 2 are now rejected.]

INFUSUM CINCHONÆ COMP. ST. B. H. Bark ℥j, orange-peel ʒij, red rose ʒiij, boiling water Oj, macerate for 2 hours, strain, and add diluted sulphuric acid ʒjss. U. S. Powdered bark ℥j, aromatic sulphuric acid fʒj, water f℥xvj; macerate for 12 hours, stirring occasionally, and strain.

INFUSUM CONII. GUY'S H. Dried hemlock ʒij, coriander seed ʒij, boiling water f℥viij. Infuse and strain. (Now rejected.)

INFUSUM CORNUS CIRCINATÆ. Dr. IVES. Coarsely powdered bark of the round-leaved dogwood ℥j, boiling water f℥xvj. Dose, f℥j to ℥ij.

INFUSUM CUSPARIÆ. L. Cusparia bark ʒv, boiling water Oj; macerate for 2 hours, and strain.

INFUSUM DAUCI. WOODVILLE. 3 spoonfuls of carrot seed (℥j SPRAGUE) in Oj of water. *Diuretic.*

INFUSUM DIGITALIS. L. Dried fox-glove leaves ʒj, boiling water Oj; macerate for 4 hours, strain, and add spirit of cinnamon f℥j. Dose, from fʒij to f℥j or f℥jss, carefully watching its effects. *Diuretic and Sedative.*

N.B. This is less than half the strength directed in L. 1824. D. directs ʒj of leaves to f℥viij of water, with f℥ss sp. of cinnamon. E. ʒij of leaves to f℥xviij of water, adding f℥ij of sp. of cinnamon. U. S. ʒj to f℥viij of water, with f℥j of tincture of cinnamon.

INFUSUM DIOSMÆ. L. (Inf. Buchu, E. & D.) Buchu leaves ℥j, boiling water Oj; macerate for 4 (2, E.) hours, and strain. D. ʒiv to f℥viij. Dose, ℥jss.

INFUSUM ERGOTÆ. PEREIRA. Bruised ergot ʒj, boiling water f℥iv; macerate till cold. For three doses.

INFUSUM ERIGERONIS CANADENSIS. Canadian fleabane ℥j, boiling water f℥xvj. *Diuretic and astringent.*

INFUSUM EUPATORII. U. S. Dried thoroughwort (Eupatorium perfoliatum) ℥j, boiling water f℥xvj; macerate for two hours, and strain. Dose, as a tonic, a wine-glassful three or four times a day. As a diaphoretic and emetic, larger doses of the warm infusion. Dr. PEEBLES gives f℥jss, warm, every half hour until perspiration and nausea, or vomiting are induced, in *Influenza.*

INFUSUM FŒNICULI. GUY'S H. Fennel seeds ʒvj, boiling water f℥xij; macerate half an hour.

INFUSUM GALLÆ. AUSTR. PH. Nutgalls ℥ij, boiling water Oj.

INFUSUM GENTIANÆ COMPOSITUM. L. *Infusum Amarum.* Gentian root ʒij, dried orange-peel ʒij, fresh lemon-peel ʒiv, boiling water Oj; macerate for an hour, and strain. E. (Inf. Gentianæ.) Gentian ʒiv, orange-peel ʒj, coriander seed ʒj, proof spirit f℥iv; pour the spirit upon the solids, in three hours add f℥xvj of cold water; and in twelve hours strain through linen or calico. D. Dried orange-peel, gentian, fresh lemon-peel, of each ʒj, boiling water f℥xij.

INFUSUM GINSENG. CHINESE form. Ginseng root ℈ij, ginger ℈j, water ℥vj. Digest in a water-bath for 2 hours, add ℈j of cinnamon, and when cold, strain.

INFUSUM GLYCYRRHIZÆ. ST. B. H. Fresh liquorice-root ℥j, boiling water Oj; macerate for 2 hours, and strain.

INFUSUM GRATIOLÆ. A. T. THOMSON. Dried hedge hyssop ʒij, boiling water f℥viij; macerate, and strain. Dose, f℥ss. *Diuretic, cathartic, and emetic.*

INFUSUM HELLEBORI FŒTIDI. WOODVILLE. Fresh stinking hellebore ʒij, (or ʒss of dry,) boiling water f℥viij; macerate for an hour, and strain. Dose, f℥j. *Vermifuge.*

INFUSUM HELMINTHOCORTI. FARR. Corsican moss ʒiv, boiling water f℥xvj. Digest 10 or 12 hours, and strain. By glassfuls, in *Cancer*, &c.

INFUSUM HEMEDESMI. Dr. ASHBURNER. Root of hemedesmus indicus ℥ij, lime water Oj; infuse in a close vessel for 12 hours.

INFUSUM HERNARIÆ. Rupture-wort ʒij, boiling water Oj.

INFUSUM HUMULI. See Infusum Lupuli.

INFUSUM HISPANICUM. BUCHAN. Foreign extract of liquorice (Spanish juice) ℈j, subcarbonate of potash ʒiij, boiling water Oij; infuse for a night, decant, and add syrup of poppies ℥ss.

INFUSUM HYSSOPI. RATIER. Hyssop leaves ʒijss, liquorice ʒij, boiling water Oij. *In catarrhal complaints.*

INFUSUM INULÆ. Elecampane root ʒv, boiling water Oj.

INFUSUM JAPONICUM. See Infusum Catechu.

INFUSUM JUGLANDIS. M. NEGRIER. Fresh walnut leaves ℥j, boiling water f℥xij; infuse till cold, and strain. Dose, f℥iv, two or three times a day.

INFUSUM JUNIPERI. PEREIRA. Juniper berries ℥j, boiling water Oj; macerate for an hour.

INFUSUM JUNIPERI [COMPOSITUM]. GUY'S H. Juniper berries ℥ijss, boiling water Oj; macerate for 2 hours, and strain; then add compound spirit of juniper fʒx, and occasionally, bitartrate of potash ℈j. Dose, f℥ij three times a day.

INFUSUM JUSTICIÆ. Root of panicled justicia ℈ij, boiling water Oj. *A powerful bitter.*

INFUSUM KRAMERIÆ. L. Rhatany root ℥j, boiling water Oj macerate for 4 hours, and strain. *Astringent.*

INFUSUM LACMI. Litmus ʒj, boiling distilled water f℥iij.

INFUSUM LAURI NOBILIS. Dr. NELIGAN. Bay leaves or berries ʒjss, boiling water f℥xij; macerate, and strain. Dose, f℥ss to f℥jss. *Stimulant.*

INFUSUM LAURO-CERASI. Dr. CHESTON. Fresh leaves of the cherry-laurel ℥iv, boiling water f℥xxxij; infuse for an hour, strain, and add clarified honey ℥iv. *For outward application to malignant ulcers.*

INFUSUM LINI COMPOSITUM. L. and E. Linseed (bruised, L., unbruised, E.) ʒvj, liquorice root ʒij, boiling water Oj; macerate near the fire for 4 hours, and strain. D. and U. S. bruised linseed ℥j, liquorice ℥ss, boiling water f℥xxxij.

INFUSUM LINI CATHARTICI. A. T. THOMSON. Dried purging flax ʒij, boiling water Oj; infuse for an hour. Dose, f℥ij? LEWIS directs a handful of the fresh plant to be infused in whey, for a dose.

INFUSUM LIRIODENDRI. Dr. WOOD. Bark of liriodendron tulipifera ℥j, boiling water f℥xvj. Dose, f℥j–ij. *Tonic, stimulant, and diaphoretic.*

INFUSUM LUPULI. L. Dried hops ʒvj, boiling water Oj; macerate for 4 hours, and strain.

INFUSUM MALAMBO. URE. Malambo bark ʒij, boiling water Oj. *An aromatic tonic.* Dose, f℥j–ij, 3 times a day.

INFUSUM MATTICONIS. Dr. H. LANE. Leaves of matico ℥j, boiling water Oj. Macerate for 2 hours, and strain. *Astringent.* Dose, ℥ss to f℥jss. *It is also used as an injection.*

INFUSUM MATTICONIS ET SENNÆ. Dr. WATMOUGH. Matico 3ij, senna ʒij, boiling water Oj. Dose, f℥jss repeatedly.

INFUSUM MELISSÆ. PLENCK. Fresh balm ʒv, boiling water Oj; infuse for ¼ of an hour.

INFUSUM MENTHÆ SIMPLEX. D. Dried mint ʒij, boiling water q. s. to produce f℥vj of strained infusion. Digest for half an hour, and strain.

INFUSUM MENTHÆ COMPOSITUM. D. Add to the last, when strained and cold, white sugar ʒij, oil of spearmint 3 drops, dissolved in comp. tincture of cardamom f℥ss.

INFUSUM MENTHÆ COMPOSITUM. [Acidum.] GUY'S H. Dried mint ℥ij, red roses ℈iv, boiling water Oj, diluted sulphuric acid fʒij, macerate for ½ an hour, strain, and add sugar ℥jss.

INFUSUM MENYANTHIS. Dried buckbean ʒv, boiling water Oj. Tonic, alterative, and cathartic. Dose, f℥j to f℥jss.

INFUSUM MILLEFOLII. Dried yarrow ʒx, boiling water Oj. In hæmorrhoidal affections, nervous debility, &c. Externally as a vulnerary.

INFUSUM NARCISSI. DUFRESNOY. Daffodil flowers from 3 to 16, boiling water Oj. *In Hooping Cough.*

INFUSUM NUCIS VOMICÆ. MANCHESTER H. Bruised nux vomica ʒj, boiling water Oj; infuse. Dose, ℥ss.

INFUSUM PAREIRÆ. L. and E. Pareira brava root ʒvj, boiling

water Oj, macerate for 2 hours, and strain. Dose, f ℥j–ij. Sir B. BRODIE prefers the decoction.

INFUSUM PERSICÆ. PEREIRA. Dried peach leaves ℥ss, boiling water Oj. Laxative and vermifuge. Dose, f ʒiv, 3 times a day.

INFUSUM PHELLANDRII. BIRD. Seeds of water-fennel ʒv, boiling water Oj. Dose, f ℥ss, to check excessive expectoration.

INFUSUM PICIS. See Aqua Picis Liquidæ.

INFUSUM PIMPINELLÆ. Root of burnet-saxifrage ℥j, boiling water f ℥xvj.

INFUSUM PRUNI VIRGINIANÆ. U. S. Wild cherry bark ℥ss, cold water f ℥xvj. Infuse for 24 hours; or it may be made by percolation. Tonic and calmative. Dose, f ℥ij.

INFUSUM QUASSIÆ. L. E. D. Quassia ℈ij [ʒj E., ℈ijss D.], boiling water Oj; macerate for 2 hours. U. S. ʒij of quassia to f ℥xvj of cold water—12 hours.

INFUSUM QUASSIÆ CUM ZINCI SULPHATE. Quassia ʒj, sulphate of zinc gr. viij, cold water f ℥viij.

INFUSUM RHEI. L. and D. Rhubarb ʒiij (D. ʒijss), boiling water Oj; macerate for 2 hours. E. Rhubarb ℥j, boiling water f ℥xviij; infuse for 12 hours, strain, and add spirit of cinnamon f ℥ij.

INFUSUM RHEI ALKALINUM. Dr. COPLAND. Rhubarb ʒij, subcarbonate of potash ʒj, boiling water Oss, macerate for 4 hours, strain, and add tincture of cinnamon ℥ss.

INFUSUM RHODODENDRI. KOELPIN. Leaves of golden-flowered rhododendron ʒij, boiling water Oss. A wine-glassful night and morning, in gout.

INFUSUM RHOIS TOXICODENDRI. SOBERNHEIM. Dried leaves of poison-oak (rhus toxicodendrum, or r. radicans) ℈ss to ℈j, boiling water f ℥vj. Dose, f ℥ss.

INFUSUM ROSÆ COMPOSITUM. L. (Inf. Rosæ, E.) Red rose petals dried ʒiij, boiling water Oj, diluted sulphuric acid f ʒjss; macerate in a glass vessel for 6 hours, strain, and add sugar ʒvj. E. directs the roses to be infused for 4 hours, and the acid and sugar to be added to the strained liquor.

INFUSUM ROSÆ ACIDUM. D. Dried rose petals ℥ss, boiling water f ℥xlviij, dil. sulphuric acid f ʒiij. Digest in a glass vessel for half an hour, strain, and add purified sugar ℥jss.

INFUSUM RUTÆ. PEREIRA. Fresh rue ℥j, boiling water Oj.

INFUSUM SABINÆ. Dr. PEREIRA. Fresh savine ʒj, boiling water f ℥viij; infuse for ½ an hour. HORN prescribes savine ʒj, camphor gr. vj, boiling water f ℥v. Dose, f ℥ss.

INFUSUM SALVIÆ. A. T. THOMSON. Dried sage leaves ℥j, boiling water Oj; macerate for ½ an hour.

INFUSUM SAMBUCI. Elder flowers ʒj to ʒiv, boiling water Ojss. Infuse and strain.

INFUSUM SANGUINARIÆ. Blood-root ℥ss, boiling water f ℥xvj. Dose, f ℥ss to f ℥j. *Emetic.*

INFUSUM SARSAPARILLÆ. U. S. Sarsaparilla ℥j, boiling water f ℥xvj; macerate for 2 hours.

INFUSUM SARSAPARILLÆ COMPOSITUM. D. Sarsap. ℥j, lime water f ℥xvj; macerate in a close vessel for 12 hours, and strain. Dr. O'BEIRNE prescribes ℥ij of sarsaparilla, ʒij of liquorice root, to Oj of lime water; to macerate 24 hours.

INFUSUM SARZÆ ALKALINUM. St. GEO. H. Sarsaparilla ℥xij, liquorice root ℥jss, solution of potash (liq. potassæ) f ℥jss, boiling water Ovss. Macerate for 24 hours, and strain. Dose, from f ℥viij to f ℥xvj daily.

INFUSUM SASSAFRAS. NIEMANN. Sassafras ℥ss, boiling water Oj; macerate for 6 hours.

INFUSUM SCOPARII. L. Broom tops ℥j, boiling water Oj; macerate for 4 hours.

INFUSUM SCUTELLARIÆ. A strong infusion of scutellaria lateriflora is employed as a preventive of hydrophobia; taken 3 times a day, for 3 or 4 months.

INFUSUM SECALIS CORNUTI. See Infusum Ergotæ.

INFUSUM SENEGÆ. E. Senega ʒx, boiling water Oj; infuse for 4 hours, and strain.

INFUSUM SENNÆ. E. Infusum Sennæ Compositum, L. Senna ʒxij (E.) or ʒxv (L.), ginger ℈iv, boiling water Oj; macerate for an hour, and strain.

INFUSUM SENNÆ COMPOSITUM. E. (Infusum Sennæ cum Tamarindis, D.) Senna ʒj (or sometimes ʒij or ʒiij), tamarinds ℥j, coriander seed ʒj, muscovado sugar ℥ss, boiling water f℥viij. Infuse for 4 hours in a covered vessel not glazed with lead, and strain.

Infusum Sennæ Tartarizatum. L. 1788. Senna ℨjss, coriander seed ℥ss, cream of tartar ʒij, boiling water f℥xvj. Macerate for an hour.

Infusum Sennæ Limoniatum. L. 1746. Senna ℥jss, fresh lemon-peel ℥j, lemon-juice ℨj, boiling water f℥xvj.

Infusum Serpentariæ. L. Virginian snake-root ʒiv, boiling water Oj; macerate for 4 hours, and strain.

Infusum Serpentariæ Compositum. Guy's H. Serpentaria ʒv, contrayerva root ʒv, boiling water Oj; macerate for 2 hours, and add tincture of serpentaria f℥ij.

Infusum Sesami. Dr. Wood. Two fresh leaves of sesamum (*benne*) infused in f℥viij of cold water form a mucilaginous demulcent drink. Dried leaves require hot water.

Infusum Simarubæ. L. Simaruba bark ʒiij, boiling water Oj; macerate for 2 hours, and strain.

Infusum Spigeliæ. U. S. Indian pink ʒiv, boiling water f℥xvj; macerate for 2 hours.

Infusum Spigeliæ cum Senna. As the last, with ʒiv of senna. Vermifuge. Dose for a child of 3 years old, from f℥ss to f℥j; for an adult, from f℥iv to f℥viij.

Infusum Solidaginis. Golden rod dried ℨj, boiling water Oj.

Infusum Tabaci. D. Tobacco leaves ʒj, boiling water f℥xvj; macerate for an hour. [Fowler's Inf. Tabaci is replaced by Vinum Tabaci, E.]

Infusum Tamarindi cum Senna. See Inf. Sennæ. Comp.

Infusum Tanaceti. Pereira. Fresh tansy ℨij [℥j Niemann], boiling water Oj. Infuse, and strain.

Infusum Thalictri Flavi. Infuse ℥ij of meadow-rue in boiling water q. s. to strain f℥xvj. (*For Hydrophobia;* to be taken in 24 hours.)

Infusum Tiliæ. See Ptisana Tiliæ.

Infusum Ulmi Fulvæ. U. S. Inner bark of slippery elm ℨj, boiling water f℥xvj; macerate for 2 hours. Demulcent, *ad libitum.*

INFUSUM URTICÆ (SEMINUM). GARBE. Nettle-seed ʒijss, boiling water f℥xviij; infuse for 3 hours, strain, and add syrup f℥ij.

INFUSUM VALERIANÆ. L. Valerian root ʒiv, boiling water Oj; macerate for 2 hours. D. ʒij to f℥viij; infuse half an hour. Dose f℥j—ij.

INFUSUM VANILLÆ. Vanilla ʒj, boiling water Oj.

INFUSUM VINCÆ MINORIS. Mr. WEATHERS. Lesser periwinkle ℥ss, boiling water Oj. Dose, f℥j 3 times a day, *in passive hæmorrhages.*

INFUSUM ZINGIBERIS. Dr. WOOD. Ginger ℥ss, boiling water f℥xvj; macerate for 2 hours.

INJECTIONES. Urethral and vaginal injections are here intended, except where otherwise stated. For intestinal injections, see Enemata.

INJECTIO ACIDI MURIATICI. Mr. WYATT. Muriatic acid 8 drops, water f℥iv.

INJECTIO ACOUSTICA. ALIBERT. Balsam of Peru ʒij, tincture of musk 4 drops, otto of roses 1 drop, decoction of St. John's wort Oj. *In Discharges from the Ear.* See also Balsamum Acousticum, and Guttæ Acousticæ.

INJECTIO ALOES. BORIES. Aloes ℈ss, muriate of ammonia gr. iv, honey of roses ℥j, fennel water ℥vj.

INJECTIO ALUMINIS. CH. Alum gr. iv, rose water ℥iv. BRANDE. Compound solution of alum fʒvj, water f℥vjss, mucilage ℥ss.

INJECTIO ALUMINÆ ACETATIS. Dr. REECE. Alum ʒj, acetate of lead ʒjss; triturate with f℥vj of boiling water, and in an hour filter.

INJECTIO AMMONIÆ. LAVAGNA. Water of ammonia 8 to 12 drops, milk ℥ij. NISATO. Water of ammonia 40 drops, barley water f℥viij, mucilage ℥ss. For 4 injections. Dr. ASHWELL. Water of ammonia fʒj, milk Oj. *In Amenorrhœa.*

INJECTIO AMMONIÆ ACETATIS. CH. Liquid acetate of ammonia f℥j, water f℥iij.

INJECTIO ARGENTI NITRATIS. The proportion of nitrate of silver, prescribed by different surgeons in injections, varies from gr. ¼th to gr. xxx to each f℥j of distilled water. Mr. ACTON uses gr. ij of nitrate in f℥viij of distilled water; and injects half a syringe-full every 4 hours for 12 times. Dr. ARNOTT uses gr. xij to f ℥j of water, and injects f ʒij, compressing the urethra 2 inches from the orifice; it should be retained half a minute. Mr. LUCAS employs from gr. x to xx to f ℥j of water. RICORD gr. viij. Dr. JEWEL (*in Leucorrhœa*) gr. iij to f ℥j of water. Glass syringes should be used.

INJECTIO ASTRINGENS. Dr. ASHWELL. Infusion of oak bark f ℥iv, powdered nutgall ʒss, tincture of catechu f ʒij.

INJECTIO CALOMELANOS. St. B. H. Calomel ʒij, mucilage f ℥jss, water Oj.

INJECTIO CERUSSÆ. CH. Compound powder of carbonate of lead (p. cerussæ comp. L. 1788,) ℈j, sulphate of zinc gr. vj, rose water ℥iv.

INJECTIO CHLORINATA. F. H. One part of liquid chlorinated soda to 12 or 16 of water. Dr. COPLAND. One fluid ounce of liquid chloride to ℥vij of camphor mixture.

INJECTIO CHLORIDI CALCIS. ROUSSE. Chloride of lime ℈j, water f ℥vij, wine of opium ℥j.

INJECTIO COPAIBÆ. CH. Copaiba balsam ʒij, mucilage ℥ss, lime water ℥iv. RICORD prescribes copaiva ʒvj—vij, decoction of poppies ℥iij. Yolk of an egg. Mix.

INJECTIO CREASOTI. Dr. ALLNATT. Creasote ♏xx, solution of potash ʒij, white sugar ʒij; rub together, and add water f ℥viij. *In Leucorrhœa.*

INJECTIO CUBEBÆ. CHEVALLIER. Ground cubebs ℥j, extract of belladonna ʒj, boiling water f ℥xvj. Infuse.

INJECTIO CUPRI ACETATIS [OLEOSA]. CH. Prepared verdigris gr. x, oil of almonds ℥iv. Dissolve by trituration, or gentle heat.

INJECTIO CUPRI AMMONIATI. Mr. FOOT. Solution of ammoniated copper 20 drops, rose water ℥iv.

INJECTIO CUPRI SULPHATIS. HUNTER. Sulphate of copper gr. iij, water f ℥iv.

INJECTIO CUPRI ET PLUMBI ACETATIS. Dr. R. REECE. Acetate of lead gr. x, acetate of copper gr. x, acetic acid ♏v, water f ℥viij.

INJECTIO ERGOTÆ. BOUDIN. Ergot ʒj, boiling water ℥viij. Infuse.

INJECTIO FERRI IODIDI. RICORD. Iodide of iron ʒss, water f℥viij.

INJECTIO FULIGINIS. M. ROGNETTA. Decoction of wood soot ℥xvj, alum ℥ss, water ℥vj. *In Leucorrhœa.*

INJECTIO GALLÆ. Tincture of nutgalls ʒj, water ʒx. Or a weak infusion.

INJECTIO HYDRARGYRI. CH. Quicksilver ʒj, mucilage ℥jss; rub together till combined, and add gradually, water f℥jss.

INJECTIO HYDRARGYRI CHLORIDI. See Inj. Calomel.

INJECTIO HYDRARGYRI BICHLORIDI. F. H. Bichloride of mercury gr. j to iv; water, or barley water, f℥xvj. ʒj of tincture of myrrh is sometimes added; others add wine of opium.

INJECTIO IODINII. VELPEAU, *in Hydrocele.* One part of tincture of iodine, to 3 parts of water; or from ʒij to ʒiij of tincture to ℥j of water, and inject ℥ss. Mr. B. COOPER says the *compound* tincture should be used. Mr. WALNE mixes from fʒj to fʒij of the tincture with fʒx of tepid water, and injects f℥j, letting it remain about 4 minutes. In *Hydarthrosis* M. BONNET injects a solution of 1 part of iodine, 2 of iodide of potassium, and 8 of water, taking care not to introduce more liquid than is withdrawn from the joint.

INJECTIO MORPHIÆ. BRERA. Morphia gr. ij, oil of almonds ℥j; triturate together.

INJECTIO OLEOSA. CH. Oil of almonds ℥iv, liquid diacetate of lead 8 drops.

INJECTIO OPIATA. CH. Tincture of opium ♏xl, water ℥iv, F. H. Wine of opium ʒj, emollient decoction Oj.

INJECTIO PLATINO-CHLORIDI SODII. HOEFER. Decoction of poppy ℥viij, chloride of platinum and sodium ʒss.

INJECTIO PLUMBI. Goulard water (Liq. Plumbi diac. dil.), or acetate of lead ℈j, water f℥viij.

INJECTIO PLUMBI OPIATA. WENDT. Extract of opium gr. jss, distilled water f℥ij, mucilage ʒij, liquid diacetate of lead 4 drops.

INJECTIO QUERCUS. Powdered oak bark ℥j, boiling water ℥xvj. Infuse.

INJECTIO TANNINI. RICHARD. Tannin ℈j, water ℥viij.

INJECTIO TEREBINTHINÆ. St. B. H. Oil of turpentine f ℥jss, olive oil f ℥xij.

INJECTIO THEÆ. CH. Green tea ʒss, boiling water ℥iv. Infuse.

INJECTIO VESICALIS. Dr. HOSKIN. *For dissolving phosphatic Calculi in the bladder.* Nitro-saccharate of lead gr. j, moistened with 5 drops of saccharic acid, and dissolved in f ʒj of distilled water. Dr. H. has since adopted the acetate of lead. M. CHEVALLIER prescribes *in lithic calculi*, carbonate of soda ʒj, soap ʒij, water f ʒxij.

INJECTIO VINI. EARLE, *in Hydrocele.* Red wine 2 parts, water 1 part. To remain in about 5 minutes.

INJECTIO ZINCI ACETATIS. Sulphate of zinc ʒj, acetate of lead ℈iv, water Ojss.

INJECTIO ZINCI CHLORIDI. M. GAUDRIOT. Liquid chloride of zinc 24 drops, water f ℥iv. Mix, and filter.

INJECTIO ZINCI SULPHATIS. Sulphate of zinc gr. viij to xx, distilled or rose water f ʒviij. [Several of the compounds under LOTIO are used as injections, properly diluted.]

IODINIUM. (Iodineum, E.) *Iodine.* Lixiviate kelp, remove the crystallizable salts by successive evaporations, dry the mother liquor, and heat the residuum with one-tenth its weight of powdered oxide of manganese, in an iron pot, stirring constantly. Dissolve it in water to obtain a solution of 1·334 sp. gr. Pass through it a current of chlorine, avoiding excess. Wash the deposit with a little water, and distil it in a glass retort. P. [For another method see Dr. PEREIRA's "Elements."]

IODIDUM AMYLI. See Amyli Iodidum.

IODOFORMUM. IODOFORM. M. CLARY. Distilled water f ʒx, rectified spirit f ʒjss, iodine ʒj, bicarbonate of soda ʒj. Heat gently in a flask, by water-bath, for 2 hours; or until yellow scales of iodoform are deposited. Collect the iodoform on a filter and wash it with a little cold water. More iodine is added to the liquid so long as it becomes decolorized by the process. Dose, about 1 grain.

JALAPINA. *Jalapine.* Mr. REDWOOD (in GRAY's Supplement) gives the following process, which was referred to in the former edition as that of BUCHNER. It may be questioned whether all the makers who supply it follow exactly the same process :—

Dissolve resin of jalap in rectified spirit, and add to it an alcoholic solution of acetate of lead, as long as a precipitate is formed. Filter, add a few drops of diluted sulphuric acid to throw down any excess of lead; filter again, and mix the clear solution with 4 or 5 times its volume of distilled water. Collect the precipitate, and dry it over a water-bath.

JULAPIUM (*vel* JULEPUM) ACIDUM. Water rendered gratefully acid by the addition of various acids, and sweetened with sugar or syrup. GUY'S H. has the following:—

Hydrochloric acid f ʒj, water Oj, sugar ℥ss.

Nitric acid ♏75, water Oij, sugar ℥jss.

Nitro-hydrochloric acid ♏70, water Ojss, sugar ℥j.

JULEPUM ANODYNUM. See Mistura Anodyna.

JULEPUM AMMONIÆ. GUY'S H. Sesquicarbonate of ammonia ℈ij, treacle f ʒiv, compound tincture of lavender f ʒiv, mint julep (jul. menthæ, GUY'S H.) f ℥xj.

JULEPUM AMMONIÆ ACETATIS. GUY'S H. Solution of acetate of ammonia, and mint water, equal parts.

JULAPIUM ANTIHYSTERICUM. F. H. Pennyroyal water ℥iv, hysteric water ℥ij, tincture of castor ʒij, fœtid spirit of ammonia ʒij, sugar ʒvj.

JULEPUM GUMMOSUM. P. Gum arabic ʒij, syrup of marshmallows ℥j, orange-flower water ʒiv, water ℥iv.

JULEPUM HYDRARGYRI BICHLORIDI COMPOSITUM. GUY'S H. Tincture of cinchona bark f ℥j, tincture of rhubarb f ʒiv, liquor of bichloride of mercury f ℥ij, distilled water f ʒiv. Dose, f ʒj to f ʒiv, twice or thrice a day.

JULEPUM IODINII COMPOSITUM. GUY'S H. Iodine gr. ij, iodide of potassium gr. xlviij, comp. tincture of lavender f ʒvj, water f ℥xj ʒij. Mix. Dose, f ℥j, twice or thrice daily.

JULEPUM LIMONIS. GUY'S H. Lemon juice and mint water, equal parts. See Limonadum.

JULEPUM MENTHÆ. GUY'S H. Peppermint water Oj, water Oss. U. C. H. *adds* spirit of nitric æther f ʒvj, syrup of senna f ℥ij.

JULEPUM OXYMELLIS COMPOSITUM. GUY'S H. Oxymel f ℥iij, nitre ʒiij, water f ℥ix. Dose, f ℥j.

JULEPUM POTASSÆ CARBONATIS. GUY'S H. Solution of carbonate of potash 1 part, mint water 11 parts.

JULEPUM POTASSÆ CITRATIS, *vulgo* JULEPUM SALINUM. GUY'S H. Julep of carbonate of potash 2 parts, lemon juice 1 part. Dose, f℥jss. See Mistura Salina.

JULEPUM POTASSÆ NITRATIS. GUY'S H. Nitre ʒiij, mint julep f℥xss, spirit of nitric æther f℈iij, syrup of lemons f℥j.

JULEPUM RHEI COMPOSITUM; Julepum Rosæ Comp.; and J. Sodæ Sulphatis. See Mistura. Other juleps will also be found under Mistura, Potio, Ptisana, &c.

JUSCULUM CUM CARNE BOVIS. Dr. SEYMOUR. *Beef Tea.* Lean beef ℔ijss (avoird. wt.?), water Oiij; simmer, without boiling, till reduced to Ojss, and strain carefully.

JUSCULUM CUM CARNE VITULI. P. Lean veal ℥iv, river water f℥xxxvj; digest with a gentle heat for 2 hours; strain when cold. In the same manner prepare *bouillons* of calves' lights, pullet, crayfish, tortoise, and frogs.

JUSCULUM CUM LIMACIBUS. P. Vine snails, deprived of their shells and intestines, washed in warm water, and cut in pieces, ℥iv, water ℔ij; simmer for 2 hours, add ʒij of Canada maidenhair; infuse for ¼ of an hour, and strain.

JUSCULUM SARZÆ. Dr. EGAN. Decoction of sarsaparilla Ojss, beef ℔ss; reduce to half. To be taken daily.

JUSCULUM VIPERINUM. L. 1746. Prepared from a middle-sized viper (freed from head, skin, and entrails,) a chicken, and ℔ij of water, S. A. *Restorative.*

KALI. See Potassa.

KERMES MINERALE. (See Antimonii Oxysulphuretum.) P. Cryst. carbonate of soda 21 parts, water 210 parts; boil in an iron vessel, and add 1 part of black sulphuret of antimony in fine powder; keep it boiling for an hour, filter whilst boiling into earthen vessels containing a very little hot water; let it cool very slowly, collect, wash, and press the precipitate, dry it with a moderate heat, pass through a silk sieve, and keep it secure from air and light. An inferior kind is prepared in the dry way, from black sulphuret of antimony ℥xvj, carbonate of potash ℥xxxij, washed sulphur ℥j. Mix accurately, and fuse in a Hessian crucible. When cold, reduce it to powder; boil it with 2 gallons of water, and proceed as above. The residue to be boiled with more water, till it yields no more kermes.

LAC AMYGDALÆ. See Mistura Amygdalæ.

LAC ASININUM FACTITIUM. *Artificial Asses' Milk.* HANN. PH. Snails 6, hartshorn shavings, pearl barley, eryngo root, each ℥ij, water ℔ij; boil to ℔j, and add syrup of maidenhair ℥j. The snails are omitted in this country.

LAC FERRATUM. Cow's milk in which red-hot iron has been repeatedly quenched.

LAC SAGO. Dr. A. T. THOMSON. Soak ℥j of sago in Oj of cold water for an hour; pour off the water, and boil the sago slowly with Ojss of milk till dissolved.

LAC CUM SEVO. GUY'S H. Suet cut small ℥j, water f℥iv; boil on a slow fire for 10 minutes, and express through linen; then add new milk ℥xvj, bruised cinnamon ʒj, sugar ℥j; boil for 10 minutes, and strain. Dose, f℥ij to f℥iv, twice a day or oftener. See also Decoctum Sevi.

LAC SULPHURIS. See Sulphur Præcipitatum.

LACTUCARIUM. The milky juice which flows from incisions in the stem of flowering lettuce, collected, and dried in the air. E. directs it to be prepared both from the *Lactuca virosa* and *Lactuca sativa.*

LAPIS DIVINUS. P. Sulphate of copper ℥iij, nitre ℥iij, alum ℥iij; fuse them together, stir in ʒj of powdered camphor, and pour it out on an oiled slab. Used in lotions, eye-waters, &c. PUTEGNAT recommends the following in recent contusions:— Alum ℥ij; sal ammoniac, verdigris, and sulphate of zinc, of each ʒj. Mix, and melt with a gentle heat. A piece of the size of a nut to be dissolved in a quart of water. The Lapis Vulnerarius of some formularies is nearly the same.

LAPIS MEDICAMENTOSUS. L. 1746. Alum, litharge and red bole, of each ℔ss; colcothar ℥iij, vinegar ℥iv. Mix, and dry.

LAUDANUM SYDENHAMI. Vinum Opii.

LAUDANUM CYDONIATUM. See Liquor Opiatus.

LILACINE. M. MEILLET. Boil the leaves, or green seed vessels of lilac in water q. s. till reduced to half, add diacetate of lead, concentrate to a thin syrup, and add calcined magnesia in excess. Evaporate to dryness, pulverize, digest the powder repeatedly in warm water (96° to 104°), and afterwards treat it with highly rectified spirit. Filter, decolorize the solution with animal charcoal, filter, evaporate to half, and set aside that crystals may form.

Limatura Ferri. See Ferri Limatura.

Limatura Stanni. Tin is sometimes divided by a file; but more usually by agitating the melted metal. See Stanni Pulvis.

Limonadum. Cut 2 lemons in slices, pour on them Ojss of boiling water, infuse for an hour in a covered vessel, then add ℥ij of sugar, and strain. Or citric acid ʒj, sugar ℥ij, water Ojss, spirit of lemon ʒj. Tartaric acid is sometimes substituted for citric.

Limonadum Aeratum. Put f℥j of syrup of lemons into each bottle and fill up with aërated water.

Limonadum Antimoniatum. It. H. Potassio-tartrate of antimony gr. ij, sugar ℥ss, lemonade Oij. A glassful every half hour.

Limonadum Lacticum. M. Lactic acid from ʒj to ʒiv, water Ojss, syrup ℥ij.

Limonadum Magnesiæ Laxativum. Mialhe. Calcined magnesia ʒij, or citric acid ʒvjss, water f℥x. Heat to boiling, and filter while hot into a pint bottle containing ℥ij of syrup of lemon-peel, and fill up with water. Contains about 3xj citrate of magnesia, equal in effect to ℥j of the sulphate.

Limonadum Oxalicum. Oxalic acid gr. x, water Oj, sugar q. s. Half this quantity in 24 hours, as a refrigerant.

Limonadum Siccum. Citric acid ʒj, sugar ℥iv, essence of lemon 8 drops. Or, white sugar ℔iv, tartaric acid ℥j, cream of tartar ʒiv, essence of lemon ʒij.

Limonadum Sulphuricum. F. H. Sulphuric acid gr. xxx, syrup of barberries ℥ij, water Oiijss. A stronger mixture is used in painters' colic. M. Gendrin. Sulphuric acid 40 drops, water Oj.

Linctus. *Common Linctus.* St. B. H. Confection of hips ℥ij, p. tragacanth ℈ijss, syrup of poppies fʒvj, water ℥ij, diluted sulphuric acid fʒss, vinegar of squills fʒiij. Mix.

Linctus Acidus. Dr. Copland. Honey of roses ʒx, muriatic acid ♏xx, syrup of red poppies ʒij.

Linctus Antimonii Sulphureti. U. C. H. Oxymel f℥j, oxymel of squills f℥j, precipitated sulphuret of antimony ℈j.

LINCTUS BORACIS. U. C. H. Borax ʒiij, honey ℥j; melt and stir together, then add syrup ℥j. Dr. COPLAND prescribes spermaceti ℈ijss, com. powder of tragacanth ʒiij, syrup of Tolu ℥j, borax ʒijss, confection of roses ʒv, syrup of marsh mallows q. s.

LINCTUS CACAO. *Crème de Tronchin.* Butter of cacao ℥ij, white sugar ℥j, syrup of capillaire ℥j, syrup of Tolu ℥j.

LINCTUS IPECACUANHÆ. Dr. COPLAND. Oil of almonds f℥j, syrup of lemon f℥j, ipecacuanha gr. vj, confection of hips ℥j, comp. powder of tragacanth ʒiij.

LINCTUS MYRRHÆ ET IPECACUANHÆ. Dr. COPLAND. Myrrh ʒj, ipecacuanha gr. vj, mucilage, syrup of marsh mallows, and oxymel of squill, each ʒvj.

LINCTUS OLEOSUS. U. C. H. Oil of almonds f℥j, syrup of poppies f℥j, tragacanth powder ʒiij.

LINCTUS OPIATUS. GUY'S H. Tincture of opium fʒij, diluted sulphuric acid fʒijss, treacle f℥viij, water f℥iij. Dose, a teaspoonful occasionally.

LINCTUS PECTORALIS. Dr. RYAN. Oxymel of squill, mucilage of acacia, and simple syrup, in equal quantities.

LINCTUS POTASSÆ NITRATIS. GUY'S H. Nitre ʒjss, honey of roses f℥j, oxymel f℥ss. A teaspoonful occasionally.

LINCTUS ROSÆ. Confection of roses ℥ij, diluted sulphuric acid fʒj, compound tincture of camphor fʒxij.

LINCTUS SCILLÆ. Oil of almonds ℥ij, oxymel of squills ℥j.

LINCTUS TEREBINTHINÆ. RECAMIER. Oil of turpentine ʒij, honey of roses ℥iv. [For other similar compounds see LOHOCH.]

LINIMENTUM ACIDI SULPHURICI COMPOSITUM. GUY'S & St. GEO. H. Sulphuric acid fʒj, oil of turpentine f℥iij, olive oil f℥iij. Sir B. BRODIE. Olive oil ℥jss, sulphuric acid ʒss. Mix, and add oil of turpentine ℥ss.

LINIMENTUM ACIDUM. Sir W. FORDYCE, *in malignant ulcerations of the throat.* Honey of roses ℥j, muriatic acid 20 drops.

LINIMENTUM ACETICUM COMPOSITUM. MID. H. Acetic acid f℥j, purified oil of turpentine f℥jss, yolk of egg q. s., distilled water f℥v. Mix.

LINIMENTUM ÆRUGINIS. L. *Oxymel Æruginis.* Verdigris ℥j, vinegar f℥vij; dissolve, strain through linen, add honey ℥xiv, and boil to a proper thickness. D. (*Oxymel Cupri Subacetatis*) *the same.*

LINIMENTUM ALBUM. *For chapped hands.* Rectified oil of turpentine ℥ij, solution of ammonia ℥ij, soap liniment ℥iij, spirit of rosemary ℥j; mix in the above order, and gradually add, with continual agitation, distilled vinegar ℥viij.

LINIMENTUM ALBUMINIS. Dr. CHRISTISON. Equal parts of white of egg and rectified spirit agitated together. *In excoriation from pressure.*

LINIMENTUM AMMONIÆ. L. & E. (Lin. Ammoniæ fortius, L. 1824.) *Volatile Liniment.* Solution of ammonia f℥j, olive oil f℥ij. Mix. D. directs only f℥ij of ammonia.

LINIMENTUM AMMONIÆ SESQUICARBONATIS. L. (Lin. Ammoniæ, L. 1788.) Solution of sesquicarbonate of ammonia f℥j, olive oil f℥iij.

LINIMENTUM AMMONIÆ COMPOSITUM. E. Dr. GRANVILLE'S *Counter-irritants.* Strong water of ammonia (density 880) f℥v, tincture of camphor f℥ij, spirit of rosemary f℥j. Mix. A weaker liniment may be made with f℥iij tincture of camphor, f℥ij of spirit of rosemary, and f℥v of strong ammonia. [Dr. GRANVILLE directs for the *milder* lotion, ʒiv of ammonia at ·872, ʒiij of spirit of rosemary distilled from the herb, and ʒj of spirit of camphor. For the *stronger*, ʒv of the same ammonia, ʒij of spirit of rosemary, ʒj of spirit of camphor. The milder is sufficient to produce vesication in a few minutes. The stronger is only employed in apoplexy, and to produce cauterization. To be applied on folded linen covered with a thick towel.]

LINIMENTUM AMMONIÆ CAMPHORATUM. CRUIKSHANK. Camphor ʒij, olive oil ℥j, water of ammonia ℥iij.

LINIMENTUM AMMONIÆ CUM TEREBINTHINA. Dr. COPLAND. Liniment of ammonia f℥jss, oil of turpentine f℥ss.

LINIMENTUM ANTHELMINTICUM. BORIES. Colocynth ʒss, ox-gall ʒiv, oil of wormwood ʒj.

LINIMENTUM ANODYNUM. D. *Linimentum Opii.*

LINIMENTUM ARCEI. See Unguentum Elemi.

LINIMENTUM BITUMINIS AMMONIATUM. Dr. KIRKLAND. Barbadoes tar ℥jss, water of ammonia ℥ss.

LINIMENTUM BELLADONNÆ. BIETT. Extract of belladonna ʒij, lime water ℥viij, oil of almonds ℥iv. *In eczema*, &c. RANQUE. Extract of belladonna ℈ij, cherry-laurel water, ℥ij, sulphuric ether ℥j.

LINIMENTUM BELLADONNÆ COMPOSITUM. GUY'S H. Extract of belladonna ℥j, soap liniment f℥viij.

LINIMENTUM BORACIS. SWEDIAUR. Borax ʒij, tincture of myrrh ℥j, distilled water ℥j, honey of roses ℥ij.

LINIMENTUM BORACIS COMPOSITUM. HARLESS. Borax ʒj, balsam of Peru ʒjss, oil of almonds ℥j, yolk of egg ʒij, white of egg ʒij. Mix.

LINIMENTUM CAJAPUTI ÆTHEREUM. TORTUEL. Camphor ʒj, oil of cajaput ʒij, æther ℥j.

LINIMENTUM CAJAPUTI STIMULANS. Dr. COPLAND. Compound camphor liniment f℥jss, soap liniment f℥jss, oil of cajaput f℥j. Dr. WILLIAMS prescribes castor oil fʒj, olive oil fʒivss, cajaput oil fʒss. To be rubbed on the chest twice a day.

LINIMENTUM CALCIS. E. Mix equal quantities of lime water, and linseed oil.

LINIMENTUM CALCIS COMPOSITUM. St. B. H. Lime water f℥viij, olive oil f℥viij, rectified spirit f℥j.

LINIMENTUM CALCIS OPIATUM. GERM. H. Lime water ʒiij, oil of almonds ʒiij, extract of opium gr. j. *For sore nipples.*

LINIMENTUM CAMPHORÆ. L. E. and D. *Oleum Camphoratum.* Camphor ℥j, olive oil f℥iv. Dissolve.

LINIMENTUM CAMPHORÆ COMPOSITUM. L. Water of ammonia f℥vijss, spirit of lavender Oj; distil Oj, and dissolve in it camphor ℥ijss. D. the same.

LINIMENTUM CAMPHORÆ CUM TEREBINTHINA. GUY'S H. Camphor liniment fʒx, oil of turpentine fʒij.

LINIMENTUM CAMPHORÆ ÆTHEREUM. WARE. Camphor ʒj, æther ʒj, oil of vipers ʒij.

LINIMENTUM CAMPHORÆ ACETICUM. BRANDE. Tincture of camphor f℥iij, acetic acid ℥j. Mix.

LINIMENTUM CAMPHORA CUM HYDRARGYRO. MANCH. H. Strong mercurial ointment ℥ij, camphor liniment Oj. Mix.

LINIMENTUM CANTHARIDIS. U. S. Powdered cantharides ℥j,

oil of turpentine f℈viij; digest for three hours in a water-bath, and strain.

LINIMENTUM CAPSICI. Dr. COPLAND. Compound camphor liniment f℥j, volatile liniment f℥j, tincture of capsicum fʒiij.

LINIMENTUM CHLORINATUM. KOPP. Solution of chloride of lime ʒvj, olive oil ℥jss. *In inveterate itch, ringworm, &c.*

LINIMENTUM COSMETICUM. QUINCY. Magistery of bismuth ʒj, oil of almonds ℥ij, spermaceti ʒiij, oil of rhodium 6 drops.

LINIMENTUM CRINISCUM. QUINCY. Labdanum ʒvj, bears' grease ℥ij, honey ℥ss, powdered southernwood ʒiij, oil of nutmeg ʒj, balsam of Peru ʒij. *To restore the hair.*

LINIMENTUM CROTONIS. PEREIRA. One part of croton oil to 5 of olive oil. Dr. CORRIGAN employs fʒj of croton oil with f℥j of oil of turpentine, or comp. camphor liniment.

LINIMENTUM DIGITALIS. Dr. ROYLE. Infusion of digitalis f℥ij, water of ammonia fʒij, oil of poppy seed f℈iv. To be rubbed on the abdomen 2 or 3 times a day. See also Lin. Diureticum.

LINIMENTUM DIURETICUM. BRERA. Squill in powder ʒj, gastric juice of a calf ℥ij. *To be rubbed on the loins in dropsy.* Dr. GUIBERT prescribes tincture of squills, of digitalis, and of colchicum, each ℥ss, camphorated oil ℥j, water of ammonia ℥ss.

LINIMENTUM HELLEBORI. DORNBLUETH. Soft soap ℥iv, hellebore powder ℥ij, hot water q. s.

LINIMENTUM HYDRARGYRI COMPOSITUM. L. Camphor ℥j, rectified spirit fʒj; rub together, and add strong mercurial ointment ℥iv, lard ℥iv, solution of ammonia f℥iv. Mix.

LINIMENTUM HYDRARGYRI NITRATIS. Sir H. HALFORD. Equal quantities of ointment of nitrated quicksilver, and oil of almonds, triturated till perfectly smooth in a glass mortar.

LINIMENTUM HUNGARICUM. SOUBEIRAN. Rectified spirit ℥xij, strong vinegar ℥vj, camphor ʒiv, mustard flour ʒiv, black pepper ʒiv, powdered cantharides ʒj, bruised garlic ʒj; macerate for some days, and filter.

LINIMENTUM IODINII. Dr. MANSON. Liniment of opium f℥j, tincture of iodine fʒj.

LINIMENTUM IODURETUM SAPONACEUM. GUIBOURT. White soap ʒx, oil of almonds ʒx, iodide of potassium ʒj, water ʒj.

Dissolve the iodide in the water, and add to it the soap and oil previously melted together. Mix. See the next.

LINIMENTUM IODURETUM GELATINOSUM. Mr. BEESLEY, of Banbury. *Gelée pour le Goître.* Dissolve by a gentle heat ʒvj or ʒvij of white soap in f℥ij of proof spirit, and add to it while yet warm, ʒiv of iodide of potassium dissolved in the same quantity of spirit, and allow it to cool slowly in wide-mouthed vials, well corked. FOY. (*Baume Hydriodaté.*) Iodide of potassium ʒiv, proof spirit ℥ij; dissolve. Dissolve also ʒvj of curd soap in ℥ij of proof spirit. Mix while still warm, and aromatize with rose or neroli, and let the mixture cool in wide-mouthed bottles, which must be kept well corked.

LINIMENTUM IPECACUANHÆ. Dr. NELIGAN. Ipecac. in fine powder ʒiv, lard ʒij, olive oil f℥jss. It is sometimes mixed with an equal quantity of Volatile Liniment. See Unguentum Ipecac.

LINIMENTUM JUNIPERI. Dr. SULLY. Oil of juniper ℥jss, lard ℥ij, oil of anise 6 drops. *In scalled heads*, &c.

LINIMENTUM MURIATICUM. F. H. Muriatic acid ʒij, balsam of Peru ʒj, water ʒvj, white wax ʒij, olive oil ℥ij.

LINIMENTUM NARCOTICUM. P. Anodyne oil (balsamum tranquillans) ℥ij, wine of opium ℥j. Mix.

LINIMENTUM NUCIS VOMICÆ. M. Tincture of nux vomica ℥j, strong ammonia ʒij. Mix.

LINIMENTUM OLEI ASELLI. Dr. BRACH. Cod-liver oil ʒj, water of ammonia ℥ss. Dr. BREFELD. (*To scrofulous ulcers.*) Cod-liver oil ʒiv, Goulard's extract of lead ʒij, yolk of egg ʒiij.

LINIMENTUM OLEI ERGOTÆ. Oil of ergot ʒj, oil of almonds, or sulphuric æther ʒiij.

LINIMENTUM OPII. L. Soap liniment f℥vj, tincture of opium f℥ij. D. 4 parts of soap liniment to 3 of tincture of opium. E. Soap ℥vj, opium ℥jss, camphor ℥iij, oil of rosemary ʒvj, rectified spirit Oij.

LINIMENTUM PHOSPHORATUM. HAMB. PH. Phosphorus gr. vj, oil of almonds ℥j; digest, and add camphor gr. x, solution of ammonia 10 drops.

LINIMENTUM PLUMBI. Mr. GAOZEY. Acetate of lead ℈ij, soft water ℔j, olive oil ℔ss.

LINIMENTUM PLUMBI OPIATUM. GUY'S H. Liquid diacetate of

lead, tincture of opium, honey of roses, each f ʒij, confection of roses ℥j.

LINIMENTUM POTASSII IODIDI. See Lin. Ioduretum Gelatinosum; and Lin. Ioduretum Saponaceum.

LINIMENTUM SAPONACEUM. U. C. H. Soft soap ℥iv, oil of turpentine f ℥j, proof spirit f ℥vj. *Liniment Savonneux*, P. consists of tincture of soap ℥j, olive oil ʒj, spirit of wine (sp. gr. ·863) ℥j.

LINIMENTUM SAPONIS COMPOSITUM. *Soap Liniment*, or *Opodeldoc*. L. and D. Hard soap ʒiij, camphor ℥j, spirit of rosemary f ℥xvj. Dissolve the camphor in the spirit, add the soap, and digest with a gentle heat, till dissolved. E. Castile soap ℥v, camphor ℥ijss, oil of rosemary f ʒvj, rectified spirit Oij. [U. S.] (In imitation of Steers' Opodeldoc.) Soap ʒiij, camphor ʒj, oil of rosemary f ʒj, oil of origanum f ʒj, rectified spirit f ℥xvj. [As this liniment is solid when Castile soap and rectified spirit are used, it is a common practice either to substitute soft soap for hard, or to use a weaker spirit. Mr. FISHER states that ⅛th of water is sufficient to preserve it liquid.]

LINIMENTUM SAPONIS AROMATICUM. GUY'S H. Soft soap ʒxij, camphor ℥iv, oil of origanum f ℥j, rectified spirit Oiij f ℥iv. Digest till dissolved. To this is occasionally added a fourth part of tincture of opium, a fifth of tincture of cantharides, or an eighth of water of ammonia.

LINIMENTUM SAPONIS CUM OPIO. D. See Linim. Opii.

LINIMENTUM SAPONIS CUM PLUMBO. CH. Soap liniment f ℥ij, liquid diacetate of lead f ʒj.

LINIMENTUM SIMPLEX. E. Olive oil f ʒiv, white wax ℥j; melt together.

LINIMENTUM SINAPIS. Dr. LEWIN. Bruised mustard-seed ℔ss, oil of turpentine ℔j; digest, strain, and add camphor ʒiv. *In imitation of Whitehead's Essence of Mustard.*

LINIMENTUM OLEI VOLATILIS SINAPIS. Dr. MEYER. Volatile oil of black mustard-seed, from 12 to 24 drops, rectified spirit ʒj. *Or*, 5 or 6 drops of the oil to ʒj of oil of almonds. M. directs, as a vesicant, equal weights of the oil and strong alcohol.

LINIMENTUM STRYCHNIÆ. Dr. NELIGAN. Strychnia ʒss, olive

oil ℥jss. Ten drops to be rubbed over the temples *in Amaurosis.*

LINIMENTUM SUCCINI. Oil of amber ℥ss, oil of cloves ℥ss, oil of olives ℥j. *The supposed form for Roche's Embrocation.*

LINIMENTUM SUCCINI OPIATUM. Rectified oil of amber ℥ij, tincture of opium ℥ij, lard ℨj. *A once celebrated remedy for cramp,* &c. BRANDE. Spirit of camphor, tincture of opium, and oil of amber, of each ℥ss.

LINIMENTUM SULPHURIS CUM SAPONE. LUGOL. Soap ℥iij, water ℨvj; dissolve by a gentle heat, and add sulphur ℨiij.

LINIMENTUM SULPHURO-SAPONACEUM. JADELOT. Sulphuret of potassium ℥iij, soap (softened with ℥j of water) ℥xvj, olive oil ℥xvj, oil of thyme ℨj. Mix. [P. omits the oil of thyme, and substitutes ℥xxxij of oil of poppies for the olive oil.]

LINIMENTUM SULPHURETI CARBONIS. GERM. H. Sulphuret of carbon ℨj, oil of almonds, or camphorated oil ℥j.

LINIMENTUM SULPHURIS IODIDI. E. WILSON. Iodide of sulphur ℨss, olive oil ℥j; triturate together.

LINIMENTUM TEREBINTHINÆ. L. Soft soap ℥ij, camphor ℥j, oil of turpentine f℥xvj. See the next.

LINIMENTUM TEREBINTHINATUM. E. Resin cerate ℥iv, oil of turpentine f℥v, camphor in powder ℥ss; mix. L. 1824. (Lin. Terebinthinæ,) and U. S. Resin cerate ℔j, oil of turpentine f℥viij. GUY'S H. Resin cerate ℥iij, oil of turpentine f℥jss. Mr. KENTISH'S *application to burns.*

LINIMENTUM TEREBINTHINÆ COMPOSITUM. U. C. H. Equal parts of oil of turpentine, and castor oil. GUY'S H. Oil of turpentine Oj, bruised mustard ℥ijss, soft soap ℥x, boiling water Oj. Macerate the seeds in the boiling water for 2 hours in a water-bath, strain, and add the turpentine and soap.

LINIMENTUM TEREBINTHINÆ ACETICUM. DR. STOKES. Oil of turpentine ℥iij, acetic acid ℨv, rose water ℥ijss, essence of lemons ℈iv, yolk of one egg. This is said to resemble Mr. ST. JOHN LONG'S celebrated liniment. *In Phthisis.* See Linimentum Aceticum Compositum.

LINIMENTUM TEREBINTHINÆ AMMONIATUM. DEBREYNE. Oil of turpentine ℥j, liquid ammonia ℨj, camphorated spirit ℥iv, lard ℥iv. *In Sciatica, &c.*

LINIMENTUM TEREBINTHINÆ VITRIOLICUM. See Lin. Acidi Sulphurici.

LINIMENTUM TRIPHARMACUM. L. 1746. Lead plaster ℥iv, olive oil ℥iv, vinegar ℥j; heat gently, and stir them till they combine.

LINIMENTUM VESICANS. Dr. MONTGOMERY, *for Children*. Compound camphor liniment f ʒiv, rectified oil of turpentine f ʒij.

LINIMENTUM VERATRIÆ. BRANDE. Veratria gr. viij, alcohol f ʒiv, soap liniment f ʒiv.

LINIMENTUM VIRIDE. Dr. CAMPBELL. Camphor ℥j, oil of olives ℥vj, water of ammonia ℥vj, extract of hemlock ℥j, spirit of ammonia ℥ij. [Some ointments have also been termed liniments. See Unguenta.]

LIQUOR ACIDI CITRICI. *Artificial Lemon Juice.* St. B. H. Citric acid ʒx, water Oj. PEREIRA. Citric acid ʒviijss, essence of lemons a few drops, water f ℥xvj.

LIQUOR ÆTHEREUS OLEOSUS. D. See Oleum Æthereum.

LIQUOR ÆTHEREUS SULPHURICUS. D. Unrectified sulphuric æther.

LIQUOR ALUMINIS COMPOSITUS. L. Alum ℥j, sulphate of zinc ℥j, boiling water Oiij. Dissolve, and filter.

LIQUOR AMMONIÆ. L. *Solution* or *Water of Ammonia.* Hydrochlorate of ammonia ℥x, lime ℥viij, water Oij. Slake the lime, put it into a retort, add the coarsely powdered hydrochlorate, then the rest of the water; and let f ℥xv distil. It may also be made by mixing 1 part of the stronger solution of ammonia with 2 parts (E. 2½) of distilled water. Sp. gr. of L. & E. 0·960, D. 0·950.

LIQUOR AMMONIÆ FORTIOR. It is made by passing gaseous ammonia, from slaked lime and sal ammoniac, into water kept very cold, till the specific gravity of the solution is ·882. E. directs it to be prepared from ℥xiij of muriate of ammonia, ℥xiij of quick-lime, slaked with f ℥vijss of water. The retort to be connected with a receiver, and this with a ℥viij bottle half filled with water, and communicating with another bottle containing f ℥viij of water. The apparatus to be furnished with safety tubes, and the receiver and bottles kept very cool. The smaller bottle contains the stronger solution, the larger the weaker, which is to be brought to ·960 by adding water, or the stronger solution, as may be required.

LIQUOR AMMONIÆ ACETATIS. *Spirit of Mindererus.* L. (Ammonia Acetatis Aqua, E. & D.) To Oiv of distilled vinegar add ℥ivss of sesquicarbonate of ammonia, or q. s. to saturate it. E. directs ℥j of carbonate of ammonia and f℥xxiv of distilled French vinegar; or so much as will remove any bitterness. D. orders one part of the carbonate to about 30 of distilled vinegar, or q. s. to saturate it, as ascertained by litmus. Dose, fʒiij to fʒxij.

Liquor Ammoniæ Anisatus. See Spiritus Am. Anis.

Liquor Ammoniæ Sesquicarbonatis. L. (Aqua Ammoniæ Carbonatis, E.) Sesquicarbonate (formerly carbonate or subcarbonate) of ammonia ℥iv, distilled water Oj. Dissolve, and filter. E. the same. D. 4 parts of the carbonate to 15 of water.

Liquor Ammoniæ Hydrosulphuretum. See Ammoniæ Hydrosulphuratum.

Liquor Anodynus Hoffmanni. See Spiritus Ætheris Compositus.

Liquor Antimonii Tartarizati. See Vinum Antimonii Potassio-tartratis, and Liquor Tartari Emetici.

Liquor Antipsoricus. Van Mons. Sulphuret of sodium ʒj, muriate of ammonia ℈ijss. Dissolve each separately in ℥vj of water, filter, and mix.

Liquor Argenti Acetatis. Hann. Ph. Acetate of silver 1 part, distilled water 19 parts.

Liquor Argenti Ammonio-chloridi. Niemann. Dissolve ℈ss of nitrate of silver in ℥ij of distilled water, and precipitate by solution of common salt q. s. Wash the precipitate, dissolve it in ℥jss of liquor ammoniæ, and add ʒiij of hydrochloric acid. Add water to make up the weight ℥ijss. Dose, 10 drops, in epilepsy, &c.

Liquor Argenti Nitratis. L. Nitrate of silver ʒj, distilled water f℥j; dissolve, and keep it in a well-stopped bottle in a dark place. This is chiefly intended as a test liquor. (See also Solutio Argenti Nit. E.) St. B. H. has under this name nitrate of silver gr. viij, rose water f℥j.

Liquor Arsenicalis. E. and U. S. As Liq. Potassæ Arsenitis, L.

Liquor Ammoniæ Arseniatis. Biett. Arseniate of ammonia gr. iv, distilled water f℥iv, spirit of angelica fʒij. Dose, as the next. There are 3 other formulæ for this solution, differing in strength from the above.

LIQUOR ARSENIATIS SODÆ. PEARSON'S Arsenical Solution. Arseniate of soda gr. iv, distilled water f ℥iv. Dose, from ♏xij to ♏xxx in the day.

LIQUOR ARSENICI PERIODIDI. WACKENRODER. Metallic arsenic in powder gr. j, iodine gr. vj, water ʒxij: digest at a gentle heat till dissolved. Evaporate the filtered solution to dryness at a moderate temperature, taking care not to raise it above 86° F. after it begins to solidify. Dissolve the salt in ℥vj of distilled water. Each ʒj contains gr. ⅛th of periodide of arsenic.

LIQUOR ARSENICI ET HYDRARGYRI HYDRIODATIS. See Liq. Hydriodatis Arsenici et Hydrargyri.

LIQUOR BARII CHLORIDI. L. *Solutio Barytæ Muriatis.* E. Chloride of barium ʒj, distilled water f ℥j. Dissolve. D. directs 1 part of muriate of barytes to 3 of water. Dose, (L.) ♏v, carefully increased to xv or xx.

LIQUOR BORACIS COMPOSITUS. Dr. COPLAND. Borax ʒvj, bitartrate of potash ℥ss, water Oj.

LIQUOR BROMINII. M. POURCHE. Bromine 1 part, distilled water 40 parts. Dose, 5 or 6 drops, 3 times a day. A stronger solution (1 part to 10) is sometimes used externally.

LIQUOR CALCIS. L. *Aqua Calcis*, or *Lime Water*. Quick-lime ℔ss, water Oxij. Add the lime, previously slaked, to the water; stir, and immediately cover the vessel, and set aside for 3 hours. Keep the mixture in stopped glass vessels, and when it is to be used take from the clear solution, [replacing what is taken out with more water, E.] D. directs the lime to be slaked with hot water, which expedites the process.

LIQUOR CALCIS COMPOSITUS. See Aqua Calcis Composita.

LIQUOR CALCIS MURIATIS. L. 1824. See Liquor Calcii Chloridi.

LIQUOR CALCII CHLORIDI. L. *Calcis Muriatis Solutio* (E.) *Aqua* (D.) Chloride of calcium (dry muriate of lime) ℥iv, [crystals ℥viij, E.] distilled water f ℥xij. Mix. D. 2 parts of the dry salt to 7 of distilled water. Dose, from ♏xv to f ʒj.

LIQUOR CALCIS CHLORINATÆ. P. Chloride [hypochlorite] of lime 1 part, water 45 parts. Triturate the chloride with successive small quantities of water, decanting and adding more till the whole is used. Mix the liquors, clear by repose or filtration, and keep it in well-stopped vessels. Each volume of the solution should contain 2 of chlorine. [A more concentrated solution, for which there is no authorized form, is usually sold in this country. Solutions of various strengths are also made for different purposes. See Gargarisma, Lotio, and Enema Calcis Chloridi.]

LIQUOR CALUMBÆ. *Concentrated Infusion of Calumba.* Calumba cut small ℥v, cold distilled water Oj; macerate for 12 hours, and press strongly. Macerate again with enough water to make up the whole Oj; filter, heat to 180° F. and again filter; and lastly, add f℥ij of rectified spirit. Other concentrated infusions may be made by a similar process, using 8 times the quantity of ingredients ordered in the Pharmacopœia for each Oj of water. But these preparations are not authorized by any Pharmacopœia. f ʒj with f ʒvij of water forms the infusion.

LIQUOR CAMPHORÆ. Camphor ℥j, alcohol ℥x; 20 drops to f℥j of water. Mr. FORDRED recommends, tincture of camphor fʒxiij, tincture of myrrh (bleached by animal charcoal) fʒss, rectified spirit f℥ij ʒijss. For camphor mixture, add f ʒiv of this liquor to f℥xvj of water. But neither of these will form an *exact* imitation of Mistura Camphoræ. SWEDIAUR directs ʒij of powdered camphor to be dissolved in f℥xxiv of water saturated with carbonic acid gas. One part of this solution with 3 of water will be about the strength of Mistura Camphoræ, L.

LIQUOR CHLORINII. See Aqua Chlorinii. *Chlore Liquide,* P., is made by saturating cold water with chlorine gas.

LIQUOR CINCHONÆ. Macerate ℥xvj of bruised yellow bark with Cj of distilled water for 24 hours. Evaporate the strained infusion at a heat not exceeding 130° till reduced to ℥iijss, then filter, and add rectified spirit ℥ss. The infusion may also be made by percolation. The following has been published as Mr. BATTLEY'S form. Macerate coarsely powdered yellow bark with twice its weight of cold distilled water, for 4 or 6 hours, and press. Repeat this twice or three times. Evaporate the mixed and filtered liquors in a warm-bath to 1·200 sp. gr.; let it settle, decant, and add proof spirit q. s. to reduce the sp. gr. of the liquid to 1·100. 28℔ of good bark yield 5℔ or 6℔ of the liquor at 1·200, containing 102 grains of quinine.

LIQUOR CUPRI AMMONIO-SULPHATIS. L. Cupri Ammoniati

Solutio. E. Ammonio-sulphate of copper ʒj, distilled water Oj; dissolve and filter. D. 1 part of the salt to 100 of water.

Liquor Cupri Sulphatis Compositus. L. 1746. *Aqua Styptica.* Sulphate of copper ℥iij, alum ℥ij, sulphuric acid ℥ij, water f℥xxiv.

Liquor Cupri cum Camphora. See Aqua Camphorata Bateana.

Liquor Disinfectans. Liq. Sodæ Chlorinatæ, and Liq. Calcis Chloridi, are so called. The name has also been applied to Sir W. Burnett's patent solution of chloride of zinc, and to a solution of nitrate of lead. These, as do sulphate of iron and several other metallic salts, absorb sulphuretted hydrogen.

Liquor Ferri Alkalini. L. 1824. Iron filings, or wire ʒijss, nitric acid f℥ij, distilled water f℥vj, solution of subcarbonate of potash f℥vj. Pour the mixed acid and water on the iron, and when the effervescence has ceased decant the clear solution. Add this gradually and at intervals, to the solution of potash, frequently stirring till the action has ceased. Set it by for 6 hours, and pour off the clear liquor. Dose, ♏xx to fʒj.

Liquor Ferri Citratis. Beral. Proceed as directed for Ferri Citras, adding distilled water to the solution to make it up f℥xvj.

Liquor Ferri Oxysulphatis. See Solutio Ferri Oxysulphatis.

Liquor Ferri Per-nitratis. See Ferri Per-nitras.

Liquor Ferri Potassio-citratis. Dr. J. Todd. Citric acid ʒxviij, carbonate of potash ʒvij, water f℥xxiv, sesquioxide of iron ʒj. Digest with a gentle heat for 24 hours, and neutralize with aromatic spirit of ammonia. fʒj contains gr. v of potash-citrate of iron.

Liquor Ferri Iodidi. U. S. Mix ℥ij of iodine with Oss of water, and add ℥j of iron filings; stir frequently, and heat the mixture gently till it assumes a greenish colour; then add f℥v of prepared honey, continue the heat for a short time, and filter. Lastly, pour distilled water in the filter till enough has passed to make up the whole fʒxx. See also Solutio Ferri Iodidi, and Syrupus Ferri Iodidi. E.

Liquor Ferri Tartarizati. Phillips. Bitartrate of potash 64 parts, soft iron filings 15 parts, water q. s. to form a soft paste. Expose to the air, stirring frequently, and adding water to keep it moist, till the action ceases; then add 7 times its weight of water, and filter. See also Solutio Ferri and Tinctura Ferri Tartarizati.

LIQUOR FOWLERI. Liq. Potassæ Arsenitis.

LIQUOR FUMANS BOYLII. Mix 4 parts of slaked lime with 2 of sal ammoniac and 1 of sulphur, and distil into a cool receiver.

LIQUOR HYDRIODATIS ARSENICI ET HYDRARGYRI. Mr. DONOVAN. Triturate 6·08 grains of metallic arsenic, 15·38 grains of quicksilver, and 50 grains of iodine, with f ʒj of alcohol till dry; mix the powder with f ℥viij of distilled water, put them into a flask with ʒss of hydriodic acid, (prepared by the acidification of 2 gr. of iodine,) and boil for a few minutes. When cold add water to make up the measure exactly f ℥viij. Dose, ♏xx to xxx. Mr. WILSON gives from 10 to 25 drops 3 times a day with meals, *in Lepra*. [M. SOUBEIRAN proposes to make the solution with 1 part of the red iodide of arsenic, 1 of red iodide (biniodide) of mercury, and 98 of water. To make f ℥viij on this principle, triturate 35 gr. of red iodide of arsenic, and 35 gr. of biniodide of mercury, with a little water, add f ℥vij of boiling water, filter the solution, and add water to make up exactly f ℥viij.]

LIQUOR HYDRARGYRI BICHLORIDI. L. *Van Swieten's Liquor.* Bichloride of mercury ℈ss, hydrochlorate of ammonia ℈ss, distilled water Oj; dissolve. It contains gr. j of sublimate in f ℥ij, or 876 gr. Dose, f ʒss to f ʒij.

LIQUOR HYDRARGYRI BICHLORIDI COMPOSITUS. *Liqueur Mercurielle Normale.* MIALHE. Distilled water ℥xvj, muriate of soda gr. xvj, muriate of ammonia gr. xvj, white of 1 egg, bichloride of mercury gr. iv. Beat the white of egg with the water, filter, dissolve the salts in the liquid, and filter again.

LIQUOR HYDRARGYRI BICYANIDI. PARENT. Bicyanide of mercury gr. viij, distilled water ʒxvj. Dose, f ʒss to f ʒij.

LIQUOR HYDRARGYRO-CYANIDI IODIDI POTASSII. M. CASTLENAU. Cyanhydrargyrate of iodide of potassium gr. iv, distilled water ℥iv. Dose, ℥ss twice a day. For outward use the quantity of the salt is from 4 to 20 grains to ℥iv of water.

LIQUOR HYDRARGYRI ET AMMONIÆ NITRATIS. WARD'S *White Drop.* Nitrate of quicksilver and ammonia in crystals 1 part, rose-water 3 parts; digest till dissolved.

LIQUOR HYDRARGYRI DEUTO-NITRATIS. P. Quicksilver ℥j, nitric acid (1·320) ℥ij; dissolve, and evaporate to ʒxviij. (*All by weight.*) A powerful caustic, giving rise to a white eschar, which does not fall off for 5 or 6 days.

LIQUOR IODINEI COMPOSITUS. E. 1841. Iodine ʒij, iodide of potassium ℥j, distilled water f℥xvj. Dissolve with gentle heat and agitation. [This is 30 times as strong as Liquor Potassii Iodidi Comp. L. A still stronger solution is directed in U. S.—viz., iodine ℈vj, iodide of potassium ℥jss, water f℥xvj.] The dose of the E. may be ♏v to xv in sugared water; of U. S. not above ♏vj.

LIQUOR MAGNESIÆ CARBONATIS. *Eau Magnésienne.* P. Crystallized sulphate of magnesia ℈vij, crystallized carbonate (subc.) of soda ℈ix; dissolve them separately in water, mix the solutions, boil as long as any gas is disengaged, let it rest, pour off the liquid, and carefully wash the precipitate; drain it, diffuse it in Oj of distilled water, charge it with 6 volumes of carbonic acid gas, and agitate the mixture frequently for 24 hours. [This solution contains about 6 gr. of carbonate of magnesia in f℥j. To make a stronger solution, as MURRAY'S, or DINNEFORD'S, the precipitate from 3 times the above quantity of salts must be used for each Oj of water, and a larger quantity of gas. By powerful pressure and agitation for some hours a solution may be procured containing 17 or 18 gr. of carbonate of magnesia in each f℥j. The dry heavy carb. of magnesia may be substituted for the moist, but is less readily dissolved.]

LIQUOR MAGNESIA CARBONATUS AERATUS. *Eau Magnésienne Gazeuse.* P. This is made as the last, but with only half the quantity of the salts; or gr. iij of carbonate of magnesia to each ounce.

LIQUOR MAGNESII CHLORIDI. Dr. LEBERT. Dissolve crystallized muriate of magnesia (chloride of magnesium) in its weight of water. Dose, ℥j, diluted: to a child (from 10 to 14) ℈iv, (by weight.)

LIQUOR MAGNESIÆ CITRATIS. Heavy carbonate of magnesia ℈v, citric acid ʒijss, syrup of orange-peel ℥j, water Oss. By corking it in a strong bottle before all the gas is escaped, an aërated laxative draught is formed.

LIQUOR MAGNESIÆ SULPHATIS. Dr. HENRY, of Dublin. Saturate cold water with sulphate of magnesia, and to ℥vij of the solution add ʒj of diluted sulphuric acid. See Solutio.

Liquor Magnesiæ Sulphatis Aeratus. See Aqua Sedlitzensis.

Liquor Magnesiæ Sulphatis cum Antimonio. Ch. Sulphate of magnesia ℥iv, tartarized antimony gr. ij, hot water f℥xvj.

Liquor Maticonis. Bruised matico leaves ʒviij, distilled water Oj, rectified spirit f℥ijss. As Liquor Calumbæ. Dose, fʒj to fʒij.

Liquor Morphiæ. Except Solutio Muriatis Morphiæ, E., there are no authorized or universally recognised standard solutions of the salts of morphia in this country, although frequently ordered in prescriptions. Several formulæ are in use, differing considerably in strength; some of them founded on those of Magendie, others intended to be of the same strength as Tinctura Opii. (See Pharmaceutical Journal, vol. 1, pages 170 and 287.) See Liq. Morphiæ Acetatis; Solutio Morphiæ Muriatis; Solutio Morphiæ Bimeconatis.

Liquor Morphiæ Acetatis. M. Acetate of morphia xvj French (equivalent to xiij English) grains, distilled water ℥j, rectified spirit ʒj, acetic acid a few drops, to render the solution complete. It is sometimes made, and the formula has been repeatedly so published, with gr. xvj of the acetate. Mr. Haden's form (adopted at Mid. H.) is acetate of morphia gr. xvj, distilled water ʒvj, distilled vinegar ʒij. But a weaker solution is frequently adopted. Some respectable establishments prepare it with gr. xij of the acetate in ℥j of liquid, which is almost exactly Magendie's strength; many put only gr. viij; and some only gr. iv or ivss, to ʒj. The latter strength is about that of laudanum. Manch H. Morphia gr. iv, distilled vinegar fʒij, distilled water fʒv, rectified spirit fʒj. Dose, ♏xx. In dispensing prescriptions, care must be taken to ascertain which of these various forms is intended.

Liquor Morphiæ Citratis. M. Pure morphiæ gr. xij (xvj French grains), citric acid gr. viij, distilled water ʒj, tincture of cochineal ʒij. For Dr. Porter's Solution, see Liquor Opii Citricus.

Liquor Morphiæ Hydrochloratis. Mid. H. Hydrochlorate (muriate) of morphia gr. xvj, rect. spirit fʒj, distilled water fʒvij. This solution is 3½ times the strength of the Ed. solution. See Solutio Morphiæ Muriatis, E.

Liquor Morphiæ Sulphatis. M. As Liq. Morphiæ Acetatis,

substituting sulphate for acetate of morphia, and diluted sulphuric for acetic acid. U. S. Sulphate of morphia gr. viij, distilled water f ℥viij. Dose of this last, f ʒss to f ʒij. Dr. COPLAND'S solution (of the strength of tincture of opium) consists of sulphate of morphia gr. iv, distilled water ℥j.

LIQUOR OPIATUS. GUY'S H. Boil gently ℥viij of powdered opium with Oij of fresh juice of crab-apples for half an hour, pour off the liquor and boil the remaining opium with Oj more juice for a quarter of an hour, strain, and press; then add to the mixed liquors bruised nutmeg ℥j, saffron ℥ss, yeast f ℥ss. Ferment for some days, macerate for 14 days, filter, and evaporate by water-bath to the consistence of thin syrup. Dose, ♏ij to x.

LIQUOR OPII ACETICUS. Mr. HOULTON. Turkey opium dried ℥ijss, diluted acetic acid ℥xxxij. Digest for 6 days with a gentle heat, and filter. Evaporate to an extract, macerate it in f ℥v of rectified spirit and f ℥xxxv of distilled water for 8 days, and filter. Of the same strength as Tinctura Opii.

LIQUOR OPII CITRICUS. Dr. PORTER'S Liq. Morphiæ Citratis. Opium ℥iv, citric acid ℥ij; triturate, and add boiling water f ℥xvj. Digest for 24 hours, and filter.

LIQUOR OPII TARTARICUS. As the last, substituting tartaric acid.

LIQUOR OPII SEDATIVUS. Mr. BATTLEY'S excellent preparation is made (according to Dr. SIGMOND) by macerating opium in distilled water for a long time at the temperature of the laboratory, and adding a little spirit to the filtered solution. Dr. CHRISTISON states that ♏xx of the solution is equal to ♏xxx of laudanum. Mr. COOLEY says it may be exactly imitated by dissolving ℥iij of hard extract of opium (prepared by percolation with temperate water) in ℥xxx of boiling distilled water, and adding to the cold and filtered solution ℥vj of rectified spirit, and water to make up exactly Oij. Other formulæ have been published; but when BATTLEY'S preparation is prescribed, his alone should be employed.

LIQUOR OPII CONCENTRATUS. Messrs. SMITH, of Edinburgh. Prepare, from ℥iv of opium, a watery extract freed from narcotine by æther (see Extr. Opii absque Narcotina); dissolve it in alcohol, evaporate the clear solution, redissolve the extract in water, and reduce the filtered solution to ℥xij. To this is added rectified spirit ʒxxij, and distilled water q. s. to make up ℥xvj. Dose, three to five drops.

LIQUOR PICIS. See Aqua Picis.

LIQUOR PLUMBI DIACETATIS. L. (Plumbi Diacetatis Solutio. E.) *Goulard's Extract of Lead.* Acetate of lead ℥xxvij, litharge ℥xvj, water Ovj; boil for half an hour, occasionally stirring, and when the liquor has cooled, add distilled water q. s. to make up Ovj, and strain it. E. The same, but one-fourth the quantity. D. (Plumbi Subacetatis Liquor.) One part of litharge boiled with twelve of distilled vinegar to eleven parts.

LIQUOR PLUMBI DIACETATIS DILUTUS. L. [Compositus, D.] *Goulard Water.* Solution of diacetate of lead f ʒjss, distilled water Oj, proof spirit f ʒij. [GUY'S H. directs f ʒij of tincture of opium, or f ʒij of spirit of camphor, to be sometimes added.]

LIQUOR POTASSÆ. L. Solution of Potassa. (*Aqua Potassæ,* E. *Aqua Potassæ Causticæ,* D.) Take of carbonate of potash ʒxv, lime ʒviij, boiling distilled water Cj. Dissolve the carbonate (subc.) of potash in Oiv of the water. Slake the lime in an earthen vessel with a little of the water, and add the rest. Mix the liquors in a close vessel, and shake them frequently till they are cold. When the carbonate of lime has subsided, decant the clear solution into well-stopped green-glass bottles. E. directs ℥iv carbonate of potassa to be dissolved in f ℥38 of water, and ℥ij of quicklime, slaked with f ℥vij of water, added in eight successive portions to the boiling solution. After standing twenty-four hours in a narrow glass vessel, draw off f ℥35 at least of clear liquid. D. directs it to be prepared from two parts of lime, two of carbonate of potash, and fifteen of water. Dose, ♏x to xxx, sometimes more, freely diluted.

LIQUOR POTASSÆ BRANDISHII. BRANDISH'S *Caustic Alkali.* American pearl ashes ℔vj, quicklime ℔ij, wood ashes prepared by burning the branches of the ash ℔ij, boiling water six old gallons (five imp.), slake the lime, add the rest of the water and the pearl ashes, and lastly stir in the wood ashes; let it stand in a covered vessel for 24 hours, and decant. To each pint add one drop of true oil of juniper berries. Keep it in stoppered bottles of green glass. Dose, ♏x to f ʒj or more in beer.

LIQUOR POTASSÆ ACETATIS. GUY'S H. Carbonate of potash ℥viij, strong acetic acid Oj, or q. s. to neutralize; then add water q. s. to make up exactly f ʒxx. Dose, f ʒj to f ʒij in infusion of juniper berries, &c.

LIQUOR POTASSÆ ARSENITIS. L. Liquor Arsenicalis, E. & D. *Fowler's Arsenical Solution.* Arsenious acid (white arsenic) in small fragments ℈iv, carbonate of potash ℈iv, distilled water f℥x; boil together in a glass vessel till dissolved. To the cold solution add, compound tincture of lavender f ʒv, and enough distilled water to make up exactly f℥xx. "Dose, ♏v three times a day. It should be given on a full stomach, and the dose reduced as soon as the conjunctiva is affected."—Mr. HUNT. [For PEARSON'S Arsenical Solution see Liq. Sodæ Arseniatis. Liqueur Arsenicale, P., contains one grain each of arsenious acid and carbonate of potash in 100 grains. DEVERGIE'S, one of each in 5000 grains. DE VALLENGER'S *Mineral Solution,* Mr. REDWOOD states, consists of two grains of arsenious acid, fʒss of hydrochloric acid, and f℥j of water.]

LIQUOR POTASSÆ CARBONATIS. L. (Liq. Pot. Subcarb., L. 1824. *Oleum Tartari.*) Carbonate of potash ℥xx, distilled water Oj; dissolve and filter. D. (Aqua Pot. Carb.) One part of carbonate to two parts of water.

LIQUOR POTASSÆ CHLORINATÆ. *Eau de Javelle.* Dissolve one part of subcarbonate of potash in eight or ten parts of water, and pass chlorine gas through it till fully saturated.

LIQUOR POTASSÆ CITRATIS. U. S. *Neutral Mixture.* Fresh lemon-juice f℥viij, carbonate of potash q. s. to neutralize the acid. Or, citric acid ʒss, oil of lemon ♏ij, water fʒviij, carbonate of potash q. s. See Mistura Salina. ELLIS'S *Neutral Solution* contains in addition gr. j of potash-tartrate of antimony in f℥ivss.

LIQUOR POTASSÆ EFFERVESCENS. L. *Aërated Potash Water.* Dissolve ʒj of bicarbonate of potash in Oj of distilled water, and supersaturate it by pressure with carbonic acid gas.

LIQUOR POTASSÆ SILICATIS. Liquamen Silicum. BATE. *Liquor* or *Oil of Flints.* Mix one part of powdered quartz with two of carbonate of potash; [or 70 parts of subcarbonate of potash, 54 of dry carbonate of soda, and 152 of fine quartzose sand;] and fuse in a Hessian crucible. Let the compound deliquesce in a damp place. Dose, from 10 to 30 drops. "It resolves the stone, and opens obstructions."—BATE.

LIQUOR POTASSII CYANIDI. LAMING. Cyanide of potassium gr. xxij, proof spirit fʒix. This is of the strength of his hydrocyanic acid, which contains gr. j of real acid in fʒj. MAGENDIE'S medicinal hydrocyanate of potash consists of cyanide of potassium dissolved in eight times its weight of distilled water.

LIQUOR POTASSII IODIDI. GUY'S H. Iodide of potassium ℥iv, distilled water f℥vij : ♏x contain gr. v of iodide of potassium.

LIQUOR POTASSII IODIDI COMPOSITUS. L. Iodide of potassium ℈ss, iodine gr. v, distilled water Oj. Dose, f ʒij to f ʒvj. [See Liquor Iodinei Compositus for E. & U. S. See also Solutio Iodinii. BOUCHARDAT'S *Eau Iodurée*, as an antidote for poisoning by vegetable alkaloids, consists of gr. iij of iodine, gr. vj of iodide of potassium, and f ℥xvj of water. To be taken by glassfuls, after the stomach has been emptied.]

LIQUOR POTASSII SULPHURETI. See Aqua Sulphureti Potassæ. D.

LIQUOR QUINÆ ACETATIS, SULPHATIS, &c. These solutions are prepared by Mr. BULLOCK from amorphous quinine, and contain gr. xij of these salts in f ʒj.

LIQUOR QUINO-ARSENICALIS. M. BOUDIN. Arsenious acid gr. j, water 4000 grains; boil, and add ℈j of sulphate of quinine, and one drop of sulphuric acid.

LIQUOR RHEI. Rhubarb cut small ℥iij, cold distilled water Oj; macerate for 12 hours, strain, and press. Macerate the rhubarb again with as much water as will make up Oj with the former, and press strongly. Filter the mixed liquors, and add f ℥ij of rectified spirit: f ʒj with f ʒvij of water forms Infusum Rhei.

LIQUOR SARZÆ. Mr. HERRING. Macerate ℥x of Jamaica sarsaparilla in Ovj of distilled water at a temperature not above 120° F., for six hours, and strain. Macerate with Ovj more water, as before. Evaporate the strained liquors in porcelain vessels, at 160°. [If reduced to f ℥x (or to f ℥ix, and f ℥j of spirit added), f ʒj mixed with f ʒvij of water forms the decoction of the usual strength. If reduced to f ℥v, f ʒj will represent f ℥ij of the decoction; if to f ℥ijss, f ℥iv. Mr. BATTLEY'S Liquor is still stronger, f ʒj representing Oss of the decoction.] See also Extractum Sarzæ Fluidum.

LIQUOR SENNÆ. To make a *concentrated infusion*, f ʒj of which shall represent f ℥j of the infusion, take ℥xv of small senna, ʒxss of bruised ginger; macerate them for 12 hours with Oij of cold distilled water; press strongly, and again macerate the senna &c. with enough water to make up f ℥xviij with the former infusion. Press strongly, filter the mixed liquids, heat them (in a loosely-corked vessel placed in water) to 180° F., and again filter. When cool, add rectified spirit f ℥ijss. To make a preparation one part of which requires three parts of water to reduce it to the strength of the infusion, take ℨvijss of senna, ℨv ℈j of ginger, and Oj of water. Proceed as above.

LIQUOR SODÆ CAUSTICÆ. *Soap Lees.* P. directs caustic soda (see Soda Pura) to be dissolved in water, so as to form a solution of 1·334 density; which indicates about 31 parts of soda pura to 68 of water.

LIQUOR SODÆ CHLORINATÆ. L. LABARRAQUE'S *Disinfecting Solution.* Liquid Chloride, or Hypochlorite of Soda. Dissolve ℔j of carbonate of soda in Oij of water. Put into a retort chloride of sodium ℥iv, and binoxide of manganese ℨiij, then add sulphuric acid ℥iv, previously mixed with f ℨiij of water, and cooled. Heat, and pass the chlorine gas first through f ℨv of water, and afterwards into the solution of carbonate of soda. [P. Diffuse ℔j of chloride of lime in ℔xx of water, and decant. Dissolve also ℔ij of carbonate of soda, in crystals, in ℔xv of water. Mix the clear solutions, and filter. It should contain twice its volume of chlorine.] Dose, ♏xx to f ʒj. It is used as a disinfectant, as chloride of lime; but is chiefly employed, in preference to the latter, as an internal remedy, and for lotions, &c.

LIQUOR SODÆ EFFERVESCENS. L. *Soda Water.* Sesquicarbonate of soda ℨj, distilled water Oj. Dissolve, and supersaturate by pressure, with carbonic acid gas. [It may be extemporaneously prepared by putting ʒss of sesquicarbonate of soda into a tumbler, and pouring on it a bottle of soda water. The ordinary soda water contains but little soda. Dr. PEREIRA.]

LIQUOR SODÆ TARTARIZATÆ EFFERVESCENS. Dr. YOUNG. Put into a soda water bottle ʒijss of carbonate of soda, ℨiij of bitartrate of potash, and Oss of water. Cork securely, and place the bottle in a cool place for 2 days.

LIQUOR TARAXACI. Dandelion roots, clean, dried, and sliced, ℨxviij; infuse for 24 hours in q. s. of cold distilled water to cover them. Press, and set aside; decant the clear liquor, and heat it to 180° F., filter whilst hot, and evaporate in a drying room, or by a current of warm air, until the product shall weigh 14 ounces; add rectified spirit ℨiv. [The quantity of spirit might perhaps be reduced.] Dose, f ʒj to f ʒiij. (Annals of Chemistry, No. 4.) See also Cremor Taraxaci.

LIQUOR TARTARI EMETICI. D. Tartarized antimony ℈j, boiling distilled water f ℥viij, rectified spirit f ℨij.

Liquor Volatilis Cornu Cervi. *Spirit of Hartshorn.* L. 1788. Distilled from hart's horns, or from bones; the volatile liquor, separated from the oil and salt which come over with it, is to be redistilled 3 times.

Liquor Volatilis Cornu Cervi Succinatus. P. Add to the last as much volatile salt of amber (Sal Succini) as will saturate it; filter, and keep in a dark place.

[See Solutio for preparations of this class which are not found under Liquor.]

Lithiæ Carbonas. Porphyrize petalite (or other mineral containing lithia) and calcine in a platina crucible, with 5 times its weight of nitrate of barytes. Mix the product with 16 times its weight of water, and add muriatic acid in excess. Evaporate the solution to dryness, heat the residue in water acidulated with muriatic acid, and filter. To the filtrate, add sulphuric acid in slight excess, filter, add ammonia, and evaporate the filtered solution to dryness. Dissolve the residue in water, treat it with carbonate of soda, wash the precipitate with a very little water, and dry it. [*As an antacid and antilithic.* Dose undetermined. Dr. Ure suggests the injection of its solution into the bladder as a solvent for uric calculi.]

Lixivium Saponarium. *Liquor Potassæ.*

Lixivum Tartari. *Liquor Potassæ Subcarbonatis.*

Lohoch Album. P. Blanched sweet almonds ʒivss, bitter almonds ℈ss, sugar ℈iv, oil of almonds ℈iv, gum tragacanth gr. xv, orange-flower water ʒiv, water ℥iv. Mix, S. A.

Lohoch Cetacei. E. 1744. Spermaceti ʒij, yolk of egg q. s.; triturate, and add gradually oil of almonds ℥ss, syrup of Tolu ℥j.

Lohoch Commune. E. 1744. Oil of almonds ℥j, syrup of Tolu ℥j, white sugar ʒij. Mix.

Lohoch Expectorans Zanetti. Kermes mineral gr. iv, manna ℥vj, oil of almonds ʒij, syrup of squills ʒij, syrup of senega ʒij. Mix. A teaspoonful every 4 hours.

Lohoch Lini. E. 1744. Fresh-drawn linseed oil ℥j, syrup of Tolu ℥j, sulphur ʒij, white sugar ʒij.

Lohoch Mannæ. E. 1744. Equal parts of manna, oil of almonds, and syrup of violets.

Lohoch Naphthalinæ. M. Dupasquier. To one common

lohoc (Lohoch Album) add from gr. viij to ℨss of naphthaline. The naphthaline must be well triturated with the gum. Dose, a tablespoonful, frequently repeated; *as an expectorant.*

LOHOCH OLEOSUM. P. Oil of almonds ʒiv, gum Arabic powder ʒiv, syrup of marsh-mallow ℥j, water ℥iij, orange-flower water ʒiv.

LOHOCH OVI. Oil of almonds ℨjss, yolk of 1 egg, syrup of marsh-mallow ℥j.

LOHOCH DE POLMONE VULPIS. *Fox's Lungs.* Powdered fox's lungs, extract of liquorice, powdered aniseed and fennel-seed, each ℥j, syrup of marsh-mallow ℥xij. The first ingredient is now usually omitted.

LOHOCH SAPONIS. E. 1744. Alicant soap ʒj, oil of almonds ℥j, syrup of Tolu ℥jss.

LOHOCH VIRIDE. Pistachio nuts (or sweet almonds) No. 14, syrup of violets ℥j, oil of almonds ℨiv, gum tragacanth gr. xv, tincture of saffron ℈j, orange-flower water ʒij, water ℥iv. [For other similar compounds, see LINCTUS.]

LOTIO ACETI. One part of vinegar to 3 of water is a common proportion for sponging: one of vinegar with one or two of water for bruises, &c.

LOTIO ACIDA. GUY'S H. Nitric acid ♏xxxviij, (or nitro-hydrochloric acid ♏xlvj,) water Oj. Tincture of opium f ℨij is occasionally added; and the quantity of acid increased 2 or 3 fold.

LOTIO ACIDI PHOSPHORICI. PEREIRA. Diluted phosphoric acid f ℥j, water f ℥x. *In Caries.*

LOTIO ACIDI HYDROCYANICI. See Lotio Hydrocyanica.

LOTIO ALKALINA. P. Subcarbonate of potash ℥ij, water (or rose-water) Oij.

LOTIO ALKALINA AMYGDALINA. DR. A. T. THOMSON. Solution of potash f ʒiv, emulsion of bitter almonds f ℥vss. [To remove the scurf in *Porrigo Furfurans;* afterwards applied twice a day diluted with warm water.]

LOTIO AD ALOPECIAM. DR. LANDERER. Bay leaves ℥ij, cloves ℨij, spirit of lavender ℥iv, spirit of origanum ℥iv. Digest for 6 days, strain, and add sulphuric æther ℥ss. Applied by friction, to prevent the hair falling off. MR. WILSON prescribes, eau de Cologne f ℥ij, tincture of cantharides f ℥ss, oil of nutmeg f ʒss, oil of lavender ♏x.

LOTIO ALUMINIS. Alum ʒj to ʒiv, water Oj.

LOTIO AMMONIÆ ACETATIS. Solution of acetate of ammonia, rectified spirit, and water (or rose-water), equal parts.

LOTIO AMMONIÆ HYDROCHLORATIS. GUY'S H. Sal ammoniac ℥j, vinegar Ojss.

LOTIO AMMONIÆ HYDROCHLORATIS SPIRITUOSA. GUY'S H. Hydrochlorate of ammonia ℥j, vinegar Oss, rectified spirit f ℥iv. MID. H. Sal ammoniac ℥j, distilled vinegar f ℥ij, rectified spirit f ℥ij, water f ℥xvj. *For contusions (when the skin is not broken), chronic tumours, chilblains, &c.*

LOTIO AMMONIÆ HYDROCHLORATIS FORTIOR. MAN. H. Muriate of ammonia ℥j, distilled vinegar f ℥xij, rectified spirit f ℥iv.

LOTIO AMMONIÆ OPIATA. Dr. KIRKLAND. Spirit of ammonia ℥iijss, water ℥iv, tincture of opium ℥ss.

LOTIO ANTIPHLOGISTICA. COPLAND. Liquid diacetate of lead ʒvj, solution of acetate of ammonia ℥iv, distilled water Oij.

LOTIO ANTIMONIALIS. Sir W. BLIZARD. Tartarized antimony ℈j, distilled water ℥j.

LOTIO ANTIPSORICA. CAZENAVE. Sulphuret of potassium ʒj, soap ʒij, water ℥viij. Dr. CULLEN. Decoction of white hellebore f ℥xvj, sulphuret of potassium ʒss. Dr. DORNBLUETH. Soft soap 125 parts, hellebore 60, hot water q. s. to form a mixture of the consistence of syrup.

LOTIO ARGENTI NITRATIS. Lotions of nitrate of silver are used of various strengths for different purposes. As, for *Bed Sores*, gr. x of the nitrate to f ℥j of distilled water applied with a camel's hair pencil 2 or 3 times a day till the skin is blackened; then only occasionally. (Mr. JACKSON, Sheffield,) for *Chilblains*, from gr. x to xxx to f ℥j of water, &c. See Injectio, &c.

LOTIO ARNICÆ. The tincture, in the proportion of from 10 to 30 drops to f ℥j of water, is used in contusions, extravasations, &c. NIEMANN prescribes the following lotion (applied cold) in acute hydrocephalus. Arnica flowers ℥ss, hot vinegar f ℥iij, boiling water f ℥v: infuse, and strain.

LOTIO ARSENICI COMPOSITA. M. LE FEBVRE, *in Cancer*. Oxide of arsenic gr. viij, distilled water f ℥xvj, extract of hemlock ℥j, liquid diacetate of lead f ℥iij, tincture of opium ʒj.

LOTIO ARSENICI ET HYDRARGYRI HYDRIODATIS. Liq. Arsen. et Hyd. f ʒj, water f ℥j.

LOTIO BELLADONNÆ. GRAEFE. Extract of belladonna ʒj, Goulard water Oj.

LOTIO BORACIS. GUY'S H. Borax ʒss, rose-water Oj. Sir A. COOPER. Borax ʒj, water ℥iij, rectified spirit ℥ss. Dr. COPLAND. Borax ʒj, rose water f ℥iij, orange-flower water f ℥iij.

LOTIO BORACIS ACIDA. Dr. ABERCROMBIE, *in Ringworm of the Scalp*. Borax ʒj, distilled vinegar f ℥ij.

LOTIO BORACIS CUM MORPHIA. Dr. MEIGS. Borax ℥ss, sulphate of morphia gr. vj, rose water f ℥viij. *In Pruritus Vulvæ.*

LOTIO BROMINII. Dr. GLOVER, to *Scrofulous Ulcers*. 20 to 30 drops of bromine to Oj of water. Others direct f ʒj of bromine to f ℥v of water.

LOTIO CALCIS SPIRITUOSA. CH. Lime-water f ℥viij, rectified spirit f ℥iv.

LOTIO CALCIS CHLORINATÆ. *For Itch.* DERHEIMS. Chloride of lime ℥j, water Oij to Oijss. Triturate and filter.

LOTIO CALCIS CHLORINATÆ CUM ACIDO HYDROCYANICO. Add to the last f ʒj of Prussic acid.

LOTIO CHLORINATA. M. Liquid chlorinated soda ℥j, water ℥x to ℥xv.

LOTIO CHLOROFORMI. Mr. TUSON. Chloric æther f ʒj—iij, water Oj. See Æther Chloricus.

LOTIO CONII ET OPII. MID. H. Extract of hemlock ʒiij, opium ʒj, boiling water Oj.

LOTIO COSMETICA. HERRMANN. Blanched almonds ℥j, orange-flower water ℥j, rose water ℥viij. Make an emulsion, strain, and add sal ammoniac ʒj, tincture of benzoin ʒijss.

LOTIO CUPRI CAMPHORATA. MID. H. Camphor ʒss, bole ʒj, sulphate of copper ℈ij, boiling water Oj. Macerate for an hour and filter. See Lotio Rubra.

LOTIO CUPRI SULPHATIS. Dr. GRAVES, *for Chilblains* and *Tinea*. Sulphate of copper gr. x, water f ℥j. Mr. LLOYD, *for Itch*, sulphate of copper ℥j, water Oj. Dr. COLEY, in *Porrigo Decalvans*, gr. xv of sulphate to f ℥j of water.

LOTIO CREASOTI CUM GALLA. Dr. NELIGAN. Creasote ♏iv, tincture of galls f ʒij, distilled water f ℥ij.

Lotio Evaporans. Copland. Æther f ℥jss, solution of acetate of ammonia f ℥jss, rectified spirit f ℥jss, rose-water f ℥iijss.

Lotio Ferri Sulphatis. Velpeau, *in Erysipelas.* Sulphate of iron ℥j, water Oj. Dr. Underwood, *for Sore Nipples,* ʒj of sulphate, to ℥viij of water.

Lotio Fuliginis. See Decoctum Fuliginis.

Lotio Gallæ. St. B. H. Bruised nutgall ʒij, boiling water Oj. Infuse, and strain. Mid. H. ʒiij to f ℥xij.

Lotio Glycerini. Mr. Startin. Glycerine ℥ss, water Oss, mix. [*To keep the skin moist in some cutaneous diseases.*]

Lotio Hydrargyri Acetatis. Acetate of mercury ℈j, distilled water Oj.

Lotio Hydrargyri Bichloridi. St. B. H. Corrosive sublimate gr. ijss, distilled water Oj, gum acacia ℥ss, Guy's H. Equal measures of solution (Liquor) of bichloride of mercury, and distilled water.

Lotio Hydrargyri Amygdalina. St. B. H. Blanch ʒiij of bitter almonds, and beat them with f ℥vj of water gradually added; strain, and add gr. iij of corrosive sublimate.

Lotio Hydrargyri Cinerea. Guy's H. *Black Wash.* Calomel ʒijss, lime-water Oj. Shake together. St. B. H. (Lotio Hydrargyri Chloridi cum Calce.) Calomel ℈ij, lime-water f ℥vj. Mid. H. Calomel ʒj, lime-water Oj, mucilage f ℥j.

Lotio Hydrargyri Flava. Guy's H. *Yellow Wash.* Corrosive sublimate gr. xxv, lime water Oj. Rub together.

Lotio Hydrargyri Bichloridi cum Calce. St. B. H. Bichloride of mercury ℈j, lime water f ℥vj.

Lotio Hydrocyanica. A. T. Thomson. Hydrocyanic acid f ʒjss, water f ℥vijss, acetate of lead gr. xvj, rectified spirit ʒij. St. B. H. Hydrocyanic acid ʒij, water f ℥vj.

Lotio Hydrocyanica Alkalina. Dr. A. T. Thomson, *in Milk Scall.* Bicarbonate of soda ʒij, milk ℥viij, hydrocyanic acid f ʒss.

Lotio Iodinii Composita. St. B. H. Iodine ʒv, iodide of potash ʒx, distilled water f ℥vj.

Lotio Iodureta Antipsorica. Cazenave. Iodide of potassium, iodide of sulphur, of each ʒjss, water ℥xxxij.

LOTIO IODO-CHLORURETA. RIGHINI. Chloride of lime ʒiv, triturate in a glass mortar, and add water ℥ijss, let it settle, filter, and add tincture of iodine ʒj. Mix, and keep it in a well-stopped bottle. [See Solutiones Iodinii.]

LOTIO LITHARGYRI, &c. See Lotio Plumbi, &c.

LOTIO MYRRHÆ. Dr. KIRKLAND. Tincture of myrrh ℥ij, lime water ℥ij. *To fungous growths.*

LOTIO MYRRHÆ COMPOSITA. CH. Honey of roses ʒij, tincture of myrrh ʒij, lime water ℥ijss.

LOTIO NIGRA. See Lotio Hydr. Cinerea.

LOTIO OPII. St. B. H. Opium ʒss, boiling water f℥vj; triturate carefully and strain. GUY'S H. directs ʒijss to Oj; to be triturated, boiled for 10 minutes, and strained.

LOTIO PICIS LIQUIDÆ. SAUNDERS. Wood tar ℥iv, lime ℥vj, water f℥xlviij; boil till half is consumed, and strain.

LOTIO PLUMBI ACETATIS. CH. Acetate of lead ʒiv, vinegar ℥iv, soft water Oij.

LOTIO PLUMBI DIACETATIS. P. Liquid diacetate of lead ʒiv, river water ℥xxx, rectified spirit ℥ij. See Liq. Plumbi Diac. Dilutus.

LOTIO PLUMBI OPIATA. Dr. CHRISTISON. Infuse gr. xxxij of opium in f℥iv of water; dissolve gr. xxxij of acetate of lead in the same quantity of water; mix the solutions, and filter them.

LOTIO PLUMBI CHLORIDI. Mr. TUSON. Chloride of lead ʒj, water Oj. To cancerous ulcers, &c.

LOTIO POTASSÆ SULPHURETI. St. B. H. Sulphuret of potash ʒij, water Oj.

LOTIO POTASSÆ CHLORATIS. Chlorate of potash ʒj, water f℥xij.

LOTIO POTASSII CYANIDI. CAZENAVE. Cyanide of potassium gr. x, emulsion of bitter almonds ℥vj. M. MALHERBE prescribes a stronger solution, ʒj of the cyanide to ℥vj of distilled water, in acute rheumatism; compresses wet with the lotion to be applied to the affected joints.

LOTIO POTASSII IODIDI. Dr. O. WARD uses ʒj iodide of potassium in from 8 to 16 ounces of water for the cure of *itch.*

LOTIO RUBEFACIENS. GERM. H. Tartar emetic ʒj, water Oj, spirit of camphor ℥ss.

LOTIO RUBRA. BATE. Sulphate of copper ʒij, red bole ℈ij, camphor ʒss, boiling water ℔ij. Strain through linen.

LOTIO SAMBUCI. F. H. Infusion of elder-flowers ℥xvj, camphorated spirit ℥ij.

LOTIO SAPONACEA. L. 1746. Rose water ℥xij, olive oil ℥iv, solution of subcarbonate of potash ℥ss.

LOTIO SODÆ CHLORINATÆ. GUY'S H. Solution of chlorinated soda ℥jss, water f℥xij.

LOTIO SODÆ HYPOSULPHITIS. Mr. STARTIN. Hyposulphite of soda ʒj—ij, alum ʒj—ij, rose water f℥vijss, Cologne water f℥ss. Apply on rag, twice a day, in the latter stage of *Acne.*

LOTIO SPIRITUS DILUTI. GUY'S H. Rectified spirit 1 part, water 5 parts.

LOTIO SPIRITUOSA CAMPHORATA. WARE. Elder flowers ℥ss, camphor ʒss, rectified spirit ℥iv. Digest 24 hours, and strain.

LOTIO STANNI. M. NAUCHE. Chloride of tin gr. j, distilled water Oij. *To Cancerous Ulcers.*

LOTIO SUCCI LIMONIS. Lemon-juice, diluted with water, is said to relieve *Pruritus Scroti.*

LOTIO TANNINI. Mr. DRUITT. Tannic acid gr. v, distilled water f℥j. To *Sore Nipples,* on lint, covered with oiled silk.

LOTIO VAPORANS. See Lotio Spiritus Diluti; and Lotio Evaporans.

LOTIO ZINCI IODIDI. Dr. ROSS. Boil from ʒj to ʒij of iodine with half its weight of zinc, in f℥viij of water, until the liquid is colourless, and filter. Applied, by means of sponge, to *Enlarged Tonsils.*

LOTIO ZINCI OXYDI. MID. H. Oxide of zinc gr. xxiv, mucilage fʒj, water fʒvij.

LOTIO ZINCI SULPHATIS. GUY'S H. Sulphate of zinc ℈j, water Oj. (U. C. H. ʒj.)

LOTIO ZINCI COMPOSITA. U. C. H. Sulphate of zinc ʒss, water Oss, Goulard water Oss. Mix, and filter.

LUPULINA. Lupuline is the yellow powder procured by rubbing and sifting the dried hops. Dose, 5 to 12 grains.

MAGNESIA. L. E. and D. Magnesia Usta. Calcined Magnesia. Calcine carbonate of magnesia for 2 hours in a strong fire, till the powder suspended in water no longer effervesces on the addition of acetic (L.) or muriatic (E.) acids. [A shorter time than 2 hours is generally sufficient; and it is injured by over-calcination, especially as an antidote to arsenic. For the latter purpose, indeed, it is better made without calcination, by adding a solution of caustic potash, or soda, to a solution of sulphate of magnesia (both cold), washing the precipitate with water, and drying it with a gentle heat.]

MAGNESIA CALCINATA PONDEROSA. Mr. R. PHILLIPS, jun. Mix solutions of 123 parts of crys. sulphate of magnesia, and 144 parts of crys. carbonate of soda; evaporate the whole to dryness, and calcine the residue till all the carbonic acid is expelled. Let it remain in water till the sulphate of soda is dissolved out, wash the magnesia, and dry it.

MAGNESIÆ CARBONAS. L. Carbonate of magnesia, [light.] Dissolve separately ℔iv of sulphate of magnesia, and ℔iv ℥viij of carbonate of soda, each in Cij of distilled water, and filter. Mix the solutions, boil with constant stirring for 15 minutes, then pour off the liquid, wash the precipitate with boiling distilled water, and dry it. [D. directs 14 parts of carbonate of potash to 25 of sulphate of magnesia. This requires longer washing.]

MAGNESIÆ CARBONAS PONDEROSA. *Heavy Magnesia.* Dr. PEREIRA. Add 1 volume of a cold saturated solution of carbonate of soda to a boiling mixture of 1 volume of saturated solution of sulphate of magnesia with 3 of water. Boil till the effervescence has ceased, constantly stirring with a spatula. Then dilute with boiling water, set aside, pour off the supernatant liquor, and wash the precipitate with hot water on a linen cloth, and dry it by heat in an iron pot.

MAGNESIÆ CITRAS. To a solution of citric acid add carbonate of magnesia, until the mixture is neutral. Wash the powder, and dry it with a gentle heat. *Laxative,* but weaker than the sulphate.

MAGNESIÆ PHOSPHAS. NIEMANN. Add to diluted phosphoric acid pure magnesia, or its carbonate to saturation. Evaporate to dryness. Dose, from 8 to 30 grains, *in Rickets.*

MAGNESIÆ SULPHAS. The commercial sulphate obtained from bittern, or from magnesian limestone, is sufficiently pure, or may be rendered so by re-crystallization.

MAGNESII BROMIDUM. To bromide of iron in solution add calcined magnesia in excess; heat the mixture, filter, and evaporate the clear solution to dryness.

MAGNESII CHLORIDUM. P. *Muriate of Magnesia.* To pure muriatic acid add carbonate of magnesia in slight excess; filter the solution, and evaporate it till the sp. gr. is 1·384, and put it, still hot, into a wide-mouthed flask to crystallize. If not required in crystals, it may be evaporated to dryness. Dose, as a laxative, ℥ij to ℥iv. (CHEVALLIER.)

MAGNESII SUPHURETUM. Fuse together 5 parts of pure magnesia and 4 of sulphur. Dose, gr. iv to xij. (JOURDAIN.)

MANGANESII CARBONAS. Wash peroxide of manganese with very dilute muriatic acid, dissolve it in strong muriatic acid, and evaporate the solution to dryness. Dissolve a portion of the residue in water, and precipitate by carbonate of soda; wash the precipitate, and digest it with a solution of the rest of the salt. Filter, and precipitate by carbonate of soda; wash the precipitate, and dry it at a gentle heat.

MANGANESII MURIAS. Saturate muriatic acid with carbonate of manganese, and evaporate to dryness by a gentle heat. Preserve it in closely stopped bottles.

MANGANESII SULPHAS. Add carbonate of manganese to dilute sulphuric acid to saturation, concentrate by a gentle heat, and set aside, that crystals may form. [It produces bilious purging and vomiting. Dose, ʒj to ʒij in Oss of water before breakfast. Mr. URE. Senna is sometimes added, to insure its purgative effect.]

MANNITA. *Mannite.* RUSPINI. Put ℔vj of common manna in ℔iij of distilled water in which the white of an egg has been beaten, and boil for a few minutes. Strain, and when cold, press the impure mannite in a cloth; mix it with its weight of water, and press again. Dissolve it in boiling water, filter into a porcelain dish, evaporate to a pellicle, and set aside to crystallize. Dose, half that of manna.

MASTICATORIA. *Masticatories.* See Pilæ Masticatoriæ.

MEL DESPUMATUM. D. *Clarified Honey.* Melt the honey in a water-bath, and remove the scum. GUY'S H. directs 4 parts of honey and 1 of water to be boiled; strained through flannel, and allowed to settle; the clear liquor to be evaporated by water-bath till the water is driven off, removing the scum.

MEL PREPARATUM. U. S. Clarified honey Oss, proof spirit Oj,

prepared chalk ℥ss; let them stand 2 hours, heat to ebullition, filter, and evaporate till its density is 1·32, when cold.

Mellitum Simplex. P. White honey ℔vj, water ℔ij; dissolve by heat, skim, and when the boiling solution attains a density of 1·261, strain through flannel.

Mel Acetatum. See Oxymel.

Mel Boracis. L. E. & D. Powdered borax ʒj, clarified honey ℥j. Mix.

Mel Chelidonii. Wendt. Mix expressed juice of greater celandine with an equal weight of honey. Dose ʒij, gradually increased to ʒiv with water. *In Glandular and Cutaneous Affections.*

Mel Colchici. Infuse one part of dried colchicum in 16 parts of water at 140° F., for 12 hours; strain, and let it settle, and boil the clear liquid with 12 parts of white honey to the consistence of syrup.

Mel Elatines. Juice of female fluellin Oiv, clarified honey ℔iv; boil to a proper thickness.

Mel Glycyrrizatum. Hamb. Ph. Liquorice root bruised ℥jss, boiling water ℥xij; infuse half an hour, strain, and boil with ℥xx of honey to the consistence of syrup.

Mel Helleboratum. L. 1746. White hellebore root ℔j, water Oiv; macerate for 3 days, boil a little, strain, and press; boil the liquor with ℔iij of honey to a syrup.

Mel Hydrargyri. Bell. Triturate ʒj of quicksilver with ℥j of honey till the globules disappear. Fouquet. Quicksilver ℈ss, chalk ℈ss, honey ℈ij. *As a dressing for Ulcers.*

Mel Hydrargyri Compositum. Allard. Honey of quicksilver ʒij, clarified honey ℥ij, oil of cloves ʒj. Mix. *To Ulcers of the Throat.*

Mel Mercuriale. E. 1744. Juice of the herb mercury, and honey, equal weights; boil to a proper consistence, removing the scum.

Mel Rosæ. L. Red rose petals dried ℥iv, boiling distilled water Oijss; macerate for 6 hours, and boil the filtered liquor with ℔v of clarified honey to a proper consistence by means of a water-bath. E. & D. nearly the same. U. S. directs the density to be 1·32.

18

MEL SALVIÆ. NEUBER. Sage leaves ℥ij, boiling water Ojss; infuse, and boil the strained liquor with ℥viij of honey to a proper consistence.

MEL SCILLÆ. SOUBEIRAN. Dried squills ℥j, boiling water ℥xvj; infuse, strain, add ℥xij of white honey, and boil to a proper consistence.

MEL SCILLÆ COMPOSITUM. Cox's Hive Syrup. Syrupus Scillæ Comp. is now substituted for it.

MEL TEREBINTHINÆ. See Electuarium Terebinthinæ.

MEL VIOLÆ. It is made either with equal quantities of boiling water, violets, and honey; or of violet juice and honey.

MELLAGO GRAMINIS. PRUS. PH. Fresh root of dog's grass is bruised with half its weight of cold water, and pressed; the juice boiled for a few moments and filtered, then evaporated to the consistence of honey.

MELLAGO TARAXACI. From fresh dandelion roots, and the young plant, in Spring, as the last.

MEZEREUM ACETATUM. Thin slices of the bark of mezereon root, soaked in vinegar for 24 hours. *Applied as a Blister.*

MERCURIUS SACCHARATUS. E. 1744. Quicksilver ʒiv, sugar-candy ʒiv, oil of juniper ♏xvj; triturate till the globules disappear.

MILLEPEDÆ PREPARATÆ. Tie millepedes in muslin, and suspend them over the vapour of heated spirit.

MISTURÆ. *Mixtures.* Under this term are placed compound liquid medicines to be taken in divided doses; including several which in some pharmacopœias are termed Juleps, Mucilages, Emulsions, Potions, &c. See also Haustus, Julapia, Ptisanæ. The usual dose of the mixture of the British pharmacopœias is f ℥j to f ℥ij, or a wineglassful. The principal exceptions will be noticed.

MISTURA ACACIÆ. L. Mucilago, E.; Mucilago Gummi Arabicæ, D. *Mucilage.* Gum arabic ℥x (E. ℥ix), water Oj. L. directs the powdered gum to be dissolved in boiling water. E. directs the gum to be dissolved in cold water, which is better, and strained through linen. Dr. CHRISTISON recommends the gum to be tied in linen. D. orders ℥iv of powdered gum to ʒiv of hot water.

MISTURA ACACIÆ. E. See Emulsio Acaciæ.

MISTURA ACIDI ACETICI. Mr. J. B. BROWN. Distilled vinegar f ʒij, syrup f ℈iv, water f ℥ij. A fourth part every 3 hours. To children, in *Scarlatina.*

MISTURA ACIDI BORACICI. CHAUSSIER. Camphor mixture ℥iv, boracic acid ʒj, syrup of orange-peel ℥j. By spoonfuls.

MISTURA ACIDI HYDROCYANICI. M. directs a Pectoral Mixture and Potion, but as the acid he employs differs from that used in England, they are omitted. For Mr. DONOVAN'S Mixture, see Haustus Hydrocyanicus.

MISTURA ACIDI OXALICI. M. NARDO. Oxalic acid gr. viij, mucilage ℥iij, syrup ℥j. By spoonfuls, *in inflammation of the fauces and digestive tube.*

MISTURA ACONITI. Dr. FLEMING, *in Gastralgia.* Tincture of aconite f ʒj, carbonate of soda ʒjss, sulphate of magnesia ℥jss, water f ℥vj. A table-spoonful when the pain is urgent.

MISTURA ÆTHERIS CAMPHORATA. BRANDE. Camphor mixture f ℥vij, sulphuric æther f ʒss, syrup of saffron f ℥ss.

MISTURA ÆTHERIS CUM TEREBINTHINA. ORFILA. *In poisoning by Nux Vomica.* Sulphuric æther ʒj, rectified oil of turpentine ʒij, white sugar ℈iv, water ℥ij. Dose, f ʒij every quarter of an hour.

MISTURA ALTHÆÆ. Decoctum Althææ. E. Marsh-mallow root [herb and root, D.] ℥iv, raisins stoned ℥ij, water Ov, boil to Oiij, and strain through calico.

MISTURA ALUMINIS. Dr. BIRD, *in Hooping Cough.* Alum gr. xxv, extract of hemlock gr. xij, syrup of red poppies f ℈ij, dill water f ℥iij. A dessert-spoonful every 6 hours.

MISTURA AMMONIACI. L. Ammoniacum ʒv, water Oj; rub the ammoniacum with the water gradually added, until they are perfectly mixed. D. directs ʒj of the gum to f ℥viij of pennyroyal water, and the mixture strained through linen.

MISTURA AMMONIACALIS. U. C. H. Gum ammoniacum ʒiij, solution of acetate of ammonia f ℥vj, spirit of nitric æther f ʒiv, mucilage of tragacanth q. s., water f ℥viij.

MISTURA AMMONIACI ACIDA. Dr. PARIS. Water f ℥iv, dilute nitric acid f ʒj, syrup ʒij, gum ammoniac ʒj. Dose, f ʒij. *Expectorant.*

MISTURA AMMONIACI ET ANTIMONII. Ammoniacum mixture

f ℥iv, antimonial wine f ʒiv, syrup of Tolu f ℥j, compound tincture of camphor f ʒiv. Mix.

MISTURA AMMONIACI FŒTIDA. St. B. H. Ammoniacum mixture f ℥viij, fœtid spirit of ammonia f ʒij.

MISTURA AMMONIÆ ACETATIS. U. C. H. Liquid acetate of ammonia f ℥iv, water f ℥viij.

MISTURA AMMONIÆ SESQUICARBONATIS. St. B. H. Sesquicarbonate of ammonia ℈ij, pimento water f ℥iv, water f ℥vj.

MISTURA AMMONIÆ MURIATIS. Sir G. LEFEVRE. Muriate of ammonia ʒj, extract of liquorice ʒiij, tartarized antimony gr. ij, distilled water ℥viij. A tablespoonful every 2 hours, *in Pleurisy, Congestion of Mucous Membranes*, &c.

MISTURA AMMONIÆ OLEOSA. St. B. H. Mixture of sesquicarbonate of ammonia f ℥vj, olive oil f ℥ij.

MISTURA AMYGDALÆ. L. Confection of almonds ℥ijss, water Oj; rub the confection with the water gradually added until perfectly mixed, and strain through linen. [When practicable it is better to make it fresh from the ingredients; peeled almonds ℥jss, white sugar ʒvj, powdered gum ʒjss; beat together, and gradually add Oj of water.] E. directs ℥ij of confection (or ʒx of peeled almonds, sugar ʒv, mucilage f ℥ss) to Oij of water.

MISTURÆ AMYGDALÆ. D. (Bitter almond mixture.) Sweet almonds, blanched, ℥jss; bitter almonds, blanched, ℈ij, white sugar ℥ss, water Oij. [BERAL directs sweet almonds ʒvj, bitter ʒij, water f ℥xvj.]

MISTURA AMYGDALINÆ. See Emulsio Amygdalæ cum Amygdalinâ.

MISTURA ANODYNA. *Julep Calmant.* P. Syrup of opium ʒij, syrup of orange flowers ʒvj, lettuce water ℥iv. Dose, f ʒiv, repeated.

MISTURA ANTIEMETICA. Dr. BARKER. Infusion of mint ℥vj, burnt brandy ℥j, compound tincture of camphor ʒj, sugar ℥ss. A tablespoonful every ¼ of an hour till the vomiting ceases. See also Mistura Effervescens.

MISTURA ANTACIDA. RYAN. Solution of potash f ʒij, lime water f ℥viij, calcined magnesia ʒj, oil of peppermint ♏v, tincture of opium f ʒj.

MISTURA ANTIHYSTERICA. Dr. PARIS. Assafœtida ʒj, peppermint water f℥jss, ammoniated tincture of valerian fʒij, tincture of castor fʒiij, æther fʒj. f℥ss every 2 hours. P. *Potion Antihysterique.* Comp. syrup of wormwood ℥j, tincture of castor ℈ss, valerian water ℥ij, orange-flower water ℥ij, sulphuric æther ʒj.

MISTURA ANTISPASMODICA. P. Syrup of orange-flowers ℥j, lime-flower water ℥ij, orange-flower water ℥ij, æther ʒss.

MISTURA ANTIMONIALIS. LAENNEC. *Julep Contrastimulant.* Tartarized antimony gr. vj, infusion of orange leaves Oj, syrup ℥ij. Dose, f℥iij every 2 hours, *in Pneumonia*, &c.

MISTURA ANTIMONII CAMPHORATA. GERM. H. Tartarized antimony gr. v, emulsion of camphor f℥x.

MISTURA APERIENS. ABERNETHY. Sulphate of magnesia ʒiv, manna ʒij, infusion of senna fʒvj, tincture of senna fʒij, mint water f℥j, water f℥ij. CHRISTISON. Tincture of senna (E.) f℥j, sulphate of magnesia ℥jss, water f℥iv, infusion of roses f℥iv. A wine-glassful every hour till it begins to operate. See also Mistura Sennæ Comp.; Mistura Magnesiæ Sulphatis, &c.

MISTURA ARMORACIÆ COMPOSITA. Dr. PARIS. Horseradish root ℥ss, mustard seed ℥ss, boiling water Oj; macerate for an hour, and to f℥vij of the strained infusion add aromatic spirit of ammonia fʒj, spirit of pimento f℥ss. *In Paralysis.*

MISTURA AROMATICA. St. B. H. Aromatic confection ʒijss, water f℥v, pimento water f℥iij. GUY'S H. Aromatic confection in powder ʒiij, mint julep f℥ix. Dose, f℥j, to which is sometimes added fʒj of tincture of calumbo.

MISTURA ASSAFŒTIDÆ. L. Assafœtida ʒv, triturate with water Oj, gradually added. [D. assafœtida ʒj, pennyroyal water f℥viij.]

MISTURA ASSAFŒTIDÆ CUM IPECACUANHA. Dr. REECE. Tincture of assafœtida fʒj, tincture of opium ♏x, ipecacuanha powder gr. x, water f℥ij. [A teaspoonful every 3 hours, in hooping cough, for a child of 2 years.]

MISTURA ASTRINGENS. PRADEL. Tannin gr. xij, syrup of rhatany ℥j, mucilage ℥j, camphor mixture ℥iv.

MISTURA BALSAMI PERUVIANI. GUY'S H. Balsam of Peru fʒiij, honey f℥ss, water f℥viij. Melt the honey in a warm mortar, add the balsam, rub together, and gradually add the water heated to about 110°.

Mistura Buchu Composita. Reece. Infusion of buchu ℥viij, tincture of buchu ℥j, tincture of cubebs ℥j. Mix. Dose, f℥j, 3 times a day.

Mistura Calumbæ Alkalina. St. B. H. Infusion of calumba f℥vijss, carbonate of soda ʒj, tincture of orange-peel ℥ss.

Mistura Camphoræ. L. *Camphor Julep.* Camphor ʒss, rectified spirit ♏x; rub together, gradually adding water Oj, and strain. [D. and L. 1788, add sugar ℥ss, rubbed with the camphor and spirit.] For Mistura Camphoræ E. See Emulsio Camphoræ.

Mistura Camphoræ cum Lacte. Dr. Cassels. Camphor in powder ʒss, milk fʒiv; triturate and add water f℥vijss.

Mistura Camphoræ cum Magnesia. E. Camphor ℈ss, carbonate of magnesia gr. xxv, water fʒvj. Mix. U. S. (*Aqua Camphoræ.*) Camphor ʒij, carbonate of magnesia ʒj, rectified spirit ♏xl, distilled water f℥xxxij. Rub the camphor with the spirit, then with the magnesia, and lastly with the water gradually added, and filter. Contains gr. iij in f℥j.

Mistura Camphoræ cum Myrrha. St. B. H. Camphor ʒss, myrrh ʒss; triturate, and gradually add water Oss. Dose, f℥jss.

Mistura Camphoræ Carbonica. Water strongly charged with carbonic acid gas, agitated with powdered camphor, and strained.

Mistura Camphoræ cum Spiritus Ætheris Nitrici. Dr. Christison. Spirit of nitric æther fʒij, camphor ℈j; dissolve, and add water f℥vj, or q. s.

Mistura Capsici. See Infusum Capsici Compositum.

Mistura Carminativa Infantilis. *Dalby's Carminative.* Carbonate of magnesia ℈ij, oil of peppermint ♏j, oil of nutmeg ♏ij, oil of aniseed ♏iij, tincture of castor ♏xxx, tincture of assafœtida ♏xv, tincture of opium ♏v, spirit of pennyroyal ♏xv, compound tincture of cardamom ♏xxx, peppermint water f℥ij. Dr. Paris.

Mistura Carminativa Antacida. Dr. Paris. Magnesia ʒss, peppermint water fʒijss, compound spirit of lavender fʒss, spirit of caraway fʒiv, syrup of ginger fʒij. St. George's H. Dill water f℥ss, comp. tincture of cardamom ♏xx, carbonate of magnesia ℈j, syrup ℥j.

MISTURA CASCARILLÆ COMPOSITA. L. Infusion of cascarilla f℥xvij, vinegar of squills f℥j, compound tincture of camphor f℥ij. The Mist. Cascarillæ C. of St. B. H. is nearly the same without the comp. tincture of camphor, the addition of which constitutes their Mist. Cascarillæ Opiata.

MISTURA CASSIÆ. F. H. *Eau de Casse.* Cassia pulp ℥ij, hot water Ojss. By glassfuls. Laxative.

MISTURA CASSIÆ ANTIMONIATA. *Eau de Casse emetisée.* FOY. Pulp of cassia ℥j; boiling water Ojss. Macerate, strain, and add sulphate of magnesia ℥j, emetic tartar gr. iij. By cupfuls, in painters' colic.

MISTURA CATHARTICA. See Mistura Sennæ, Mistura Aperiens, &c.

MISTURA CETACEI. GUY'S H. Spermaceti ʒvj, yolk of 1 egg; beat them well together, and add syrup of Tolu f℥jss, pennyroyal water Oj. Dose, f℥j, to which is sometimes added nitre gr. x, or comp. tincture of camphor ♏xxx. See Emulsio Cetacei for another form.

MISTURA CETRARIÆ. Dr. A. T. THOMSON. Decoction of Iceland moss f℥vijss, diluted sulphuric acid fʒj, syrup fʒiv, tincture of opium ♏xl. A wineglassful 3 times a day, *in Phthisis.*

MISTURA CHLORIDI CALCIS. Dr. REID. Tincture of calumba fʒij, chloride of lime gr. x, syrup f℥ss, water f℥iijss. Dose, f℥ss every hour.

MISTURA CHLORINII. MID. H. Solution of chlorine (H.) fʒiij, water f℥xij. Dr. WATSON prescribes f℥ij of the solution to Oj of water. Dose, a tablespoonful, or more according to age, *in Scarlatina,* &c.

MISTURA CINNAMOMI COMPOSITA. GUY'S H. Cinnamon powder ʒj, carbonate of magnesia ʒij, rhubarb ʒj, dill water f℥xij. Dose, f℥ss to f℥j.

MISTURA CINCHONÆ. Dr. COPLAND. Confection of roses ℥ss, boiling decoction of bark f℥viij; triturate, and in 10 minutes add diluted sulphuric acid fʒjss, spirit of nutmeg fʒiv. Occasionally sulphate of magnesia may be added.

MISTURA COCCI ALKALINA. Dr. ALLNATT. Cochineal ℈j, subcarbonate of potash ʒj, boiling water ℥viij. Dose, a teaspoonful 3 times a day, *in Hooping Cough.* [See also Syrupus Cocci Alkalinus. The earliest form I have met with for this popular remedy is that of Dr. LOBB (Medicinal Letters, 1765). Salt of wormwood ℈j, cochineal ℈ss, water ¼ of a pint, white sugar to the taste. Dose, from a teaspoonful to a tablespoonful, according to age.]

MISTURA COLCHICI. SCUDAMORE. Magnesia ʒjss, peppermint water f ℥iij, vinegar of colchicum f ʒiv, syrup of orange-peel f ʒiv. A tablespoonful every 3 hours; *in acute Gout.* SOBERNHEIM. Carbonate of potash ʒj, vinegar of colchicum q. s. to saturate it; spirit of nitric æther ʒj, spirit of juniper ℥j, water f ℥vj. A spoonful every 2 hours; *in Dropsy after Scarlatina.*

MISTURA CONII COMPOSITA. GUY'S H. Extract of hemlock ʒj, carbonate of soda ʒjss, decoction of liquorice f ℥xj, spirit of pimento f ʒvj. Dose, f ℥j to f ℥ij. Myrrh mixture is sometimes substituted for decoction of liquorice.

MISTURA COPAIBA. GUY'S H. Copaiva f ʒiij, solution of carbonate of potash f ʒjss; rub together, and gradually add decoction of barley f ℥viij, spirit of nitric æther f ʒiij. Dose, ℥j—ij, 3 times a day. St. B. H. Copaiva f ʒiij, mucilage f ℥iij, water f ℥iv, pimento water f ℥ij. CHARING CROSS H. Copaiva ℥ss, powdered cubebs ℥ss, spirit of nitric æther f ʒij, liquor of potash f ʒjss, tincture of henbane f ʒiij, water f ℥viij. Other forms in use are, copaiva ℥ss, powdered gum ʒj, tincture of cubebs f ʒv, syrup f ʒiv, peppermint water f ℥vj : or, copaiva f ʒij, mucilage ʒvj, mint water f ℥v, tincture of capsicum ♏xij. For 4 doses.

MISTURA COPAIBÆ BENZOINATA. Mr. SODEN. Benzoic acid ʒj, balsam of copaiva ℥ss, yolk of egg, q. s., camphor mixture f ℥vij. Dose, ℥j, twice a day in *dysuria senilis.*

MISTURA COPAIBÆ CUM HEMEDESMO. Copaiva ℥ij, yolks of 2 eggs; triturate, and add syrup of Hemedesmus Indicus ℥ij, white wine ℥iv.

MISTURA COPAIBÆ VINOSA. FULLER. Copaiva ℥ij, yolks of 2 eggs; triturate, and add syrup of Tolu f ℥ij, white wine f ℥iv.

MISTURA CORNU USTI. L. 1824. *Decoctum Album.* Burnt hartshorn ℥ijss, gum arabic ʒx, water Oiij, boil to Oij, constantly stirring, and strain.

MISTURA CORNUS CIRCINATÆ. REECE. Alkaline extract of round-leaved dogwood ʒij, tincture of the same f ʒvj, water f ℥vij.

MISTURA CREASOTI. E. Creasote ♏xvj, acetic acid ♏xvj, comp. spirit of juniper f ℥j, syrup f ℥j, water f ℥xiv. Dose, f ʒj.

MISTURA CRETÆ. L. Prepared chalk ℥ss, refined sugar ʒiij, mucilage f ℥jss, cinnamon water f ℥xviij. Mix. D. Ppd. chalk ℥ss, sugar 3iij, mucilage f ℥jss, water f ℥xvj. E. Pr. chalk ʒx, sugar ʒv, mucilage f ℥iij, spirit of cinnamon f ℥ij, water Oij. See Pulvis pro Mist. Cretæ.

MISTURA CRETÆ ASTRINGENS. U. C. H. Prepared chalk ℥ss, mucilage f ℥jss, water f ℥viij, infusion of catechu f ℥viij, tincture of kino ℥j.

MISTURA CRETÆ OPIATA. GUY'S H. Comp. powder of chalk with opium ʒiij, mint julep f ℥ix.

MISTURA CUBEBÆ. Powdered cubebs ℥j, sugar ʒij, mucilage ℥ij, cinnamon water ℥vj. Dose, f ℥ss to f ℥jss.

MISTURA CUPRI SULPHATIS. Mr. CHAVASSE, *in Hooping Cough.* Sulphate of copper gr. j, syrup of poppies ℥j, aniseed water ℥iij. Dose, ♏xl to f ʒij.

MISTURA DEMULCENS. A. T. THOMSON. Mucilage f ℥ij, oil of almonds f ℥ss, syrup of poppies f ℥ss, citric acid q. s. to render it gratefully acid. Dose, f ʒij occasionally.

MISTURA DIURETICA. SWEDIAUR. Spirit of nitric æther ℥j, vinegar of squills f ℥j, juniper water f ℥iij, spirit of horse-radish f ℥ij, syrup of ginger ℥ij. Dose, f ℥j. GERM. H. Oxymel of colchicum ℥ij, liquor of acetate of ammonia ℥ij, parsley water ℥vj.

MISTURA EFFERVESCENS. P. *Potion Gazeuse, Rivieri.* Dissolve 3ss of bicarbonate of potash in ℥ij of water, and add ʒiv of syrup of lemon-peel. Mix also ℥ss of lemon-juice with ℥j syrup of lemon-juice, and ℥j of water. Mix an equal quantity of each, and give it while effervescing.

MISTURA ELATERII. Dr. FERRIAR. Elaterium gr. j, spirit of nitric æther f ℥ij, tincture of squills f ℥ss, oxymel of colchicum f ℥ss, syrup of buckthorn f ℥j. Dose, f ʒj 3 times a day, in water.

MISTURA EMETINÆ. *Melange Vomitif.* M. Coloured emetine gr. iv, infusion of orange-leaves f ʒxviij, syrup of orange-flowers ℥ss; or *(Potion Vomitive).* Pure emetine gr. j, infusion of lime flowers f ℥iijss, acetic acid ♏viij, syrup of marsh-mallows, f℥j. A table-spoonful every quarter of an hour, till it vomits.

MISTURA EMETICA EXCITANS. COPLAND. Sulphate of zinc ℈ij, peppermint water f℥ivss, ipecacuanha wine f℥ss, tincture of serpentary f℥ss, tincture of capsicum ♏xl, oil of chamomile ♏xij. A 3d or 4th part at short intervals till it operates.

MISTURA ERGOTINÆ. BONJEAN. Ergotine (Extractum Ergotæ Aquosum) gr. xvj, water ℥iij, syrup of orange-flowers ℥j. By spoonfuls, every 3 hours, in hæmorrhage; or repeated every quarter of an hour to excite expulsive pains.

MISTURA FERMENTI. NEUMANN. Yeast ℥ij, clarified honey ℥j, water fʒviij. Dose, ʒss to ʒj every hour.

MISTURA FERRI AROMATICA. D. Cinchona bark in coarse powder ʒj, calumba sliced ʒiij, cloves bruised ʒij, iron filings ʒss; digest for 3 days in a close vessel with peppermint water q. s. to produce ʒxij of strained liquor; add comp. tincture of cardamoms ʒiij, tincture of orange-peel ʒiij.

MISTURA FERRI COMPOSITA. L. & E. Myrrh bruised ʒij, [sub] carbonate of potash ʒj; rub them in a mortar with spirit of nutmeg fʒj, and add, still rubbing, rose water fʒxviij, sugar ʒij, and lastly, sulphate of iron in fine powder ℈ijss. Put the mixture immediately into a proper glass bottle, and close it. D. nearly as L. GUY'S H. substitutes decoction of liquorice for the rose water and sugar.

MISTURA FERRI CUM ALOES. U. C. H. Compound mixture of iron fʒv, compound decoction of aloes fʒiij.

MISTURA FUSCA. Dr. WOOD'S brown Cough Mixture. Extract of liquorice ʒij, gum arabic ʒij, boiling water f℥iv. Dissolve, and add antimonial wine fʒij, laudanum ♏xx. Dose, a spoonful occasionally.

MISTURA GENTIANÆ COMPOSITA. L. Compound infusion of gentian fʒxij, infusion of senna fʒvj, compound tincture of cardamoms fʒij. [If Alexandria senna is used it should be freed from Argel leaves.]

MISTURA GUAIACI. L. & E. Guaiacum resin ʒiij, sugar ℥ss; rub together, adding first mucilage of acacia f℥ss, and lastly cinnamon water f℥xix. [xixss, E.]

MISTURA GUAIACI AMMONIATA. GUY'S H. Guaiacum resin ʒiij, solution of sesquicarbonate of ammonia fʒv, decoction of barley f℥xij.

MISTURA GUMMOSA. Julep Gommeux, P. Gum arabic ʒij, orange-flower water ʒiv, water ℥iij, syrup of marsh-mallow ℥j.

MISTURA HÆMATOXYLI. ST. B. H. Extract of logwood ʒiij, boiling water f℥vij; strain, and add tincture of cinnamon fʒvj, tincture of catechu fʒij. Dose, ℥j, every 6 hours.

MISTURA HEMEDESMI. MID. H. Bruised root of Hemedesmus Indicus (country or scented sarsaparilla) ʒx, extract of liquorice ℈ss, distilled water f℥x. Digest for 12 hours, heat the strained liquor to 180° and strain again. One-third 3 times a day. Mr. H. BELLINAYE prescribes solution of potash (liquor potassæ) fʒss to fʒj, orange-flower water f℥j, syrup of hemedesmus ℥v. Take f℥j, 3 times a day in barley water. *Gonorrhœa.*

MISTURA HORDEI, E. As Decoctum Hordei Compositum. L.

MISTURA HYDRARGYRI. Dr. D. DAVIES. Confection of quicksilver gr. xxxij, mucilage f℥j, syrup fʒvj, cinnamon water fʒij.

MISTURA HYDRARGYRI BICHLORIDI. See Julepum Hydr. Bichloridi.

MISTURA HYDROCYANICA SIMPLEX. U. C. H. Emulsion of bitter almonds f℥viij, hydrocyanic acid ♏xx.

MISTURA HYDROCYANICA COMPOSITA. U. C. H. Add to the last, tartrate of potash ʒiij.

MISTURA IODINII CUM DECOCTO GRAMINIS. M. Decoction of dog-grass Ojss, iodide of potassium ʒss, syrup of mint ℥ij. To be taken by glassfuls in 24 hours.

MISTURA IODINII CUM SARZA. M. Decoction of sarsaparilla Ojss, iodide of potassium ʒj, syrup of orange ℥ij.

MISTURA IPECACUANHÆ ALKALINA. Dr. R. PEARSON, *in Hooping Cough.* Ipecac. wine ♏xl, tincture of opium eight drops, subcarbonate of soda gr. xvj, water fʒxiv, syrup fʒij. When the cough is abated, substitute myrrh gr. viij for the ipecac. Dose, a teaspoonful to children two or three years old.

MISTURA IPECACUANHÆ CUM SENNA. GUIBOURT. Ipecac. ʒj, senna ʒij, boiling water ℥vj; infuse for 12 hours, strain, and add oxymel of squills ℥j, syrup of hyssop ℥j. *For Hooping Cough.* By spoonfuls.

MISTURA [VINI] IPECACUANHÆ. Dr. CHEYNE. Ipecac. wine

f ʒiij, syrup of Tolu f ʒv, mucilage f ℥j. A teaspoonful every hour or two, for children threatened with *Croup* or *Bronchitis.*

MISTURA JALAPÆ COMPOSITA. U. C. H. Infusion of senna f ℥vj, extract of jalap ʒss, tartrate of potash ʒiv, oil of ginger ♏xx.

MISTURA LAXATIVA. *Napoleon's Medicine.* CORVISART. Soluble cream of tartar (see Potassæ Boro-tartras) ℥j, tartar emetic gr. ss, sugar ℥ij, water Ojss.

MISTURÆ MAGNESIÆ. GUY'S H. Carbonate of magnesia ʒiij, mint water ℥viij, water f ℥iv. Dose, f ℥j once, twice, or thrice a day; adding occasionally, tincture of calumba f ʒss; or, wine of colchicum ♏xv to ♏xxx.

MISTURA MAGNESIÆ BICARBONATIS. Liquid bicarbonate of magnesia f ℥xij, syrup of orange-peel f ʒjss, comp. tincture of cardamoms f ʒjss, aromatic spirit of ammonia f ʒiv, syrup of ginger f ʒiv.

MISTURA MAGNESIÆ CUM MAGNESIÆ SULPHATE. GUY'S H. Sulphate of magnesia ℥ij, carbonate of magnesia ʒij, mint water f ℥viij, water f ℥iv.

MISTURA MAGNESIÆ SULPHATIS CUM ANTIMONIO. CH. Sulphate of magnesia ℥iv, potash-tartrate of antimony gr. ij, water Oj.

MISTURA MENTHÆ COMPOSITA. St. GEORGE'S H. Confection of roses ℥j, mint water f ℥viij, diluted sulphuric acid f ʒjss. Dose, f ℥j–ij.

MISTURA MENTHÆ SULPHURICA. St. B. H. Mint water, distilled water, each f ℥vijss, diluted sulphuric acid f ʒij. Dose, f ℥jss.

MISTURA MONESIÆ. Dr. NELIGAN. Extract of monesia ℈ij, water f ℥vijss, compound tincture of cardamoms f ℥ss.

MISTURA MOSCHI. L. Musk ʒiij, triturate it with white sugar ʒiij, gum acacia ʒiij, and gradually add rose water Oj.

MISTURA MOSCHI AMMONIATA. Mr. WHITE. Musk mixture f ℥vj, liquor of ammonia f ʒss, comp. spirit of lavender f ʒj, spirit of juniper ʒj.

MISTURA SEMINUM MOSCHI. REECE. Tincture of musk seeds (seeds of Hibiscus Abelmoschus) f ℥j, aromatic spirit of ammonia f ʒiij, compound spirit of lavender f ʒiv, camphor mixture f ℥vj. Dose, f ℥ss to f ℥j.

MISTURA MUCILAGINOSA. GUY'S H. Oil of almonds f ʒij, mucilage f ℥iv; rub together with syrup f ʒj, then gradually add water f ℥vjss, diluted sulphuric acid f ʒss. Dose, f ʒss. Compound tincture of camphor f ʒiij, or syrup of poppies f ʒvj, may be occasionally added.

MISTURA MYRRHÆ. GUY'S H. Myrrh ʒiij, cold decoction of liquorice f ℥ix; rub together, and strain. Dose f ℥j, to which may be sometimes added carbonate of soda gr. xij; or diluted sulphuric acid ♏xv, or compound tincture of camphor f ʒss.

MISTURA NAPHTHÆ MEDICINALIS. Dr. NELIGAN. Pyro-acetic spirit f ʒij, comp. tincture of cardamom f ʒvj, water f ʒvij. Dose, f ʒiv every 4 hours.

MISTURA OLEI. St. B. H. Oil of almonds f ℥jss, mucilage of acacia f ℥jss, water f ʒv. Mix. GUY'S H. Olive oil f ℥j, solution of carbonate of potash f ʒss, mint water f ʒvij.

MISTURA OLEI AMMONIATA. GUY'S H. Olive oil f ʒj, solution of sesquicarbonate of ammonia f ʒj, mint water f ʒvij.

MISTURA OLEI CUM MANNA. St. B. H. Oily mixture (Mist. Olei) f ʒviij, manna ʒjss. Dose, f ʒjss.

MISTURA OLEI LINI COMPOSITA. St. B. H. Linseed oil, mucilage, comp. tincture of rhubarb, of each f ʒvj, diluted pimento water f ʒvj. Dose f ʒjss.

MISTURA OLEI CUM RHEO. GUY'S H. Linseed oil, and tincture of rhubarb, of each f ʒj. Shake together. Dose, f ʒij to f ʒiv.

MISTURA OLEI JECORIS ASELLI. Cod liver oil f ʒiv, solution of carbonate of potash f ʒss, peppermint or other water f ʒvij, syrup of orange-peel f ℥ss. Dose, f ℥jss to f ℥iij. FEHR prescribes, for rickety children, ℥j of the oil, ʒij of the solution, ℥j of syrup of orange-peel, and 3 drops of oil of calamus. Dose, f ʒj–ij, night and morning.

MISTURA OLIBANI. GUY'S H. Olibanum ʒiv, honey f ʒvj, decoction of barley f ℥xj. Dose, f ℥j to f ℥ij.

MISTURA OPIATA. NEW YORK H. Tincture of opium f ʒij, liquid acetate of ammonia f ℥iv, water f ℥iv.

MISTURA OPII CUM ANTIMONIO. Dr. GRAVES. Tartarized antimony gr. iv, tincture of opium f ʒj, camphor mixture f ℥viij. Dose, f ℥ss to f ℥j, *in Delirium Tremens*, and the advanced stage of nervous fever, with extreme debility.

Mistura Phosphori. Soubeiran. Phosphorated oil ʒij, powdered gum acacia ʒij, peppermint water ℥iij, syrup ℥ij. Mix the gum with ʒx of the water, and this with the oil, and gradually add the others.

Mistura Pimpinellæ. Sobernheim. Infusion of burnet saxifrage ℥v, anisated spirit of ammonia ʒij, syrup of seneka ℥j. Mix. A spoonful every 2 hours, *in Inveterate Catarrhs.*

Mistura Platini Chloridi. Hoefer. Perchloride of platinum gr. iv, distilled water f℥iij, sugar ʒij. Dose, fʒiv, 3 or 4 times a day.

Mistura Potassæ cum Calce. Sir G. Blane. Solution of potash fʒij, lime water f℥vj. Dose, f℥ss to f℥j, in beef tea.

Mistura Potassæ Supertartratis. U. C. H. Cream of tartar ℥j, borax ʒij, boiling water q. s. to dissolve them. To f℥x of the cooled solution add nitre ʒij, oxymel f℥ij.

Mistura Potassii Bromidi. M. Lettuce-water ℥iij, bromide of potassium (hydrobromate of potash) ℈ss, syrup of marsh-mallow ℥j. To be taken by spoonfuls, in 24 hours.

Mistura [Potio] Potassii Cyanidi. M. Lettuce-water ℥ij, cyanide of potassium gr. ss to gr. jss, syrup of marsh-mallow ℥j. Dose, ʒiv, every 2 hours.

Mistura Potassii Iodidi. M. *Solution Atrophique.* Lettuce-water ℥viij, mint water ʒij, iodide of potassium ʒiv, syrup of marsh-mallow ℥j. Dose, fʒiv morning and evening, *in hypertrophy of the heart, &c.* From ʒj to ʒij of tincture of digitalis is occasionally added. Cazenave prescribes iodide of potassium ʒij, distilled water ℥xvj, syrup ℥ij. Two or three spoonfuls *per diem.*

Mistura Purgans. *Apozema Purgans.* P. Senna ʒij, rhubarb ʒj, boiling water ℥iijss; digest for half an hour, strain, and press; and dissolve in the strained infusion by a gentle heat, manna ℥ij, sulphate of soda ʒiv.

Mistura Purgans. Sydenham. Tamarinds ℥ss, senna ʒij, rhubarb ʒjss, water ℥vj; boil to ℥iij, and add manna ℥j, syrup of roses ʒj.

Mistura Purgans Amara. Dr. Gall. Infusion of senna f℥vj, extract of dandelion ʒj, tartar emetic gr. ss. For other purging mixtures, see Mistura Sennæ; Haustus Sennæ; Mistura Jalapæ, &c.

MISTURA QUASSIÆ. U. C. H. Infusion of quassia f ℥xv, compound spirit of lavender f ℥ss.

MISTURA QUINÆ MURIATIS. Dr. NELIGAN. Muriate of quinine gr. xij, diluted muriatic acid ♏v, distilled water f ℥vij, syrup of orange flowers f ʒj. Dose, f ʒj.

MISTURA QUINÆ TARTARICA. BOUCHARDAT. Sulphate of quinine gr. xv, tartaric acid ℈j, water ℥ix, syrup f ℥iij.

MISTURA QUINÆ ET CAFFEI. *Café Quininé.* Prepare ʒv of infusion from ʒiv of ground coffee by percolation, and add gr. xxiv of sulphate of quinine, and ℥iv of sugar. Dose, a tablespoonful. The coffee conceals the bitterness of the quinine.

MISTURA RHEI COMPOSITA. GUY'S H. Rhubarb powder ℥j, carbonate of soda ℥ij, tincture of orange-peel f ʒjss, decoction of liquorice f ʒxss. Dose, f ʒss to f ʒj, two or three times a day. Dr. GREGORY'S Mixture. Peppermint water Oj, rhubarb ℥j, calcined magnesia ℥jss, ginger ℈j. Dose, f ʒss.

MISTURA RHEI APERIENS. BRANDE. Rhubarb ℈ij, tartrate of potash ʒj, peppermint water f ʒvj, tincture of senna f ʒss, syrup of ginger f ʒss. Dose, f ʒjss.

MISTURA RICINI. See Emulsio Purgans cum Oleo Ricini.

MISTURA [JULEPUM] ROSÆ. GUY'S H. Infusion of roses f ʒvj, sulphate of magnesia ℥vj, pimento water f ʒij.

MISTURA ROSÆ LAXANS TONICA. Dr. BAILEY. Infusion of roses ʒxv, tincture of cascarilla ʒj, sulphate of magnesia ℥vj.

MISTURA SALINA. *Neutral* or *Saline Mixture.* A common form for this mixture is equal parts of lemon-juice and water, neutralized with carbonate of potash, (℈j of carbonate or 24 grains of bicarbonate to f ʒj of the mixture.) See Liquor Potassæ Citratis, U. S. Dr. COPLAND prescribes under this name—Camphor mixture f ʒivss, liquid acetate of ammonia f ʒiij, nitre ℈ij, spirit of nitric æther f ℥iij, syrup of lemons f ℥ij. Dose, f ʒj.

MISTURA SALINA CARDIACA. BATH H. Subcarbonate of soda ʒjss, water Ovijss, diluted sulphuric acid f ʒj. Mix, and add aromatic confection ʒiij, spirit of peppermint ℥iij.

MISTURA SALINA CUM FERRO. GUY'S H. Sulphate of magnesia ℥v, sulphate of soda ℥v, sulphate of iron gr. ij, warm water Oij. Dose, Oss early in the morning, and repeated in an hour if required.

MISTURA SARSAPARILLÆ COMPOSITA. Sir C. SCUDAMORE. Root-bark of sarza ʒiij, lime water fʒxij; macerate for 12 hours, strain; add syrup of sarza fʒvj, Brandish's alkaline solution fʒij to fʒiij, tincture of orange, or of gentian fʒij to fʒiij, iodide of potassium gr. ix to xij.

MISTURA SCAMMONII. E. Resin of scammony gr. vij, unskimmed milk f℥iij; triturate the resin with a little of the milk, and gradually with the rest. See Emulsio Purgans cum Scammonio.

MISTURA SCILLÆ. *Potio Scillitique*, P. Oxymel of squills ʒiv, hyssop water ℥iij, peppermint water ℥j, spirit of nitric æther ʒss; for 2 doses. U. C. H. Oxymel of squills f℥j, syrup of poppies f℥j, water f℥iv.

MISTURA SCILLÆ COMPOSITA. St. B. H. Vinegar of squills fʒij, solution of acetate of ammonia f℥jss, compound spirit of horse-radish f℥jss, diluted pimento water f℥ivss. Dose, f℥ij three times a day.

MISTURA SCILLÆ CUM VALERIANA. KIMBEL. Powdered valerian ʒij, oxymel of squills ℥j, tincture of opium 20 drops, water ℥j; mix. A teaspoonful every hour, in *Croup*, after an emetic of ipecacuanha.

MISTURA SENEGÆ. JADELOT'S Anti-Croupal Mixture. Infusion of seneka ℥iv, syrup of ipecacuanha ℥j, oxymel of squills ʒiij, tartar emetic gr. jss. By spoonfuls, every quarter of an hour till vomiting is produced.

MISTURA SENNÆ COMPOSITA. St. B. H. Infusion of senna f℥vijss, tincture of senna f℥ss, sulphate of magnesia ℥jss; mix. U. C. H. Infusion of senna f℥x, sulphate of magnesia ℥j, tincture of senna f℥ss, compound tincture of cardamoms f℥ss. Dr. CHRISTISON recommends a mixture of equal parts of infusion of senna (E.), and of a solution of ℥j of sulphate of magnesia in f℥viij of water. A wineglassful every two hours until it begins to operate. Other approved formulæ are—Infusion of senna f℥xivss, tincture of senna f℥jss, sulphate of magnesia ℥iv, carbonate of ammonia ℈j; mix. Infusion of senna f℥xss, tartrate of potash ʒxij, manna ʒiv, tincture of senna f℥j, aromatic spirit of ammonia fʒij. Dose, f℥jss. See Haustus Senna Co., and Mistura Aperiens.

MISTURA [JULEPUM] SODÆ SULPHATIS. GUY'S H. Sulphate of soda ℥j, carbonate of soda ʒij, mint water f℥viij. Dose, f℥j.

MISTURA SODII CHLORIDI COMPOSITA. GUY'S H. Lemon-juice with as much common salt as it will dissolve. Dose, f ℥ss to f ℥j.

MISTURA SPIRITUS VINI GALLICI. L. French brandy f ℥iv, cinnamon water f ℥iv, yolks of two eggs, refined sugar ℥ss, oil of cinnamon ♏ij. Mix.

MISTURA STRYCHNIÆ. M. Pure strychnine gr. j, distilled water f ℥ij, white sugar ʒij, acetic acid three drops, [f ʒj contains 1-16th of a grain of strychnia.]

MISTURA TEREBINTHINÆ. Mr. CARMICHAEL, *in Iritis.* Rectified oil of turpentine f ʒj, yolk of one egg; triturate together, and gradually add emulsion of almonds f ℥iv, syrup of orange f ℥ij, comp. spirit of lavender f ʒiv, oil of cinnamon four drops. Dose, f ℥j three times a day.

MISTURA TEREBINTHINÆ VENETÆ. CLOSSIUS. Venice turpentine ʒj or ʒjss, yolk of egg q. s. Triturate, and add gradually peppermint water f ℥ivss.

MISTURA VALERIANÆ. St. B. H. Valerian bruised ʒij, boiling water Oss; macerate for an hour, strain, and add powdered valerian ʒiv.

MISTURA VERMIFUGA. COPLAND. Valerian ʒij, wormseed ʒiv, boiling water f ℥viij; infuse for an hour, strain, and add assafœtida ʒj triturated with yolk of egg. DESLANDES. Alcoholic extract of pomegranate root bark ʒvj, triturate in a mortar, gradually adding lemon-juice ℥ij, mint water ℥ij, lime-flower water ℥ij. By spoonfuls, for *Tape-worm.*

MISTURA VINI. GUY'S H. White wine f ℥vj, yolks of two eggs, sugar ℥ss, oil of cinnamon three drops. Dose, f ʒj.

MISTURA ZINCI COMPOSITA. Dr. COPLAND. Sulphate of zinc gr. iv to vj, infusion of roses f ℥vijss, ipecacuanha wine ʒjss, extract of lettuce f ʒss, syrup of Tolu f ʒij.

MITHRIDATIUM. *Confectio Damocratis.* L. 1746. Cinnamon ʒxiv, myrrh ʒxj, agaric, spikenard, ginger, saffron, seeds of treacle-mustard, frankincense, Chio turpentine, of each ʒx, zedoary, mace, camel's hay, long pepper, seeds of hartwort, French lavender, hypocistus juice, storax, opoponax, galbanum, oil of mace, castor, of each ℥j, mountain poly, scordium, cubebs, white pepper, seeds of Cretan carrot, bdellium, of each ʒvij, Celtic nard, gentian, Cretan dittany, red rose, parsley seed, cardamom seed, fennel seed, gum arabic, opium, of each ʒv, root of sweet-flag, valerian, aniseed, sagapenum, of each ʒiij, spignel, St. John's wort, catechu, bellies of scincks, of each ʒijss, clarified honey triple the weight of all the rest. Mix the opium, dissolved in wine, with the gums (previously strained), melted with the expressed oil of nutmegs and turpentine; gradually add the honey, and then the other species reduced to powder. It contains gr. j of opium in ℥ss. See Theriaca.

MONESIA. An astringent extract imported from South America, obtained from the Buranheim bark. See Extractum Monesiæ.

MORPHIA. *Morphine,* or *Morphia.* L. Dissolve ℥j of hydrochlorate of morphia in Oj of distilled water, then add to the solution fʒv of solution of ammonia mixed with f℥j of distilled water, and shake them together. Wash the precipitate with distilled water, and dry it by a gentle heat. [To procure it directly from the opium MOHR directs concentrated infusion of opium to be mixed with milk of lime (in which the lime is 1-4th the weight of the opium employed), the mixture heated to boiling, filtered while boiling hot through linen, and pulverized sal ammoniac added in excess. As it cools, the morphia is precipitated. One grain is considered equal to 6 grains of opium.]

MORPHIÆ ACETAS. L. Morphia ʒvj, acetic acid fʒiij, distilled water f℥iv; mix the acid and water, and pour it on the morphia to saturation. Let the solution evaporate by a gentle heat, that crystals may be formed. Dose, ⅛th to ¼th grain.

MORPHIÆ BIMECONAS. Dissolve 200 grains of meconic acid in hot water (without boiling), and add 310 grains (or q. s.) of morphia. Evaporate the solution to dryness with a gentle heat.

MORPHIÆ HYDRIODAS. Dr. A. T. THOMSON. Mix strong solutions of 2 parts of hydrochlorate of morphia, and 1 part or rather more of iodide of potassium. Wash the precipitate with a little cold water, press it between folds of blotting paper, redissolve in hot water, and leave it to crystallize.

MORPHIÆ HYDROCHLORAS. L. *Muriate,* or *Hydrochlorate of Morphia.* Macerate ℔j of sliced opium in Oiv of distilled water for 30 hours, bruise it, digest 20 hours longer, and press it; repeat this 2 or 3 times with the residuum, and evaporate the mixed liquors at 140° to the consistence of syrup. Add Oiij of distilled water, and when the dregs have subsided, decant, and gradually add ℥ij of chloride of lead dissolved in Oiv of boiling distilled water, till nothing more is precipitated.

Pour off the liquor, wash the residue with distilled water, and evaporate the mixed liquors by a gentle heat as before, and set aside that crystals may be formed. Press these in a cloth, dissolve them in Oj of distilled water, and digest with ℥jss of animal charcoal, at 120°, and strain. Lastly, having washed the charcoal, evaporate the liquors carefully that pure crystals may be produced. To the liquor poured off the first crystals add Oj of water, and drop in, frequently shaking it, sufficient solution of ammonia to throw down all the morphia; wash this, saturate with hydrochloric acid, and digest with ℥ij of animal charcoal, and strain. The charcoal being washed, cautiously evaporate the liquors that pure crystals may be obtained. E. directs ℥xx of opium to be exhausted with distilled water, and to the clear infusion, moderately concentrated and boiling, ℥j of muriate of lime to be added. The clear liquid is sufficiently concentrated to form a solid mass on cooling, which is strongly pressed in a cloth, redissolved in warm water, a little pulverized white marble added, and the liquid filtered, and acidulated with muriatic acid. It is then concentrated for crystallization, and the crystals pressed as before. Repeat the process of solution, &c., until a snow-white mass be obtained. [Dr. A. T. THOMSON mixes the softened opium with clean sand, and exhausts it by percolation with cold water, precipitates the concentrated solution with diacetate of lead, adds to the clear solution diluted sulphuric acid in slight excess, and decomposes the solution with chloride of barium. See Pharmaceutical Journal, vol. i., p. 457. U. S. directs it to be made with morphia and muriatic acid, as Morphiæ Sulphas.] Dose, from gr. ⅛th to ¼th.

MORPHIÆ NITRAS. A. T. THOMSON. Add morphia in slight excess to very dilute nitric acid, filter, concentrate by gentle evaporation, and set aside that crystals may form.

MORPHIÆ PHOSPHAS. As the last, substituting dilute phosphoric for nitric acid.

MORPHIÆ SULPHAS. U. S. Morphia ℥j, distilled water f℥viij; mix, and add sufficient diluted sulphuric acid to neutralize the morphia. Evaporate by water-bath, and dry the crystals which form in cooling, on bibulous paper.

MORPHIA TARTRAS. A. T. THOMSON. Saturate a solution of tartaric acid with morphia, concentrate by evaporation, and set aside that crystals may form. By using an excess of acid, an acid tartrate is formed.

MORSULI. See Trochisci.

MOSCHUS ARTIFICIALIS. See Oleum Succini Oxydatum.

MOXA. The Chinese moxas are made from the downy leaves of a species of wormwood. Various substitutes are used, as the pith of the sun-flower; cotton wool (enveloped in muslin), lint, calico, or unsized paper, soaked in solutions of nitrate, chromate, or chlorate of potash, or of diacetate of lead, and rolled up into small cones, or cylinders. Dr. OSBORNE uses quick lime enclosed in a hoop of card, and moistened with water.

MUCILAGO ACACIÆ. E. Mucilago Gummi Arabici, D. *Mucilage.* See Mistura Acaciæ.

MUCILAGO ALTHÆÆ. P. Althæa root ℥j, boiling water ℥vj; digest for 6 hours, and strain.

MUCILAGO AMYLI. E. & D. As Decoctum Amyli, L.

MUCILAGO CYDONIÆ. See Decoctum Cydoniæ.

MUCILAGO FŒNUGRECI. Digest ℥j of fœnugreek seed with Oss of water for 12 hours, boil, and strain with pressure.

MUCILAGO GLYCYRRHIZÆ. From liquorice root; as Muc. Althææ.

MUCILAGO LINI. P. Linseed ℥j, boiling water ℥vj; digest for 6 hours, stirring now and then, and strain.

MUCILAGO MERCURIALIS PLENKII. Quicksilver ʒj, gum arabic ʒij, water ℥j. Mix.

MUCILAGO SALEPI. See Gelatina Salepi.

MUCILAGO SASSAFRAS. Boil ʒj of pith of sassafras twigs with ℥xvj of water, and strain.

MUCILAGO TRAGACANTHÆ. E. & D. Tragacanth ʒij, boiling water f℥ix (f℥viij, D.); macerate for 24 hours, triturate, and express through linen or calico. U. S. One part of gum to 16 of water. P. One part to 8.

NAPHTHA. This name has been applied to many kinds of inflammable liquids, several of which have been employed medicinally. But the *medicinal naphtha* lately introduced by Dr. HASTINGS as a remedy for consumption, is *Acetone,* or Pyroacetic spirit. It is made by distilling acetate of lime, and redistilling the product over lime till its boiling point becomes constant. Or it may be procured by passing the vapour of acetic acid through a tube heated to dull redness, and rectifying the product as before. The dose, to commence, is 12 or 15 drops 3 times a day in water; after a few days it may be gradually increased as the patient can bear it. It is also used in *Rheumatism.*

NAPHTHALINA. Naphthaline is a product of the distillation of coal, and is deposited from the rectified oil of coal tar. For medicinal use it may be purified by dissolving it in alcohol, and crystallizing. Dose, gr. ss, frequently repeated as a stimulating expectorant.

NARCOTINA. Digest the residue of opium left in making the extract by cold water, with acetic acid, add ammonia to the solution, dissolve the precipitate in hot alcohol, decolorize by animal charcoal, and crystallize by refrigeration. *Antiperiodic?* Dose, gr. iij, 3 times a day.

NITRUM FULMINANS. See Pulvis Fulminans.

OLEA DESTILLATA. L. Olea Volatilia, E. *Distilled Volatile,* or *Essential Oils.* The general directions are to put the herbs, flowers, seeds, &c., into an alembic, with as much water as will cover them, and distil into a large receiver kept cold. (L.) The proper proportion of water varies for each article, and must in all instances be such as to prevent the matter being empyreumatized before the whole of the oil is carried over. (E.) A regulated temperature, not much exceeding 212°, should be maintained by steam, or a bath of oil, or solution of muriate of lime. Sometimes the materials are suspended in network in or over the water in the still. A proper vessel for collecting the oil is described in E. 1839 & 1841. [Essential oils are directed to be prepared from the fruits of Anise, Caraway, and Juniper (L. E. & D.), of Dill (E.), and Fennel (E. & D.); from Pimento berries (L. & D.); from the flowers of Chamomile (L. & E.), Lavender (L. E. & D.), Elder? (L.), Rue (E.) and unblown Cloves (E.); from the fresh tops of Rosemary (L. & E.), and Savin (E. & D.); from the fresh herbs (flowering, D.) of Mint, Peppermint, Pennyroyal, and Marjoram (L. E. & D.); and from Sassafras root (E.), wood and bark (D.) A few others will be noticed below.]

OLEA EXPRESSA. OLEA FIXA. *Expressed* or *Fixed Oils* are obtained from certain fruits and seeds by expression, or sometimes by decoction.

OLEA EMPYREUMATICA. Oily fluids produced in the destructive distillation of various vegetable and animal substances, either alone, or mixed with clean sand to divide the substance, and expose it more effectually to the heat.

OLEA MEDICATA. OLEA COCTA *vel* INFUSA. Oils medicated by infusion or decoction. They are mostly prepared by digesting, or gently boiling, the fresh leaves or flowers of various plants in olive oil till they become crisp, taking care that the temperature does not rise above the boiling point of water, which it is apt to do when the moisture is nearly all expelled. The oil is then pressed out, and strained. Several will be noticed below; but where no directions are given, 1 part of the herb to 2 or 3 of oil may be used. A few animal substances are treated in the same way. MM. ROSE and SIEBERT propose to obtain the medicated oils from *dried* plants; they reduce them to coarse powder, moisten them with a little spirit, and after a few hours' digestion, put them in a percolator and pour olive oil over them.

OLEUM ABSINTHII. The *Essential Oil* is obtained by distilling 1 part of fresh wormwood with 3 of water. The *Medicated Oil* by digesting it with 8 parts (P.), or 3 parts (E. 1744,) of olive oil.

OLEUM ÆTHEREUM. L. Rectified spirit ℔ij, sulphuric acid ℔iv; mix cautiously, distil till a black froth appears, remove the retort, separate the lighter supernatant liquor, and expose it to the air for a day; then wash it by agitation with f℥j of solution of potash mixed with f℥j of water, and separate the æthereal oil which subsides. [D. directs one-half of what remains in the retort, after distilling sulphuric æther, to be distilled with a gentle heat.]

OLEUM AMMONIATUM. Linimentum Ammoniæ.

OLEUM AMYGDALÆ. D. Bruise fresh almonds in a mortar, and express the oil without heat.

OLEUM AMYGDALÆ AMARÆ DESTILLATUM. P. The cake of bitter almonds (from which the fixed oil has been expressed without heat) is mixed into a thin paste with cold water, and after 24 hours, subjected to distillation. The oil comes over with the water, and falls to the bottom. [This oil contains a considerable but variable proportion of hydrocyanic acid, and is consequently highly poisonous. It is more used by confectioners, cooks, and perfumers, than in medical practice. The dose is stated to be from ¼th to ½ a drop.]

OLEUM AMYGDALÆ AMARÆ DEPURATUM. LIEBIG states that the crude distilled oil of bitter almonds may be deprived of its hydrocyanic acid by mixing it with peroxide of mercury, and after a few days' contact, redistilling the oil. A mixture of perchloride of iron and slaked lime is economically substituted for the peroxide; Mr. GRINDLEY, however, found it insufficient; but succeeded by employing it in combination with the peroxide.

OLEUM ANETHI, from Dill Seeds; Oleum Anisi, from Aniseed; Oleum Fœniculi, from sweet fennel seed; see Olea Destillata.

OLEUM ANIMALE. See Oleum Cornu Cervi.

OLEUM ANTHEMIDIS. Distilled from chamomile flowers. The imported oil is probably from a different species. A medicated oil is also made by digesting the flowers with 8 times their weight of olive oil. P.

OLEUM ARMORACIÆ. By distilling fresh horse-radish root with 2-3ds of its weight of water, redistilling the oil with water, separating it and digesting with muriate of lime. It appears to be identical with volatile oil of black mustard.

OLEUM ASELLI. See Oleum Morrhuæ.

OLEUM ASPHALTI. From Asphaltum; as Ol. Succini.

OLEUM AURANTII CORTICIS. As Oleum Limonum.

OLEUM AURANTII FLORUM. P. *Neroli.* Orange flowers ℔x, water ℔xxx; put the flowers, enclosed in a wire vessel, into an alembic containing boiling water; put on the head immediately, and distil as long as any oil comes over; the oil is separated in the usual way, and preserved in well-closed bottles, shaded from the light. [An oil is also obtained from the leaves.]

OLEUM BALSAMINÆ. Balsam apple (deprived of seeds) ℥j, oil of almonds ℥iv. Digest and strain.

OLEUM BELLADONNÆ. P. Fresh leaves of Belladonna ℔j, olive oil ℔ij; bruise the leaves, and heat them with the oil over a slow fire, till the moisture of the herb is dissipated, digest for 2 hours, strain with pressure, and filter.

OLEUM BENZOINI. From benzoin (after the acid has been sublimed); as Oleum Succini.

OLEUM BERGAMII. From bergamot peel, as Oleum Limonum.

OLEUM BETULÆ. A tarry oil, from the bark of birch.

OLEUM BEZOARDICUM. WEDEL'S oil. Camphor ℈ij, oil of almonds f℥ij, oil of bergamot ʒss, alkanet root, q. s. to colour it.

OLEUM BUBULUM. U. S. *Neatsfoot Oil.* By boiling the feet with water, and skimming off the oil.

OLEUM BUXI EMPYREUMATICUM. L. 1746. Distilled from fragments of boxwood in a retort, with a sand-bath, gradually increased in heat. *Anodyne*, *anti-spasmodic*, and *diaphoretic.* Dose, 10 to 20 drops. (JOURDAN says 4 or 5 drops in *gonorrhœa.*) *It relieves tooth-ache.*

OLEUM CACAO CONCRETUM. *Beurre de Cacao.* The cacao nuts are beaten to a paste (see Chocolata) and heated for a short time in a water-bath with 1-10th of their weight of water; then inclosed in a hempen bag, and quickly pressed between tinned plates heated by boiling water. The oil is purified by melting it, and filtering it through paper in a funnel kept warm.

OLEUM CAJAPUTI. Distilled from the leaves previously macerated with water.

OLEUM CAMPHORÆ. The liquid camphor, obtained by piercing the young camphor tree, is so termed in India.

OLEUM CAMPHORATUM. Linimentum Camphoræ.

OLEUM CAMPHORÆ NITRICUM. FEE. Pulverized camphor 208 grains, nitric acid ℥j, dissolve without heat, and decant the oil.

OLEUM CANNABIS. Expressed from hemp seed.

OLEUM CUM CANTHARIDIBUS. P. Cantharides in coarse powder 1 part, olive oil 8 parts; digest for 6 hours in a closed vessel, by water-bath, strain with pressure, and filter. [See Linimentum Cantharidis, U. S.]

OLEUM CARDAMOMI; Oleum Carui; Oleum Caryophylli; see Olea Destillata.

OLEUM CASSIÆ. As Oleum Cinnamomi.

OLEUM CERÆ. Distil bees'-wax, mixed with sand, and rectified by repeated distillations. Diuretic; dose, 2 to 4 drops.

OLEUM CHARTÆ. BATE. *Paper* or *rag oil.* Pyrothonide. Burn paper on a cold tin plate, and collect the oily liquid which condenses on it. It is also made by distilling paper or linen rag. It is used in *tooth ache* and *skin diseases;* and was formerly esteemed in ophthalmies.

OLEUM CHENOPODII. U. S. Distilled from the seeds of Chenopodium Anthelminticum. Dose, 4 to 8 drops, with treacle or milk, for 3 nights in succession, for children; for adults, ʒss. *Vermifuge.*

Oleum Cinnamomi. P. Bruised cinnamon bark ℔x, water ℔xx; macerate for 2 days, and add common salt ℔ij; distil till the water comes over clear. In 24 hours decant the water, return it to the still, and repeat this as long as any oil comes over. Let it rest for 24 hours, decant the watery liquid, and preserve the oil in well-stopped bottles.

Oleum Citri, and Ol. Citri florum. Oil of cedrat. From the peel and flowers of citron; as Ol. Limonis.

Oleum Colocynthidis. From the pulp, by digestion, as the other infused oils. See Olea Medicata. Externally in *Rheumatism* and *Neuralgia.*

Oleum Conii. P. As Oleum Belladonna.

Oleum Copaibæ. E. Copaiva ℥j, water Ojss; distil, and remove the oil, preserving the water; when most of the water has passed over, heat it, return it to the still, and resume the distillation; repeat this till no more oil comes over.

Oleum Coriandri. Coriander seed 4 parts, water 16, salt 1 part. Distil.

Oleum Cornu Cervi. Dippel's Animal Oil. It accompanies the ammoniacal liquor (Liq. Volatilis Cornu Cervi) in the distillation of hartshorn or bones. It is rectified by redistillation.

Oleum Crotonis. P. The seeds of croton tiglium (freed from their coats, Guibourt) are ground, placed in a hempen bag, and pressed between warm tinned plates. A further quantity is obtained from the marc, by heating it with rectified spirit, pressing, and distilling off the spirit. Both require to be filtered after standing a fortnight, and are then mixed. Dose, one to two drops.

Oleum Cubebæ. E. By distilling the ground berries in water.

Oleum Cucurbitæ. Expressed from the seeds of the pumpkin. *A soothing application to Piles.*

Oleum Digitalis. P. As Oleum Belladonnæ.

Oleum Ergote. Dr. Wright. From coarsely-powdered ergot of rye, by percolation with æther, and allowing the æther to evaporate spontaneously; or by digesting the ergot in solution of potash at 120° or 150°, diluting the liquid with half its weight of water, neutralizing by sulphuric acid, and distilling by an oil-bath. [Dose, 20 to 50 drops in *Hæmorrhage;* 10 drops every three hours in *Diarrhœa;* and locally in *Rheumatism, Toothache,* &c. An inferior oil is obtained by pressing powdered ergot, placed in muslin, between iron plates heated to 212°. An empyreumatic oil is also obtained by distilling it alone.]

OLEUM EUPHORBIÆ LATHYRIS. From the seeds of caper spurge, by expression. *Purgative.* Dose, three to ten drops.

OLEUM EXCESTRENSE. *Exeter Oil.* GRAY. Green oil ℔xvj, euphorbium, mustard-seed, castor, pellitory, of each ℥j; digest and strain. [The original form is more complex. The following is also used:—Rape oil Ojss, green oil Oss, oils of wormword, rosemary, and origanum, of each ʒss.]

OLEUM FŒNUGRÆCI. P. An infused oil of fœnugreck seeds; as Oleum Cantharidis.

OLEUM FILICIS MARIS. Dr. PESCHIER. Macerate the buds of male fern in æther, and distil off the æther from the tincture by a water-bath. Dose, from 10 to 30 drops, in sugar, almond emulsion, or wafer paper, for *Tape-worm.*

OLEUM FORMICARUM. Digest ℥iv of ants in ℥xvj of olive oil with a gentle heat, and strain.

OLEUM GAULTHERIÆ. Distilled from the leaves of partridgeberry (Gaultheria procumbens).

OLEUM GUAIACI. An empyreumatic oil is distilled from the wood, as Oleum Buxi. A fragrant oil is obtained by steeping the shavings in salt and water for some months, and distilling.

OLEUM HEDEOMÆ. U. S. Distilled from American pennyroyal.

OLEUM HYOSCYAMI. P. From fresh henbane; as Oleum Belladonnæ. An oil is also obtained by expression from the seeds.

OLEUM HYPERICI. L. 1746. Picked flowers of St. John's wort ℥iv, olive oil ℥xxxij; digest till the oil is well tinged.

OLEUM HYSSOPI. Distilled from fresh hyssop.

OLEUM JATROPHÆ. Expressed from the seeds of jatropha curcas, or physic nuts; as Oleum Crotonis.

Oleum Jecoris Aselli. See Oleum Morrhuæ.

Oleum Juglandis. Expressed from walnuts, as Oleum Amygdalæ.

Oleum Juniperi. Distilled from juniper berries, the seeds of which should be well crushed. The foreign oil is said to be distilled from the wood.

Oleum Lateritium. L. 1746. Quench red-hot bricks in olive oil, break them, distil in a retort with a gradually increased heat, and separate the oil from the accompanying liquid.

Oleum Lathyris. *Oil of Spurge.* From the seeds of euphorbia lathyris. *Purgative.* Dose, four to ten drops.

Oleum Laurinum. P. Fresh bay-berries are crushed, heated gently, placed in a hempen bag, and quickly pressed. If *dried* berries are used, they must be ground, then steamed, and pressed between warm plates. *Externally as a gentle stimulant.*

Oleum Lauro-cerasi. P. Distilled from the leaves of cherry-laurel, as Oleum Aurantii Florum. The leaves should be gathered in summer. It contains prussic acid, and is, consequently, poisonous.

Oleum Lavandulæ. From the flowers, as the other Olea Destillata. The oil which first comes over is most esteemed.

Oleum Liliorum. L. 1746. White lily flowers ℔j, olive oil ℔iij; boil slowly till the flowers become crisp, then strain, and press out the oil.

Oleum Limonum. P. The yellow portion of the peel is grated off the fruit, and the oil expressed. An inferior kind is obtained by distillation as directed for Ol. Aurantii Florum. Oils are obtained by both methods from the peel of bergamot, citron, sweet and bitter orange, all of which are preferably prepared by expression.

Oleum Lini. By expressing bruised linseed between warm plates.

Oleum Lumbricorum. E. 1744. Washed earthworm ℔ss, olive oil Ojss, white wine Oss. Boil gently till the wine is consumed, and press, and strain.

Oleum Marjoranæ, from sweet marjoram; Oleum Menthæ, from mint; Oleum Menthæ Piperitæ, from peppermint; Oleum Pulegii, from penny-royal: as the other distilled oils.

Oleum Meliloti. From the flowering tops of melilot; as Ol. Absinthii (infusum).

Oleum Monardæ. U. S. Distilled from horsemint, Monarda punctata. *Rubefacient.*

Oleum Morrhuæ. Oleum Jecoris Aselli. *Cod-Liver Oil.* The imported oil is prepared by exposing the livers to the heat of the sun, in tubs, till putrefaction takes place, drawing off the oil, and boiling the livers to obtain more oil. In this country, the bland, pale, straw-coloured variety obtained from the fresh livers by a similar process to that described below, has been found to produce all the therapeutical effects attributed to the more offensive kinds above noticed, and is less liable to disagree. Mr. Donovan directs the livers to be heated over a slow fire, and constantly stirred till they break down into a pulp; when the temperature has risen to 150° F., the pulp is placed in canvass bags, and in 24 hours the oil which drains out is separated from the watery liquor which accompanies it. Dose, f ʒss to f ʒjss, three times a day, in *Scrofula, Consumption, Chronic Rheumatism, Chronic Skin Diseases,* &c. *It is applied externally in Rheumatic and Neuralgic Affections,* &c.

Oleum cum Mucilaginibus. L. 1746. Fresh marsh-mallow root ℔ss, linseed ℥iij, fœnugreek seed ℥iij, water ℔ij, olive oil ℔iv. Boil the bruised root and seeds in the water for half an hour, add the oil, and boil till the water is dissipated.

Oleum Myristicæ. The essential oil is obtained by distillation; the *concrete* oil, called *oil of mace,* by expression.

Oleum Myrrhæ. An empyreumatic oil is obtained from myrrh, as ol. succini. An oil *per deliquium* was formerly made by putting myrrh into a boiled egg from which the yolk had been removed, and placing it in a cellar.

Oleum Olivæ. Expressed from crushed olives; an inferior kind is made by boiling the pressed paste with water.

Oleum Opiatum. Neuber. Opium ʒj, infused oil of henbane ℥xvj; digest with a moderate heat, and strain. U. C. H. directs ℈j of opium to f ℥ij of olive oil.

Oleum Ophioglossi. From adder's-tongue, as Ol. Belladonnæ.

Oleum Ovorum. P. Heat the yolks of eggs gently till the moisture is dissipated, and exhaust them by æther in a stoppered displacement apparatus; distil the product in a water-bath, heat the residue till the viscous matter coagulates, and strain. It may also be obtained by pressing the evaporated yolks between warmed tin plates.

OLEUM OXYGENATUM. Expose olive oil in a wide receiver to chlorine gas slowly evolved.

OLEUM PALMÆ. Expressed from the fruit of the Elais Guineensis.

OLEUM PAPAVERIS. *Huile Blanche.* From poppy seeds, as Oleum Amygdalæ.

OLEUM PETRÆ. *Rock Oil,* or *Oil of Petroleum.* The name is also given to the following mixture: [GRAY] Oil of turpentine ℥viij, Barbadoes tar ℥iv, oil of rosemary ʒiv.

OLEUM PHOSPHORATUM. PRUS. PH. Digest gr. xij of phosphorus with ℨj of oil of almonds, by the aid of warm water and agitation. M. directs ʒj of sliced phosphorus to be macerated without heat, in a dark place, with ℨij of the oil, for 14 days. Dose, 4 or 5 drops in a mucilaginous liquid.

OLEUM PICIS LIQUIDÆ. *Oil* or *Spirit of Tar.* It is obtained by distilling tar; and rectified by repeated distillation.

OLEUM PIMENTÆ, from allspice; OLEUM PIPERIS, from black peppercorns; see Olea Destillata.

OLEUM PLUMBAGINIS EUROPÆÆ. The bruised root is digested with olive oil at 212°. It cures *Itch,* but irritates the skin.

OLEUM PURGANS. VAN MONS. Scammony ℈iv, oil of almonds ℥iv; digest with a moderate heat. Dose, ℨss.

OLEUM RAIÆ. From the liver of the skate; as Ol. Morrhuæ.

OLEUM RHEI. FULLER. Digest powdered rhubarb with oil of almonds for 12 hours, and filter.

OLEUM RHODII. P. From rosewood (Convolvulus Scoparius), as Oleum Cinnamomi.

OLEUM RHOIS TOXICODENDRI. Digest 1 part of fresh leaves of poison-oak with 2 of olive oil for 24 hours in water bath, and strain. *In frictions, for paralysis,* &c.

OLEUM RICINI. P. Reduce the picked seeds to a paste in a mill, enclose it in hempen bags, and express the oil very slowly. Clarify it by filtering in a warm place. To obtain it *colourless* the seed-coats must be previously removed. [DR. WOOD says it is clarified in America by heating it with water till the latter boils, separating the oil, and again heating it with a little water until the latter is driven off. Dose, ℨss, or from ʒiij to ʒxij.]

Oleum Rosæ. P. As Oleum Aurantii Florum.

Oleum Rosatum. E. 1744. Digest ℔j of fresh roses with ℔iij of olive oil. P. directs the bruised petals of pale roses to be macerated for 3 days with 4 parts of olive oil, and strained with pressure. The decanted oil to be digested with 3 successive quantities of roses. But *the perfumed rose oil* is generally made by colouring olive or almond oil with alkanet root, and scenting it with otto.

Oleum Rosmarinæ, and Ol. Sabinæ; see Olea Destillata.

Oleum Rutæ. E. Distilled from the leaves and unripe fruit. An infused oil (P.) is made as Ol. Absinthii.

Oleum Sambucinum. An infused oil is prepared from the flowers of elder, as Oleum Anthemidis, P. L. directs an oil to be distilled from the flowers, but the quantity obtainable is very trifling.

Oleum Sambuci Viride. From the fresh leaves of elder with olive or rape oil, as Oleum Belladonnæ.

Oleum Sabinæ. As the other Olea Destillata.

Oleum Sassafras (from the bruised root, E.; and bark, D.) and Oleum Santali Flavi; as Oleum Cinnamomi.

Oleum Sinapis Expressum. From black mustard-seed, or from its bran; as Oleum Lini.

Oleum Sinapis Volatile. Distilled from black mustard-seed; as Oleum Amygdalæ Amaræ. *It is an active rubefacient.*

Oleum Solani. P. From garden nightshade; as Oleum Belladonnæ.

Oleum Spicæ. Distilled from spike lavender. A mixture of oil of turpentine with oil of lavender, coloured with alkanet, is also sold under this name.

Oleum Stramonii. As Oleum Belladonnæ.

Oleum Strychninatum. Cunier. Linimentum Strychniæ.

Oleum Succini. L. [Rectificatum. D.] Put amber into an alembic, and distil, by the gradually-increased heat of a sand-bath, an acid liquor, oil, and salt. Redistil the oil a second and a third time [with water, D. & U. S.] *Antispasmodic.* Dose, ♏v to x.

OLEUM SUCCINI OXYDATUM. *Artificial Musk.* Put into a cup f℥j of oil of amber, and add to it, drop by drop, f℥iijss of strong nitric acid; let it stand for 36 hours, then separate and wash the resinous matter. *Antispasmodic and nervine.* Dose, gr. v to x. For children gr. ss to gr. j.

OLEUM SULPHURATUM. L. 1824. *Balsam of Sulphur.* Washed sulphur ℥ij, olive oil f℥xvj; to the oil heated in a large vessel, gradually throw in the sulphur, and stir constantly till they combine.

OLEUM SULPHURATUM ANISATUM. Originally made by dissolving sulphur in oil of aniseed, but now usually made by adding oil of aniseed to the balsam of sulphur, previously warmed.

OLEUM SULPHURIS RULANDI. ZWELFER. Rose oil (by infusion) ℔ij, rectified oil of turpentine ℥iij, sulphur ℥iij; heat by a sand-bath until they combine.

OLEUM TABACI. From fresh tobacco leaves, as Oleum Belladonnæ.

OLEUM TANACETI. By distillation from the fresh tops of tansy.

OLEUM TARTARI PER DELIQUIUM. Subcarbonate of potash is allowed to deliquesce in a damp place, and the clear liquid poured off.

OLEUM TEREBINTHINÆ. D. Common turpentine is distilled in a copper alembic with about an equal weight of water.

OLEUM TEREBINTHINÆ PURIFICATUM. L. Oil of turpentine Oj, water Oiv, [Oij, D.] Let the oil cautiously distil. [Dr. PEREIRA states that the oil is purified by redistilling it from a solution of caustic potash. It is sold under the name of Camphine.]

OLEUM TEREBINTHINÆ PURIFICATUM. Dr. NIMMO'S method. Agitate the oil with an eighth part of alcohol, and pour off the spirit; repeat this 3 or 4 times.

OLEUM TEREBINTHINATUM ACOUSTICUM. Mr. MAULE. Oil of almonds f℥iv, oil of turpentine ♏xl.

OLEUM TIGLII. See Oleum Crotonis.

OLEUM TRITICI. BATE. It is made by strongly expressing bruised wheat between hot iron plates. It is useful in some skin diseases, chilblains, &c. Mr. WISE, of Maryport, found it efficacious in *Tinea Capitis*. The Colne wheat yields most oil. Another kind of wheat oil is prepared by digesting wheat with olive oil; and sometimes a mixture of fixed oils is sold for it.

OLEUM VALERIANÆ. PRUS. PH. Valerian root 1 part, water 8 parts; distil, and separate the oil. It contains valerianic acid, the quantity of which is increased by exposure to the air.

OLEUM VINI. See Oleum Æthereum.

OLEUM VIRIDE. Bay leaves, rue, origanum, sea wormwood, of each ℥iij, olive oil Oij; digest till the herbs are crisp, press and strain. Green oil of elder is sometimes substituted for it.

OLEUM VITRIOLI. Sulphuric acid was formerly so called, because distilled from sulphate of iron (green vitriol) calcined to whiteness.

OLEO-SACCHARA. See Elæo-sacchara.

OPIUM TORREFACTUM. ZWELFER. Heat thin slices of opium on an iron plate, over a slow fire, so long as it emits vapour, taking care that it is not burnt.

OXYDA. *Oxides*. See their several bases.

OXYGENIUM. P. *Oxygen Gas*. Heat chlorate of potash in a small retort or flask of green glass, as long as gas is disengaged, and collect the gas in a proper apparatus. [The process is much expedited by mixing the chlorate with an eighth part of black oxide of manganese.]

OXYMEL. L. 1824. *Mel Acetatum*. Clarified honey 24 parts, distilled vinegar 16 parts; boil together to a proper consistence. L. 1836 directs clarified honey ℔x, strong acetic acid Ojss; but this has been found too acid.

OXYMEL ÆRUGINIS. Oxym. Cupri Acetatis, D. See Linimentum Æruginis.

OXYMEL ALLII. L. 1746. Sliced garlic ℥jss; bruised caraway and fennel seed, each ʒij, boiling vinegar f℥viij; macerate, strain, and make an oxymel with clarified honey ℥x.

OXYMEL COLCHICI. D. Vinegar of colchicum f℥xvj, clarified honey ℔ij; boil to the consistence of syrup. Dose, fʒj, gradually increased to fʒij.

OXYMEL NARCISSI. VAN MONS. Vinegar of narcissus (made with 1 part of fresh flowers of daffodil to 8 of vinegar) 1 part, white honey 4 parts. Dissolve. Dose, a teaspoonful. *In Hooping Cough* and *Spasmodic Asthma.*

OXYMEL PECTORALE. BRUNS. PH. Elecampane root ℥j, orris root ℥ss, water ℥xxxvj; boil to ℥xxiv, strain, and add honey ℥xvj, gum ammoniac ℥j, dissolved in vinegar ℥viij, and boil to an oxymel.

OXYMEL SCILLÆ. L. Clarified honey ℔iij, vinegar of squills Ojss; boil to a proper consistence. Dose, f ʒss to f ʒij.

OXYSACCHARUM. See Syrupus Aceti.

OXYSACCHARUM DIGITALIS. MARTIUS. Dried fox-glove ℥j, distilled vinegar ℥viij; digest with a gentle heat, strain with pressure, and add white sugar ℥x; dissolve and filter.

PANACEA MERCURIALIS. Calomel digested with rectified spirit, and dried.

PANES BISCOCTI MERCURIALES. OLIVIER'S *biscuits* are said to contain, in each biscuit of ʒij, gr. ⅙th of the dried precipitate obtained by mixing a solution of 77 grains of corrosive sublimate with the white of two eggs beaten up with ℔j of water.

PANES BISCOCTI PURGANTES. F. H. Jalap in fine powder ʒj, flour ℥j, 2 eggs, sugar ℥j; make them into three biscuits.

PANES BISCOCTI SCAMMONII. Fine scammony ʒj, Spanish soap gr. v, white sugar ℈ij; triturate to a fine powder, and form into 10 cakes, with ℥j of biscuit powder and a few drops of water.

PANIS FERRI LACTATIS. CAP. Bread, containing one grain of lactate of iron in each ounce.

PANNUS VESICATORIUS. See Tela Vesicatoria.

PASTA ADHESIVA. SCHWILGUE. Make a paste with flour and vinegar, and mix it with an equal quantity of melted pitch, and apply it to the scalp on linen, to eradicate the hair by removing it after a few days. For *Tinea Capitis.* MORRISON directs ℔ij of ale to be mixed with ℥vj of flour, and set on the fire; and ℥ix of powdered resin stirred in, till they form a smooth paste.

PASTA ALTHÆÆ. *Pate de Guimauve.* P. Decorticated marshmallow root ℥iv, water Oiv; macerate for 12 hours, strain, and add ℔ijss of picked gum arabic, and ℔ijss of refined sugar: dissolve, strain, and evaporate to the thickness of honey, constantly stirring, and add gradually the whites of 12 eggs well beaten with ℥iv of orange water. Evaporate with constant stirring till the paste is so firm as not to adhere to the hands. The Codex of 1836 substitutes water for decoction of althæa, and terms the compound *Pate de Gomme.*

PASTA CARICARUM. CADET. Mix pulp of figs with 4 times its weight of powdered sugar, and roll it out. Dry it in a stove for 24 hours, and divide it into squares.

PASTA CAUSTICA. See Caustica Zinci.

PASTA DACTYLIFERA. *Pate de dattes.* Dates ℥xvj, picked gum Senegal ℔iv, white sugar ℥xxxij, orange-flower water ℥ij, water q. s. Proceed as for Pasta Jujubæ.

PASTA EPILATORIA. Mix 2 parts of slaked lime with 3 of water, and saturate with sulphuretted hydrogen. A layer a line in thickness denudes the scalp in 3 minutes.

PASTA ESCHAROTICA ARSENICALIS. The Pulvis Escharoticus Arsenicalis moistened with mucilage at the time of using.

PASTA ESCHAROTICA CUPRI SULPHATIS. M. PAYAN. Powdered sulphate of copper made into a soft paste with yolk of egg.

PASTA GLYCYRRHIZÆ ALBA. *Pâte de réglisse Blanche.* As Pasta Althææ, substituting liquorice root for marsh-mallow root.

PASTA GLYCYRRHIZÆ FUSCA. *Pâte de réglisse brune.* Extract of liquorice ℥iij, gum arabic ℥xlviij, white sugar ℥xxxij, water Oiv. Dissolve the liquorice in the water, strain, add the sugar and gum, and evaporate very gently to a firm consistence. Pour it on an oiled slab.

PASTA GLYCYRRHIZÆ OPIATA. P. *Pâte de réglisse opiacée.* Add to the last gr. xv of extract of opium.

PASTA GLYCYRRHIZÆ NIGRA. P. *Pâte de réglisse noire.* Dissolve ℔j of extract of liquorice (Italian juice) in ℔iv of cold water, strain, and add picked gum arabic ℔ij, refined sugar ℔j. Evaporate gently, constantly stirring, to a proper consistence; spread it on an oiled slab. It may be aromatized with 24 drops of oil of aniseed, mixed with ʒj of powdered orris root.

PASTA GUMMI. *Pâte de Gomme.* See Pasta Althææ.

PASTA JUJUBÆ. P. *Jujube Paste* or *Lozenges.* Jujube fruit

℔j, water ℔iv; boil for half an hour, strain, let it settle, and decant. Dissolve ℔vj of picked and washed gum arabic in ℔viij of cold water, and strain. Clarify the decoction of jujubes with the whites of 4 eggs, mix it with ℔v of sugar and the mucilage, and heat it till it boils, stirring constantly with a wooden spatula. Then keep it lightly boiling, without stirring, till reduced to the consistence of soft extract; and add orange-flower water ℥vj, place the pan in another vessel, filled with boiling water. In 12 hours remove the scum, and pour the matter into tin moulds, and finish the evaporation in a stove heated to 104° F. [The jujubes are now generally omitted. GUIBOURT.]

PASTA LICHENIS. Iceland moss ℔j, water q. s.; heat nearly to boiling, reject this liquor, and boil the moss for an hour in fresh water; strain and press; add to the decoction, gum arabic ℔v, white sugar ℔iv, dissolve by a gentle heat, and evaporate over a slow fire to a firm paste. Spread it on a slab slightly oiled, and when cold, carefully wipe off the oil, and enclose it in a box.

PASTA LICHENIS OPIATA. P. To ℥xvj of the last add gr. viij of extract of opium.

PASTA AD PERNIONES. SWEDIAUR. Blanched bitter almonds ℥viij, honey ℥vj, camphor ℈iv, flour of mustard ℈iv, burnt alum ʒij, olibanum ℈ij, yolks of 3 eggs. Mix.

PASTA PECTORALIS. *Pâte Pectorale de* REGNAULD. In a decoction of ℥iv of the pectoral flowers (species bechicæ), dissolve ℥xxiv of gum, and ℥xx of white sugar, and add f ʒjss of tincture of Tolu. Strain the solution, and evaporate it to a proper consistence.

PASTA PIPERIS. See Confectio Piperis Nigri.

PASTA TORMENTILLÆ. M. MORIN, *for Whitlow*. Powdered tormentil root mixed into a paste with white of egg, and applied on linen.

PASTA TORMENTILLÆ COMPOSITA. *Pâte contre les Epididymites.* DESRUELLES. Linseed meal ℥iv, powdered tormentil ℥iv, mercurial ointment ℥j, extract of belladonna ʒj, oil of hemp-seed q. s. To be spread on cloth, and the testicle enveloped in it.

PASTA VIENNENSIS. *Vienna Paste* is Potassa cum Calce. Instead of employing it in the usual form of a soft paste, M. FIL-

HOS melts together 2 parts of caustic potash and 1 of lime in an iron ladle over a quick fire, and casts it into warm moulds (as in making lunar caustic); they are afterwards covered with wax, and kept in well-corked glass tubes; or they are cast in leaden tubes of convenient size (from 2 to 3 inches long, and from 1 to 6 lines wide), both to preserve them, and for convenience of applying them.

PASTA ZINCI. See Causticum Zinci. (CANQUOINS.)

PASTILLI ODORATI. *Aromatic Pastils.* P. Benzoin ℥ij, balsam of Tolu ʒiv, labdanum ʒj, yellow sandal wood ℈iv, charcoal ℥vj, nitre ℈ij, mucilage of tragacanth q. s. Mix and divide into conical pastils. Those Pastilli of which sugar is the basis, are placed under TROCHISCI.

PEDILUVIUM ACIDUM—Alkalinum—Salis. See Balneum Acidum —Alkalinum—Maris.

PEDILUVIUM IRRITANS. AUGUSTIN. Bruised horse-radish root ℥ij to ℥iv, hot water Oiv, or q. s.

PEDILUVIUM SINAPIS. Mix ℥iv of flour of mustard with a little cold water, and add hot water q. s.

PHILONIUM LONDINENSÆ. See Confectio Opii.

PHLORIDZINUM. *Phloridzine* is prepared from the fresh root-bark of the apple, pear, cherry, or plum, by boiling it with rectified spirit, straining, distilling off most of the spirit, and allowing the residue to cool; or from the watery decoction, decolorized by oxide of lead (any excess of which may be removed by a few drops of sulphuric acid), and evaporating the filtered liquid. Its properties and uses are similar to those of Salicine. Dose, gr. x. to xv.

PHOSPHORUS. Mix 12 parts of powdered bone-ash with 24 of water, and gradually add 10 parts of sulphuric acid, stirring it constantly; then add sufficient water to form a thin pulp, and leave it at rest for 24 hours; filter, adding water to the pulp as long as it passes acid, and evaporate the liquors to the consistence of honey. Mix this with 1 part of vegetable charcoal, dry the mixture thoroughly in an iron or copper vessel heated to dull redness, and distil the dry mass in an earthen retort, receiving the product into water. To purify the phosphorus, tie it in chamois leather and plunge it into water heated to 122° F., and without removing it from the water, force the softened phosphorus through the leather by twisting it with pincers.

The phosphorus melted in hot water is to be drawn up into slightly conical glass tubes, from which, when cool, it is removed, and preserved under water in well-closed bottles, shaded from the light.

PICROTOXINA. Dr. KANE. Treat an alcoholic extract of the seeds of Cocculus Indicus with water as long as anything is dissolved; then add muriatic acid, and set aside that crystals may be deposited. *Poisonous.*

PILÆ MASTICATORIÆ. *Masticatories.* QUINCY. Mastic ℥iij, pellitory ʒij, stavesacre seeds ʒij, angelica root ℈ss, cubebs ʒj, nutmeg ʒj, wax q. s. to make it into balls. AUGUSTIN. Mastic, white wax, pellitory, each ʒss; mix and divide into 3 masticatories. HARTMAN. Mastic ℈j, pellitory ʒj; mix, by heat, and form 2 masticatories. In India a mixture of betel leaf, areka nut, and lime is used.

PILULÆ. Pill masses should be of such a consistence that the pills may be easily moulded, and yet retain their rounded form. Those which contain volatile oils should not be kept long. The dry ingredients are to be reduced to powder, and the whole to be well-mixed and beaten into a uniform mass. When soap is ordered, Castile (olive-oil-soda) soap is intended. To *silver* pills, introduce into a small dry gallipot, a leaf or two of silver, then the pills (taking care that their surface is sufficiently moist), and placing over them another leaf of silver. Cover the gallipot with the hand, and give the whole a sudden rapid circular motion. Pills may be coated with *gelatine* by the following method: prepare by heat, a strong solution of equal parts of pure gelatine and jujube paste, about the consistence of treacle. Fix the pills on the points of long slender pins, dip them in the warm jelly, after removing any skin which may have formed on its surface. As each pill is withdrawn from the jelly, wave it in the air to cool it, and then fix the head of the pin in sand, stiff paste, or other support. When 50 or 60 are done, the pins may be withdrawn, previously warming them by placing the centre of each for a moment in the flame of a taper.

PILULÆ ACONITI. Dr. TURNBULL. Alcoholic extract of aconite gr. j, liquorice powder gr. xij, syrup q. s.; for six pills.

PILULÆ ÆTHIOPICÆ. E. 1744. Quicksilver ℈vj, honey ʒiv; triturate, and add oxysulphuret of antimony ℈iv, guaiacum ʒiv; mix.

PILULÆ EX ALLIO. E. H. Garlic, soap, millepedes, each ℈j; mix, for 36 pills.

Pilulæ Alöes. E. Socotrine aloes, soap, of each equal parts, confection of roses q. s. [U. S. (and St. B. H., Pil Aloes cum Sapone) equal weights of aloes and soap, with water q. s. Some prefer the fine Barbadoes aloes.] Dose, gr. x to xxx.

Pilulæ Alöes Compositæ. L. Aloes ℥j, extract of gentian ℥ss, oil of caraway ♏xl, syrup q. s. Dose, gr. v–xv.

Pilulæ Alöes et Assafœtidæ. E. Aloes, assafœtida, soap, of each equal parts, confection of roses q. s. Dose. gr. x to xv.

Pilulæ Alöes Dilutæ. Dr. M. Hall. Barbadoes aloes, soap, extract of liquorice, treacle, of each equal parts; dissolve them in water, strain, and evaporate to a pilular consistence.

Pilulæ Alöes et Ferri. E. Sulphate of iron three parts, Barbadoes aloes two parts, aromatic powder six parts, confection of roses eight parts; make a mass, to be divided into five-grain pills.

Pilulæ Alöes et Ipecacuanhæ. Dr. Baillie. Aloes ℈j, ginger ʒss, ipecacuanha gr. viij, syrup q. s. In 16 pills; one before dinner, daily.

Pilulæ Alöes cum Mastiche. (*Grains de Vie, de Mesue. Pilules* Antecibum of the old French Pharmacopœia. *Dinner Pills.*) Aloes ʒvj, mastic ʒij, red rose petals ʒij, syrup of wormwood q. s. To be divided into three-grain pills. [There are many other formulæ for these pills; the rose petals are often omitted, and sometimes rhubarb is substituted for them. The Paris Codex of 1837 has replaced these pills by a very different compound. See Pilulæ Dictæ Antecibum.]

Pilulæ Alöes cum Myrrha. L. E. & D. *Pil. Rufi.* Aloes (Socotrine or E. I., E.; hepatic, D.) ℥ij, saffron ℥j, (ʒss, E.) myrrh ℥j, syrup (conserve of roses, E.) q. s.

Pilulæ Alöes cum Rheo. Dr. Buchan. Aloes ʒj, rhubarb ʒj, soap ʒij; mix, for 80 pills.

Pilulæ Aloeticæ. Guy's H. Aloes ʒiij, soap ʒj, oil of peppermint ♏x, water q. s.; for 60 pills.

Pilulæ Alöes Rosatæ. *Pilules Angeliques. Grains de Sante.* Aloes ℥iv, dissolve in juice of roses ℥iv, of borage ℥ij, of chicory ℥ij; evaporate to an extract, and add rhubarb ʒij, agaric ʒj; divide into gr. jss pills.

Pilulæ Alöes et Zingiberis. D. Hepatic aloes ℥j, ginger ʒj, soap ʒiv, oil of peppermint ʒss. Mix.

Pilulæ Aloës et Terebinthinæ. Bois. Boiled turpentine ℥ij, aloes ʒss; in 40 pills.

Pilulæ Alterantes Plummeri. See Pil. Hydrargyri Chloridi Compositæ.

Pilulæ Aluminis Helvetii. Alum ʒij, dragon's blood ʒj, honey of roses q. s.; divide into 48 pills.

Pilulæ Aluminis Opiatæ. Capuron. Catechu ʒij, alum ʒj, opium ℈j, syrup of red roses q. s. In five-grain pills; dose, one or two.

Pilulæ Analepticæ. Dr. James's Pills. James's powder ʒj, guaiacum ʒj, pill of aloes and myrrh ʒj, syrup q. s. Divide into four-grain pills.

Pilulæ Andersonis. P. (Scot's Pills.) Aloes ʒvj, camboge ʒvj, oil of aniseed ʒj, syrup q. s. Mix, and divide into four-grain pills.

Pilulæ Angelicæ. *Frankfort Pills.* Guibourt. Aloes ℥j; dissolve in clarified juice of pale roses ℥j, of succory ℥ss, of borage ℥ss; evaporate to an extract, and add rhubarb ʒss, agaric gr. xv. Mix, and divide into pills of two grains each; silver them.

Pilulæ Anodyne. F. H. Extract of opium gr. iij, camphor gr. vj, syrup q. s.; for six pills.

Pilulæ Anodyne Mercuriales. Dr. A. T. Thomson, in *Acute Rheumatism.* Calomel gr. j, tartarized antimony gr. j, opium gr. jss; make a pill, to be taken at bedtime.

Pilulæ Dictæ Antecibum. P. *Dinner Pills.* Aloes ℥vj, extract of cinchona ʒiij, cinnamon ℥j, syrup of wormwood q. s. (These are substituted for the Pil. Aloes et Mastiches.) Dose, gr. vj or more.

Pilulæ Anthelminticæ. Phœbus. Iron filings ℥ss, assafœtida ʒjss, oil of tansy 10 drops, extract of wormwood q. s. for 80 pills, 6 pills three times a day. Bresmer's are—Aloes ℥ss, tansy ʒss, oil of rue nine drops. In 12 pills.

Pilulæ Antidysentericæ. Lyons' H. Pure alumina, extract of green walnut shell, equal parts; mix, and divide into three-grain pills.

Pilulæ Anticephalalgicæ. Broussais. Extract of belladonna gr. xv, extract of henbane gr. xv, extract of lettuce ʒss, extract of opium gr. vj, butter of cacao ʒiv; for 120 pills; one, night and morning. [Dr. Wilson Philip's pills for *Nervous Headache*—Rhubarb ʒss, nutmeg ℈ss, extract of chamomile ℈j, oil of peppermint q. s. In 30 pills. Dose, 3 pills, twice a day.]

Pilulæ Antiepilepticæ. Recamier. Oxide of zinc gr. ix, camphor gr. vj, extract of belladonna gr. vj; in 12 pills. Podreca. Indigo gr. lxxv, assafœtida gr. xv, castor gr. viij; in 20 pills, one every hour.

Pilulæ Antineuralgicæ. Marchal de Calvi. Sulphate of quinine gr. xij, extract of valerian gr. xv, extract of opium gr. iij, powdered orange leaves gr. xv, powdered cinnamon gr. xv, syrup of belladonna q. s.; in 30 pills, one every hour.

Pilulæ Antiarthriticæ. See Pil. Colchici, Pil Colocynthidis et Colchici, and Pil. Sodæ Laxantes.

Pilulæ Antimonii Comp. St. B. H. Tartarized antimony gr. j, guaiacum ʒss, pill of aloes and myrrh ʒss, treacle q. s.; make 16 pills.

Pilulæ Antimonii Opiatæ. Guy's H. Tartarized antimony gr. j, opium gr. ij, treacle q. s. for 4 pills. They are sometimes made with a double quantity of opium, and occasionally gr. j of calomel is added to each pill. Dose, one or two.

Pilulæ Antisyphiliticæ. See Pilulæ Hydrargyri Bichloridi, &c.

Pilulæ Arabicæ Mercuriales. The following pills are employed in the celebrated *Traitement Arabique* (see Electuarium Arabicum):—Quicksilver ʒss, bichloride of mercury ʒss; triturate carefully together, and add of senna, pellitory root, and agaric, each ʒj, honey q. s.; divide into pills of three or four grains each; two, daily.

Pilulæ Argenti Iodidi. Dr. Patterson. Iodide of silver, nitrate of potash, of each gr. x; rub together into a very fine powder, and add liquorice powder ʒss, white sugar ℈j, mucilage q. s. to form a mass to be divided into 40 pills; one, three times a day.

Pilulæ Aromaticæ. L. 1746. Compound powder of aloes ℥iij, balsam of Peru ℥ss, syrup of orange-peel q. s.

Pilulæ Argenti Ammonio-Chloridi. Serre. Ammonio-chloride of silver gr. j, orris powder gr. ij, conserve q. s.; to be divided into 14 pills.

PILULÆ ARGENTI NITRATIS. St. B. H. Nitrate of silver gr. xij, liquorice powder xxiv, treacle q. s.; mix, and divide into 12 pills. GUY'S H. Crystallized nitrate of silver, extract of gentian, powdered calumba, of each gr. xij. Mix, accurately, and divide into 12 pills; one, twice a day, or oftener.

PILULÆ ARSENICI. P. Pil. Asiaticæ. *Tanjore Pills.* White arsenic gr. j, black pepper gr. xij; triturate for a long time, and add acacia gum gr. ij, water q. s. Divide into 15 pills. [The CODEX says 12 pills; but we have put 15 to allow for the difference between French and Troy grains. Each pill contains 1-15th of a grain of arsenic, which is very nearly the proportion contained in the formula generally adopted. Arsenious acid gr. lv, black pepper ℥ix, gum arabic q. s. In 800 pills. It is very erroneously given in the *Formulaires* of RICHARD; (7th ed.) and EDWARDS and VAVASSEUR, (4th ed.) "The original Indian recipe is very indefinite." Dr. PEREIRA.]

PILULÆ ARSENICI. Dr. BARTON. White arsenic gr. ij, opium gr. viij, soap gr. xxxij, in 32 pills. (1-16th gr. of arsenic in each.)

PILULÆ ARSENICI IODIDI. Dr. NELIGAN. Iodide of arsenic gr. ij, manna ℈ij, mucilage q. s. In 20 pills. One 3 times a day, in *Psoriasis* and *Lepra*.

PILULÆ ASSAFŒTIDÆ. Assafœtida, galbanum, myrrh, of each 3 parts, confection of roses 4 parts or q. s. Mix. GUY'S H. Assafœtida ℥iij, soap ʒj, water q. s. for 60 pills.

PILULÆ ASSAFŒTIDÆ COMPOSITA. GUY'S H. Assafœtida ℈ss, ipecacuanha, and squill in powder, each gr. j, water q. s.; for 3 pills.

PILULÆ ASTRINGENTES. CAVARRA. Pure tannin gr. vj, gum arabic gr. xij, sugar ℥j, syrup q. s. Mix, and divide into four-grain pills. [See also Pil. Tannini, Pil. Aluminis, Pil. Zinci Sulphatis, &c.]

PILULÆ AURI OXYDI. M. Oxide of gold gr. v, extract of mezereon ʒij. Mix accurately, and divide into 60 pills.

PILULÆ AURI SODA MURIATIS. M. Soda-muriate of gold gr. j, extract of mezereon ℥j; in 60 pills.

PILULÆ BALSAMICÆ. MORTON. Powdered millepedes ʒxviij, gum ammoniacum ʒix, benzoic acid ℥vj, saffron ʒj, balsam of Tolu ℥j, anisated balsam of sulphur ℥vj, or q. s.

Pilulæ Barii Chloridi. Walsh. Chloride of barium gr. xv, mucilage of tragacanth and powdered marsh-mallow root q. s.; in 200 pills, 3 daily, increased to 12.

Pilulæ Bebeerinæ. Dr. Maclagan. Sulphate of bebeerine gr. xxiv, aromatic confection q. s. Make 16 pills; two every 4 hours, as an anti-periodic.

Pilulæ Benedictæ. Fuller's *Bennet Pills.* Aloes ℥ss, senna ʒij, assafœtida, galbanum, and myrrh, each ʒj, sulphate of iron ʒvj, saffron ʒss, mace ʒss, oil of amber 40 drops, syrup of mugwort q. s. to form a mass. Dose ℈j, every, or every other night.

Pilulæ Benzoes. Dr. Paris. Benzoic acid gr. xij, extract of poppies gr. xviij. Mix, for 6 pills. Dose, one pill. *Expectorant.*

Pilulæ Bruciæ. M. Brucia gr. xij, confection of roses ʒss; in 24 pills, silvered. Dose, one pill.

Pilulæ Calcis. Mr. Stephen's *remedy for Stone.* Lime (from shells of eggs and snails) made into a mass with soft soap, and divided into three-grain pills.

Pilulæ Calcis Chloridi. Dr. Copland. Chloride of lime gr. viij to xvj, compound powder of tragacanth ʒjss, syrup q. s., make 24 pills; two twice a day.

Pilulæ e Calomelane. U. C. H. Calomel ʒij, rhubarb ʒjss, confection of senna q. s.; make 50 pills. See Pil. Hydrargyri Chloridi.

Pilulæ Calomelanos Compositæ. E. & D. See Pil. Hydrargyri Chloridi Compositæ.

Pilulæ Calomelanos et Opii. E. Calomel 3 parts, opium 1 part, confection of roses q. s. Beat into a mass, to be divided into pills, each containing gr. ij of calomel.

Pilulæ Calomelanos et Rhei. U. C. H. Calomel ʒj, rhubarb ʒiv, water q. s.; in 60 pills.

Pilulæ Cambogiæ Compositæ. L. & D. Gamboge ʒj, aloes ʒjss, ginger ʒss, soap ʒij. Mix. E. (Pil. Cambogiæ,) Gamboge, aloes (E. I. or Bbd.), and aromatic powder, of each, 1 part; soap 2 parts, syrup q. s.

Pilulæ Cambogiæ et Scammoniæ. U. S. Gamboge ℥j, scammony ℥ss, nitrate of potash ʒj, soap ʒij. Mix for 400 pills.

Pilulæ Camphoratæ. U. C. H. Extract of valerian ʒij, assafœtida ʒj, camphor ℈j; in 30 pills.

Pilulæ Camphoræ cum Thridace. Ricord. Camphor, and extract of lettuce, of each ℈ijss. In 20 pills; 4 to 6 daily. *Anaphrodisiac.*

Pilulæ Cantharidis. St. B. H. Cantharides gr. vj, extract of gentian ℈ij. Mix, for 12 pills. One 3 times a day.

Pilulæ Cantharidis Opiatæ. Cantharides gr. xviij, opium xxxvj, camphor gr. xxxvj, confection of hips q. s. Mix, and divide into 36 pills.

Pilulæ Capsici. St. B. H. Powdered capsicum gr. xxiv, extract of gentian gr. xvj. Mix, and divide into 12 pills. One 3 times a day.

Pilulæ Capsici cum Rheo. Guy's H. Capsicum ʒj, rhubarb ʒij, treacle q. s. Mix, and divide into 60 pills; 2 or 3 to be taken before dinner.

Pilulæ Catharticæ Compositæ. U. S. Compound extract of colocynth in powder ℥ss, extract of jalap ʒiij, calomel ʒiij, gamboge ℈ij. Mix, for 180 pills. Dose, 1, 2, or 3 pills.

Pilulæ Cetrarinæ. Dr. Neligan. Cetrarine gr. xxiv, extract of calumba ʒss; in 12 pills; one every 4 hours, as a *Febrifuge.*

Pilulæ Cevadillæ. Equal parts, sabadilla and honey, in five-grain pills. Dose for an adult 4 to 6 pills; for a child 1 or 2. *Vermifuge.*

Pilulæ Chiraytæ. Reece. Extract of chirayta ʒij, dried subcarbonate of soda ℈j, ginger gr. xv. Mix, for 36 pills. 2 twice a day.

Pilulæ Cocciæ. E. 1744. Pilulæ Colocynthidis Compositæ.

Pilulæ Cochiæ Minores. L. 1677. Aloes, scammony, and colocynth, of each ℥j; oil of cloves ℈ij; syrup of buckthorn and of wormwood q. s.

Pilulæ Cœruleæ. By *blue pills* we understand Pilulæ Hydrargyri; but in some of the continental pharmacopœias (as those of Portugal and Germany) the Pil. Cupri Ammoniatæ are so termed.

Pilulæ Colchici. Sir C. Scudamore. Acetic extract of colchicum ʒj, powdered marsh-mallow root q. s. Divide into 40 pills.

PILULÆ COLCHICI CUM OPIO. St. GEO. H. Acetic extract of colchicum gr. ij, compound ipecacuanha powder gr. v, in 2 pills, for a dose.

PILULÆ COLOCYNTHIDIS SIMPLICIORES. L. 1746. *Pil. ex Duobus.* Colocynth ℥ij, scammony ℥ij, oil of cloves ʒij, syrup of buckthorn q. s.

PILULÆ COLOCYNTHIDIS. E. [—Compositæ, D.] Aloes ℥j, scammony ℥j, colocynth ʒiv, sulphate of potash ʒj, [soap ʒij, D.] oil of cloves ʒj, rectified spirit [treacle, D.] q. s.

PILULÆ COLOCYNTHIDIS ET CALOMELANOS. St. B. H. Compound extract of colocynth ʒj, calomel gr. xij, treacle q. s. Make 12 pills.

PILULÆ COLOCYNTHIDIS ET HYOSCYAMI. E. Compound colocynth pill 2 parts, extract of henbane 1 part, rectified spirit q. s. Mix, and divide into five-grain pills.

PILULÆ COLOCYNTHIDIS ET COLCHICI. BOUCHARDAT. Compound extract of colocynth ℈j, extract of colchicum ʒj, extract of opium gr. j. Mix, and divide into 18 pills. Dose, one or more according to their purgative effect. Substituted for *Lartigue's Gout Pills.* A similar compound, termed Sir H. HALFORD'S *Gout Pills.* Acetic extract of colchicum gr. ijss, Dover's powder, and comp. ext. of colocynth each gr. jss, in each pill.

PILULÆ COLOCYNTHIDIS CUM OLEO CROTONIS. Sir B. BRODIE. Comp. extract of colocynth ℈ijss, soap ℈ss, croton oil one drop. In 12 pills—one or two every or every other night.

PILULÆ COLOCYNTHIDIS FERROSÆ. Sir J. WYLIE. Compound extract of colocynth ʒiij, assafœtida, soap, inspissated ox-gall, ammonio-chloride of iron, and extract of celandine, each ʒj, tartarized antimony gr. ix, oil of chamomile 30 drops, syrup q. s. to form a mass, to be made into two-grain pills.

PILULÆ COLOCYNTH. CUM SCAMMONIO. St. B. H. Colocynth ℈ss, scammony ℈ss, confection of roses q. s. To form 12 pills.

PILULÆ CONII. STOERCK. Extract of hemlock ℥ss, powdered hemlock q. s. To form a mass, to be divided into three-grain pills. One night and morning, gradually increased.

PILULÆ CONII COMPOSITÆ. L. Extract of hemlock ʒv, ipecacuanha ʒj, mucilage q. s. Dose, gr. v, or from ij to viij.

PILULÆ CONII CUM HYDRARGYRO. GUY'S H. Extract of hemlock gr. iv, mercurial pill gr. j. Mix. One pill once a day or oftener.

PILULÆ COPAIBÆ. U. S. and MIALHE. Balsam of copaiva ℥ij, fresh calcined magnesia ʒj. Mix and set aside, stirring occasionally, till it acquires the consistence of a pill mass, which is to be divided into 200 pills. [This does not always succeed even with pure copaiba. M. FAURE recommends the addition of 1-6th Bordeaux turpentine. For present use copaiva will require nearly its own weight of magnesia. Five parts of copaiva and three of carbonate of magnesia form a suitable proportion for pills.]

PILULÆ COPAIBÆ CUM CERA. J. F. SIMON. White wax ʒj, copaiva ʒij. Melt together, and add powdered cubebs ʒiij. Mix.

PILULÆ CORNUS CIRCINATÆ. REECE. Extract of round-leaved dogwood ʒjss, ginger gr. x, dried subcarbonate of soda gr. x; in 24 pills.

PILULÆ CREASOTI. WOLFF. Creasote ʒj, powdered althæa root ʒj, extract or powder of liquorice ʒj, water q. s.; for 120 pills, each containing half gr. of creasote. PITSCHAFT prescribes, against vomiting in pregnancy, creasote gr. iij, powdered henbane gr. xij; in 12 pills—one 3 times a day.

PILULÆ CROTONIS CUM QUINA. CAVENTOU. Croton oil soap ℈j, sulphate of quinine ℈j, extract of borage (or dandelion) q.s. for 20 pills, one for a dose.

PILULÆ CROTONIS CUM HYDRARGYRO. Dr. NELIGAN. Croton oil soap gr. iij, extract of henbane gr. xxiv, mercurial pill gr. xxiv, oil of pimento ♏xij. Divide into 12 pills; dose, 2 at bedtime.

PILULÆ CUPRI AMMONIATI. E. Ammoniated copper, in fine powder, 1 part; bread-crumb 6 parts; solution of carbonate of ammonia q. s. Beat it into a pill mass—to be divided into pills containing gr. ss of ammoniated copper in each.

PILULÆ CUPRI SULPHATIS. BRANDE. Sulphate of copper gr. iij, bread-crumb ʒj. Mix, for 24 pills; one 3 or 4 times a day. SWEDIAUR. Sulphate of copper gr. xvj, bread-crumb ℈iv, solution of carbonate of ammonia q. s.; make 96 pills.

PILULÆ CYNARÆ. Extract of artichoke ʒss, sarsaparilla powder ℈j, oil of sassafras 1 drop. In 12 pills. One 3 times a day in *Rheumatism.*

PILULÆ CUM CYNOGLOSSO. P. Root-bark of hounds-tongue ℨiv, henbane seed ʒiv, soft extract of opium ʒiv, myrrh ʒvj, olibanum ʒv, saffron ʒjss, castor ʒjss, syrup of opium q. s. Mix. Contains gr. j of extract of opium in gr. viij. The original formula of NICOLAUS contained *styrax*, and seems to have been the origin of Pil. Styracis Compositæ as well as of this compound.

PILULÆ DELPHINIÆ. TURNBULL. Delphine gr. j, extract of henbane gr. xij, extract of liquorice gr. xij. Mix, and divide into 12 pills.

PILULÆ DIAPHORETICÆ. Dr. A. T. THOMSON. Tartarized antimony, opium, and calomel, each gr. j; confection of roses q. s. In 2 pills, at bedtime. See Pil. Antimonii Comp.

PILULÆ DIGITALIS ET SCILLÆ. E. Digitalis one part, squill one part, aromatic electuary two parts, confection of roses q. s. Mix, and divide into pills of 4 gr. each.

PILULÆ DIGITALINÆ. *Granules of Digitaline.* HOMOLLE. Digitaline gr. xv, refined sugar ʒxijss. Mix accurately, and form into 1000 granules, S. A. From 4 to 6 may be given in 24 hours.

PILULÆ DIGITALINÆ COMPOSITÆ. FALKEN. Digitaline gr. ¾, squill gr. 75, pure scammony gr. 75. Mix by long trituration, and form a mass with syrup of gum. Divide into 100 pills, and silver them. Give 2 pills, then 4, and afterwards 6 daily, in *Dropsy, with disordered circulation.*

PILULÆ EX DUOBUS. E. 1744. Pil. Colocynthidis Simpliciores.

PILULÆ ECPHRACTICÆ. L. 1746. Aromatic pill ℥iij, rhubarb ℥j, extract of gentian ℥j, sulphate of iron ℥j, subcarbonate of potash ℥ss, syrup of roses q. s.

PILULÆ ECPHRACTICÆ CUM ACULEO. E. 1744. Aloes, extract of black hellebore, scammony, each ℥j, ammoniacum ℥ss, guaiacum ℥ss, sulphate of potash ʒij, oil of juniper ʒj, syrup of buckthorn q. s.

PILULÆ EMETICÆ. SWEDIAUR. Sulphate of copper ℈j, ipecacuanha ℈j, syrup q. s. Divide into five-grain pills.

PILULÆ AD EPILEPSIAM. CHARING CROSS H. Extract of jalap gr. xv, extract of aloes gr. xv, sulphate of zinc ʒss, disulphate of quinine ʒss, soap gr. vj, tincture of ginger q. s.; divide into 30 pills.

PILULÆ ERGOTÆ COMPOSITÆ. LALLEMAND. Ergot, aloes, and rue, of each gr. viij. In twelve pills; one, three times a day, in *Amenorrhœa.*

PILULÆ ERGOTINÆ. BONJEAN. Ergotine (watery extract of ergot) gr. xxiv, liquorice powder ℈ij. In 24 pills; six in the day.

PILULÆ FELLIS BOVINI. Dr. CLAY. Inspissated oxgall may be formed into four-grain pills alone, or as follows:—Inspissated gall ℥ij, oil of caraway ♏x, carbonate of magnesia q. s. Divide it into 36 pills; two pills, three times a day, in *Costiveness, Deficiency of Bile,* &c. The *desiccated* oxgall is conveniently formed into a pill mass with spirit.

PILULÆ FERRI CUM ABSINTHIO. *Pilulæ Martiales.* SYDENHAM. Levigated iron ʒj, extract of wormwood q. s. [SWEDIAUR substitutes the black oxide for the powdered filings.]

PILULÆ FERRI AMMONIATI. JUSTAMOND. Ammonio-chloride of iron ʒiij, mucilage q. s. Mix, and divide into 60 pills. Dr. COPLAND. Am. iron ℥j, aloes ℥ss, extract of gentian ℥ss; in 30 pills. U. C. H. Ammon. iron ℥j, sagapenum ℈ijss, galbanum ℈ijss, aloes ℈j, aromatic confection q. s. In 50 pills.

PILULÆ FERRI AMMONIO CITRATIS. BERAL. Ammonio-citrate of iron ʒj, sugar ʒiij, mucilage q. s. Mix, divide into pills of three grains each, and silver them.

PILULÆ FERRI ARSENIATIS. BIETT. Arseniate of iron gr. iij, extract of hop ʒj, powdered althæa root ʒss, syrup of orange q. s.; mix accurately, and divide into 48 pills. Dose, one, daily.

PILULÆ FERRI BROMIDI. M. Bromide of iron, gr. x, conserve of roses gr. xviij, gum acacia gr. xij. Mix accurately, and divide into 20 pills.

PILULÆ FERRI CHLORIDI. BIETT. Hydrochlorate (protochloride) of iron gr. xij, powdered gentian gr. xxiv; in 12 pills. From 1 to 4 daily.

PILULÆ FERRI COMPOSITÆ. L. & D. Myrrh powdered ℥ij, carbonate of soda ℥j; rub together, add sulphate of iron ʒj, rub them again, then beat them in a warm mortar, with ℥j of treacle, until incorporated.

PILULÆ FERRI CARBONATIS. E. Saccharated carbonate of iron four parts, conserve of roses one part, beat into a mass, and divide into five-grain pills. These are similar to VALLET'S

Pills. U. S. Dissolve separately ℥iv of sulphate of iron, and ℥v of cr. carbonate of soda in f℥xvj of boiling water, to which f℥j of syrup has been added. Mix the solutions, and leave them in a closely-stoppered bottle that the carbonate of iron may subside. Wash this repeatedly with warm water and syrup (f℥j to f℥xvj) till tasteless; press it in flannel; mix it immediately with ℥ijss of clarified honey, and reduce the mass to a pilular consistence by water-bath. Dr. BLAUD'S Pills are made by triturating in an iron mortar ʒiv of sulphate of iron, ʒiv of subcarbonate of soda, and ʒss of tragacanth. To form a mass to be divided into 96 pills.

PILULÆ FERRI CUM ALOE. BRANDE. Sulphate of iron ℈j, carbonate of potash ℈j, myrrh ʒj, aloes ʒss. Mix, and divide into 30 pills. See Pil. Aloes et Ferri. The Philadelphia Col. of Pharm. give the following as a substitute for Hooper's Pills: —Barbadoes aloes ℥j, dried sulphate of iron ʒij, extract of hellebore ʒij, myrrh ʒij, soap ʒij, canella and ginger each ʒj, water q. s. In pills 2½ grains each.

PILULÆ FERRI PROTOCHLORIDI. F. H. Protochloride of iron gr. xij, powdered gentian gr. xxiv. In 12 pills. One to four daily.

PILULÆ FERRI ET CONII. Dr. A. T. THOMSON. Sesquioxide of iron ʒj, extract of hemlock ʒj; mix, and make 24 pills. Two twice a day in *Scrofula*, &c.

PILULÆ FERRI ET COPAIVÆ. Balsam copaiva ʒjss, red oxide of iron ʒiij. Mix, and divide into 200 pills. One before each meal, increased to 9 or 10 daily; in *Incontinence of Urine*.

PILULÆ FERRI FŒTIDÆ. St. B. H. Subcarbonate of iron gr. xv, comp. galbanum pill ʒss, treacle q. s. to make 12 pills. Dose 3 pills, 3 times a day.

PILULÆ FERRI CUM GENTIANA. GUY'S H. Sesquioxide of iron, soft extract of gentian, powdered ginger, of each, ʒjss; for 60 pills; 2 twice or thrice a day.

PILULÆ FERRI IODIDI. Mr. LESLIE. Agitate 127 grains of iodine, ℥ss of stout iron wire, with 75♏ of water in a strong stoppered bottle, until the froth becomes white; triturate the liquid immediately with ʒij of powdered sugar for a few minutes, and add gradually the following mixed powders: liquorice ℥ss, gum arabic ʒjss, flour ʒj. Divide the mass into 144 pills. Each contains gr. j of iodide of iron. CALLOUD prescribes sulphate of iron gr. xxiv, iodide of potassium gr. xxxij; triturate, and add bread-crumb ʒss, powdered althea q. s. Divide into 36 pills, each containing 3-4ths of a grain of dry or one grain of hydrated iodide of iron, and nearly half a grain of sulphate of potash. [There are several other formulæ, but the above are probably the best. LUGOL'S pills contain a quarter of a grain, and DUPASQUIER'S 3-4ths of a gr. of iodide in each.]

PILULÆ FERRI LACTATIS. CAP. Lactate of iron gr. xv, marshmallow root powder gr. xv, honey q. s. to form a mass for 20 pills.

PILULÆ FERRI PERCYANIDI COMPOSITÆ. JOLLY. Prussian blue gr. xviij, sulphate of quinine gr. xij, extract of opium gr. j, conserve of roses q. s. Mix, and make 12 pills; one every 3 hours, in *neuralgia.*

PILULÆ FERRI SUBPHOSPHATIS. CARMICHAEL. Subphosphate of iron ʒss to ℈ij, pure potash or soda gr. iij, extract of aloes gr. iv, liquorice ℈j, white of egg q. s.; for 12 pills.

PILULÆ FERRI SULPHATIS. E. Dried sulphate of iron 2 parts, extract of taraxacum 5 parts, conserve of roses 2 parts, liquorice powder 3 parts. Beat them together, and divide into five-grain pills. [U. S. substitutes extract of gentian for extract of dandelion.]

PILULÆ SULPHATIS FERRI COMPOSITÆ. E. 1817. Sulphate of iron ℥j, extract of chamomile ℥jss, oil of peppermint ʒj, syrup q. s. to form a mass.

PILULÆ FERRI ET QUINÆ IODIDI. BOUCHARDAT. Fresh protoiodide of iron ʒjss, disulphate of quinine gr. xviij, honey ℈j, liquorice powder q. s. Mix, and make 60 pills; from 2 to 6 daily in *chlorosis.*

PILULÆ FILICIS. PESCHIER. Extract of male fern (oleum filicis) ℈j, powdered fern ℈ss, conserve of roses, q. s. In 12 pills.

PILULÆ FŒTIDÆ. See Pilulæ Assafœtidæ, and Pil. Galbani Compositæ.

PILULÆ FULIGINIS. Dr. NELIGAN. Extract of soot ʒss, compound galbanum pill ℈j, oil of valerian ♏x. In 12 pills, two 3 times a day in *hysteria.* Dr. FULLER prescribed wood-soot ʒjss, carbonate of ammonia ʒss, tar q. s. In five-grain pills.

PILULÆ FULIGOKALI SULPHURATI. DESCHAMPS. Sulphurated

fuligokali ʒv, starch ℈ijss, tragacanth gr. viij, syrup q. s. Make 100 pills, and cover them with two or three coats of tragacanth. The pills of simple fuligokali are made in the same way, but do not require to be covered with gum.

PILULÆ GALBANI COMPOSITÆ. L. & D. *Pilulæ Gummosæ.* Galbanum ℥j, myrrh ℥jss, sagapenum ℥jss, assafœtida ℥ss, syrup [treacle, D.] q. s.

PILULÆ GUMMOSÆ ALKALINÆ. Mr. HULSE. Choice myrrh ℈jss, sagapenum ʒjss, galbanum ʒj, assafœtida ʒss. Triturate in an iron mortar with carbonate of potash ʒij, add brown sugar ʒij, and beat together in a uniform mass.

PILULÆ GALBANI CUM FERRO. GUY'S H. Comp. galbanum pill ʒiij, sesquioxide of iron ℈jss, water q. s. Make 60 pills.

PILULÆ GALBANI CUM ZINCO. GUY'S H. Comp. galbanum pill ℈iv, sulphate of zinc ʒj. Mix, make 60 pills. Dose, 1 or 2 twice a day.

PILULÆ GENTIANINÆ. F. H. Gentianine gr. v, conserve of roses and liquorice powder to form a mass for 6 pills.

PILULÆ GLYCYRRHIZÆ ET ALOES. BENEDICTUS FAVENTIUS. Extract of liquorice ℈ij, aloes ʒj, hound's-tongue pill (Pil. cum Cynoglosso, P.) ʒss, syrup of violets q. s. [℈j Pil. Styracis Comp. may be substituted for Pil. cum Cynoglosso.]

PILULÆ GUAIACI. St. B. H. Guaiacum resin ʒj, treacle q. s. In 18 pills. Dose, 3 pills, 3 times a day.

PILULÆ GUAIACI COMPOSITÆ. U. C. H. Guaiacum, calomel, oxysulphuret of antimony, and extract of hemlock, of each ℈j, copaiba q. s. Make into pills of 3 grains each. ST. B. H. Guaiacum gr. x, ipecacuanha gr. j, opium gr. j, treacle to form a mass for 4 pills.

PILULÆ GUMMI ELASTICI. BOUIS. *Caoutchouc Pills.* Cut India-rubber with scissors into small squares, weighing 3 or 4 grains; moisten them with syrup of Tolu, and shake them in a box with a mixture of powdered sugar and gum. Let them dry. Mr. HALLER gives gr. jss, and gradually increases the dose to 3 or 4 grains, in *consumption.*

PILULÆ HYDRAGOGÆ. P. *Bontius' Pills.* Aloes ℥j, gamboge ℥j, gum ammoniac ℥j, white vinegar ℥vj; dissolve by heat, strain, and evaporate to a pilular consistence. Divide into four-grain pills.

Pilulæ Hydrargyri. L. E. & D. Quicksilver ℈ij, confection of red rose ʒiij, liquorice powder ℈j, [Extract, D.] Rub the mercury with the confection till the globules can no longer be perceived, then add the liquorice, and beat all together till incorporated.

Pilulæ Hydrargyrosæ. P. Quicksilver ʒvj, honey ʒvj; triturate till the quicksilver is extinguished, and add aloes ℈vj, rhubarb ℈iij, scammony ℈ij, black pepper ʒj, honey q. s. Mix; 4 gr. contain 1 of quicksilver. [The Pil. Mercuriales Laxantes, E. 1744; Pil. Mercuriales, L. 1746; and those of Belloste, Borelot, and Barberousse, are very similar compounds.]

Pilulæ Hydrargyri Aloeticæ. Bories. Quicksilver ℥jss, lard ℥j; triturate accurately, and add powdered socotrine aloes sufficient to form a mass; to be divided into four-grain pills. Dose, 4 pills in the morning for *tape-worm.*

Pilulæ Hydrargyri cum Aloe. Brande. Mercurial pill ʒj, aloes ʒss. Mix, and divide into 24 pills.

Pilulæ Hydrargyri Camphoratæ. U. C. H. Calomel ℈ij, guaiacum ʒij, camphor ℈ss, copaiva q. s. Divide into two-grain pills.

Pilulæ Hydrargyri cum Colocynthide. U. C. H. Extract of colocynth, soap, and mercurial pill, of each equal parts; in four-grain pills.

Pilulæ Hydrargyri cum Conio. U. C. H. Quicksilver ʒj, mucilage of tragacanth ʒvj; rub till the quicksilver is extinguished, and add extract of hemlock ʒj. Make into three-grain pills. See Pil. Conii cum Hydrargyro.

Pilulæ Hydrargyri et Cretæ Compositæ. St. B. H. Equal weights of quicksilver with chalk, and comp. ipecac. powder; made into pills of 5 grains each.

Pilulæ Hydrargyri Ferruginosæ. Dr. Collier. Sesquioxide of iron ʒj, quicksilver ʒij, confection of red rose ʒiij; rub together till the globules disappear. It is made in a few minutes.

Pilulæ Hydrargyri cum Hyoscyamo. U. C. H. Mercurial pill ʒj, extract of henbane ʒiij; make 60 pills.

Pilulæ Hydrargyri cum Rheo. Guy's H. Mercurial pill ʒj, rhubarb ℈j; mix for 24 pills. U. C. H. (Pil Hyd. Compositæ.) Mercurial pill ʒij, rhubarb ℈j, confection of senna q. s.; for 30 pills.

PILULÆ HYDRARGYRI CUM SCILLA. St. B. H. Mercurial pill gr. xv, dried squill gr. iij; in 3 pills. See Bolus Scillæ cum Hydrargyro.

PILULÆ [UNGUENTI] HYDRARGYRI. BIETT. Mercurial ointment, powdered sarsaparilla, each ʒj; mix, and divide into 48 pills. From 1 to 4 daily. LAGNEAU directs mercurial ointment ℈iv, powdered marsh-mallow root ʒj; in 40 pills.

PILULÆ HYDRARGYRI CUM STEARINO. Mr. WRIGHTSON. Pure stearine ʒj; rub it in a mortar, and add quicksilver ʒiv; triturate for 10 minutes, and add confection of roses ʒiij, flour ʒiij, powdered gum ʒj, otto of roses 1 drop. As a substitute for Pil. Hydrargyri.

PILULÆ HYDRARGYRI CUM SAPONE. SEDILLOT. Mercurial ointment ʒij, soap ℈iv, liquorice powder ℈v; in four-grain pills.

PILULÆ HYDRARGYRI ACETATIS. KEYSER. Acetate of mercury, manna, gum acacia, of each ℈j, rose water q.s.; to form a mass for 80 pills.

PILULÆ HYDRARGYRI ACETATIS OPIATÆ. CARMICHAEL. Acetate of mercury, opium, camphor, of each ʒss, syrup of poppies q. s. For 30 pills.

PILULÆ HYDRARGYRI CHLORIDI MITIS. U. S. *One-grain Calomel Pills.* Calomel ʒiv, powdered gum arabic ʒj, syrup q. s. Mix, and divide into 240 pills.

PILULÆ HYDRARGYRI CHLORIDI COMPOSITÆ. L. Pil. Calomelanos Comp. [E. and D.] *Plummer's Pills.* Calomel ʒij, oxysulphuret of antimony ʒij; rub together, then with guaiacum resin ʒiv, and treacle ʒij, [ʒiv, E., q. s. D.,] that it may form a mass. [To be divided into five-grain pills, E.]

PILULÆ HYDRARGYRI SUBMURIATIS CUM CONIO. St. B. H. Calomel gr. vj, extract of hemlock ʒj; mix, for 12 pills. One 3 times a day.

PILULÆ HYDRARGYRI CHLORIDI CUM OPIO. See Pil. Calomelanos cum Opio.

PILULÆ HYDRARGYRI SUBMURIATIS [CHLORIDI] CUM SCILLA. Sir A. COOPER. Calomel gr. xij, mercurial pill gr. xxiv, squill gr. xxxvj; in 12 pills.

PILULÆ HYDRARGYRI BICHLORIDI. *Pil. Majores Hoffmanni.* There are several formulæ for these pills, varying in the proportion of bichloride of mercury. The following are some of the more usual:—GUY'S H. Bichloride of mercury gr. xv, muriate of ammonia gr. xx.; rub together, then with boiling water f ℥iv, and add sufficient bread-crumb to form 120 pills. Dose, from one pill to two, once, twice, or oftener daily. Each pill contains 1-8th of a grain of sublimate. St. GEO. H. Bichloride gr. x, gum acacia ℥ij; triturate together, accurately, and add bread-crumb ℈ijss; divide into 60 pills. Dose, one pill. NIEMANN. Bichloride of mercury gr. xv, distilled water ʒj; triturate carefully, and add bread-crumb ʒvj; mix accurately, and divide into 180 pills, each containing 1-12th of a grain of sublimate. BRERA. Sublimate gr. j, alcohol q. s. to dissolve it, bread-crumb q. s. to form a mass; divide it into eight pills. DZONDI. Sublimate gr. xij, water q. s.; dissolve, and add bread-crumb and white-sugar q. s. to form a mass for 240 pills, each containing 1-20th of a grain of sublimate. HUFELAND'S pills contain 1-30th of a grain in each.

PILULÆ HYDRARGYRI BICHLORIDI CUM ACONITO. M. GIBERT. Extract of aconite gr. xij, powder of opium gr. ij, sublimate gr. ij; mix accurately, and divide into eight pills.

PILULÆ HYDRARGYRI BICHLORIDI CUM CONIO. KOPP'S *Anti-herpetic Pills.* Bichloride of mercury gr. iij, dissolve in alcohol q. s., and add extract of hemlock ʒj; mix, and make 60 pills; six pills to be taken in the day, and the quantity gradually increased to nine or ten.

PILULÆ HYDRARGYRI BICHLORIDI CUM GLUTINE. Sublimate gr. j, fresh vegetable gluten gr. xv, powdered gum arabic gr. iv, powdered althæa root gr. viij; triturate the sublimate with the gluten, and add the rest. Divide into ten pills.

PILULÆ HYDRARGYRI BICHLORIDI CUM GUAIACO. DUPUYTREN. Extract of guaiacum gr. xxxvj, extract of opium gr. viij, corrosive sublimate gr. iij. Rub the sublimate with a little syrup, mix the whole accurately, and divide into 24 pills.

PILULÆ HYDRARGYRI ET QUINÆ CHLORIDI. HAMILTON. Double chloride of mercury and quinine gr. xv, opium gr. vj, bread-crumb q. s.; mix carefully and divide into 30 pills; one 3 times a day, to produce salivation.

PILULÆ HYDRARGYRI IODIDI. L. Iodide (proto-iodide) of quicksilver ʒj, confection of hips 3iij, ginger ʒj; mix. [Another mode of exhibiting this remedy is: Compound calomel pill ℈j, iodide of potassium ʒss; make 12 pills; one every night. M. directs them to be made in the same manner as the Pilulæ Deuto-iodidi Hydrargyri.]

PILULÆ HYDRARGYRI PROTO-IODIDI COMPOSITÆ. BIETT. Proto-iodide of mercury ℈ss, extract of guaiacum ℈j, extract of lettuce ℈ij, extract of sarza q. s.; make 72 pills. Take one, and afterwards two, daily. RICORD. Iodide of mercury gr. j, extract of lettuce gr. j, extract of hemlock gr. ij; in each pill. Dr. BARBOUR. Iodide of mercury ℈j, aloes ʒss, dried sulphate of iron ʒss, myrrh ʒss, oil of savin 20 drops. In 24 pills, one 3 times a day, in *Amenorrhœa.*

PILULÆ HYDRARGYRI DEUTO-IODIDI. M. Deuto-iodide (biniodide) of quicksilver gr. j, extract of juniper gr. xij, powdered liquorice q. s.; for 10 pills.

PILULÆ HYDRARGYRI ET POTASSII IODIDI. PUCHE. Iodide of potassium gr. viij, biniodide of quicksilver gr. viij, syrup of gum q. s.; rub together, and add sugar of milk gr. lxiv. Divide into 32 pills. MIALHE directs iodide of potassium gr. vj, proto-iodide of quicksilver gr. vj, extract of opium gr. xij. Mix the salts accurately, then the extract, and divide into 24 pills.

PILULÆ HYDRARGYRI PROTOXYDI. Mr. TYSON. Protoxide of mercury (Tyson's) ℈j, confection of roses ʒiij, powdered chamomiles ʒss; mix. [Recommended as a substitute for *blue pill.*]

PILULÆ HYDRARGYRI OXYDI RUBRI. Red oxide of mercury and opium, of each ʒj, syrup q. s.; for 60 pills. Formerly in GUY'S H. PH., but now rejected. Some add camphor ʒj.

PILULÆ HYDRARGYRI PHOSPHATIS. BIETT. Phosphate of mercury ℈ss, extract of fumitory ʒj; mix, and make 48 pills. Dose, 1 or 2 daily.

PILULÆ HYDRARGYRI PHOSPHATIS COMPOSITÆ. COPLAND. Phosphate of mercury gr. ix, tartarized antimony gr. j, opium gr. vj, confection of hips q. s. In 6 pills; one at bedtime.

PILULÆ HYDRARGYRI HAHNEMANNI. F. H. Hahnemann's soluble mercury (see Hydrargyri Precipitatum Nigrum) ℈j, gum arabic ʒss, sugar ʒss. Mix, and divide into 30 pills.

PILULÆ HYDRARGYRI PROTO-NITRATIS. *Pilules de Sainte-Marie* Powdered proto-nitrate of mercury gr. vijss, extract of liquorice ℈ss; mix accurately, and divide into 60 pills. Dose, one 4 times a day.

PILULÆ HYDRARGYRI SUBSULPHATIS. CH. Subsulphate of mercury ʒj, opium ʒj, syrup q. s. Mix, and divide into 60 pills.

PILULÆ HYOSCYAMI ET ZINCI. *Pilules de Meglin.* P. Extract of henbane ℥j, extract of valerian ℥j, oxide of zinc ℥j. Mix, and form it into three-grain pills.

PILULÆ IODINII. BRERA. Iodine gr. j, liquorice powder ℈j, elder rob q. s.; for 8 pills.

PILULÆ IODOFORMI. BOUCHARDAT. Iodoform ʒss, extract of wormwood q. s.; mix, and divide into 36 pills. One 3 times a day, in *scrofulous affections*, &c.

PILULÆ IPECACUANHÆ COMPOSITÆ. L. Compound ipecacuanha powder ʒiij, fresh dried squill ʒj, ammoniacum ʒj, mucilage q. s. Mix.

PILULÆ IPECACUANHÆ CUM CONIO. St. B. H. Extract of hemlock ʒj, ipecacuanhæ gr. xij; mix, and make 12 pills. Dose, 1 every 6 hours.

PILULÆ IPECACUANHÆ ET OPII. E. Compound ipecacuanha powder 3 parts, confection of roses 1 part. Mix, and divide into pills of 4 grains each.

PILULÆ JALAPÆ. E. 1783. Extract of jalap ʒij, aromatic powder ʒj, syrup q. s., to make a mass.

PILULÆ JALAPÆ COMPOSITÆ. Jalap, rhubarb, soap, of each ℥j, calomel ℈xx, tartarized antimony gr. xxviij. Mix.

PILULÆ JALAPÆ ALKALINÆ. REECE. Alkaline extract of jalap ʒjss, ginger gr. x, in 24 pills. Dose, three occasionally.

PILULÆ SAPONIS JALAPÆ. PHŒBUS. Soap of jalap ʒj, powdered jalap ℈j. Mix.

PILULÆ JALAPÆ CUM CALOMELANE. ALIBERT'S *Purgative Pills.* Resin of jalap ʒj, calomel ʒj, soap ʒj, oil of orange-peel 6 drops. Make 60 pills.

PILULÆ JATROPHÆ. Dr. BARHAM. Decorticated seeds of jatropha gossypifolia ʒiij, camboge, extract of colocynth, and scammony, each ʒj. Make 90 pills. Dose, 1, 2, or more.

PILULÆ LACTUCARII. Dr. DUNCAN. Lactucarium gr. xij, liquorice powder ℈ij. Mix, and make 12 pills.

PILULÆ LUPULINÆ. M. The powder triturated forms a sufficiently tenacious mass for pills, without any addition. [CHEVALLIER. Lupuline ℥ijss, gum acacia ℥j, extract of chicory q. s.; make into four-grain pills.]

PILULÆ MANGANESII MURIATIS. NIEMANN. Muriate of manganese ℈ij, gum arabic ℈ij, liquorice ℈j. Mix.

PILULÆ MATTHÆI. *Pil. Pacificæ.* E. 1744. Castor ℥ij, saffron ℥j, opium ℥j, soap of turpentine ℥iij, copaiva q. s.

PILULÆ MEGLIN. See Pil. Hyoscyami et Zinci.

PILULÆ MORPHIÆ. M. Morphine gr. j, conserve of roses q. s. for 4 pills. MIALHE. Acetate of morphine gr. j, conserve of orange flowers gr. xvj; in 8 pills.

PILULÆ MORPHIÆ COMPOSITÆ. ROUGIER. Sulphate of morphia gr. ij, cyanide of potassium gr. iv, mucilage q. s.; make 24 pills. One every 6 hours; in *neuralgia.*

PILULÆ MOSCHI. F. H. Musk ℥j, oxide of zinc ʒss; in 36 pills. One every 3 hours.

PILULÆ MYRRHÆ. GUY'S H. Myrrh ℥iijss, soap ℥ss, water q. s.; make 60 pills. Take 2 to 4 twice or thrice a day.

PILULÆ MYRRHÆ COMPOSITÆ. U. C. H. Myrrh ℥jss, subcarbonate of iron ℥ss, soap ℥j, aromatic confection q. s. For 30 pills.

PILULÆ NUCIS VOMICÆ. M. The resinous extract formed into pills of gr. j each, with or without confection of roses.

PILULÆ NUCIS VOMICÆ CUM ALOE. Dr. COPLAND. Pill of aloes and myrrh ℈iv, extract of nux vomica gr. x; mix accurately, and divide into 36 pills. One or two night and morning.

PILULÆ OLEI CROTONIS. Dr. REECE. Oil of croton seeds 6 drops, soap ℥ss, oil of caraway 8 drops, liquorice powder q. s. For 12 pills. Dose, 2 or more. Dr. COPLAND prescribes oil of croton 6 drops, pill of aloes and myrrh ℥jss, soap ℈j, liquorice powder q. s. In 30 pills. Dose, 2 or 3.

PILULÆ OLEI ERGOTÆ. Oil of ergot, powdered althæa root, yolk of egg, of each gr. xv; in 20 pills.

PILULÆ OPII. E. *Pil. Thebaicæ.* Opium 1 part, sulphate of potash 3 parts, conserve of roses 1 part; mix, and divide into five-grain pills. They contain twice as much opium as those of the Phar. of 1817. U. S. powdered opium ℥j, soap gr. xij, water q. s.; make 60 pills.

PILULÆ OPII COMPOSITÆ. CH. Purified opium ʒj, camphor ʒjss, tartarized antimony gr. xv, syrup q. s.; for 60 pills.

PILULÆ PAPAVERIS CUM IPECACUANHA. Ipecac. ʒj, extract of poppies ʒiv; mix, and divide into 60 pills. One pill once or oftener in the day.

PILULÆ PAULLINIÆ. Dr. GAVRELLE. Each pill contains gr. jss of the extract. 4 to 5 daily.

PILULÆ PERPETUÆ. Metallic antimony (regulus) cast into pills.

PILULÆ PECTORALES. E. 1746. Ammoniacum ʒiv, benzoin ʒiij, myrrh ʒij, saffron ʒj, anisated balsam of sulphur ʒss, syrup of Tolu q. s. Dr. LATHAM'S cough pills; comp. ipecac. powder ʒj, fresh squill ℈j, ammoniacum ℈j, calomel gr. iv; in 20 pills. One 3 times a day.

PILULÆ PICIS. Tar ʒj, elecampane powder q. s. to form a mass. DR. WOOD recommends flour and tar. Dr. SEYMOUR. Tar ℈ij, liquorice powder ℈j; in 16 pills. 2 or 3 pills 3 times a day.

PILULÆ PICIS NIGRÆ. Dr. WARDLEWORTH. Black pitch ʒj, powdered gum arabic ʒss; mix, and divide into 20 pills. Two every night, in hæmorrhoidal diseases.

PILULÆ PIGMENTI INDICI. MICHEL. Indigo gr. xij, opium gr. jss, extract of valerian gr. xviij, extract of bark gr. xviij; in 20 pills. 4 in the day. *In traumatic epilepsy.*

PILULÆ PIPERINÆ. IT. H. Piperine gr. xxiv, crumb of bread q. s.; make 12 pills. One every 2 hours as a febrifuge.

PILULÆ PIPERINÆ CUM HYDRARGYRO. Dr. HARTLE. Blue pill gr. j, piperine gr. ij, sulphate of quinine gr. ij, syrup to form a pill.

PILULÆ PLATINI BICHLORIDI. Dr. HŒFER. Bichloride of platina gr. vijss, extract of guaiacum ʒj, liquorice powder q. s.; divide into 20 pills. Dose, 1 pill 3 times a day.

PILULÆ PLUMBI OPIATÆ. E. Acetate of lead 6 parts, opium 1 part, conserve of roses 1 part; mix, and divide into four-grain pills.

PILULÆ PLUMBI IODIDI. COTTEREAU. Iodide of lead ʒss, confection of roses q. s.; mix, and divide into 120 pills. In scrofula, schirrous tumours, &c. Dose, 1 (gradually increased to 5) night and morning.

PILULÆ PLUMMERI. See Pil. Hydrargyri Chloridi Compositæ.

PILULÆ POTASSII IODIDI. PIERQUIN. Iodide of potassium 3ijss, water ℥iij, crumb of bread q. s. Make 150 pills: 2 morning and night.

PILULÆ PURGANTES. See Pil. Aloes, Catharticæ, Colocynthidis, Crotonis, Jalapæ, &c.

PILULÆ PURGANTES STIMULANTES. Dr. ROBINSON. Extract of aloes ℨj, balsam of Peru gr. x, oil of caraway 10 drops, scammony ℨss; mix, for 20 pills. For sluggish bowels of old persons. Dose, 2 pills.

PILULÆ PURGANTES CUM FELLE. Dr. COPLAND. Inspissated ox-gall 3j, aloes ℨj, compound extract of colocynth ℈j, soap ℈j; mix, and divide into 36 pills.

PILULÆ QUERCETANI. Compound colocynth pill gr. xlviij, calomel gr. xij; in 12 pills.

PILULÆ QUINIÆ SULPHATIS. U. S. Sulphate of quinine ℥j, powdered gum acacia ℨij, syrup q. s. Make 480 pills. Dose, 1 to 5 pills. 12 pills equal to ℥j of bark. Dr. WOOD.

PILULÆ QUINÆ SULPHATIS CUM GENTIANA. Disulphate of quinine ℈j, extract of gentian ℈ij; mix, for 20 pills.

PILULÆ QUINÆ COMPOSITÆ. RYAN. Sulphate of quinine gr. xij, extract of gentian ℈j, compound rhubarb pill ℈ij, blue pill gr. vj; mix, and make into 12 pills; 1 three times a day.

PILULÆ QUINÆ CUM CAMPHORA. COPLAND. Camphor in powder ℈j, sulphate of quinine ℈ij, pill of aloes and myrrh ℨjss, syrup of ginger q. s. Make 40 pills. 1 twice a day.

PILULÆ QUINÆ FERRO-PRUSSIATIS. DONOVAN. Hydrocyanoferrate of quina gr. xxiv, mucilage q. s.; make 12 pills. Dose, 2 pills.

PILULÆ AD RABIEM. WERLHOF. Cantharides in fine powder gr. j, belladonna gr. ij, calomel gr. ij, camphor gr. iv, mucilage q. s.; make 6 pills. Three, twice a day, in Hydrophobia.

PILULÆ RHATANIÆ ET RHEI. REECE. Extract of rhatany ℨj, extract of rhubarb ℈ij, ginger ℈j; in 24 pills.

PILULÆ RESOLVENTES. *Pilules Fondantes.* F. H. Soap ℨiij, ammoniacum ℨj, rhubarb ℨj, aloes gr. x, assafœtida ℨss, tincture of saffron q. s. Mix, and divide into three-grain pills.

Dan. Ph. Rhubarb ʒij, acetate of soda ʒij, inspissated ox-gall ʒij, mucilage q. s.

Pilulæ Rhei. E. Rhubarb 9 parts, acetate of potash 1 part, conserve of roses 5 parts. Beat into a proper mass, and divide into five-grain pills. U. S. Rhubarb ʒvj, soap ʒij, water q. s.; for 120 pills.

Pilulæ Rhei Compositæ. L. Rhubarb ℥j, aloes ʒvj, myrrh ʒiv, soap ʒj, oil of caraway f ʒss, syrup quant. suf. Mix.

Pilulæ Rhei Compositæ. E. 1841. Rhubarb 12 parts, aloes 9, myrrh 6, soap 6, oil of peppermint 1, conserve of roses 5. They may also be made without the oil of peppermint. Before 1839 the form was: rhubarb ℥j, aloes ʒvj, myrrh ʒiv, oil of peppermint ʒss, syrup of orange q. s. [The Pil. Rhei Comp. of the Hospitals are very different. St. B. H.: Rhubarb ʒss, scammony gr. viij, antimonial powder gr. viij, syrup of ginger q. s. Mix, and make 12 pills. Dose, 3. Guy's H. See Pil. Rhei cum Soda.]

Pilulæ Rhei et Carui. Dr. Kitchener's *Peristaltic Persuaders.* Turkey rhubarb ʒij, syrup ʒj, oil of caraway ♏x. Mix, and divide into 40 pills. Dose, 1, 2, or 3 pills.

Pilulæ Rhei et Anthemidis. *Speediman's Pills.* Rhubarb, aloes, myrrh, extract of chamomiles, of each ʒj, oil of chamomiles 12 drops. Into four-grain pills.

Pilulæ Rhei Balsamicæ. Swediaur. Powdered rhubarb, and gum acacia, equal parts; balsam copaiva q. s., to form a mass.

Pilulæ Rhei et Ferri. E. Dried sulphate of iron 4 parts, extract of rhubarb 10 parts, conserve of roses 5 parts. Mix, and divide into five-grain pills.

Pilulæ Rhei cum Opio. St. B. H. Rhubarb gr. ix, opium gr. j, water q. s. For 2 pills.

Pilulæ Rhei cum Soda. U. C. H. Rhubarb, dried soda, each ʒjss, syrup q. s.; in 30 pills. Guy's H. (Pil. Rhei Comp.) Rhubarb, dried carbonate of soda, extract of gentian, of each ʒjss. Mix, and make 60 pills.

Pilulæ *seu* Extractum Rudii. E. 1783. Black hellebore root ℥ij, colocynth ℥ij, water Oiv; boil to Oij, strain, evaporate to consistence of honey; add aloes ℥ij, scammony ℥j, remove from the fire, and add sulphate of potash ℈ij, oil of cloves ʒj.

PILULÆ RUFI. See Pil. Aloes cum Myrrhâ.

PILULÆ SAGAPENI COMPOSITÆ. L. Sagapenum ℥j, aloes ʒss, syrup of ginger q. s.

PILULÆ SALICINÆ. JOY. Salicine gr. xij, extract of gentian gr. xij, liquorice powder q. s.; for 6 pills.

PILULÆ SALICINÆ LAXANTES. Salicine ℈j, compound rhubarb pill ℈ij; mix, and make 12 pills.

PILULÆ SAPONIS COMPOSITÆ. L. *Pil. Saponis cum Opio.* Opium powdered ʒiv, soap ℥ij. Mix. 5 grains contain 1 of opium. [U. S. (Pil. Opii.) Opium ʒj, soap gr. xij; beat them with water, and divide into 60 pills.]

PILULÆ CUM SAPONE. P. Soap ℥iv, althæa root ℥ss, nitre ʒj. Mix.

PILULÆ SCAMMONII. Dr. COPLAND. Scammony gr. xv, white sugar gr. x; rub together, and add oil of caraway ♏iv.

PILULÆ SCAMMONII COMPOSITÆ. GUY'S H. Scammony, extract of henbane, gamboge, compound extract of colocynth, and soap, of each gr. xij, water q. s.; make 12 pills. Dose, 2 to 3. ST. B. H. Scammony gr. xxiv, aloes gr. xij, gamboge gr. xij, ginger ℈j, treacle q. s. For 12 pills.

PILULÆ SCILLÆ CUM AMMONIACO. ST. B. H. Powdered squills gr. xij, ammoniacum gr. xlviij, water q. s. Make 12 pills.

PILULÆ SCILLÆ. E. Squill in fine powder 5 parts; ammoniac, ginger, and soap, each 4 parts; conserve of roses 2 parts. Make a uniform mass, and divide into five-grain pills.

PILULÆ SCILLÆ COMPOSITÆ. L. & D. Powdered squill ʒj, ginger ʒij, [ʒiij, D.] ammoniacum ʒij, soap ʒiij, syrup [treacle, D.] q. s.

PILULÆ SCILLÆ CUM CROTONE. Mr. SELWYN. Croton oil ♏vj, compound squill pill ℈ij, compound extract of colocynth ℈ij; in 18 pills. Three twice a week, in *Dropsy*.

PILULÆ SCILLÆ CUM HYDRARGYRO. GUY'S H. Oxide of quicksilver ℈j, compound squill pill ʒiv; mix, and divide into 60 pills.

PILULÆ SCILLÆ CUM OPIO. GUY'S H. Powdered opium gr. xx, compound squill pill ʒiv; mix, and divide into 60 pills. Dose, 3 every night.

Pilulæ Scillæ cum Zingibere. D. 1807. Powdered squill ʒj, ginger ʒij, oil of aniseed 10 drops, jelly of soap q. s.

Pilulæ Sedativæ. U. C. H. Extract of henbane ℈j, camphor ʒj, alcohol ♏iij. Make 20 pills.

Pilulæ Sennæ. Hufeland. Senna p. ʒj, extract of dandelion q. s. Mix, and make 30 pills. Dose, 5 to 8.

Pilulæ Sennæ Compositæ. The comp. powder of senna formed into pills.

Pilulæ Smuckeri. Galbanum ʒj, sagapenum ʒj, soap ʒj, rhubarb ʒjss, tartar emetic gr. xvj, liquorice juice ʒj. Mix.

Pilulæ Sodæ cum Sapone. E. 1817. Dried subcarbonate of soda ʒij, soap ʒjss, syrup q. s. [Dr. Beddoes. Dried subc. of soda ʒj, soap ℈iv, oil of juniper 10 drops, syrup of ginger q. s. Make 30 pills.]

Pilulæ Sodæ cum Hyoscyamo. Dr. Copland. Dried subcarbonate of soda ℈ijss, rhubarb ʒj, extract of henbane ℈ij. In 36 pills.

Pilulæ Stomachicæ. E. 1744. Replaced by Pilulæ Rhei Comp. The name is also given to Pil. Aloes et Mastiches, and Pil. Antecibum. P. Dr. H. Smith's *Stomachic Pills* are, sagapenum, rhubarb, aloes, aromatic powder, of each ʒj, oil of peppermint and of cloves, each 10 drops, balsam of Peru q. s. Divide into four-grain pills. 3 to 6 daily.

Pilulæ Strychniæ. M. Strychnine gr. ij, confection of dog-rose ʒss; mix, divide into 30 pills, and silver them.

Pilulæ Styracis Compositæ. L. (Pil. e Styrace, D.) Strained storax ʒiij, opium ʒj, saffron ʒj; mix. [E. (Pil. Styracis) directs ʒij of storax, and the mass to be divided into four-grain pills.]

Pilulæ Tabaci. Augustin. Powdered tobacco gr. xxiv, confection of roses q. s.; mix, and form 72 pills. Dose, 2 to 4 daily till nausea is produced. *In Dropsy.*

Pilulæ Tannini. Cottereau. Tannic acid ʒss, conserve of roses q. s. Make 18 pills. 1 every hour, in hæmoptysis.

Pilulæ Terebinthinæ. P. Boiled turpentine (see Terebinthina Cocta) is softened by warm water, and formed into pills, which must be rolled in powdered starch.

Pilulæ Terebinthinæ cum Rheo. Guy's H. Chio turpentine

ʒj, rhubarb ℈j, soap ʒss; mix, and make 30 pills. CLINE. Boiled turpentine ʒij, rhubarb ʒj; in 36 pills.

PILULÆ THEBAICÆ. E. See Pilulæ Opii.

PILULÆ TIGLII. CHARING CROSS H. Oil of croton tiglium ♏iij, oil of caraway ♏iij, bread-crumb q. s. In 3 pills. See Pil. Olei Crotonis.

PILULÆ TONICÆ BACHERI. P. Alkaline extract of hellebore ʒij, extract of myrrh ʒij, powdered holy thistle ʒj; mix, and divide into four-grain pills.

PILULÆ TONICÆ STAHLII. Levigated iron ʒj, gum ammoniac ʒj, extract of lesser centaury ʒj, syrup of fumitory q. s.

PILULÆ TONICÆ APERIENTES. COPLAND. Sulphate of quinine ℈j, pill of aloes and myrrh ℈ij, extract of gentian ʒj; mix, for 30 pills.

PILULÆ VALERIANÆ COMPOSITÆ. DUPUYTREN. Valerian ʒss, castor ℈j, oxide of zinc ℈j; mix for 18 pills. Dose 3 pills 3 times a day.

PILULÆ VERATRIÆ. M. Veratria gr. ss, gum acacia gr. vj, syrup q. s. for 6 pills. Dr. TURNBULL. Veratria gr. j to ij, extract of henbane gr. vj, liquorice powder gr. xij; mix accurately, and make 12 pills.

PILULÆ VERMIFUGÆ. PESCHIER. Ethereal extract of male fern 30 drops, extract of dandelion ʒj, powdered gum acacia q. s.; mix, and make 30 pills.

PILULÆ ZINCI SULPHATIS. CH. Sulphate of zinc ʒij, Venice turpentine q. s.; mix, and make 60 pills.

PILULÆ ZINCI CUM GENTIANA. Sulphate of zinc ʒss, extract of gentian ʒij, powdered calumba q. s. Make 30 pills.

PILULÆ ZINCI ET MYRRHÆ. Dr. PARIS. Sulphate of zinc gr. x, myrrh ʒjss, confection of roses q. s. Make 20 pills.

PILULÆ ZINCI VALERIANATIS. BOUDET. Valerianate of zinc gr. ix, tragacanth ʒss; mix, and divide into 12 pills. One night and morning.

PIPERINUM. P. *Piperine.* Treat alcoholic extract of white pepper with a solution of caustic potash (containing one part of potash in 100); wash the residue with cold water, dissolve it in alcohol, filter through a little animal charcoal, and let the solution evaporate spontaneously in a warm place. Purify the crystals by redissolving and crystallizing. *Febrifuge.* Dose, two to five grains, or from 12 to 24 or 30 grains in 24 hours.

PLATINI BICHLORIDUM. Dissolve platina in nitro-muriatic acid, and evaporate the solution to dryness by a gentle heat. Dose, gr. ss to gr. jss.

PLATINO-CHLORIDUM SODII. *Chloride of Platina and Sodium.* Mix solutions of 6 parts of chloride of sodium, and 17 parts of bichloride of platina, and evaporate that crystals may be produced. Dose, gr. j to gr. iij. [They are used for the same purposes as the salts of gold.]

PLUMBAGINA. *Plumbagine.* Dr. O'SHAUGHNESSY. Mix an æthereal tincture of the root-bark of plumbago rosea with water, distil off the æther, boil, and filter the liquid while hot, and set it aside to crystallize.

PLUMBI ACETAS. L. Acetate (or sugar) of lead. Powdered litharge ℔iv ℥ij, acetic acid Oiv, distilled water Oiv. Dissolve by a gentle heat, filter, and evaporate that crystals may form. [E. directs, Oij pyroligneous acid, Oj of water, and ℥xiv litharge. D. Carbonate of lead and distilled vinegar.]

PLUMBI DIACETAS. See Liquor Plumbi Diacetatis.

PLUMBI CARBONAS. *White Lead,* or *Ceruss.* It may be procured by adding any alkaline carbonate to a solution of acetate or nitrate of lead, and washing the precipitate.

PLUMBI CHLORIDUM. L. Dissolve ℥xix of acetate of lead in Oiij of boiling water, and ℥vj of chloride of sodium in Oj of water; mix the solutions, and when cold wash the precipitate with distilled water, and dry it.

PLUMBI CYANIDUM. To a solution of acetate of lead add hydrocyanic acid as long as it occasions a precipitate, which must be well washed with distilled water, and dried with a gentle heat. [Dr. R. D. THOMPSON proposes to procure hydrocyanic acid from this cyanide. Put 130 grains of cyanide of lead into a stoppered bottle, and add f ʒvj of diluted sulphuric acid, previously mixed with f ʒxviij of distilled water; agitate the bottle for some time, then let the mixture settle, and decant off the clear liquid.]

PLUMBI IODIDUM. L. Acetate of lead ℥ix, iodide of potash ℥vij; dissolve the former in Ovj of distilled water, and filter; add it to the latter dissolved in Oij of water; wash the precipitate, and dry it. [E. directs ℥j each of iodide of potassium and nitrate of lead, to be dissolved separately in f ℥xv of distilled water, the solutions mixed, and the resulting powder washed, and boiled in three gallons of water with f ℥iij of pyroligneous acid; let any undissolved matter subside, maintaining the temperature near the boiling point, and pour off the clear liquor, from which the iodide of lead will crystallize on cooling. Dose, from a quarter to half a grain or more, but chiefly used externally.]

PLUMBI NITRAS. E. Litharge ℥ivss, diluted nitric acid Oj; digest with a gentle heat, filter, and set aside to crystallize; concentrate the residual liquor to obtain more crystals.

PLUMBI OXYDUM SEMIVITREUM. Melted lead is exposed to a current of air till oxydized, and the oxide fused by a stronger heat.

PLUMBI OXYDUM HYDRATUM. Solution of diacetate of lead Ovj, distilled water Ciij, solution of potash Ovj, or sufficient to precipitate the oxide. Mix, and wash the precipitated oxide till nothing alkaline remains.

PLUMBI OXYDUM RUBRUM. *Red Lead.* It is obtained by heating massicot or litharge in a reverberatory furnace till by absorbing oxygen it assumes a red colour.

PLUMBI SACCHARAS. Mix one part of sugar with two parts of nitric acid, diluted with ten of water, and apply heat as long as reaction takes place; neutralize by chalk, filter, and add to the filtered solution acetate of lead as long as any precipitate is formed; wash this and dry it.

PLUMBI NITRO-SACCHARAS. Dissolve saccharate of lead in cold nitric acid diluted with 19 parts of water; filter, evaporate, and set aside, that crystals may form. Dr. HOSKINS proposed a solution of this salt (one grain with five drops of saccharic acid to ℥j of water) *as a solvent for Phosphatic Calculi.*

PLUMBI TANNAS. Dr. FANTONETTI. To a concentrated infusion of oak-bark add a solution of acetate of lead drop by drop; wash the precipitate, and dry it. A purer tannate is obtained by substituting a solution of pure tannic acid for infusion of oak-bark.

POMATUM. Originally *Apple Ointment,* but now applied to lard, or mixed fats, carefully washed and scented. [The *Pommades* of the French Codex are combinations of prepared lards, or mixed fats, with various vegetable or mineral substances. In this work they are placed under the head UNGUENTA, *Ointments*, which term the French pharmacists restrict to those containing *resinous* substances.]

POTASSA PURA. Potassa Fusa. See Potassæ Hydras.

POTASSA CUM CALCE. L. Rub together equal parts of hydrate of potash and quicklime, and keep them in a well-stopped bottle. E. & D. direct solution of potash to be evaporated in a clean iron vessel to one-fourth, and enough quicklime added to form a stiff paste. See Pasta Viennensis, for *Caustique de Filhos.*

POTASSÆ ACETAS. L. Acetic acid f℥xxvj, distilled water f℥xij; mix, and add carbonate of potash ℔j, or to saturation, and filter. Evaporate carefully in a sand-bath to dryness. D. directs distilled vinegar; and the salt to be liquefied by cautiously raising the heat. E. orders pyroligneous acid. Dose, ℈j to ʒij. *Diuretic.*

POTASSÆ ARSENIAS. *Arsenias Kali.* D. White arsenic (arsenious acid) ℥j, nitrate of potash ℥j; pulverize separately, mix, and heat them in a glass retort to dull redness. Dissolve the residuum in ℔iv of boiling distilled water, evaporate, and set aside to crystallize. Dose, gr. 1-16th to 1-8th.

POTASSÆ ANTIMONIAS. Washed diaphoretic antimony. See Antimonium Calcinatum.

POTASSÆ ARSENITIS LIQUOR. See Liq. Potassæ Arsenitis.

POTASSÆ BORAS. Mix 6 parts of boracic acid with 5 of bicarbonate of potash; heat them to redness in a crucible, dissolve the salt, filter the solution, and evaporate it to dryness.

POTASSÆ CARBONAS. L. Formerly *P. Subcarbonas.* Dissolve ℔ij of impure carbonate of potash (American pearlash) in Ojss of distilled water, and filter; then evaporate in a suitable vessel, and when it begins to thicken, stir constantly till the salt concretes. D. nearly the same.

POTASSÆ CARBONAS PURUM. E. Pure carbonate of potash is most readily obtained by heating crystallized bicarbonate to redness in a crucible, but more cheaply by dissolving bitartrate of potash in 30 parts of boiling water, separating and washing the crystals which form on cooling, heating them in a loosely-covered crucible, breaking down the mass, and roasting it in an oven for 2 hours with occasional stirring; lixiviating the product with distilled water, and evaporating the filtered solution to dryness with constant stirring. D. (Potassæ carb. e Tartari crystallis) directs this process to be performed in silver vessels.

Potassæ Bicarbonas. L. Carbonate of potash ℔vj, distilled water Cj, dissolve, pass carbonic acid gas through the solution till fully saturated; heat it gently, and set aside, that crystals may be produced. Pour off the liquor, and dry them. E. Take of carbonate of ammonia, in fine powder ℥iijss; carbonate of potash ℥vj; triturate them thoroughly together, with a very little water, to form a smooth pulp. Dry this at a temperature not exceeding 140°, triturating occasionally towards the close, till a fine powder be obtained, free from ammoniacal odour. D. nearly as L.

Potassæ Chloras. Graham. Mix 2 parts of carbonate of potash with 1 of quicklime, and expose to a current of chlorine. When saturated, heat the mixture gently, digest it in water, and separate the chlorate from the filtered liquid by crystallization. Dose gr. v to xv.

Potassæ Citras. Saturate a solution of citric acid with carbonate or bicarbonate of potash, and evaporate to dryness. This deliquescent salt is rarely used except in solution. See Liquor Potassæ Citratis. A mixture of the acid and bicarbonate, each separately dried, is sometimes kept. 10 parts of the acid require 14½ of the bicarbonate. But the name Potassæ Citras, or acidulated or citrated Kali, is often improperly given to a mixture of tartaric acid, bicarbonate of soda, sugar, and essence of lemon.

Potassæ Hydras. L. Potassa Fusa. *Caustic Potash.* Evaporate solution of potash in an iron vessel, until, the ebullition having ceased, the hydrate of potash liquefies; pour this into proper moulds. D. Pour it on an iron plate, and when cold, cut it into proper pieces, which must be immediately put into closely-stopped vials. [A purer kind is obtained by dissolving this in alcohol, and evaporating the clear solution in a silver basin.]

Potassæ Hydriodas. D. See Potassi Iodidum.

Potassæ Hydrocyanas. See Potassii Cyanidum. But Magendie's *Hydrocyanate de Potasse medicinal* consists of cyanide of potassium dissolved in 8 times its weight of distilled water. It soon decomposes.

Potassæ Murias. See Potassii Chloridum.

POTASSÆ NITRAS PURIFICATUM. Nitre of commerce is purified by recrystallization. D. Dissolve common nitre in twice its weight of boiling water, and set it aside to crystallize. [Neither chloride of barium nor nitrate of silver should throw down any precipitate from its solution.]

POTASSÆ NITRAS FUSA. *Mineral Crystal.* Sal Prunella. Melt nitrate of potash in a Hessian crucible, and cast it on a smooth surface, or in moulds. P. directs 1-128th part of sulphur to be added to the nitre in fusion.

POTASSÆ SILICAS. Mix 1 part of powdered quartz or flint, or of fine siliceous sand, with 2 parts of subcarbonate of potash, and fuse them in a Hessian crucible. Dissolve the mass in water, filter the solution, and evaporate it to dryness. Dose, gr. x to xv, in 6 or 8 ounces of water, twice a day, *to dissolve gouty concretions.* MR. URE.

POTASSÆ SUPEROXALAS. To form a *binoxalate,* neutralize 1 part of oxalic acid with carbonate of potash, add to the neutral salt another part of acid, and crystallize; a *quadroxalate* is made by dissolving the binoxalate in hydrochloric acid, and crystallizing. Poisonous.

POTASSÆ SULPHAS. Ignite ℔ij of the salt (Sal Enixum) which remains after the distillation of nitric acid till the excess of sulphuric acid is expelled; boil it in two gallons of water till a pellicle floats, and having strained the liquor, set it aside that crystals may form; having poured off the liquor, dry them. D. directs the residuary salt to be dissolved in water, and the excess of acid neutralized with carbonate of potash; E. with marble. Dose, gr. x to ℈ij. In doses of a few drachms it sometimes acts as an irritant poison.

POTASSÆ BISULPHAS. L. Dissolve ℔ij of the salt which remains after the distillation of nitric acid in Ovj of boiling water; add to it ℔j (f℥vij fʒj, E.) of sulphuric acid, boil down the solution, and set it aside to crystallize. D. Mix 1 part of sulphuric acid with 6 of water, saturate it with carbonate of potash, add another part of sulphuric acid, and evaporate, that crystals may form on cooling. Dose, gr. x to ʒj properly diluted.

POTASSÆ SULPHAS CUM SULPHURE. E. *Sal Polychrest.* Mix equal parts of nitrate of potash and sulphur; throw the mixture in small successive portions into a red-hot crucible, and when cool, reduce the salt to powder, and preserve it in well-closed bottles. [This differs from the Potassæ Sulphas, which is, however, often substituted for it.] Dose ʒss to ʒj.

POTASSÆ SULPHURETUM. D. See Potassii Sulphuretum.

POTASSÆ TARTRAS. L. and E. *Soluble Tartar.* Carbonate of potash ℥xvj, boiling water Ovj; dissolve, add bitartrate of potash in powder ℔iij, and boil; strain the solution, boil it down till a pellicle floats on the surface, and set aside, that crystals may form. Having poured off the solution, dry these, and again evaporate, that more may be obtained. D. by the same process from 5 parts of carbonate of potash, 14 of bitartrate, and 45 of water.

POTASSÆ BITARTRAS. *Cream of Tartar.* Obtained from the crude tartar deposited by wines, by solution and crystallization. The crystals are again dissolved in boiling water containing charcoal and clay. When these have subsided, the clear solution is drawn off and left to crystallize.

POTASSÆ AMMONIO-TARTRAS. *Tartarum Solubile Ammoniacale.* NIEMANN. Dissolve bitartrate of potash in hot water, and add carbonate of ammonia to saturation. Evaporate the solution to dryness with a gentle heat, or set the concentrated solution aside that crystals may form.

POTASSÆ ET SODA TARTRAS. E. See Sodæ Potassio-tartras.

POTASSÆ BORO-TARTRAS. P. *Soluble Cream of Tartar.* Bitartrate of potash in powder ℥iv, boracic acid in crystals ℥j, water ℔ij; put them into a silver basin, boil till most of the water is evaporated, and continue the evaporation with a regulated heat, stirring incessantly. When the matter becomes very thick, take it up in portions, flatten them, and place them in a stove till sufficiently dry; reduce them to powder, and preserve it in well-stopped bottles. [LIEBIG recommends 47½ parts of cream of tartar and 15½ of boracic acid; the solution to be evaporated in a water-bath.] See Tartarum Boraxatum.

POTASSÆ BI-ZINCAS. FREMY. To a saturated solution of oxide of zinc in solution of potash add a little alcohol, which throws down the salt in crystals.

POTASSII BROMIDUM. L. To Ojss of distilled water add ℥j of iron filings, and then ℥ij of bromine. Set aside for half an hour, stirring occasionally; then apply a gentle heat, and when the liquid becomes greenish, add ʒxvij of carbonate of potash, dissolved in Ojss of water. Filter, wash what remains with

Oij of boiling water, and filter again; then evaporate the mixed solutions, that crystals may form. Dose, 2 to 5 grains.

POTASSII CHLORIDUM. *Muriate of Potash. Sal Sylvii.* To a solution of carbonate of potash add muriatic acid to saturation; concentrate the solution by evaporation, and leave it to cool slowly, that crystals may form.

POTASSII CYANURETUM. U. S. *Cyanide of Potassium*, or *Hydrocyanate of Potash.* Let ℥viij of ferro-prussiate of potash be thoroughly dried with a moderate heat, then introduced into an earthen retort, having its beak loosely stopped, and exposed to a red heat for two hours, or as long as gas escapes. Withdraw the retort from the fire, close the orifice with lute, and leave it till quite cold; then break the retort, reduce the black mass to powder, and put it into a ℥xij bottle with ℥vj of water. Agitate it occasionally for half an hour, then filter, evaporate the filtered solution rapidly to dryness, and keep the dry salt in closely-stopped bottles. [The watery solution of this salt can scarcely be evaporated without undergoing decomposition. The process in P. is nearly as U. S.; but when the gas ceases to escape, the heat is increased for a quarter of an hour; the tube is then closed with lute, the openings of the furnace closed, and the whole allowed to cool. The retort is then broken, and the upper layer of pure fused salt removed from lower dark matter, and preserved for use.] Mr. DONOVAN states that an iron quicksilver bottle, furnished with a curved tube dipping half an inch into water in a cup, answers the purpose very well. LIEBIG'S process is—take 8 parts of ferro-prussiate of potash in powder, dry it sharply, mix it with 3 parts of dried pure carbonate of potash; fuse together, and when the mass is fluid, stir it occasionally with a glass rod until it becomes perfectly colourless; allow it to settle, and pour off the clear fused salt on a marble slab. This contains 1-8th of cyanate of potash. *Poisonous.* Dose, 1-8th to 1-4th of a grain. Dissolved in 8 times its weight of distilled water, it forms MAGENDIE'S *Medicinal Hydrocyanate of Potash.*

POTASSII SULPHOCYANIDUM. Digest a watery solution of cyanide of potassium with sulphur, of which it takes up a third of its weight. Filter, and evaporate.

POTASSII IODIDUM. L. Mix ℥vj of iodine with Oiv of distilled water, and add ℥ij of iron filings, stirring frequently for half an hour; apply a gentle heat, and when a greenish colour appears, add ℥iv of carbonate of potash dissolved in Oiv of water, and strain. Wash the residue with Oij of boiling water, again strain, and evaporate the mixed liquors, that crystals may be formed. [The process of E. is nearly the same; but with ℥v of iodine, ℥iij of iron wire, and ℥ij ʒvj of dry carbonate of potash. The salt obtained by evaporation is then crystallized from a solution in less than its weight of boiling water, or twice its weight of boiling rectified spirit.] D. directs a current of sulphuretted hydrogen to be passed into a mixture of iodine and water, and the resulting hydriodic acid saturated with carbonate of potash, the filtered solution evaporated, and the residual salt taken up with rectified spirit, and the solution evaporated for crystals. MOHR mixes ℥xvj of iodine with 6 or 8 pints of water, and gradually adds powdered sulphuret of barium till the solution becomes colourless, stirring constantly. The solution is then heated to the boiling point, ℥xj of sulphate of potash added, the liquid boiled for a quarter of an hour, and filtered. The clear solution is then evaporated for crystals. Dose, 2 to 15 grains. Some practitioners give still larger doses; but Dr. CHAMBERS says 2 grains twice or thrice a day will serve every purpose the salt is capable of effecting.

POTASSII SULPHURETUM. L. and E. *Liver of Sulphur.* Mix together one part of sulphur and four of carbonate of potash; heat them in a crucible until they have united. [When cold, it is to be broken into fragments, and kept in well-closed vessels, E.] Potassæ Sulphuretum. D. the same.

POTESTATES SUCCINI. QUINCY. *Powers of Amber.* Oil of amber ℥j, carbonate of ammonia ℥ss, alcohol ℥viij; digest until dissolved.

POTIO ANTISPASMODICA, ANODYNA, &c. See Mistura.

POTUS; Drinks. PTISANÆ; Ptisans. *Tisanes* of the P. Codex. These are nearly synonymous, and include the aqueous infusions, decoctions, or solutions, which are so slightly medicated as to be taken *ad libitum.* Some of them are merely dietetic, and form the ordinary drink of the patient. The more active Ptisans will be found among the Decoctions and Infusions; others among the Juleps.

POTUS APERIENS. COPLAND. Manna ʒjss, cream of tartar ℥ss, whey Oij.

POTUS HORDEATUS. To Oj of barley water add ʒj of nitre, or ʒj of cream of tartar, or ℥ss of gum arabic, or f℥j of lemon-juice, or fʒj of diluted sulphuric acid, with f℥j of syrup. P.

Barley water is made by boiling ʒvj of pearl barley with Oiv of water to Oij, and infusing in it ʒiij of liquorice.

Potus Imperialis. One lemon sliced, ℥ss cream of tartar, white sugar ℔ss, hot water Oiij. Infuse half an hour, and strain. See also Limonadum.

Potus Regalis. *King Cup.* Brande. The rind of 1 or 2 lemons cut very thin, and macerated in Oij of cold water for 6 or 8 hours.

Ptisana Avenæ. E. From groats, as Ptisana Oryzæ.

Ptisana Antimonialis. Brera. Lemonade Oij, tartar emetic gr. ij, sugar q. s.

Ptisana Anti-catarrhalis. Pierquin. Aniseed ʒij, elecampane root ℈j, boiling water Oj; infuse, strain, and add honey ℥ij.

Ptisana Arnicæ. P. As Ptisana Sambuci.

Ptisana Asparagi. P. Asparagus root ℥j, liquorice root ʒiij, boiling water Oij; infuse 4 hours, and strain. Ptisans are prepared in the same way from various roots, barks, &c.

Ptisana Boraginis. Dried borage leaves ʒiij, boiling water Oij; infuse for an hour, and sweeten to the taste. [Ptisans are made in the same manner, from the leaves of maidenhair, blessed-thistle, succory, orange, heart's-ease, field scabious, and male speedwell.]

Ptisana Cassiæ. P. Cassia pods ℥ij; slit them, mix the pulp with Oij of warm water, and strain.

Ptisana Gummosa. *Eau de Gomme.* P. Picked gum arabic ʒv, water Oij; dissolve without heat, and strain.

Ptisana Hordei. Infuse ʒiij of liquorice root in Oij of hot barley water.

Ptisana Lactis. See Serum Lactis.

Ptisana Lichenis Hibernici. Decoction of carrageen Oijss, syrup of gum ℥iij.

Ptisana Lichenis Islandici. Steep ℥j of Iceland moss for 12 hours in cold water; then boil it in Oijss of fresh water to Oj, and add ℥j of syrup of althæa.

Ptisana Lini. *Linseed Tea.* See Infusum Lini.

Ptisana Limonis. See Limonadum.

PTISANA MELLIS. See Hydromel.

PTISANA ORYZÆ. P. *Rice Water.* Infuse ʒiij of liquorice root in Oij of a decoction of ʒv of washed rice.

PTISANA ORYZÆ CITRATA. AUGUSTIN. Washed rice ℥j, water ℔iv; boil, strain, add barley sugar ℥ss, lemon-juice ℥j.

PTISANA PANIS. *Decoctum Album.* P. Prepared hartshorn ʒij, bread-crumb ʒvj, gum acacia ʒij, water Oij; boil for half an hour, strain through a coarse sieve, and add white sugar ℥j, orange-flower water ℥ss.

PTISANA PECTORALIS. Dates and jujubes (stoned) each ℥ss, figs ℥ss, raisins ℥ss; boil in water q. s. to strain Oij.

PTISANA REGALIS. See Apozema dictum Ptisana Regalis. P.

PTISANA RHŒADOS. From the flowers, as Ptisana Sambuci.

PTISANA ROSÆ CUM LACTE. Conserve of roses ℥j, new milk Oj; rub together, and strain.

PTISANA SALEPI. Boil ʒj of salep in f℥xvj of water, and strain.

PTISANA SAMBUCI. P. Elder flowers ʒj, boiling water Oj¾; macerate for half an hour, and strain.

PTISANA SARZÆ. See Decoctum Sarzæ.

PTISANA TAMARINDORUM. Pulp of tamarind ℥j, hot water Oij.

PTISANA TILIÆ. P. Lime flowers ʒij, boiling water Oj¾; macerate for half an hour, and strain. In the same way prepare Ptisans of roses, violets, mallows, &c.

PTISANA TARTARICA. Syrup of tartaric acid ℥ij, water Ojss.

PULPÆ. Pulps are the soft parts of plants separated from the harder parts by pressing them through a hair sieve. The general directions of the L. college are, "Press the pulpy fruits that are ripe and fresh through a hair sieve, without boiling them. Put pulpy fruits, if unripe, or if ripe and dry, in a moist place to soften; then press the pulps through a hair sieve; boil them afterwards over a slow fire, and lastly evaporate the water in a water-bath, until the pulps become of a proper consistence." D. and E. 1817, direct the dried or unripe fruits to be softened by boiling them in a little water; other authorities by steaming them. Few of the pulps require a separate notice.

PULPA CAROTÆ. P. Carrot roots are reduced to a pulp by means of a rasp. The tubers of potato, bulbs of garlic, and root of patience dock, are pulped in the same way.

PULPA CASSIÆ. Bruise the pods, wash out the pulp with boiling water, and press it first through a sieve with large holes, afterwards through a hair sieve, and evaporate as above directed.

PULPA CONII. P. Fresh hemlock is beaten in a marble mortar to a fine paste, and pressed through a hair sieve. All fresh leaves and flowers may be pulped in the same manner.

PULPA PRUNORUM. L. As directed for dried fruits. P. & U. S. direct the prunes to be softened by steam, and (the stones being removed) the fruit beaten in a marble mortar, and pressed through a hair sieve. Dates and jujubes are pulped by the same method, and the bulbs of lily, onion, and squill, the roots of marsh-mallow, &c.

PULPA ROSÆ CANINÆ. The ripe hips are picked, deprived of their seeds and hairs, and pulped in the usual way. P. directs them to be put into an earthen pan, moistened uniformly with white wine, and left in a cool place, stirring them occasionally till they become soft; they are then beaten and pressed through a sieve.

PULPA TAMARINDORUM. P. & U. S. Put the tamarinds into an earthen pan with a small quantity of water, and digest them at a gentle heat till uniformly softened, then pass the pulp through a hair sieve.

PULVERES. Few of the *simple powders* require special notice. The dry ingredients of the *compound powders* having previously been separately pulverized and passed through a sieve, the whole should be uniformly mixed by trituration in a shallow mortar, and again sifted.

PULVIS ABSORBENS. SPAN. PH. Carbonate of magnesia ℥iv, dried subcarbonate of soda ℈j, ginger ℈j; mix.

PULVIS ACONITI COMPOSITUS. VOGLER. Extract of aconite gr. j, oxysulphuret of antimony gr. j, magnesia gr. x; mix.

PULVIS ACIDI BENZOICI COMPOSITUS. Dr. PARIS. Benzoic acid gr. iij, myrrh gr. x, compound tragacanth powder gr. xij; mix. Dr. COPLAND. Benzoic acid gr. vj, camphor gr. ij, white sugar ℈j; mix.

PULVIS ÆRUGINIS CUM CALOMELANE. CH. Prepared verdigris ʒj, calomel ʒj; mix. *For external use.*

PULVIS ÆRUGINIS COMPOSITUS. MID. H. As Pulvis Sabinæ Compositus.

PULVIS ALÖES COMPOSITUS. L. & D. (Pulv. Alöes cum Guaiaco, L. 1787.) Aloes (hepatic, D.) ℥jss, guaiacum resin ℥j, compound powder of cinnamon ʒiv; mix.

PULVIS ALÖES CUM CANELLA. D. Hiera Picra. Hepatic aloes ℔j, canella ℥iij; pulverize separately, and mix.

PULVIS ALOETICUS CUM FERRO. L. 1788. (*Vice* Pil. Ecphracticæ.) Aloes ℥jss, myrrh ℥ij, sulphate of iron ℥j, dried extract of gentian ℥j.

PULVIS ALTERATIVUS. Dr. PLUMMER. Equal parts of calomel and golden sulphur of antimony, levigated together. [It alters by keeping.]

PULVIS ALTERATIVUS. Mr. CLINE. Sarsaparilla ℥j, carbonate of soda ʒij, Peruvian bark ʒiij; mix, for 16 doses.

PULVIS ALUMINIS COMPOSITUS. E. Pulvis Stypticus. Alum ℥iv, kino ℥j; mix. See Pulvis Stypticus.

PULVIS ALUMINIS CUM CAPSICO. Dr. TURNBULL. Alum three parts, concentrated tincture of capsicum one part; mix, dry, and triturate again. *Applied to the Tonsils.*

PULVIS ALUMINIS GUMMOSUS. FRANKEL. Alum, gum tragacanth, in equal parts. VOGT. Gum acacia ʒiv, alum ℈ij. *As local applications to Sore Breasts,* &c.

PULVIS ALUMINIS OPIATUS. BOUCHARDAT. Alum ʒj, sugar ʒj, opium gr. iv; mix, for 12 powders; two or three daily, in *Obstinate Diarrhœa* and *Passive Hæmorrhages.*

PULVIS ALUMINIS SACCHARATUS. Alum ʒj, sugar ʒj; mix. To be blown into the throat.

PULVIS AMBERGRISEÆ MOSCHATUS. BAT. PH. Ambergris ʒvj, musk ʒj, oil of cinnamon ℈ij, refined sugar ℥xjss; mix.

PULVIS AMMONIATUS AROMATICUS. P. LEAYSON'S Ammoniacal Collyrium. Muriate of ammonia ʒj, slaked lime ℥j, charcoal gr. xv, cinnamon gr. xv, cloves gr. xv, bole ʒss. Put them into a bottle, and moisten with a little water.

PULVIS AMYLI ET SODÆ. DEVERGIE'S Alkaline Powder. Mix

one part of carbonate of soda in fine powder, with ten of white starch. *For external use in some skin diseases.*

Pulvis Anthelminticus. Guibourt. Sulphate of iron ʒss, tansy ʒj, worm-seed ʒjss; mix. Dose, gr. ix. Bouchardat. Corsican moss ʒv, worm-seed ʒv, calomel gr. xlv; mix. Dose, gr. vij to xx.

Pulvis Anthemidis Compositus. U. C. H. Chamomile ℥j, rhubarb ℥ss, ginger ʒss. St. Geo. H. Chamomile, calumbo, and ginger, of each gr. vij.

Pulvis Anthemidis cum Antimonio. Morton. Chamomile ℈j, subcarbonate of potash ℈ss, calx of antimony ℈ss; mix. *In Intermittents.*

Pulvis Anthemidis cum Aloe. Dr. Heberden. Chamomile gr. x, long pepper gr. iij, aloes gr. j.

Pulvis Anthrakokali Simplex. Poyla. Anthrakokali gr. ij, liquorice powder gr. v; mix, for one dose.

Pulvis Anthrakokali Compositus. Anthrakokali gr. ij, washed sulphur gr. iv, liquorice powder gr. ij. For a dose, in some skin diseases. Oxysulphuret of antimony gr. ss, is sometimes substituted for sulphur.

Pulvis Anticatarrhalis. Germ. H. Sulphur ʒij, cream of tartar ʒvj, golden sulphur of antimony gr. xv; in 16 powders.

Pulvis Antiepilepticus. E. 1744. White dittany, pœony, valerian, mistletoe of the oak, equal parts. Behrends. Valerian ʒiv, magnesia, muriate of ammonia, oil of cajeput, of each ℈j. A teaspoonful three times a day. Dr. Paris says the following was used successfully by a Dutch empiric:—Sulphur ℈j, sulphate of potash gr. x, rhubarb gr. v, nutmeg gr. ij; mix. Germ. H. Oxide of zinc gr. xvj, carbonate of magnesia gr. xlviij, oleo saccharum of cajeput ʒiij; mix, for eight doses. *Poudre de Ragolo.* Valerian ℥jss, orange leaves ʒiv, magnesia ℈ij, oil of cajeput ℈ij. As Behrends'. Pasquier prescribes —Wall-crop ℈ss, gum acacia ℈ss. One to four powders daily for eight times. Sommer's Specific consists of—Wall-crop gr. vj to ℈ss, oleo-saccharum of mint gr. viij. One, morning and evening, for six times. See also Pulvis Artemisiæ Saccharatus. The *Poudre de Guttète* consists of mistletoe two parts, white dittany two, pœony root and seeds each two, prepared coral one, elk's hoof two, seeds of orache two. Given in doses of a few grains in *Convulsions of Infants*, or in larger doses for *Epilepsy.*

PULVIS ANTIGASTRALGICUS. *P. Antispasmodicus.* GUIBOURT. Cyanide of zinc gr. iij, calcined magnesia gr. xxiv, cinnamon gr. xij; mix, for six doses.

PULVIS ANTIHÆMORRHOIDALIS. GERM. H. Sulphur ℥ij, tartrate of potash ℥j, oleo-saccharum of lemon ʒvj. A teaspoonful two or three times a day.

PULVIS ANTILYSSUS. Dr. MEAD. Ash-coloured ground liverwort ℥ss, black pepper ʒij; mix, and give a fourth part every morning, for four times. *To prevent Hydrophobia.*

PULVIS ANTILYSSICUS ORMSKIRKIANUS. Elecampane ʒj, chalk ℥iv, bole ʒiij, alum gr. x, oil of anise five drops; mix.

PULVIS ANTILYSSICUS TUNQUINENSIS. Sir G. COBB'S Tonquin Powder. Musk gr. xvj, cinnabar gr. xlviij; to be mixed and washed down with arrack or other spirit. Three doses to be given on three alternate days, and three more on the next three changes of the moon. [The last three formulæ have been celebrated as preventives of *Hydrophobia*, but are not now relied on. The following, according to Dr. ASMUS, has the repute of having been long in use without an instance having occurred of hydrophobia after using it:—Prepared crabs'-eyes ℥ij, gentian ℥ij, red bole ℥j, myrrh ℥ss; reduce it to an impalpable powder, and give three times as much as can be taken up on the point of a knife for three successive mornings.]

PULVIS ANTIMONII COMPOSITUS. L. Pulvis Antimonialis. E. & D. Sesqui-sulphuret of antimony ℔j, hartshorn shavings ℔ij, (an equal quantity, E.) mix, and throw them into a crucible (an iron pot, E.) red hot in the fire, and stir constantly till vapour no longer rises. Rub what remains to powder, and put it into a proper crucible. Then apply fire, and slowly increase it that it may be white-hot for two hours. Rub the residue into a very fine powder.

PULVIS ANTIMONII CUM CAMPHORA. Dr. MURSINNA. Camphor ℥ss, ipecacuanha ℈ss, oxysulphuret of antimony ℈ss, white sugar ʒvj; mix accurately and divide into 12 doses.

PULVIS ANTIMONII TARTARIZATI COMPOSITUS. U. C. H. Prepared oyster shells ℥j, tartarized antimony gr. xvj, nitrate of potash ℥ij.

PULVIS ANTIMONII PROTOXYDI COMPOSITUS. Mr. TYSON. Protoxide of antimony (Tyson's) gr. ij, sulphate of potash gr. ix, precipitated phosphate of lime gr. ix; mix, for 4 doses.

PULVIS ANTIMONIALIS SULPHURATUS. HUFELAND. Prepared oyster shells 3xj, sulphur 3iv, black sulphuret of antimony ʒiij; mix, calcine in a covered crucible for an hour, and powder.

PULVIS ANTIPERIODICUS ANTIMONIALIS. SICHEL. Sulphate of quinine ʒij, antimonial æthiops ʒij; mix, and divide into 24 powders. Dose, from 2 to 8 in the day.

PULVIS ANTIPHLOGISTICUS. HUFELAND. Nitre, potassio-tartrate of soda, and sulphate of potash, of each equal parts.

PULVIS ANTIPSORICUS. *Poudre de Pihorel.* Sulphuret of lime pulverized and divided into packets of ʒss each. One of them, mixed with a little oil, and rubbed into the palms of the hands night and morning, is said to cure the *Itch.* The following are used in the same way:—F. H. Flowers of sulphur ℥j, acetate of lead ℥j, sulphate of zinc 3iv; mix. Also, equal parts of sulphur and charcoal.

PULVIS ANTISPASMODICUS. JOURDAN. Valerian ℥j, oxide of zinc ℈j, musk gr. viij. Mix. See also Pulv. Zinci cyanidi. This name also belongs to Pulv. Antiepilepticus.

PULVIS ARGENTI COMPOSITUS. SERRE. Chloride of silver gr. j, washed orris powder gr. ij. Used in frictions, as Pulvis Auri Compositus.

PULVIS AROMATICUS. E. Cinnamon, cardamom, and ginger, in equal parts; mix, and reduce to a very fine powder. D. Cinnamon ℥ij, cardamom ℥j, ginger ℥j, long pepper ʒj. [Dupuytren's *Poudre Aromatique,* for external use, consists of ℥iv each of thyme, sage, and rosemary, and ℈j each of sal ammoniac and camphor.] For L. See Pulv. Cinnamomi Comp.

PULVIS ARSENICALIS. See Pulvis Escharoticus Arsenicalis, and Pulv. Calomelanos Arsenicalis.

PULVIS ARTEMISIÆ SACCHARATUS. BRESLER. Powdered mugwort root ℥iij, sugar ℥vj. A teaspoonful 4 times a day in *chorea, epilepsy,* &c.

PULVIS ASARI COMPOSITUS. E. 1817. Asarabacca leaves 3 parts, marjoram leaves 1 part, lavender flowers 1 part; rub them together to a powder. D. Asarabacca ℥j, lavender ʒj. See Pulvis Sternutatorius for other forms.

PULVIS AURI. P. Triturate leaf gold with 10 or 12 times its weight of sulphate of potash till bright particles are no longer visible; pass it through a sieve, mix with boiling water, wash what remains on the filter, and dry in a stove.

PULVIS AURI COMPOSITUS. Auro-chloride of sodium (soda muriate of gold) gr. j, lycopodium, starch, or washed orris powder ℈j; mix. A 15th part, gradually increased to an 8th part, of this powder to be rubbed on the gums.

PULVIS AURI ET FERRI. Dr. BUCKLER, *as an Antidote for Corrosive Sublimate.* Pulverized gold ℈ij, clean levigated iron filings ℈ij, gum acacia powder ℨss; mix, for one dose; to be given in water acidulated with a few drops of diluted sulphuric acid.

PULVIS BASILICUS. BATE. Equal parts of calomel, calx of antimony, cream of tartar, and scammony, carefully triturated together. BATE directs *ceruss* of antimony, made by deflagrating the *metallic* antimony with nitre. The following is sometimes substituted:—Calomel ℥j, scammony ℨj, cream of tartar ℥j, jalap, ginger, and antimonial powder, of each ℈j. So also is Pulvis Scammonii cum Calomelane.

PULVIS BELLADONNÆ COMPOSITUS. HECKER. Belladonna gr. j to iij, musk gr. v, camphor gr. v, white sugar ℥ss; mix, for 8 powders. KOPP. Belladonna root gr. ij, ipecac. gr. ij, sulphur gr. xxxij, sugar of milk gr. xxxij. Mix, and divide into 8 powders. 3 daily, in *Hooping Cough.*

PULVIS BELLADONNÆ SACCHARATUS. WETZLER. Belladonna root gr. xv, pure sugar ℨj; mix, for 60 powders. One twice a day, or oftener, according to the age; in *Hooping Cough*, &c.

PULVIS BENZOICUS ASTRINGENS. GEIGEL. Benzoic acid gr. xv, tannin gr. xv, sugar ℥ijss; mix, and divide into 20 packets. One every two hours to children of 3 years old, *in the convulsive period of Hooping Cough.*

PULVIS BENZOICUS CAMPHORATUS. SAUNDERS. Benzoic acid gr. vj, camphor gr. vj, sugar ℨj; in 6 powders.

PULVIS BISMUTHI COMPOSITUS. GUY'S H. Trisnitrate of bismuth ℥j, compound powder of tragacanth ℥ij; mix. Dose, from gr. x to xx twice or thrice a day.

PULVIS E BOLO COMPOSITUS, and P. e Bolo cum Opio, are replaced by P. Cretæ Comp., and P. Cretæ Comp. cum Opio.

PULVIS BUXI VERMIFUGUS. Mr. PERFECT. Dried leaves of tree box ℥j, white sugar ℥ss; triturate to a powder. Dose, for a child of 4 months, gr. viij; of 6 to 8 months gr. xv to xx; of 12 months ℈j; twice or thrice a day.

PULVIS CALAMINÆ CUM MYRRHA. St. B. H. Equal parts of calamine and myrrh. *For sprinkling ulcers.*

PULVIS CALAMINÆ COMPOSITUS. MID. H. Calamine pp. ʒvj, nitric oxide of mercury ʒij. Mix.

PULVIS CALOMELANOS ARSENICALIS. DUPUYTREN. One part of arsenious acid, intimately mixed with 199 parts of calomel. These are the proportions according to SOUBEIRAN, and HENRI, and GUIBOURT; but they are differently stated by other authorities. PEREIRA, 1 part to 99; RICHARD, 4 parts to 96; MIALHE, 1 to 58, &c.

PULVIS CALUMBÆ COMPOSITUS. Calumba ℥j, rhubarb ℈iv, dried carbonate of soda ℈ij, ginger ʒj. See the next.

PULVIS CALUMBÆ ET SODÆ. U. C. H. Calumba ʒj, sesquicarbonate of soda ℥iij, rhubarb ℥j.

PULVIS CALUMBÆ ET FERRI. Dr. COPLAND. Potash-tartrate of iron gr. x to xv, calumba gr. xij to xx. Mix.

PULVIS CAMPHORÆ. P. Camphor is readily pulverized by triturating it with the addition of a few drops of rectified spirit.

PULVIS CAMPHORÆ NITRATUS. CALLISEN. Nitrate of potash ʒj, camphor gr. xv, tartarized antimony gr. j. Mix for 6 powders.

PULVIS CANTHARIDIS CUM CAMPHORA. AUGUSTIN. Cantharides gr. iv, camphor gr. viij, sugar of milk ℈iij; mix, to form a fine powder, and divide into 6 doses.

PULVIS CARBONATIS CALCIS COMPOSITUS. E. 1817. Prepared chalk ℥iv, cinnamon ʒjss, nutmeg ʒss. Mix.

PULVIS PRO CATAPLASMATE. D. Linseed meal 1 part, oatmeal 2 parts. GUY'S H. Linseed meal 1 part, ground bran 2 parts.

PULVIS CEPHALICUS. See Pulvis Asari Co. and P. Sternutatorius.

PULVIS CERUSSÆ COMPOSITUS. L. 1788. Carbonate of lead ℥v, sarcocol ℥jss, tragacanth ℥ss. Mix. *For outward use.*

PULVIS CETACEI. Spermaceti is pulverized as camphor, by the aid of a few drops of spirit.

PULVIS CETACEI CUM SACCHARO. One part of spermaceti with two of sugar candy. Pectoral.

PULVIS E CHELIS COMPOSITUS. L. 1788. *Gascoign's Powder.* Prepared crab shells ℔j, prepared chalk ℥iij, prepared coral ℥iij. Mix.

PULVIS CINCHONÆ CUM ANTIMONIO. *Pulvis Febrifugus.* BRERA. Yellow Peruvian bark ℥j, tartarized antimony gr. ij, opium gr. j; mix, for 4 doses.

PULVIS CINCHONÆ LAXANS. CLEGHORN. Peruvian bark ʒiv, sulphate of magnesia ℈vj. Mix, for 4 doses. One every 2 hours, *in the intermissions.*

PULVIS CINCHONÆ COMPOSITUS. GENEVA PH. Peruvian bark ℥j, rhubarb ℈jss, muriate of ammonia ℈jss. Mix. [There are many other combinations of cinchona in the Foreign Formularies; as, with an equal weight of magnesia, of rhubarb, or carbonate of soda; with half its weight of valerian; with 1-12th of camphor; with 1-8th or 1-6th of ginger or cinnamon.]

PULVIS CINCHONÆ CUM MYRRHA. Dr. KIRKLAND. Equal parts of myrrh and bark. *For outward use.*

PULVIS CINNABARIS CUM RHEO. HEBERDEN, *for Ascarides.* Red sulphuret of mercury ʒss, rhubarb ʒss; mix.

PULVIS CINNAMOMI COMPOSITUS. L. *Pulvis Aromaticus.* Cinnamon ℥ij, cardamom ℥jss, ginger ℥j, long pepper ℥ss; mix. For E. & D. See Pulvis Aromaticus.

PULVIS CITRICUS. See Limonadum Siccum.

PULVIS COLCHICI COMPOSITUS. HADEN. Powdered colchicum 3 parts, sulphate of potash 4, bicarbonate of potash 3 parts; mix. Dose, from gr. viij to ʒj, in *Rheumatism, Gout,* and inflammatory diseases and painful diseases generally.

PULVIS CONFECTIONIS AROMATICÆ—Opii—Piperis. See Confectio Aromatica—Opii—Piperis.

PULVIS CONTRA AMENORRHŒAM. TSUHIERCHKI. Extract of yew gr. vj, calomel gr. iij, white sugar ℈ss, oil of savine 4 drops; mix, for 4 doses. One, night and morning.

PULVIS CONTRA RACHITEM. TEMPLE. Black oxide of iron gr. xviij, rhubarb gr. xviij, sugar ℈j; mix, and divide into 6 doses. One, morning and night.

PULVIS CONTRAYERVÆ COMPOSITUS. L. 1824. Contrayerva root ℥v, prepared oyster shells ℥xviij; mix.

PULVIS CORNACHINI. P. & E. 1744. *Warwick's Powder.* Scammony, diaphoretic antimony, cream of tartar, in equal parts. Triturate together.

PULVIS CORNU USTI CUM OPIO. L. 1824. *Pulvis Opiatus.* Opium ʒj, burnt hartshorn ℥j, cochineal 3j; mix carefully. One grain of opium in 10.

PULVIS CRETÆ COMPOSITUS. L. Prepared chalk ℥vj, cinnamon ℥iv, tormentil ℥iij, gum acacia ℥iij, long pepper ℥ss; mix. (gr. j of opium in ℈ij.) E. Prepared chalk ℥iv, cinnamon ʒjss, nutmeg ʒj. Mix.

PULVIS CRETÆ COMPOSITUS CUM OPIO. L. E. & D. Compound chalk powder ℥vjss, (℥vj, E.) opium ℈iv; mix very accurately.

PULVIS PRO MISTURA CRETÆ. Prepared chalk ℥iv, white sugar ℥iij, acacia gum ℥v, oil of cinnamon fʒjss; mix. [℈ij of this powder to each f℥j of water forms the Mistura Cretæ of the Pharmacopœia.] GUY'S H. (Pulvis Cretaceus.) Prepared chalk ℥iv, powdered gum ℥iv, white sugar ℥iij. To Oj of water add ʒxiv of the powder.

PULVIS CUBEBÆ CUM ALUMINE. Dr. MATTHIEU. Cubebs ℥ij, alum ʒiv; mix, for 9 doses; 3 daily in *Gonorrhœa.*

PULVIS DENTIFRICIUS. *P. Dentifricium.* P. Red bole ℥iij, coral ℥iij, sepia bone ℥iij, dragon's blood ℥jss, cochineal ʒiij, cream of tartar ℥ivss, cinnamon 3vj, cloves ʒj. All to be very finely powdered and mixed. A few more forms for Tooth Powders are added. PITSCHAFT: Aromatic calamus ʒiv, charcoal ʒj, soap ʒj, oil of cloves ♏xij. DESCHAMPS: Venetian talc ℥iv, bicarbonate of soda ℥j, carmine gr. v, oil of mint gr. x. HAMB. PH. Charcoal 4 parts, cinchona 2, myrrh 1. RUS. PH.: Cinchona ℥ij, orris ℥j, muriate of ammonia ℥ss, catechu ʒvj, myrrh ʒvj, oil of cloves ♏vij. *Camphorated Chalk* is made by mixing 1 part of finely pulverized camphor, with from 3 to 7 parts of prepared or precipitated chalk.

PULVIS DEPILATORIUS. PLENK. Quicklime ʒxij, starch ʒx, yellow sulphuret of arsenic ʒj; to be mixed with water when used, and the paste left on to dry. RAYER'S (*without arsenic*). Lime ʒj, carbonate of potash ℥ij, charcoal ʒj.

PULVIS DIAPENTE. E. 1744. Aristolochia root, gentian, bay berries, myrrh, ivory dust, each ℥ij. Mix.

PULVIS DIATESSARON. E. 1744. As Diapente, omitting the ivory dust.

Pulvis Digestivus. Klein. Tartrate of potash ʒiij, rhubarb ʒj, sulphur ℈ij, orange-peel ℈ss, magnesia ℈ss. Mix. A tea-spoonful 3 times a day, *in hepatic obstructions.*

Pulvis Diureticus. P. Acacia gum ℥ij, pure sugar ℥ij, nitrate of potash ℥j, althæa root ℥j. Mix.

Pulvis Doveri. See Pulvis Ipecac. Compositus.

Pulveres Effervescentes. E. *Soda Powders.* Tartaric acid ℥j, divide it into 16 powders. Bicarbonate of soda 534 grains, (or bicarbonate of potash 640 grains;) divide it into 16 parts; keep the acid and alkaline powders in separate papers of different colours. [The more usual proportions are 25 or 26 grains of tartaric acid, and 30 or 32 of bicarbonate of soda.]

Pulveres Effervescentes Aperientes. *Seidlitz Powders.* Tartarized soda ʒij, bicarbonate of soda ℈ij; mix. The other paper contains ʒss of tartaric acid. Or the soda may be increased to ℈ijss, and the acid to ℈ij. [Dr. Barker recommends—Bisulphate of potash 73 grains, bicarbonate of soda 43 grains; to be dissolved separately, and mixed when taken.]

Pulveres Effervescentes cum Ferro. Dried sulphate of iron ʒss, white sugar ʒiij, tartaric acid ʒjss; mix, and divide into 12 powders. Bicarbonate of soda ʒij, white sugar ʒiij; mix, and divide into 12 powders. One of each to be dissolved in half a glassful of water, then mixed, and drank immediately.

Pulveres Effervescens cum Zingibere. *Ginger Beer Powders.* Ginger ʒj, bicarbonate of soda ʒvj, refined sugar ʒxx, essence of lemon 6 drops. Mix, and divide into 12 powders. The other papers contain ʒss of tartaric acid in each. To be taken as the last.

Pulvis Ecphracticus. Selle. Chamomile, rhubarb, carbonate of potash, magnesia, sulphur, oleosaccharum of fennel, of each equal parts.

Pulvis Eccoproticus. Germ. Ph. Bitartrate of potash ℥j, carbonate of magnesia ℥ss, sulphur ℥ss, nitrate of potash ʒij. Mix. Dose, ʒj to ʒiij.

Pulvis Elaterii Compositus. Guy's H. Extract of elaterium gr. iv, bitartrate of potash ℈v, ginger ℈j. Mix them well. Dose, from gr. v to xxx.

Pulvis Elaterinæ Compositus. Dr. G. Bird. Elaterine gr. iv, bitartrate of potash ʒx ℈ij. Triturate till thoroughly mixed. ℈ss contains 1-16th of a grain of elaterine.

PULVIS EMETICUS. GUY'S H. Ipecacuanha 20 parts, tartar emetic 1 part. Dose, from 5 to 30 grains.

PULVIS ERRHINUS. See Pulvis Sternutatorius.

PULVIS ESCHAROTICUS ARSENICALIS. P. Red sulphuret of mercury ʒiv, dragon's blood ℈iv, levigated arsenious acid ʒij. Mix accurately. [This is the *Poudre du frère Cosme*, but contains more arsenic than other authorities direct. The Codex of 1818 directed only ℈j of white arsenic to ʒviij of dragon's blood, and ℥ij of vermilion. This is the formula of DUBOIS and of PATRIX. ROUSSELOT directs 1 part of white arsenic, 8 of dragon's blood, and 8 of cinnabar. The original formula is said to be white arsenic gr. v, cinnabar ʒss, burnt shoe-leather gr. xv. To be moistened, at the time of using, with saliva or mucilage.] See Causticum Anticancrosum.

PULVIS ESCHAROTICUS ALUMINOSUS. SHARP'S *Pulvis Angelicus.* Burnt alum and red precipitate, equal parts.

PULVIS EUPHRASIÆ. FULLER. Powdered eyebright ℈iij, mace ʒj. Mix; half a teaspoonful before meals.

PULVIS FEBRIFUGUS. CHARING CROSS H. Potassio-tartrate of antimony ʒss, sulphate of potash ℥j, liquorice powder ℥jss. Mix accurately. Contains gr. j of emetic tartar in ℈ij. See also Pulv. Cinchonæ cum Antimonio.

PULVIS FERRI COMPOSITUS. See Pulvis Tonicus. Dr. NELIGAN. Saccharated carbonate of iron ℈ss, myrrh gr. xxiv, aromatic powder ʒss; mix, for 12 doses. *In protracted Infantile Diarrhœa.*

PULVIS FERRI ET IPECACUANHÆ. Dr. ASHWELL. Carbonate of iron gr. viij, ipecac. gr. j, quicksilver with chalk gr. ij. Once or twice a day, in *Anæmia.*

PULVIS FERRO-CARBONICUS. DAUVERGNE. Sulphate of iron 10 parts, charcoal 35 parts; mix. Externally, in *Sycosis Menti.*

PULVIS FŒNICULI COMPOSITUS. *Pulvis Galactopœus.* BRUNSW. PH. Carbonate of magnesia ℥j, fennel seed ℥ss, orange-peel ℈ij, white sugar ℈ij; reduce each to a fine powder, and mix.

PULVIS FULMINANS. BATE. Nitre ʒivss, salt of tartar ℈jss, sulphur ʒij. Mix. Dose, as a diuretic and deobstruent, ℈j to ℈ij. But more frequently used to produce a loud explosion, ℈ss being heated in an iron ladle, or shovel.

Pulvis Fumalis. Russ. Ph. Olibanum, mastic, amber, of each 3 parts; styrax 2, benzoin 1, labdanum 1. See Fumigatio Balsamica.

Pulvis Glutenis Emulsivus. Taddei. Fresh vegetable gluten ℥x, soap ℥ij, water Oj; dissolve, evaporate the solution, dry it on plates, and reduce to powder. As an antidote to corrosive sublimate.

Pulvis Guaiaci Compositus. Burdach. Guaiacum resin ʒij, sulphur ʒij, cream of tartar ʒiv, oil of fennel 6 drops. Dose, a teaspoonful. Hufeland. Guaiacum ʒvj, extract of aconite gr. xxiv, oil of valerian gr. xxiv, golden sulphur of antimony gr. xxiv, calomel gr. xxiv, white sugar ʒiv; mix, for 24 doses.

Pulvis Guaiaci Opiatus. Peraire. Guaiacum 3j, orange leaves ʒss, acetate of morphia gr. $\frac{3}{4}$; mix, and divide into 6 powders. One every two hours, in *articular rheumatism.*

Pulvis Gummo-mercurialis. Dr. Mouton. Calomel ʒj, gum acacia ʒiv. *For external use.*

Pulvis ad Guttetam. See Pulvis Antiepilepticus.

Pulvis Hæmostaticus. Bonafoux. Resin 3iv, acacia gum ʒj, charcoal ʒj; mix. Mialhe. Alum, gum, tragacanth, and tannin, of each 3ij; mix.

Pulvis Hydrargyri. Dr. D. Davies. Equal parts of confection of quicksilver and liquorice powder, rubbed together.

Pulvis Hydrargyri Compositus. U. C. H. Quicksilver with chalk ℈ij, calumba ℈ij, rhubarb ℈j; in 12 powders.

Pulvis Hydrargyri Sulphureti Compositus. U. C. H. Ethiop's mineral ℥ij, nitre ℥j; mix.

Pulvis Hydrargyri cum Magnesia. U. C. H. Gray oxide of quicksilver ʒj, magnesia 3ij.

Pulvis Iodinii cum Calomelane. Calomel gr. viij, iodine gr. j, white sugar ℈iv; mix, and divide into 16 powders. [If the calomel be first rubbed with the iodine, biniodide of mercury is formed; if with the *sugar*, a protoiodide results. The former is the more active.] Seyffer prescribes biniodide of mercury gr. j, alcohol 3 drops, hydrosublimed calomel gr. viij; triturate, and add refined sugar ℈x. Mix, and divide into 40 powders. One three times a day for a child of 6 years, in *acute hydrocephalus.*

PULVIS IPECACUANHÆ COMPOSITUS. L. E. & D. *Dover's Powder.* Ipecacuanha ʒj, hard opium ʒj, sulphate of potash ℥j; mix, by long trituration. [The Pulvis Doveri (P.) comes nearer to the original form. It consists of sulphate of potash ℥iv, nitrate of potash ℥iv, ipecacuanha ℥j, liquorice root ℥j, extract of opium ℥j.]

PULVIS IPECACUANHÆ CUM ANTIMONIO. GUY'S H. See Pulvis Emeticus.

PULVIS IPECACUANHÆ CUM POTASSÆ NITRATE. U. C. H. Comp. ipecacuanha powder ʒj, nitrate of potash ℥j, mix.

PULVIS IPECACUANHÆ CUM RHEO. GUY'S H. Ipecacuanha ʒj, rhubarb ʒij; mix. Dose, gr. iij to v, twice or oftener daily. U. C. H. Ipecacuanha ℥ss, rhubarb ℥ij, prepared chalk ℥ij.

PULVIS JACOBI. The Pulvis Antimonii Compositus (L.) is intended to resemble Dr. James's fever powder, but is not exactly identical with it. It is not known in what respect the processes differ. The following has been published in America (on the authority of Dr. R. E. Robinson) as the genuine recipe, derived from the family; but it does not agree with the results of analysis. Tartarized antimony ℈j, prepared burnt hartshorn ℈v, calx of antimony ℈v; mix, and put gr. xxj in each powder.

PULVIS JALAPÆ COMPOSITUS. L. Jalap ℥iij, bitartrate of potash ℥vj, ginger ʒij, mix. [E. & D. & U. S. omit the ginger.]

PULVIS JALAPÆ CUM HYDRARGYRO. GUY'S H. Jalap ʒiv, calomel ʒj, ginger ʒj; mix. Dose, gr. xv to xxx in the morning.

PULVIS JALAPÆ CUM MAGNESIÆ. SPAN. PH. Equal weights of jalap, cream of tartar, and magnesia, mixed by long trituration.

PULVIS JALAPÆ AURANTIATUS. *Sucre Orangé purgatif.* Jalap ℥ij, cream of tartar ℥j, refined sugar ℥xiij, oil of orange-peel ʒij; mix. Dose, ʒj to ʒij.

PULVIS JALAPÆ CUM IPECACUANHA. Dr. PARIS. Jalap gr. xv, ipecacuanha gr. v, oil of cinnamon 2 drops. BRANDE. Ipecacuanha gr. ij, jalap gr. x, calomel gr. j; for 1 dose.

PULVIS JUSTICIÆ COMPOSITUS. Dr. AINSLIE. Powdered root of panicled justicia gr. x, rhubarb gr. vj, black pepper gr. viij. To be taken at bedtime, in *dyspepsia.*

PULVIS KERMETIS CUM CAMPHORA. GERM. H. Kermes mineral gr. iij, camphor gr. vj, white sugar ʒij; mix, for 12 doses.

PULVIS KERMETIS CUM IPECACUANHA. F. H. Kermes gr. ij, ipecacuanha gr. ij, crab's eyes ℈ij, gum acacia ℈ij; mix, for 12 doses, in *Hooping Cough.*

PULVIS KINO COMPOSITUS. L. & D. Kino ʒxv, cinnamon ʒiv, opium ʒj; rub them separately into a very fine powder, and mix. Dose, gr. v to xx.

PULVIS LENITIVUS. KLEIN. Orange-peel ʒss, rhubarb ʒss, tartrate of potash ʒss, oil of cajeput ♏iij; mix.

PULVIS LIENTERICUS, COPLAND. Compound powder of tragacanth ʒiij, rhubarb ʒiij, compound powder of ipecacuanha ʒj, quicksilver with chalk ʒj. Mix. Dose, gr. v to ʒss.

PULVIS MAGNESIÆ. P. Magnesia in squares is pulverized by rubbing them on a hair sieve placed over a sheet of paper. The powder should be then passed through a finer sieve.

PULVIS MAGNESIÆ TARTARICUS. SW. PH. Tartaric acid ℥j, heavy carbonate of magnesia ℥j, refined sugar ℥iv, oil of peppermint 18 drops. The powders should be well dried before mixing, and the compound kept from the air. VAN MONS directs, carbonate of magnesia ℥ij, tartaric acid ℥ij, cinnamon ʒj.

PULVIS MOSCHI COMPOSITUS. RUSS PH. Musk 8, valerian 10, camphor 3.

PULVIS E MYRRHA COMPOSITUS. L. 1788. Myrrh, savin, rue, and castor, of each ℥j. Mix.

PULVIS MYRRHÆ CUM NITRO. DR. PARIS. Myrrh gr. xij, ipecacuanha gr. vj, nitrate of potash ʒss. In 4 doses; one every 4 hours.

PULVIS NEPHRITICUS. FULLER. Powdered roots of smallage and saxifrage each ʒij, crab's eyes ʒj, sulphate of potash ℈iij, sal prunelle ℈ij, oil of juniper 4 drops. Mix. ℈j to ʒj. *Diuretic.*

PULVIS NITRO-CAMPHORATUS. SWEDIAUR. Nitre gr. x, camphor gr. iv, gum arabic gr. xxiv; mix, for 2 or 3 doses.

PULVIS NUCIS VOMICÆ COMPOSITUS. VOGT'S *Stomachic Powder.* Nux Vomica gr. xviij, ipecacuanha gr. xxiv, rhubarb ʒj, prepared oyster shell gr. xlviij, oleo-saccharum of mint ʒj. Mix, and divide into 12 powders.

PULVIS OPIATUS. E. 1813. Opium ʒj, prepared carbonate of lime ʒix. Mix accurately.

PULVIS AD PARTUM. E. 1774. Borax ʒiv, castor ʒjss, saffron ʒjss, oil of cinnamon 8 drops, oil of amber 6 drops; mix. Dose, ℈j to ℥ss. [This name, and that of *Pulvis Parturifaciens*, have also been given to powdered ergot.] SCHMIDT'S *Poudre Ocytique* is ergot, borax, and oleo-saccharum of chamomile, of each gr. viij; divided into 6 powders. One every quarter of an hour.

PULVIS PANCHYMAGOGUS. FULLER. Cream of tartar ℥ss, senna ℥j, rhubarb ʒvj, scammony ʒij, mace ℥ss; beat them all into a powder. Dose ℈ij to ʒj.

PULVIS PAULLINIÆ COMPOSITUS. Dr. GAVRELLE. Paullinia ʒj, compound cinnamon powder ʒiv. Mix.

PULVIS PEPTICUS. FULLER. Coriander seed ℥ss, aniseed ℈iv, sweet fennel ℈iv, nutmeg ʒss, cinnamon ℈j, cloves ℈j, long pepper ℈ss, white sugar ℥j. Mix, and divide into 16 doses. One after meals.

PULVIS PIPERIS. U. C. H. Chamomile ℥ss, prepared oyster shells ʒij, long pepper ℈iijss, aloes ℈j; mix.

PULVIS PIPERIS CUBEBÆ COMPOSITUS. U. C. H. Cubebs ʒj, subcarbonate of soda ℥iij.

PULVIS POTASSÆ NITRATIS COMPOSITUS. U. C. H. Nitre ℥ij, supertartrate of potash ʒiv, tartarized antimony gr. iv; mix.

PULVIS PURGANS. See Pulv. Jalapæ, &c.; Pulv. Rhei, &c.; Pulv. Scammonii, &c.

PULVIS PURGANS ANTHELMINTICUS. BOERHAAVE. Jalap gr. xij, (or agaric gr. viij,) Æthiop's mineral gr. xij; for one dose. DUPUYTREN. Jalap ʒss, rhubarb gr. vj, calomel gr. ij; mix for a dose. See Pulvis Vermifugus.

PULVIS QUERCUS MARINÆ. D. Yellow bladder-wrack, in flower, is dried, cleansed, and heated in a crucible with a perforated lid till vapours cease; and the carbonaceous residue reduced to powder. Dose, gr. x to ʒij.

PULVIS QUINÆ CUM ANTIMONIO. GOLA. Tartarized antimony gr. iij, sulphate of quina gr. x. Mix, for 6 doses.

PULVIS QUINÆ AERATUS. Dr. MEIREU. Tartaric acid gr. xv, disulphate of quina gr. jss; mix, and add bicarbonate of soda gr. xviij, refined sugar ʒss. Mix, for one dose, between the fits of *intermittent fever*.

PULVIS QUINÆ CUM MORPHIA. M. Disulphate of quinine gr.

ij to vj, sulphate of morphia gr. ss to gr. j; mix, for 3 or 4 doses.

PULVIS RESOLVENS STAHLII. Antimonial powder, nitre, prepared crab's eyes, in equal parts. RICHTER. Oxysulphuret of antimony gr. vj, calomel gr. vj, hemlock powder ℥ss, white sugar ʒij; mix, for 6 doses.

PULVIS RHEI COMPOSITUS. E. *Gregory's Powder.* Calcined magnesia ℥xij, rhubarb ℥iv, ginger ℥ij. Some private formulæ for Gregory's Powder contain chamomile. Ginger ʒj, powdered chamomile ʒij, rhubarb ʒiv, magnesia ℥j. [The compound rhubarb powders of the Hosp. are different. U. C. H. Rhubarb ʒj, calomel ℈j, tartarized antimony gr. j. In 6 powders. GUY'S H. Dried soda ʒj, rhubarb ʒj, calumba 3ij. Dose, gr. x to xx. ST. B. H. As Pulv. Rhei Salinus.]

PULVIS RHEI CUM HYDRARGYRO. GUY'S H. Rhubarb 3iv, calomel ʒj, ginger 3j. Mix. Dose, gr. x to xxx.

PULVIS RHEI CUM HYDRARGYRO ET CRETA. GUY'S H. Rhubarb 3ij, quicksilver with chalk gr. xlviij. Dose, gr. iij to xiv. The addition of ipecacuanha gr. xxiv forms Pulv. Rhei cum Hydr. et Ipecac.

PULVIS RHEI CUM MAGNESIA. Rhubarb ʒj, carbonate of magnesia ʒij.

PULVIS RHEI OPIATUS. ST. B. H. Rhubarb gr. xv, compound chalk powder with opium ʒss.

PULVIS RHEI SALINUS. GUY'S H. Rhubarb ʒj, sulphate of potash ʒij. Mix, and give from gr. x to 3j every morning. FORDYCE. Rhubarb and sulphate of potash, each ℈ss. SAUNDERS. Rhubarb ʒss, sulphate of potash gr. x, scammony gr. viij, oil of fennel 1 drop. ST. B. H. Rhubarb gr. x, sulphate of potash ʒss.

PULVIS RHEI USTI. See Rheum Ustum.

PULVIS SABINÆ CUM ÆRUGINE. J. HUNTER, *for Warts.* Equal weights of savine and verdigris.

PULVIS SALEPI. P. The tuberous roots of orchis (orchis mascula, and some other species) are macerated in cold water for 24 hours, rubbed with a coarse cloth, dried, and reduced to powder by contusion.

PULVIS SALICINÆ COMPOSITUS. DR. NELIGAN. Salicine ℈ij,

aromatic powder 3j; mix, for 12 powders. [A substitute for the salts of quinine.]

PULVIS SALINUS COMPOSITUS. E. and D. Muriate of soda ℥iv, sulphate of magnesia ℥iv, sulphate of potash ℥iij; dry the salts separately, and triturate them together. Dose, ʒij to ʒiv.

PULVIS SALINUS ANTICHLORICUS. Dr. STEVENS. Chlorate of potash gr. vij, muriate of soda ℈j, carbonate of soda ʒss; mix, for 1 dose. Dr. O'SHAUGHNESSY. Phosphate of soda gr. x, chloride of sodium gr. x, carbonate of soda gr. v, sulphate of soda ℈ss; mix for 1 dose.

PULVIS SAPONIS. Soap, in thin shavings or scrapings, is dried gradually in a warm place, and afterwards rubbed to powder. [This should be done, not merely as a matter of convenience in dispensing, but in order to neutralize, by exposure to the air, any excess of caustic alkali which the soap may contain; the presence of which may be detected by the gray colour which it communicates to calomel.]

PULVIS SARZÆ CUM CINCHONA. See Pulvis Alterativus.

PULVIS SCAMMONII COMPOSITUS. L. and D. Scammony ℥ij, dried extract of jalap ℥ij, ginger ℥ss; mix. E. Mix equal parts of scammony and bitartrate of potash; and triturate them together to a fine powder. Dose of L., gr. x to xx; of E. gr. xx to xxx.

PULVIS E SCAMMONIO CUM ALÖE. L. 1788. Scammony ʒvj, dried extract of jalap 3xij, ginger ʒiv, aloes 3xij. Mix.

PULVIS E SCAMMONIO CUM CALOMELANE. L. 1788. Scammony ʒiv, calomel ʒij, white sugar 3ij. Mix.

PULVIS SCAMMONII CUM FULIGINE. *Poudre d'Ailhaut.* Scammony 3j, wood-soot 3jss, resin ʒij. Mix. Dose, ʒss. *A once fashionable purgative.*

PULVIS SCILLÆ. D. Remove the membranous integuments from the bulb of the squill, cut it into thin slices, dry it at a heat between 90° and 100°, reduce it to powder, and keep it in bottles with ground glass stoppers.

PULVIS SCILLÆ COMPOSITUS. GUY'S H. Dried squill ℥j, bitartrate of potash ℥ix; mix. Dose, gr. x to xxx, twice or thrice a day. U. C. H. Squill ʒj, ipecacuanha ʒj, sugar ℥iv; make a powder. SWED. PH. Squill 3j, nitre ʒiij, cream of tartar ʒiv, aromatic powder ʒij. GUIBOURT. Squill 1, sulphur 2, white sugar 3; mix. Dose, gr. xv to xxiv.

PULVIS E SCORDIO COMPOSITUS. L. 1746. Bole ℥iv, scordium ℥ij, cinnamon ℥jss, styrax, tormentil, bistort, gentian, dittany, galbanum, gum acacia, red rose petals, each ℥j, long pepper ℥ss, ginger ℥ss; make a powder.

PULVIS E SCORDIO CUM OPIO. Add to the preceding ʒiij, of dry strained opium, and powder it with the other ingredients.

PULVIS SENNÆ COMPOSITUS. L. 1824. Senna ℥ij, bitartrate of potash ℥ij, scammony ℥ss, ginger ʒij; mix. Dose, ℈j to ʒj.

PULVIS SODÆ COMPOSITUS. U. C. H. Dried soda ℥j, rhubarb ʒiv, ginger ℈j. Mix.

PULVIS SODÆ CUM HYDRARGYRO. GUY'S H. Dried carbonate of soda ʒv, calomel ʒj, compound chalk powder ʒx. Mix. Dose, gr. viij to xvj.

PULVIS SODÆ MURIATIS COMPOSITUS. RUSH. Muriate of soda ℥ij, cochineal ℈ij; triturate together. Dose, ʒss before breakfast, *as a vermifuge.*

PULVIS SODÆ SULPHATIS COMPOSITUS. *Sel de Guindre.* Dried sulphate of soda ʒxviij, nitrate of potash ʒss, potash-tartrate of antimony gr. j. A third part to be taken in water or herb broth.

PULVIS SPECIFICUS ASTRINGENS. COLBATCHE'S *Specific.* Liquid chloride of iron (Liquor Ferri Perchloridi) ℥iv, acetate of lead ℥iv; evaporate to dryness. Dose, gr. iv to gr. x.

PULVIS SPLANCHNICUS. FULLER. Ash bark ℈ss, rhubarb gr. v, spikenard gr. ij, saffron gr. ij, long pepper gr. j; make a powder. Twice a day, in *visceral obstructions,* &c.

PULVIS SPONGIÆ. D. Beat the sponge, cut it into small pieces, and burn it in a covered iron vessel until it becomes black and friable; finally reduce it to powder. [If over-burnt its efficacy is impaired; it should only be burnt to a *brown black.*]

PULVIS SPONGIÆ COMPOSITUS. CLARUS. Burnt sponge ʒiv, carbonate of magnesia ʒij, nitre ʒij, white sugar ʒij; mix. Dose, a teaspoonful three times a day. RUST. Burnt sponge ℥ss, digitalis gr. iv to viij, oleo-saccharum of fennel ʒij; mix, for 12 doses. *Poudre de Sency* consists of 20 parts of burnt sponge, 1 of sal ammoniac, and 1 of vegetable charcoal. Dose, gr. xv, three times a day.

PULVIS STANNI. D. and P. Melt pure tin in an iron ladle, pour it into a warm iron mortar, and triturate it lightly with a warm pestle; separate the powder by a sieve, and treat the remainder as before.

PULVIS STERNUTATORIUS. (See Pulvis Asari Comp.) PRUS. PH. Marjoram ℥iij, true marum ℥j, lily of the valley ℥jss, orris ℥j; mix. BOELI'S *Cephalic Snuff.* Valerian ʒij, tobacco ʒij, oil of lavender 3 drops, oil of marjoram 3 drops; mix. PEARSON. Asarabacca ʒjss, marum ʒjss, hellebore 3j; make a very fine powder. Hellebore, with 4 or 5 parts of starch or orris powder, is also used. ST. ANGE. Asarabacca ℥j, hellebore ℈j. MIALHE. Sugar candy ℥j, veratrine gr. j to ij; mix exactly.

PULVIS STERNUTATORIUS MERCURIALIS. WARE. Yellow subsulphate of mercury gr. j, liquorice powder gr. viij. A fourth part to be snuffed once or twice a day.

PULVIS STERNUTATORIUS CUM QUINA. RADIUS. Snuff ℥j, disulphate of quinine gr. xv. *In intermittent headache.*

PULVIS STRYCHNIÆ COMPOSITUS. BRERA. Strychnine gr. j, black oxide of iron ʒj, sugar ʒiij; mix. This should be divided, in the first instance, into 12 or 16 doses. There is no authorized formula in this country for Pulv. Strychniæ Comp.

PULVIS STYPTICUS HELVETII. Equal parts of dragon's blood and alum, melted together, and powdered.

PULVIS E SUCCINO COMPOSITUS. L. 1746. Amber 3x, gum arabic ʒx, juice of hypocistis ʒv, balaustines ʒv, catechu ʒv, olibanum ʒiv, strained opium ʒj. Mix.

PULVIS SULPHURIS COMPOSITUS. RATIER. Sulphur ℥j, cream of tartar ℥j, white sugar q. s. VAN MONS. *Antidysenteric Powder.* Sulphur ℥j, fennel seed ʒj, white sugar ℥ij, gum arabic ℥ij; mix. SWEDIAUR. *Pectoral Powder.* Sulphur ℥ss, liquorice ℥j, orris ʒij, benzoic acid ℈j, white sugar ℥ij, oil of anise and fennel each 10 drops. The *Lausanne Compound,* according to Mr. Ince, consists of cream of tartar, carbonate of magnesia, precipitated sulphur, each ℥ss, nitre ʒjss, sugar of milk ℥j, oleo-saccharum of peppermint ℥ss.

PULVIS SULPHURIS NITRATUS. U. C. H. Equal parts of nitre and sulphur.

PULVERIS TEMPERANS STAHLII. P. Sulphate of potash ℥ix, nitrate of potash ℥ix, red sulphuret of mercury ℥ij; mix.

PULVIS TESTACEUS CERATUS. E. H. Melt bees'-wax, and stir in gradually as much prepared oyster shells as it will receive. Dose, ʒj.

PULVIS TONITRUANS. See Pulv. Fulminans.

PULVIS TRAGACANTHÆ COMPOSITUS. L. Tragacanth ℥jss, gum acacia ℥jss, white starch ℥jss, white sugar ℥iij; powder separately, and mix.

PULVIS DE TRIBUS. See Pulvis Cornachini. The same name is given by RECAMIER to a mixture of gentian ℥ss, bistort ʒij, pœony ʒij.

PULVIS UVÆ URSI COMPOSITUS. Dr. FERRIAR. Uva ursi ʒij, cinchona ʒij, opium gr. iij; make 6 doses. One twice a day, washed down with lime water. CHARING CROSS H. Uva ursi ℥jss, carbonate of magnesia ʒij, sesquicarbonate of soda ʒij.

PULVIS UVULARIS. FULLER. Catechu ℈j, balaustines ℈j, alum gr. x, long pepper gr. x; powder and mix. To be blown upon the uvula.

PULVIS VANILLÆ. *Poudre de Vanille.* Vanilla is reduced to powder by cutting it in pieces and triturating it with refined sugar. P. directs twice its weight of sugar; SOUBEIRAN 4 times. The quantity required depends on the state of the pods. GUIBOURT directs *Poudre de Vanille Sucrée* to be made with one part of vanilla to eleven of sugar.

PULVIS VERMIFUGUS. P. Corsican worm-moss ℥j, worm-seed ℥j, rhubarb ℥ss; mix. E. H. Scammony ʒj, calomel ʒj, rhubarb ʒiij. (The doses of the above are not given.) BAUME. Quicksilver ʒiij, Æthiop's mineral ʒij, white sugar ʒviij; triturate till the mercury disappears. Dose, gr. v to ℈j twice a day. P. 1818. Æthiop's mineral ʒj, scammony ʒj; mix. SWEDIAUR. Tin filings ʒij, sulphate of iron gr. v; mix, for 6 doses. One every two hours. GERM. H. Male fern gr. xxiv, gamboge gr. ij.

PULVIS VIENNENSIS. Potassa cum Calce.

PULVIS VISCI COMPOSITUS. *Poudre de Carignan. Poudre de guttète* (pulvis antiepilepticus) ℥viij, amber ℥xij, coral ℥iv, sealed earth ℥iv, kermes mineral ʒiij, ivory black ʒiij. Mix.

PULVIS ZINCI CYANIDI COMPOSITUS. GUIBOURT. Cyanidi of zinc gr. iij, calcined magnesia gr. xxiv, cinnamon gr. xij; mix, for 6 doses. *In cramp of the stomach.*

PULVIS ZINCI SULPHATIS COMPOSITUS. ST. B. H. Sulphate of zinc ʒiv, sulphate of copper ʒiv, dried alum ʒiv, camphor ʒjss. Mix.

QUASSINA. *Quassine.* WIGGERS. Evaporate a decoction of quassia to 2-3ds the weight of the wood; add slaked lime, and in 24 hours filter. Evaporate, dissolve the extract in rectified spirit, and again evaporate.

QUINA, *vel* QUININA. *Quinine, Quina,* or *Quinia.* To a solution of disulphate of quinine add solution of ammonia sufficient to throw down the quinine; wash this with warm distilled water, and dry it. To procure it in *crystals,* dissolve it in the smallest possible quantity of alcohol, and let it evaporate spontaneously in a warm place.

QUINA IMPURA. Coloured Quinine. *Quinine Brute.* Exhaust Peruvian bark by boiling it in water acidulated with muriatic acid, neutralize the decoction with milk of lime, dry the precipitate, and boil it repeatedly with rectified spirit. Mix, and filter the solution, and distil off the spirit. The residue is impure quinine, which M. TROUSSEAU regards as preferable to the sulphate.

QUINA AMORPHA. (Quina Informis, NELIGAN.) *Amorphous,* or *Uncrystallizable Quinine.* LIEBIG. By adding a solution of carbonate of potash or of soda to the mother water, from which sulphate of quinine has crystallized, a precipitate is thrown down, which, when washed and gently dried, forms *Quinoidine* or *Chinoidine.* Dissolve this by digestion with pure sulphuric æther, decant the ethereal solution, and evaporate it with a very gentle heat. Amorphous quinine remains, which may be neutralized with diluted acids to form the salts; which are not crystallizable, and are commonly used in solution. Its uses and doses are the same as those of the ordinary salts of quinine. For Mr. BULLOCK's *patent* process, see Pharmaceutical Journal, vol. vi. page 271.

QUINÆ ACETAS. P. Mix 100 parts of quinine with 150 of distilled water, heat the mixture, and add as much acetic acid as will dissolve the quinine, and render the solution slightly acid. Filter boiling, and set aside to crystallize. Concentrate the residuary liquor for more crystals.

QUINÆ ARSENIAS. BOURIERES. Dissolve ʒjss of arsenic acid in ℥vj of water, add ʒv of pure quinine, and boil till the quinine is dissolved. Let the clear solution cool, that crystals may form, which purify by recrystallization. Dose, 1-5th of a grain.

QUINÆ CITRAS. P. As the acetate, substituting citric for acetic acid.

QUINÆ ET FERRI CITRAS. See Ferri et Quinæ Citras.

QUINÆ FERRO-PRUSSIAS. P. Boil 100 parts of quinine, and 31 of ferro-prussiate of potash, with 2500 of distilled water for a few minutes. Let the solution cool, separate the oily compound, and wash it with a little water. It may be crystallized by dissolving it in boiling alcohol, and cooling. [M. PELOUZE regards it as merely sulphate of quinine with a little Prussian blue.]

QUINÆ ET FERRI IODIDUM. BOUCHARDAT. Pour a strong solution of acid sulphate of quinine into a fresh solution of iodide of iron. Collect the precipitate, dry it quickly by pressing it between blotting paper, and keep it from the air.

QUINÆ IODIDUM. RIGHINI. Add, by drops, a solution of 24 parts of iodide of potassium in 8 of water, to a strong solution of 20 parts of bisulphate of quinine. Wash the precipitate quickly, and dry it in the shade.

QUINÆ HYDRIODAS IODURETA. BOUCHARDAT. Into an acid solution of quinine pour a solution of iodide of iron containing a slight excess of iodine. Boil the precipitate in alcohol, and filter while hot. The salt is deposited in fine scales.

QUINÆ ET HYDRARGYRI CHLORIDUM. See Hydrarg. et Quinæ Chloridum.

QUINÆ KINAS. It may be made by saturating kinic acid with quinine; or by the mutual decomposition of sulphate of quinine and kinate of lime. [Kinate of lime is a residuary product in manufacturing sulphate of quinine. Kinic acid is obtained from it by carefully adding to its solution enough oxalic acid to throw down the lime; and evaporating the filtered liquid to the consistence of syrup.]

QUINÆ LACTAS. PRINCE L. L. BONAPARTE. Saturate lactic acid with quinine, and leave the solution in a shallow vessel, to evaporate spontaneously in a warm room till crystals are produced. [The Prince recommends this, and all the salts of quinine, to be made by adding a strong alcoholic solution of quinine to a *cold* solution of the acid.]

QUINÆ MURIAS *vel* HYDROCHLORAS. P. Disulphate of quinine 10 parts, chloride of barium 3 parts; dissolve separately in boiling distilled water, mix the solutions, filter, evaporate till crystals begin to form on the surface, and set aside to crystallize. [It may also be made by saturating dilute muriatic acid with quinine.]

QUINÆ NITRAS. P. Nitrate of quinine is made in the same way as the muriate, substituting nitrate of barytes for chloride of barium.

QUINÆ PHOSPHAS. Saturate dilute phosphoric acid with quinine, concentrate the solution, and crystallize by refrigeration.

QUINÆ SULPHAS. There are two sulphates of quinine, differing in the proportion of acid they contain. Some confusion exists in the names by which they are distinguished. *Quinæ Disulphas*, L., is the Quinæ Sulphas of the E., D., P., U. S., and other pharmacopœias; the subsulphate, or basic sulphate of KANE, &c.; and the neutral sulphate of SOUBEIRAN, GUIBOURT, and other continental pharmacists. This is the *Sulphate of Quinine* of commerce, and the kind in general use. The other sulphate is the *Neutral Sulphate* of KANE, BULLOCK, &c.; and the bisulphate, or acid sulphate of SOUBEIRAN, GUIBOURT, and others.

QUINÆ DISULPHAS. L. (Quinæ Sulphas, E.) *Sulphate of Quinine.* Mix Cvj of distilled water with ℥iv ʒij of sulphuric acid, boil it in ℔vij of yellow cinchona bark for an hour, and strain. Boil what remains in a similar mixture for an hour, strain; lastly, boil the bark in Cviij of distilled water for 3 hours, and strain. Wash the remaining bark repeatedly with boiling distilled water. To the mixed liquors add moist oxide of lead to saturation. Pour off the supernatant liquor, and wash the deposit with distilled water. Boil the liquors for a quarter of an hour, and strain; then gradually add solution of ammonia to throw down the quinine. Wash this until nothing alkaline is perceptible, saturate it with ℥iv ʒvj of sulphuric acid diluted with water; digest with ℥ij of purified animal charcoal, strain, and having washed the charcoal thoroughly, evaporate the mixed liquors cautiously that crystals may be produced. E. directs the bark to be first boiled with carbonate of soda, and afterwards with the acidulated water. The acid liquor is concentrated, filtered, and decomposed with carbonate of soda; the impure quinine washed, neutralized by sulphuric acid, and crystallized from the filtered solution. The salt is purified by digesting it with animal charcoal, and crystallizing. D. The acidulated decoction is treated with lime, and the quinine extracted from the precipitate by rectified spirit, and neutralized by sulphuric acid. Dr. PEREIRA states that the following method is usually followed by *manufacturers:* coarsely pulverized yellow bark is boiled repeatedly in water acidulated with sulphuric or muriatic acid, and powdered slaked lime added until the liquor is sensibly alkaline. The precipitate is drained, pressed, powdered, and digested in rectified spirit. The filtered tincture is distilled, and the brown viscid residuum carefully saturated with very dilute sulphuric acid, filtered and set aside to crystallize. The coloured salt thus obtained, is drained, compressed, dissolved in water, decolorized by digestion with animal charcoal, recrystallized, and carefully dried. [This is the salt of quinine most frequently employed. The dose is from one grain to five.]

QUINÆ SULPHAS NEUTRALIS. *Soluble Sulphate of Quinine.* Dissolve ℥j of disulphate of quinine in distilled water acidulated with f℈ss of sulphuric acid, by the aid of heat; filter while hot, and crystallize by refrigeration.

QUINÆ SULPHO-TARTRAS. By evaporating the solution (see Solutio Quinæ Sulpho-tartratis) to dryness.

QUINÆ TANNAS. To a solution of any soluble salt of quinine add a solution of tannic acid. Wash the precipitate with a little cold water, and dry it. Dose, &c., as the other salts of quinine.

QUINÆ TARTRAS. P. As the acetate, substituting tartaric for acetic acid.

QUINÆ VALERIANAS. PRINCE L. L. BONAPARTE. To a cold solution of valerianic acid, in distilled water, add a concentrated solution of quinine in highly rectified spirit to saturation, and let it evaporate spontaneously, or by the aid of a very moderate heat, that crystals may be produced. WITTSTEIN directs 3 parts of recently precipitated quinine to be boiled with 1 of valerianic acid and 60 of water, and the solution to be filtered hot, and set aside that crystals may form. Dry the crystals under 122° F. Dose, gr. ss every 2 hours, in *epilepsy, hemicrania,* &c.

RADIX ANGELICÆ CONDITA. *Candied Angelica.* Slice the fresh roots, removing the pith, and soak them for 2 days in water several times changed; boil them a little and pour off the water; cover them with a syrup to the height of 2 inches. After a day or two, boil them gently if necessary. In the same manner are candied the roots of Eringo, Elecampane, &c.; and the peels of orange, lemon, and citron.

RHAMNINA. *Rhamnine.* Boil in water the cake left after pressing buckthorn berries, filter while hot, and set the liquor aside. Boil what is deposited in alcohol, filter, and set aside to crystallize. The crystals may be purified by macerating them first in cold water, then in a little cold weak spirit, and afterwards boiling them in alcohol with animal charcoal, and filtering.

RESINA ALOES. L. 1746. Boil aloes in 8 parts of water; set aside for a night, wash and dry the resin which will be found at the bottom of the vessel.

RESINA CANNABIS. See Extractum Cannabis. A purer resin (*cannabine*) is thus prepared by Messrs. Smith, of Edinburgh. The dried plant (*gunjah*) is bruised and repeatedly macerated in warm water, then in a solution of carbonate of soda (containing of this salt half the weight of the plant), and afterwards well washed with water, pressing the plant after each operation. It is then dried and digested with rectified spirit, to which cream of lime, containing an ounce of lime to each pound of gunjah, has been added. To the filtered tincture, add sulphuric acid in slight excess, again filter, distil off most of the spirit, add to the residue 3 or 4 times its bulk of water, evaporate the remaining spirit in a porcelain dish, pour off the watery liquid, wash the resin with water, and dry it. 2-3ds of a grain acted as a powerful narcotic.

RESINA CINCHONÆ. P. As Resina Jalapæ.

RESINÆ COPAIBÆ. See Extractum Copaibæ.

RESINÆ JALAPÆ. P. Macerate the powdered root with repeated portions of rectified spirit till exhausted, filter and distil the mixed tinctures; mix the residue with 20 or 30 times its weight of warm water, wash the resinous matter, and dissolve it in a little rectified spirit; then spread it on plates, and dry in a stove until it becomes brittle. MOUCHON directs 1 part of ivory black to be put into a percolator, and over it 2 parts more, mixed with an equal weight of jalap powder; rectified spirit is then poured on till a tincture is obtained, equal in weight to the jalap, and twice its volume of water added to separate the resin, which is treated as above.

RESINA NUCIS VOMICÆ. See Extractum Nucis Vomicæ.

RESINÆ SCAMMONII. See Extractum Scammonii.

RESINA TURPETHI. As Resina Jalapæ.

RHEUM USTUM. Mr. HOBLYN. Heat powdered rhubarb in an

iron vessel, with constant stirring, till it becomes nearly black; then smother it in a covered jar. Dose, gr. v to x, as an astringent in *diarrhœa*.

ROB. The inspissated juices of fruits. See Extractum Sambuci, &c.

RUBIGO FERRI. Iron filings are moistened with water, and exposed to the air till rusted; then triturated with water, and prepared as chalk. The precipitated sesquioxide is now more generally used in pharmacy. See Ferri Sesqui-oxydum, and Ferrugo.

SACCHARA. Medicated sugars, or Saccharides (*Saccharures* and *Sacchorolés pulverulents* of BERAL), are usually made by moistening refined sugar with a strong alcoholic, æthereal, or aqueous solution of a medicinal substance, drying it very gradually, and afterwards reducing it to powder; or are mere mixtures of sugar with other dry substances. A mixture of an essential oil with sugar, is termed Oleo-saccharum (which see), and by BERAL, *Saccharolé oleulique*.

SACCHARUM ALUMINATUM. PRUS. PH. Equal parts of alum and white sugar triturated together.

SACCHARUM BELLADONNÆ. GUIBOURT. Tincture of belladonna (made with one part of powdered leaves to five of rectified spirit) ʒj, refined sugar ℥x; triturate them together, dry in the air, and then, by a moderate heat in a stove; reduce again to a powder, and pass it through a sieve. 50 grains are equal to 1 of the dried leaves; other authorities direct 8 parts of sugar to 1 of tincture. *Saccharures* of Castor, Digitalis, Ipecacuanha, Henbane, Hemlock, and Squill, are prepared in the same manner.

SACCHARUM CINCHONÆ. GUIBOURT. Resinous extract of bark ʒij, refined sugar ℥xx. Dissolve the extract in the smallest possible quantity of alcohol, and proceed as above.

SACCHARUM CHONDRI. MOUCHON. Concentrate a decoction of carrageen to the consistence of thick syrup, add 4 times as much sugar as of the moss, and finish the operation on a sand-bath, stirring constantly till dry.

SACCHARUM CORNU CERVI. Jelly of hartshorn shavings 4 parts, syrup 3 parts; mix, and evaporate to dryness.

SACCHARUM FERRI CITRATIS. BERAL. Liquid citrate of iron (see Liquor Ferri Citratis,) ʒj, white sugar ℥xj; mix, dry in a stove, and pulverize with a drop or two of oil of lemon. Dose, ʒj to ʒij, daily.

SACCHARUM FERRI CARBONATIS. See Ferri Carbonas Saccharatum.

SACCHARUM FERRI IODIDI. Dr. A. T. THOMSON. Expose syrup of iodide of iron in a shallow vessel in a warm stove, till it crystallizes. Rub the crystals to powder.

SACCHARUM HELMINTHOCORTI. M. DELESCHAMPS. To a clear and concentrated decoction of ℔j of Corsican moss, add ℔ij of white sugar, coarsely powdered, and evaporate, as Sach. Lichenis.

SACCHARUM JALAPÆ. Tincture of jalap ʒj, white sugar ℥j; triturate together, dry in a stove by a gentle heat, and again triturate.

SACCHARO-KALI. BLONDEAU. Bicarbonate of soda ℈viij, refined sugar ℥viij, carmine to colour; mix.

SACCHARUM LICHENIS. M. ROBINET. Iceland moss ℔j, refined sugar ℔j; macerate the moss in water to extract the bitterness; express, boil in water, strain, settle, decant, add the sugar, evaporate to dryness with a gentle heat, constantly stirring, and powder.

SACCHARUM MARTIS. *Mars. Saccharatus.* E. 1744. Put clean iron filings into a brass kettle suspended over a gentle fire, and add by little and little, twice their weight of sugar boiled to a candy, agitating continually.

SACCHARUM MERCURII. See Mercurius Saccharatus, and Æthiops Saccharatus.

SACCHARUM MERCURII COMPOSITUM. BRUNS. PH. Quicksilver ʒiv, sugar ℥ij; triturate till the globules disappear, and add jalap ʒiv.

SACCHARUM CUM MOSCHO. GAUGER. Triturate ℥j of musk with ℥j or ℥jss of alcohol, and gradually add ℥iij of refined sugar. Set the mixture in a warm situation till dry, and triturate it with more sugar, if required, to make up the weight, ℥iv.

SACCHARUM NITRATUM. FULLER. Nitre ℥j, refined sugar ℥iij.

SACCHARUM ROSACEUM. L. 1746. Red rose petals and refined sugar reduced to powder, of each ℔j; mix, and moisten it with water to form tablets, to be dried with a gentle heat. E. 1744, directs it to be made with juice of red roses.

SACCHARUM CUM VANILLA. *Poudre de Vanille.* See Pulvis Vanillæ. But a weaker compound, prepared from the tincture as Saccharum Jalapæ, is commonly intended when *saccharure* or *saccharolé* de Vanille is directed.

SACCHARUM CONDITUM. *Sugar Candy* is prepared by slowly evaporating syrup in vessels having threads stretched across for the crystals to form on.

SACCHARUM HORDEATUM. *Barley Sugar* was directed to be made by boiling sugar in barley water until it became ductile; it is now only prepared by confectioners. Penidium was made by rapidly drawing out melted sugar and twisting it.

SACCHARUM LACTIS. *Sugar of milk.* Clarify whey by white of egg, and carefully evaporate the strained liquid by a gentle heat, that it may crystallize on cooling. Purify by animal charcoal and repeated crystallizations.

SACCHARUM VANILLÆ ET CARYOPHYLLI. From the tinctures, as Saccharum Jalapæ.

SACCULI. *Sachets.* Little bags containing dry substances, commonly in coarse powder, used as local applications. Sometimes they are moistened with spirits, &c.

SACCULUS AMMONIACALIS. Equal parts of sal ammoniac and quicklime are mixed, and sprinkled between cotton wadding, which is to be quilted in muslin.

SACCULUS ANODYNUS. QUINCY. Chamomiles ℥j, bay berries ℥j, lavender flowers ℥ss, henbane seed ʒj, opium ʒj. To be dipped in hot spirits.

SACCULUS ANTIPHTHISICUS. Dissolve ℥j of aloes in ℥xij of strong decoction of rue. Fold a large piece of soft muslin in eight folds, large enough to cover the chest and part of the stomach. Steep it in the decoction and dry it in the shade. Wear it on the chest constantly. A celebrated domestic remedy for consumption. [It is more properly a breast-plate than a sachet.]

SACCULUS LATERALIS. FULLER. Bay-berries, cumin seed, fœnugreek seed, chamomiles 1 handful each; common salt and bran each 2 handfuls. Make 2 bags, to be applied hot alternately.

SACCULUS RESOLVENS. Dr. BRESLAU. Iodide of potassium

ʒijss, muriate of ammonia ℥ijss. Powder separately, mix, and put it into a linen bag. TANCHOU prescribes, for tumours of the breast:—Iodide of potassium ℈iv, burnt sponge ʒijss, muriate of ammonia 3x, muriate of soda ʒijss. DUMERIL directs ʒj each of sulphate of lime, sulphate of iron, and muriate of ammonia.

SACCULUS SPONGII. *Collier de Morand.* Muriate of ammonia, muriate of soda, burnt sponge, of each ℥j; mix, sprinkle the powder on a piece of cotton wool, and quilt between muslin, in the form of a cravat. To be worn constantly in goitre or bronchocele, renewing it every month.

SACCULUS STOMACHICUS. FULLER. Mint ℥ss, wormwood, thyme, red roses each ʒij, balaustines, angelica root, caraway seed, nutmeg, mace, cloves each ʒj. Coarsely powder the ingredients, and put them in a bag; to be moistened with hot red wine when applied. *For flatulence,* &c.

Those which are merely employed as *perfumes* do not belong to the present work.

SAL ABSINTHII. L. 1746. Burn wormwood in an iron vessel for some hours, boil the ashes with water, filter and evaporate to dryness. [Salt of wormwood is now considered identical with that obtained from the ashes of other plants; consequently subcarbonate of potash is usually sold for it.]

SAL AERATUS. Bicarbonate of potash, prepared by placing a solution of the subcarbonate near a brewer's vat, is known by this name in the United States.

SAL AMMONIACUS. See Ammoniæ Hydrochloras.

SAL AMMONIACUS VOLATILIS. See Ammoniæ Sesquicarbonas.

SAL ACETOSELLÆ. Formerly made by evaporating clarified juice of wood-sorrel; now by adding 7 parts of subcarbonate of potash to a solution of 13 of oxalic acid, and evaporating the solution that it may crystallize. See Potassæ Superoxalas.

SAL ESSENTIALIS CINCHONÆ. See Extractum Cinchonæ Siccum.

SAL CORNU CERVI. An impure carbonate of ammonia, produced in distilling hartshorn or bones.

SAL ENIXUM. The crude bisulphate of potash which remains in the retort after distilling nitric acid.

SAL POLYCHRESTUM GLASERI. See Potassæ Sulphas cum Sulphure.

SAL PRUNELLÆ. Fused nitrate of potash. See Potassæ Nitras Fusa.

SAL SUCCINI PURIFICATUS. L. 1788. Salt of amber (see Acidum Succinicum) ℔ss, water ℔j; boil, and set aside to crystallize.

SAL TARTARI. *Salt of Tartar*. See Potassæ Carbonas.

SALICINE. P. To a strong clear decoction of willow bark add milk of lime; filter, evaporate the liquor to a syrupy consistence, add alcohol to separate the gummy matter, filter, distil off the spirit, evaporate the residuum, and set aside to crystallize. KANE directs willow bark to be boiled four times in water, the decoction to be evaporated to three times the weight of the bark, the filtered liquor evaporated to the consistence of syrup, and set aside to crystallize. The crystals may be purified by animal charcoal if necessary. *Tonic and Febrifuge.*

SANTONINUM. *Santonine.* M. CALLOUD. Boil wormseed in water, and add to it milk of lime. Strain and press; boil the marc with more water, and again press. Mix the decoctions, and when clear, concentrate the liquor by evaporation. Clarify, and strain, and evaporate further, then pour it into an earthen vessel, and add muriatic acid in slight excess. In 24 hours, collect the precipitate, wash it with a little weak spirit; press, and dry it. Dose, 4 to 6 grains, *as a vermifuge.*

SAPO AMYGDALINUS. P. Solution of caustic soda (at 1·334) ℥x, oil of almonds ℥xxj; add the ley to the oil in small portions, stirring frequently; leave the mixture for some days at a temperature of from 64° to 68° F., stirring occasionally, then put it into moulds till sufficiently solidified. It should be exposed to the air for some weeks before it is used.

SAPO ANIMALIS. Beef marrow boiled with 2 parts of water, and half of soda ley; when saponified add one-fifth of salt, stir, remove the soap from the surface, and place it in moulds.

SAPO ANTIMONIALIS. *Sapo Stibiatus.* PRUS. PH. Dissolve ℥j of oxysulphuret of antimony in liquor potassæ q. s. Dilute with 3 times the quantity of water, add ℥vj of scraped soap, and evaporate to a pilular consistence.

SAPO CAMBOGIÆ. SOUBEIRAN. Mix 1 part of gamboge with 2 of soap, and dissolve it in a little spirit, and evaporate to a pilular consistence.

SAPO GUAIACINUS. PRUS. PH. Caustic soda ℥j, guaiacum resin

℥vj, aquæ ℥iv; boil for four hours, replacing the water as it evaporates, and reduce to a due consistence.

Sapo Hydrargyri. M. Herbert. Dissolve ℥iv of quicksilver in its weight of nitric acid, without heat; melt in a porcelain basin, by water-bath, ℥xviij of veal suet, and add the solution, stirring the mixture till the union is complete. To ℥ivss of this ointment add ℥ij of solution of caustic soda (density 1·330), and grind the mixture on a porphyry slab till a soap is formed, which is completely soluble in water. For external use, alone or dissolved in water, in some *Cutaneous diseases.*

Sapo Jalapinus. Prus. Ph. Resin of jalap, hard soap p. æq.; dissolve in rectified spirit q. s., and evaporate to a due consistence, stirring constantly. Dose, gr. x to xv.

Sapo Olei Jecoris Aselli. Deschamps. Cod-liver oil ℥ij, caustic soda ʒij, water ʒv; dissolve the soda in the water, and mix it with the oil. An ioduretted soap is made by mixing with ℥j of the above, ʒj of iodide of potassium dissolved in ʒj of water.

Sapo Potassæ Hydriodatis. See Linimentum Ioduretum.

Sapo Saturni. Bristol Infirmary. Boil ℔j of white soap in Oiv of rain water, when the soap is dissolved add ℥j of camphor pulverized with spirit, and mixed with ℥ij of liquid diacetate of lead; stir the whole till cold.

Sapo cum Sulphure. *Savon Sulphureux.* Franck. Soap ℥iv, sulphur ℥iv, oil of bergamot ʒss, water q. s.

Sapo Terebinthinæ. P. *Starkey's Soap.* Equal parts of subcarbonate of potash, oil of turpentine, and Venice turpentine, triturated together till they combine.

Sapo Tiglii. M. Croton oil 2 parts, solution of caustic soda (sp. gr. 1·330) 1 part; triturate together without heat till they combine; put it into paper moulds, and after a few days slice, and preserve in a well-stopped bottle. Dose, gr. j to iij.

Saponinum. *Saponine.* Boil the root of soapwort with proof spirit, filter the solution while hot, and when cold collect the precipitate, which may be purified by digestion with animal charcoal. [The same name is applied to a composition for cleaning gloves—an abuse of language greatly to be deprecated.]

Scilla Cocta. Remove the outer coat from the bulb, and bake the squill in flour until tender.

SERUM LACTIS. *Whey.* Infuse dried calf's stomach in 12 parts of water for 10 or 12 hours; to Oij of milk add ʒiij or q. s. of the infusion, and heat gently till the curd is formed; then strain without pressure. It may be clarified as the next.

SERUM LACTIS [cum Acido Tartarico]. P. Milk Oij; boil it, adding by small quantities a solution of 1 part of tartaric acid in 8 of water, q. s.; when coagulated, strain without pressure. Replace the whey on the fire, after mixing with it rather more than half the white of an egg previously beaten up with a little cold water, and when it boils, add a little cold water, strain through a sieve, and filter. [Whey is also prepared by means of vinegar, lemon or orange juice, cream of tartar, &c.]

SERUM ALUMINOSUM. L. 1746. Milk Oj, alum ʒij; boil, and strain.

SERUM ANTISCORBUTICUM. L. 1746. Milk Oj, scorbutic juices ℥iv; boil, and strain.

SERUM LACTIS CEREVISIATUM. Boil Oj of milk with ℥iv of good beer, and strain.

SERUM CHALYBEATUM. BRUNS. PH. Repeatedly quench red-hot iron in whey.

SERUM NITROSUM. Boil ʒij of nitre in Oj of milk, and strain.

SERUM PURGANS. GERM. H. Manna ℥ij, cream of tartar ʒiv, clarified whey ℥vj; a third part every 2 hours.

SERUM SINAPIS. Milk Oj, water Oj, bruised mustard seed ℥jss; boil till curdled, and strain.

SERUM CUM TAMARINDIS. Tamarinds ℥j, whey ℔j; boil, and strain.

SERUM VINOSUM. SWEDIAUR. Milk ℔ij, water ℔ij, rhenish wine ℥jss; boil, strain, and clarify.

SERUM LACTIS COMPOSITUM. BRUNS. PH. Acidulous whey Ojss, lemon-juice ℥j, vitriolated conserve of roses ʒvj. Mix.

SERUM LACTIS PULVERATUM. Sugar of milk ʒij, white sugar ℥j, gum arabic ℥ss. Mix.

SERUM DICTUM DE WEISSE. Senna ℥ss, sulphate of magnesia ℥ss, elder flowers, tops of St. John's wort, yellow bed-straw, of each a pinch. Infuse for 12 hours in Oviij of clarified whey. Dose, ℥xvj, *to diminish the secretion of milk.*

SMILACINA. *Smilacine.* Boil sarsaparilla in rectified spirit, distil off two-thirds, filter, concentrate, and set aside to crystallize. Purify the crystals by digestion with animal charcoal, and re-crystallize.

SODA PURA. *Caustic Soda.* P. Crystallized subcarbonate of soda ℥xx, quicklime ℥viij, water Ovj. Boil for half an hour, strain, evaporate rapidly in a silver dish to dryness, and melt as directed for Potassa Fusa.

SODÆ ACETAS. D. Saturate distilled vinegar, or diluted wood vinegar, with carbonate of soda, evaporate to 1·276, and set aside to crystallize. [It is usually obtained by decomposing acetate of lime (made by saturating crude pyroligneous acid with chalk) by sulphate of soda. Dose, ℈j to ʒj, as a diuretic; in larger doses, as a cathartic.]

SODÆ ARSENIAS. P. Nitrate of soda 100 parts, arsenious acid 116 parts; mix exactly, heat to redness in a hessian crucible, treat the residue with water, add carbonate of soda to the solution till it is alkaline, evaporate and crystallize. If the mother liquor is not alkaline, add more carbonate of soda, and again evaporate. Dose, 1-16th to 1-8th of a grain.

SODÆ BENZOAS. Heat benzoic acid and water, and add carbonate of soda q. s. to neutralize the acid; filter, evaporate, and crystallize.

SODÆ BIBORAS. The native borax (tincal) is refined by calcination, solution, and crystallization. Borax is also made from the native boracic acid by saturating it with carbonate of soda.

SODÆ CARBONAS. L. (Sodæ Subcarbonas. L. 1824.) Boil ℔ij of impure carbonate of soda (washing soda) in Oiv of distilled water, filter while hot, and set aside that crystals may form.

SODÆ CARBONAS EXSICCATA. L. E. & D. Expose the crystallized carbonate of soda to heat till it is dried, and afterwards raise the heat to redness. Lastly, reduce it to powder. D. directs it to be done in a silver vessel.

SODÆ SESQUICARBONAS. L. Dissolve 4 parts of the crystallized (sub-) carbonate in 7 of water, and pass carbonic acid through it till saturated. Drain and squeeze the sesquicarbonate which falls, and dry it with a very gentle heat. [Dissolve more carbonate in the liquor, and proceed as before.] This salt, as usually sold, is rather a bicarbonate than a sesquicarbonate. The small quantity of neutral carbonate it contains may be removed by causing a little distilled water to percolate through it. D. nearly as L. For E. see the next article.

SODÆ BICARBONAS. E. Carbonic acid is passed into a vessel containing a mixture of 1 part of crystallized and 2 of dried carbonate of soda, till gas is no longer absorbed; and the salt dried at a heat not exceeding 120° F. To procure the carbonic acid gas, fill with fragments of marble a glass jar, open at the bottom and tubulated at top; close the bottom so as to keep in the marble without preventing the free passage of a fluid; and having connected the tubulature by a bent tube and corks with an empty bottle, and this with the vessel containing the soda, immerse the jar in diluted muriatic acid.

SODA CHLORINATA. Dr. CHRISTISON. Pass chlorine gas (from 8 parts of black oxide of manganese, 10 of chloride of sodium, 14 of sulphuric acid, and 10 of water) into a vessel containing 19 parts of dried carbonate of soda mixed with 1 part of water. When the air of the apparatus is expelled, the junctions should be secured. See Liquor Sodæ Chlorinatæ.

SODÆ HYDROSULPHAS CRYSTALLIZATA. *Sulfure de sodium cristallisé.* P. Prepare a solution of caustic soda at 120°, and pass into it sulphuretted hydrogen, till no more gas is absorbed; leave the solution in close vessels till crystals form; drain them, and keep them in well-stopped bottles. *Used in preparing some mineral waters.*

SODÆ HYPOSULPHIS. Hyposulphite of Soda. P. Dissolve ℥x of cry. carbonate of soda in Oj of distilled water; add ʒx of sulphur, and pass sulphurous acid gas in excess into the liquid. Boil the mixture for a few moments in a glass matrass, filter, and evaporate the liquor to 1-3d of its volume; then set it aside in a cool place, that the salt may crystallize. [It is used in skin diseases in doses of ℈ss to ʒj or more. Dupasquier says it is not poisonous, and that it resembles sulphate of soda in its action, and may be taken in the same doses.]

SODÆ MURIAS PURUM. E. Evaporate a filtered solution of common salt, skim off the crystals as they form, wash them quickly with a little cold water, and dry them.

SODÆ PHOSPHAS. E. Bones burnt to whiteness and powdered ℔x, sulphuric acid Oij f℥iv; mix, add gradually Ovj of water; digest for three days, replacing the water which evaporates; add

Ovj of boiling water, and strain through linen; pass more boiling water through the mass on the filter till it comes away nearly tasteless. Let the impurities subside in the united liquors, pour off the clear fluid and concentrate to Ovj. Let it settle; boil the clear liquor, and add carbonate of soda (dissolved in boiling water) till the acid is neutralized. Set the solution aside to crystallize. More crystals may be obtained by evaporating the remaining liquor, adding carbonate of soda in slight excess. Preserve the crystals in well-closed vessels. Dose, ʒiv to ℥j as a laxative; or from ℈j to ʒss 3 times a day in uric gravel.

SODÆ SULPHAS. *Glauber's Salt.* L. Dissolve ℔ij of the salt left in the distilling muriatic acid in Oij of boiling water; saturate with carbonate of soda, evaporate, and crystallize. E. directs the excess of acid to be neutralized with marble. [The commercial sulphate of soda (being a product in making sal ammoniac) frequently contains sulphate of ammonia. To purify it, add to a hot solution a little subcarbonate of soda, and boil for a few minutes. Strain the solution, and set it in a cool place to crystallize. More crystals may be obtained from the remaining liquor by evaporating it at a gentle heat; or it may be used for dissolving a fresh portion of the salt.]

SODÆ BISULPHAS. Mix 10 parts of dried sulphate of soda with 7 of strong sulphuric acid. Heat the mixture gently in a crucible.

SODÆ POTASSIO-TARTRAS. L. Soda Tartarizata. L. 1824. Potassæ et Sodæ Tartras. E. *Rochelle Salts.* Carbonate of soda ℥xij, boiling water Oiv; dissolve, and gradually add ℥xvj of bitartrate of potash in fine powder. Filter the solution, apply a gentle heat till a pellicle floats upon the surface, and set aside that crystals may form. Dry these, and evaporate the liquor for more. D. directs 5 parts of carbonate of soda to 7 of bitartrate of potash.

SODA TARTARIZATA EFFERVESCENS. *Acidulated Alkali.* Bicarbonate of soda ℥iv, tartaric acid ℥iv, refined sugar ℥xij, essence of lemon fʒss. The powders to be separately dried at a moderate temperature, and the whole uniformly mixed. [The above is one from the many private formulæ that might be given. It is to be regretted that the name of a pharmacopœial preparation (soda tartarizata) is sometimes given to this compound.]

SODII AURO-TERCHLORIDUM. See Auro-chloridum Sodii.

SODII BROMIDUM. As Potassii Bromidum.

SODII CHLORIDUM. See Sodæ Murias.

SODII IODIDUM. Sodæ Hydriodas. By decomposing iodide of iron by carbonate of soda, and evaporating the filtered solution with a gentle heat, that crystals may be produced by cooling. It is very deliquescent.

SODII PLATINO-BICHLORIDUM. See Platino-chloridum Sodii.

SODII SULPHO-ANTIMONIATUM. SCHLIPPE'S *Antimonial Salt.* STRASB. PH. Cryst. carbonate of soda 9 parts, water 40 parts; dissolve, and to the boiling solution add prepared sulphuret of antimony 4 parts, sulphur 1½, milk of lime (with 2½ parts of lime to 7 of water) 10 parts. Boil for 2½ hours, filter, and crystallize.

SOLUTIO. *Solution.* This term is used as synonymous with LIQUOR. If the preparation sought for cannot be found under the one, look under the other.

SOLUTIO ACIDI CITRICI. Citric acid ℥j, water ℥xv. This is about the strength of lemon-juice. See Succus Limonis.

SOLUTIO ACIDI TARTARICI. U. C. H. Tartaric acid ʒj, syrup f℥j, water f℥xvj.

SOLUTIO ACONITINÆ. Dr. TURNBULL. Aconitine gr. viij, rectified spirit f℥j. Externally, by a sponge on the unbroken skin, *in neuralgia and rheumatic affections.*

SOLUTIO ALKALINA CAUSTICA. BRANDISH'S *Caustic Alkali,* or *Alkaline Solution.* American pearlash ℔vj, quicklime ℔ij, wood-ashes made from the branches of the ash ℔ij, boiling water Cvj. Slake the lime, add the rest of the water and the pearlash; lastly, stir in the wood-ashes. Let it stand in a covered vessel for 24 hours, and pour off the clear liquid. To each Oj add 1 drop of true oil of juniper. Keep it in green-stoppered bottles.

SOLUTIO AMYGDALINÆ. See Emulsio Amygdalæ cum Amygdalinâ.

SOLUTIO ANTISCROFULOSA. AUGUSTIN. Muriate of barytes ʒss, muriate of iron ʒss, distilled water ℥j. CLARUS. Ammoniated iron ℈j, muriate of barytes ℈j, water ℥ij. Dose, 20 to 30 drops, two or three times a day.

SOLUTIO ARGENTI NITRATIS. E. (*Test.*) Nitrate of silver ℈ij, distilled water 1600 grains. Dissolve, and preserve in well-closed bottles. For L. see Liquor Argenti Nitratis.

SOLUTIO ARGENTI AMMONIATI. E. (*Test.*) Nitrate of silver 44 grains, distilled water f ℥j; dissolve, and add gradually aqua ammoniæ till the precipitate, at first thrown down, is very nearly but not entirely redissolved.

SOLUTIO ARSENIATIS AMMONIÆ. BIETT. See Liquor Arsen. Ammoniæ. A weaker solution is sometimes employed. Dr. NELIGAN. Arseniate of ammonia gr. jss, distilled water ℥iij, spirit of angelica ʒvj. Dose, from f ʒj to f ʒiij.

SOLUTIO ARSENIATIS SODÆ. See Liquor Ars. Sodæ.

SOLUTIO ATROPIÆ. Mr. WILDE. Atropia gr. j, rectified spirit ♏iij, diluted nitric acid ♏j, distilled water f ʒj. This forms No. 1; Nos. 2 and 3 contain respectively 2 and 3 grains of atropia. One drop applied to the conjunctiva of the lower lid dilates the pupil. Mr. W. W. COOPER's solution for the same purpose consists of atropia gr. ij, rectified spirit f ʒj, water f ʒvij.

SOLUTIO AD BALNEUM BARETGINENSE. P. Crystallized hydro-sulphate of soda ℥ij, carbonate of soda ℥ij, muriate of soda ℥ij, water ℥x; mix, and preserve it in a well-closed bottle.

SOLUTIO BARYTÆ NITRATIS. E. (*Test.*) Nitrate of barytes 40 grains, distilled water 800 grains. Dissolve, and keep in well-closed bottles.

SOLUTIO BARII CHLORIDI. L. See Liquor Barii Chloridi.

SOLUTIO BEBEERINÆ. Dr. RODIE's *Solution* contains impure sulphate of bebeerine, but the quantity is not known. The dose is from 20 to 30 drops.

SOLUTIO BELLADONNÆ. HAHNEMANN's *Prophylactic Solution.* Extract of belladonna gr. iij, distilled water (or cinnamon water) ℥j. Dose, 3 drops twice a day to a child under 12 months, and 1 drop more for every year above.

SOLUTIO BROMINII. M. POURCHE. *For internal use.* Bromine f ʒj, distilled water f ℥v; mix. Dose, 5 to 6 drops. [*For external use,* f ʒiv of bromine to f ℥v of water.]

SOLUTIO CALCII CHLORIDI. Solutio Calcis Muriatis. E. See Liquor Calcii Chloridi.

SOLUTIO CALCIS CHLORINATÆ. See Liquor Calcis Chlorinatæ.

SOLUTIO CALCIS CHLORIDI SPIRITUOSA. CHEVALLIER. Chloride of lime ʒiij, distilled water ℥ij, rectified spirit ℥ij; mix, and filter.

SOLUTIO CAMPHORÆ CARBONICA. SWEDIAUR. Water saturated with carbonic acid gas ℔ij, powdered camphor ʒiij.

SOLUTIO CAMPHORÆ ET MYRRHÆ. SWEDIAUR. Camphor ʒj, myrrh ʒj; rub together, and add gradually ℔j of hot distilled water. When cold, filter.

SOLUTIO CAUSTICA COPAIBÆ *vel* CUBEBÆ. Dr. CATTELL. Oil of cubebs or copaiva ℥ij, solution of potash ℥j, water q. s. As an injection.

SOLUTIO CARBONIS SULPHURETI. OTTO. Sulphuret of carbon ʒij, alcohol ℥j. Dose, 4 drops every 4 hours.

SOLUTIO CHLORINII. E. & D. See Aqua Chlorinii. MIDDL. H. Chlorate of potash ʒij, hydrochloric acid f℥ij, water f℥ij. Dissolve. [Dr. MAITLAND recommends doubling the quantity of water, which is insufficient to dissolve the chlorate and retain the chlorine.] Of this solution add fʒiij to f℥xij of distilled water, for a mixture. [Dr. WATSON says, add f 3ij to Oj of water, and give a tablespoonful or two, according to the age, frequently.] *In Scarlatina.*

SOLUTIO CONII. Dr. PARIS. *For Inhaling.* Extract of hemlock ʒj, tincture of hemlock fʒj, warm water (at 120° F.) Oss. To be used 3 or 4 times a day.

SOLUTIO COPAIBÆ. Dr. SIGMOND. Copaiva ℥xij, calcined magnesia ℥vj; mix, and digest them in Oj of proof spirit; filter, and add f℥ss of spirit of nitric æther.

SOLUTIO COPAIBÆ ALKALINA. Copaiva ℥ij, solution of potash f℥iv, distilled water ℥x; boil together, and when cooled to 140° F. add spirit of nitric æther f℥j. Separate the clear solution from the sediment and what floats on the surface. Dr. CHRISTISON directs ℥jss of aqua potassa and no water. Mr. BELL. Balsam of copaiva 2 parts, solution of potash or soda 8 parts, water 7 parts. Boil for a quarter of an hour, and add sweet spirit of nitre 1 part.

SOLUTIO CREASOTI. The *watery* solution consists of 1 part of creasote to 80 of water. A weaker solution, from 3 to 6 drops to Oj of water, is used for preserving pathological specimens. The alcoholic solution consists of 1 part of creasote to 16 [LAENNEC says 10] parts of rectified spirit.

SOLUTIO CUPRI SULPHATIS COMPOSITUS. *Aqua Styptica.* E. 1817. Sulphate of copper ℥iij, alum ℥iij, water ℥xxxij, sulphuric acid ℥jss. Dissolve the sulphate by heat, filter, and add the acid.

SOLUTIO DELPHINIÆ. Dr. TURNBULL. Delphinia ℈j, rectified spirit f℥ij. *For outward use.*

SOLUTIO ELATERINÆ. Dr. G. BIRD. Elaterine gr. iv, rectified spirit f℥iv. Dr. DUNCAN adds 16 drops of nitric acid; f℈ss contains gr. 1-16th of elaterine.

SOLUTIO ERGOTÆ ÆTHEREA. Dr. G. O. REES. As Essentia Secalis Cornuti Ætherea. Dose, ♏v to viij in *Menorrhagia;* from ♏xv to xxx, *to puerperal women.*

SOLUTIO ESCHAROTICA. FRIEBURG. Camphor ℈ss, corrosive sublimate ℈j, rectified spirit ℥j. See also Hydrargyri deutonitras liquidus.

SOLUTIO FERRI. U. C. H. Tartarized iron ℈iij, distilled water f℥ij; make a solution.

SOLUTIO FERRI AMMONIO-TARTRATIS. AIKIN. Ammonio-tartrate of iron gr. xxxij, distilled water ʒvij, rectified spirit ʒj.

SOLUTIO FERRI CITRATIS, and SOLUTIO FERRI POTASSIO-CITRATIS. See Liquor, &c.

SOLUTIO FERRI IODIDI. E. 1839. Iodine 190 grains, clean iron wire 100 grains, distilled water f℥vj. Boil together in a narrow-necked matrass for about an hour, until the liquid becomes colourless, filter (keeping it hot), and add boiling distilled water to make up f℥vj. Put it immediately into ℥j stoppered bottles, each containing a piece of iron wire. [This has been since replaced by Syrupus Ferri Iodidi, but is retained here as furnishing a convenient solution for dispensing; ♏xij contain gr. j of iodide of iron.] DUPASQUIER's Normal Solution is made with one part of iodine, two of iron, and eight of water, digested at 160° F. till colourless.

SOLUTIO FERRI SESQUI-IODIDI. Dr. OBERDOERFFER. Iodine ʒiv, iron ʒjss, water ℥j; digest in a flask until a greenish solution is obtained; dilute with water f℥iv, filter two or three times, add iodine ʒij, and water to make up f℥x. (It contains gr. j of iodine in about ♏xiij.)

SOLUTIO FERRI OXYSULPHATIS. Mr. TYSON. Sulphate of iron ʒij or ʒiij, nitric acid ʒiij; triturate together for 15 minutes, and add gradually distilled water ℥jss. Dose, five to twelve drops.

Solutio Ferri Pernitratis. See Ferri Pernitras.

Solutio Ferri Sulphatis. See Lotio Ferri Sulphatis. M. Dauvergne employs a solution of from one to two parts of the crystallized sulphate to eight parts of water, as a lotion for *Mentagra*.

Solutio Gambogiæ Alkalina. Van Mons. Gamboge ʒss, solution of carbonate of potash ℥ss.

Solutio Hydrargyri Ammonio-Nitratis, Sol. Hydr. Deuto-Nitratis, Sol. Hydr. Cyanidi. See Liquor, &c.

Solutio Hydrargyri Deuto-Iodidi. M. The *Alcoholic Solution:* Deuto-iodide of mercury gr. xij, rectified spirit f℥jss. Dose, 10 to 15 drops. *Æthereal Solution:* With sulphuric æther, in the same proportion.

Solutio Hydrargyri Iodidi. M. Iodide of mercury gr. viij, sulphuric æther f℥j.

Solutio Ætherea Iodinii. M. Iodine ℈ij, rectified æther f℥jss.

Solutiones Iodinii *vel* Ioduretæ. Lugol's Solution of Iodine. —*Ioduretted Waters*, Nos. 1, 2, and 3: Iodine gr. jss, ij, and ijss, water Oj. *Drops:* Iodine ℈j, iodide of potassium ℈ij, water f3ix. *Lotions*, &c.: Iodine gr. jss to iij, iodide of potassium gr. iij to vj, water Oj. *Rubefacient:* Iodine one part, iodide of potassium two, water 12. *Caustic:* Iodine one, iodide of potassium one, water two.

Solutio Iodinii cum Conio. Dr. Scudamore's Solution *for Inhaling*. Iodine gr. vj, iodide of potassium gr. vj, rectified spirit ʒij, water ℥v 3vj. From ʒss to 3v of this solution, with ʒss of tincture of hemlock, to be added to warm water (120° F.) in a glass inhaler, and used twice a day. [The preserved juice (succus conii) is often substituted for the tincture of hemlock. Two-thirds of the ingredients are first put into the inhaler, and the rest added when half the time for inhaling has elapsed.]

Solutio Iodhydrargyratis Potassii. Dr. Channing. Iodide of potassium gr. iijss, biniodide of mercury gr. ivss, distilled water f℥j. Dissolve first the iodide of potassium, and then the iodide of mercury, in the water. Dose, two to five drops three times a day. [Puche's consist of gr. vj of each salt in

℥viij of water. LIMOUSIN—LAMOTHE'S, gr. xij of iodhydrargyrate of potassium in ℥xvj of water.]

SOLUTIO MAGNESIÆ CARBONATIS. See Liquor Magn. Carbonatis.

SOLUTIO MAGNESIÆ SULPHATIS. For Dr. HENRY'S, see Liquor. A convenient solution for dispensing is one containing ℥j of the salt in f℥ij.

SOLUTIO MAGNESIÆ SULPHATIS COMPOSITA. U. C. H. Sulphate of magnesia ℥j, sulphate of soda ℥j, water ℥vj.

SOLUTIO MORPHIÆ ACETATIS—CITRATIS—SULPHATIS; see Liquor, &c.

SOLUTIO MORPHIÆ BIMECONATIS. [There is no standard formula; it is made about the same strength as Tinctura Opii. The following contains one grain in 84♏:—] Bimeconate of morphiæ ℈ss, rectified spirit f ʒj, distilled water f ʒxiij.

SOLUTIO MORPHIÆ MURIATIS. E. Muriate of morphia ʒjss, rectified spirit f ℥v, distilled water f ℥xv; dissolve with a gentle heat. It contains one grain of muriate of morphia in 106 minims, and is intended to be the same strength as tincture of opium. Dr. CHRISTISON'S solution was nearly the same—Muriate of morphia gr. x, distilled water gr. 1000. But a stronger solution, founded on MAGENDIE'S solutions of the acetate and sulphate, is used in many respectable establishments, containing gr. viij, gr. xij, or gr. xvj of the muriate in f ℥j of water, with a little rectified spirit. The solution used at Apothecaries' Hall contains 16 grains in ℥j. Until some uniform standard is adopted, it is desirable that physicians should specify the strength of the solution they prescribe. See Liquor Morphiæ.

SOLUTIO MYRRHÆ ALKALINA. SWEDIAUR. Subcarbonate of soda ʒj, myrrh ℥ij, boiling water ℥viij. Digest in a water-bath for two days, frequently stirring, and strain.

SOLUTIO OLEI CARYOPHYLLI. Alcohol Caryophyllatum. CH. Oil of cloves ʒj, alcohol ʒiij. *Applied to carious bones.*

SOLUTIO PHOSPHORI ÆTHEREA. M. Sliced phosphorus gr. v, rectified æther ℥j; mix, set the bottle in a dark place for three or four days, shaking occasionally, and decant.

SOLUTIO POTASSÆ. See Liquor Potassæ.

SOLUTIO POTASSÆ ALCOHOLICA. POL. PH. Hydrate of potash ℥j, alcohol ℥vj.

SOLUTIO POTASSÆ CHLORATIS. Dr. COPLAND. Chlorate of potash ʒj, distilled water f ℥xij.

SOLUTIO POTASSII CYANIDI. For LAMING'S, see Liquor Pot. Cyanidi. M. directs a stronger solution (*Hydrocyanate de potasse medicinal*). Cyanide of potassium ʒj, distilled water ℥j. It will not keep.

SOLUTIO POTASSI IODIDI. M. and Dr. GAIRDNER. Iodide of potassium ʒss (Dr. MANSON, gr. xxiv), distilled water ℥j. Dr. COINDET adds iodine gr. viij. See Liquor Potassii Iodidi and Liq. Pot. Iod. Comp.

SOLUTIO POTASSII SULPHURETI. See Aqua Sulphureti Potassæ.

SOLUTIO QUINÆ ARSENIATIS. BOUDIN. Arseniate of quinine gr. j, water Oj. Dose, from f ℥ij to ℥iv.

SOLUTIO QUINÆ SULPHO-TARTRATIS. RIGHINI. Disulphate of quinine ʒiv, tartaric acid ʒivss, distilled water f ℥ij; make a solution, of which from ♏xv to ʒj may be given in the day.

SOLUTIO QUINÆ ET FERRI. Dr. MEIGS. Citrate of iron ʒij, sulphate of quinine ʒss, water ℥j. Dose, 20 to 30 drops.

SOLUTIO QUINÆ AMORPHÆ ACETATIS, &c. Mr. BULLOCK'S solutions of the salts of amorphous quinine contain gr. xij of the salt in f ʒj of solution. The sulphate is most frequently employed.

SOLUTIO SAPONIS ÆTHEREA. PELLETIER. White soap 3v, camphor ʒv, oil of thyme ℈ij, acetic æther ℥v.

SOLUTIO SODÆ CARBONATIS. *Sodæ Carbonatis Aqua.* D. Crystallized subcarbonate of soda ℥j, water f ℥xvj, or q. s. to form a solution whose sp. gr. is 1024.

SOLUTIO SODÆ PHOSPHATIS. E. (*Test.*) Crystallized phosphate of soda gr. 175, distilled water f ℥viij.

SOLUTIO STANNI CHLORIDI. NAUCHE. Chloride of tin gr. j, distilled water f ℥xlvj. Dose, f ℥ss daily in gum water. And as a lotion to cancerous ulcers.

SOLUTIO STRYCHNIÆ ACETATIS. Dr. A. T. THOMSON. Strychnine gr. j, distilled vinegar f 3j. Of this solution ♏v, containing 1-12th of a grain of strychnia, may be given at first, and the dose cautiously increased. Or this solution may be diluted with f ʒix of water, and f ʒj given. Dr. NELIGAN dissolves one grain of strychnine in f ʒij of spirits, with 2 drops of acetic or other acid, and gives ♏x (1-12th of a grain of strychnia); but there is no authorized formula.

Solutio Zinci Acetatis. E. 1817. Sulphate of zinc ℨj, acetate of lead ʒiv; dissolve each separately in ℥x of distilled water, mix, and filter.

Solutio Zinci Ætherea. Hufeland. Chloride of zinc ℨiv, alcohol ℥j, sulphuric æther ℥ij.

Solutio Zinci Alkalina. Dr. A. T. Thomson. Sulphate of zinc gr. xxiv, solution of potash f ʒxij.

Solutio Zinci Sulphatis. E. 1817. Sulphate of zinc gr. xvj, water f ℥viij, dilute sulphuric acid ♏xvj.

Solutio Veratriæ. M. Veratria gr. j, distilled water f ℥ijss. Dr. Turnbull's *Solution for external use* is veratria ℈j, rectified spirit ℥xij. [Other solutions will be found under Liquor, and several *alcoholic* solutions under Tinctura.]

Sparadrapum cum Cera. *Toile de Mai.* P. White wax ℥viij, oil of almonds ℥iv, Venice turpentine ℥j; melt together, and dip into it strips of linen cloth, which are to be passed between wooden rules to remove the superfluous plaster. Spread on paper it forms waxed paper.

Sparadrapum Commune. *Common spread plaster.* P. directs, under this name, Emp. Gummosum spread on linen, which is the *Sparadrap* of the hospital of Paris. With us, the Empl. Plumbi and Emp. Resinæ are commonly used. See Empl. Resinæ.

Sparadrapum Elemi. See Charta pro Fonticulis.

Sparadrapum Epispasticum. See Charta Epispastica. It may be spread on sarcenet or linen.

Sparadrapum Icthyocollæ. See Emplastrum Icthyocollæ.

Sparadrapum Opii. M. Schæufelle. On a piece of black sarcenet, of a close and strong texture, properly stretched, spread with a brush 3 layers of extract of opium, softened with water to the consistence of treacle, and mixed with a sixth part of powdered gum. Keep the plaster dry.

Sparadrapum Vesicans. *Taffetas Vesicant.* P. Exhaust powdered cantharides by percolation with sulphuric æther; distil off the æther to obtain a thick oily extract. To ℥iv of this oil add ℥viij of yellow wax; melt with a very gentle heat, and spread it on waxed cloth. [It may also be spread upon oiled silk, isinglass plaster, paper, or other material. It should be carefully kept from the air. See Tela Vesicatoria.]

SPECIES. Mixtures of dried plants, or parts of plants, in a divided state, which, for convenience, are kept mixed for use. The *Compound Powders* (which are sometimes included under this name) are mostly placed under PULVERES.

SPECIES AMARÆ. P. *Bitter Herbs.* Dried tops, of lessor centaury, and wormwood, and leaves of germander, in equal quantity.

SPECIES ANTHELMINTICÆ. P. Dried flowering tops of tansy, and wormwood, and chamomile flowers, in equal parts.

SPECIES AROMATICÆ. P. (*Espèces Vulneraires.*) Dried leaves of sage, thyme, wild thyme, hyssop, water mint, origanum, and wormwood, of each ℥j; mix.

SPECIES PRO CONF. AROMATICÆ. See Conf. Arom.

SPECIES PRO CONF. OPII. See Conf. Opii.

SPECIES ASTRINGENTES. P. Bistort root ℥j, tormentil root ℥j, pomegranate bark ℥j.

SPECIES BECHICÆ. Dried flowers of mallow, catsfoot, coltsfoot, and petals of red poppy, each ℥j; mix. The Fructus Bechici are—Dates (stoned) ℥j, jujubes ℥j, figs ℥j, raisins ℥j.

SPECIES CORDIALES. *The 4 Cordial Flowers.* L. 1720. Flowers of borage, bugloss, roses, and violets.

SPECIES DIURETICÆ. P. (*The 5 opening roots,* E. 1744.) Dried roots of sweet fennel, butcher's broom, smallage, asparagus, and parsley, of each ℥j. [*The 5 lesser opening roots* are, Dog-grass, madder, eryngo, caper, and restharrow.]

SPECIES EMOLLIENTES. P. Dried leaves of mallow, marsh-mallow, great mullein, groundsel, and wall pellitory, of each ℥j; mix. *The 5 emollient herbs,* E. 1744. Mallow, marsh-mallow, mercury, pellitory, and violet. [Farinæ Emollientes, *Emollient meals* (P), consist of the meals of linseed, rye, and barley, in equal parts.]

SPECIES FUMALES. See Pulvis Fumalis, and Fumigatio Balsamica.

SPECIES NARCOTICÆ. Dried leaves of belladonna, stramonium, black nightshade, and henbane, in equal parts.

SPECIES DICTÆ QUINQUE HERBÆ CAPILLARES. 5 *capillary herbs.* L. 1720. Black and white maidenhair, spleen-wort, harts-tongue, and golden maidenhair.

SPECIES DICTÆ RADICES APERIENTES. As Species Diureticæ.

SPECIES PRO FOTU. See Species Emollientes. GRAY'S *Herbæ pro Fotu.* Southernwood, sea wormwood, and chamomile, each 2 parts, bay leaves 1 part. Boil ℥iijss in 6 pints of water.

SPECIES RESOLVENTES. HUFELAND. Tops of milfoil, fumitory, roots of madder, dog-grass, dandelion, and soap-wort, equal parts. The *Resolvent Meals,* Farinæ Resolventes, P., are those of fœnugreek, beans, lupines, and tares, in equal quantities.

SPECIES DICTÆ SEMINA FRIGIDA. P. (*The* 4 *cold seeds,* L. 1720.) Seeds of water melons, gourds, cucumbers, and melons, of each ℥j. *The* 4 *lesser cold seeds,* L. 1720, are those of succory, endive, lettuce, and purslain.

SPECIES DICTÆ SEMINA CALIDA. *The* 4 *greater hot seeds,* L. 1720. Aniseed, caraway-seed, cumin-seed, and fennel-seed. *The* 4 *lesser:* Seeds of bishop's-weed, stone parsley, smallage, and wild carrot.

SPECIES SUDORIFICÆ. P. Rasped guaiacum, cut sarsaparilla, sliced china root, of each ℥j.

SPECIES PRO THEA. Male speedwell, ground ivy, coltsfoot, of each ℥xij, balm and sage, of each ℥ij; mix. *Faltrank,* Thea Helvetica, P., contains 16 other herbs.

SPIRITUS. *Spirits.* Under this head are placed distilled spirits, simple and compound; with a few alcoholic solutions, and æthereal spirits. The spirit which forms the basis of these compounds is not prepared by pharmacists, but is a separate branch of manufacture. The Colleges, however, have indicated, by their densities, the strength of the spirits to be employed. See Spiritus Rectificatus, Spiritus Tenuior, and Alcohol. These are the degrees of strength used in this country; but in France a spirit intermediate between rectified and proof spirit is used in many preparations, the density of which is about 863. In preparing the distilled spirits, the seeds &c. are to be bruised; the E. P. and other Ph. direct previous maceration for 2 or more days.

SPIRITUS ABSINTHII. Wormwood ℥v, proof spirit Oj; distil by a vapour-bath f℥xvj.

Spiritus [*vel* Aqua] Absinthii Composita. L. 1720. Dried wormwood ℔ss, cardamom seed ℥ss, coriander seed ℥jss, brandy Cj; distil.

Spiritus Ætheris Acetici. Acetic æther ℥j, rectified spirit ℥iij.

Spiritus Ætheris Muriatici. *Dulcified Spirit of Salt.* E. 1744. To 3 parts of rectified spirit in a large vessel gradually add 1 part of muriatic acid; digest for some days, and distil cautiously in a sand-heat.

Spiritus Ætheris Nitrici. L. *Sweet Spirit of Nitre.* Rectified spirit ℔iij, nitric acid (sp. gr. 1·5) ℥iv; add the acid gradually to the spirit, and mix; then let f℥xxxij distil. E. directs it to be made by adding one measure of hyponitrous æther to 4 of rectified spirit. D. Nitric acid ℥ij, rectified spirit f℥xvj: distil ℥xij. [The density of the L. preparation is ·834; E. ·847. U. S. directs ℔ij of nitre in coarse powder to be mixed with 9½ old pints (Ovijss) of rectified spirit in a large retort, and ℔jss of sulphuric acid gradually poured in, and digested for two hours with a gentle heat. The heat is then raised and a gallon distilled; add to the distilled liquor f℥xvj proof spirit, and ℥j of carbonate of potash, and redistil.]

Spiritus Ætheris Sulphurici. L. 1824, and E. Rectified æther f℥viij, rectified spirit f℥xvj; mix.

Spiritus Ætheris Sulphurici Compositus. L. *Hoffman's Anodyne Liquor.* Sulphuric æther f℥viij, rectified spirit f℥xvj, æthereal oil f℈iij; mix.

Spiritus Ætheris Aromaticus. L. 1824. Cinnamon ʒiij, cardamom seed ʒjss, long pepper ʒj, ginger ʒj, spirit of sulphuric æther f℥xvj. Macerate for 14 days in a stoppered bottle, and strain.

Spiritus Alexiterius. Aqua Alexiteria Spirituosa. L. 1746. Mint ℔ss, angelica leaves ℥iv, tops of sea wormwood ℥iv, proof spirit Cj, (o. m., Ovjss imp.) water q. s.; distil Cj (o. m., Ovjss imp.)

Spiritus Ammoniæ. L. Hydrochlorate of ammonia ℥x, carbonate of potash ℥xvj, rectified spirit Oiij, water Oiij; distil Oiij. D. Dissolve by heat ℥iijss of [sesqui-] carbonate of ammonia in Oijss of rectified spirit. [E. directs the ammonia from powdered muriate of ammonia ℥viij, quicklime ℥xij, water f℥vjss, to be passed into Oij of rectified spirit. It differs from the L. and D., being a solution of *caustic* ammonia in the place of the *carbonate*. This was also the case in that of L. 1809, and the present U. S.]

SPIRITUS AMMONIÆ AROMATICUS. L. *Spirit of Sal Volatile.* Hydrochlorate of ammonia ℥v, carbonate of potash ℥viij, cinnamon ʒij, cloves ʒij, lemon-peel ℥iv, rectified spirit Oiv, water Oiv. Mix, and let Ovj distil. [Some manufacturers substitute nutmegs for cloves, the latter occasioning the spirit to become coloured.] E. Spirit of ammonia f℥viij, oil of lemon fʒj, oil of rosemary fʒjss. D. Spirit of ammonia f℥xxxij, oil of lemon 3ij, nutmegs ʒiv, cinnamon ʒiij; macerate for 3 days, and distil ℥xxiv.

SPIRITUS AMMONIÆ COMPOSITUS. L. 1787. Spirit of ammonia ℥xxxij, oil of lemon ʒij, oil of nutmeg ʒij; mix.

SPIRITUS AMMONIÆ FŒTIDUS. L. As Spiritus Ammoniæ, adding to the other ingredients ℥v of assafœtida. E. Spirit of ammonia f℥xss, assafœtida ℥ss; digest for 12 hours, and distil f℥x, by vapour-bath. D. Sp. of ammonia f℥xxxij, assafœtida ʒx; macerate for 3 days, and distil f℥xxiv.

SPIRITUS AMMONIÆ SUCCINATUS. See Tinctura Ammonia Composita.

SPIRITUS ANISI. L. Aniseed ℥x, proof spirit Cj, water Oij; distil Cj.

SPIRITUS AMMONIÆ ANISATUS. PR. P. Rectified spirit ℥xxiv, water of ammonia (density ·960) ℥vj, oil of aniseed ℥j; mix.

SPIRITUS ANISI COMPOSITUS. D. & L. 1787. Aniseed ℔ss, angelica seeds ℔ss, proof spirit Cj, water Oij, distil Cj.

SPIRITUS ARMORACIÆ COMPOSITUS. L. & D. Horse-radish root ℥xx, dried orange-peel ℥xx, nutmegs ʒv, proof spirit Cj, water Oij. Let Cj distil.

SPIRITUS AURANTII. P. Yellow of fresh orange-peel ℔j, spirit of wine (at ·863) ℔vj; macerate 2 days, and distil by water-bath to dryness.

SPIRITUS BERGAMII. From fresh bergamot-peel, as Sp. Aurantii.

SPIRITUS BRIONIÆ COMPOSITUS. E. 1744. Briony ℔ss, valerian ℥ij, pennyroyal ℥iij, rue ℥iij, mugwort ℥ss, feverfew flowers ℥ss, savin tops ℥ss, outer rind of orange ℥j, lovage seed ℥j, brandy Cj; distil. [*Aqua Hysterica* the same, omitting the briony.]

SPIRITUS CALAMI AROMATICI. P. Calamus root ℔j, spirit of wine (at ·863) ℔viij; macerate for 4 days, and distil nearly to dryness.

SPIRITUS CARYOPHYLLI. P. From Cloves, as Sp. Calami.

SPIRITUS CAMPHORÆ. *Tinctura Camphoræ.* L. Camphor ℥v, rectified spirit Oij; dissolve.

SPIRITUS CARDAMOMI. L. 1746. Cardamom seed ℥iv, proof spirit Cj, water q. s.; distil Cj, (o. m.)

SPIRITUS CARUI. L. Caraway seed ℥xxij, proof spirit Cj, water Oij; mix, and distil Cj. E. Bruised caraway ℔ss, proof spirit Ovij; macerate for 2 days in a covered vessel; add water Ojss, and distil off Ovij.

SPIRITUS CASSIÆ. E. Cassia in coarse powder ℔j. Proceed as for spirit of caraway.

SPIRITUS CINNAMOMI. L. Oil of cinnamon ʒij, proof spirit Cj, water Oj; distil Cj. [Formerly made from the bark, ℥xv of which may be substituted for the oil. E. directs Ovij to be distilled from ℔j of cinnamon, as Sp. Carui.]

SPIRITUS COCHLEARIÆ. P. Fresh leaves of scurvy grass ℔ix, rectified spirit ℔vj; distil ℔v.

SPIRITUS COCHLEARIÆ COMPOSITUS. P. Fresh scurvy-grass ℔v, spirit (density ·863) ℔vj, horse-radish ℥viij; distil ℔v.

SPIRITUS COLCHICI AMMONIATUS. *Tinctura Colchici Composita.*

SPIRITUS COLONIENSIS. See Aqua Coloniensis.

SPIRITUS CORNU CERVI. See Liquor Volatilis C. C.

SPIRITUS FORMICARUM. PRUS. PH. Ants ℔j, rectified spirit ℔j, water ℔ij; distil ℔ij.

SPIRITUS FULIGINIS. L. 1746. Distilled from wood-soot, as Liq. Vol. C. C. An alcoholic spirit is also made from 1 part of wood-soot, 5 of proof spirit, 15 of water; distil 4 parts.

SPIRITUS JUNIPERI COMPOSITUS. L. Juniper berries ℥xv, caraway seed ℥ij, fennel seed ℥ij, proof spirit Cj, water Oij; distil Cj. E. nearly the same, with 2 days' maceration.

SPIRITUS LAVANDULÆ. L. & E. Fresh lavender flowers ℔ijss, rectified spirit Cj [water Oij, L.]; distil Cj [Ovij, E.] D. directs proof spirit, and Ov to be distilled. [As a perfume various additions are usually made.]

Spiritus Lavandulæ Compositus. E. Spirit of lavender Oij, spirit of rosemary f ℥xij, cinnamon in coarse powder ℥j, bruised cloves ʒij, nutmeg ʒiv, red sandal-wood f ʒiij. Digest for 7 days, and strain. D. directs f ℥xlviij of sp. of lavender, f ℥xvj of sp. rosemary, ℥ss of nutmeg and cinnamon, ʒij of cloves, f ℥j of red saunders. [For L. see Tinctura Lavandulæ Composita.]

Spiritus Limonis. P. As Spiritus Aurantii.

Spiritus Marjoranæ. From sweet marjoram, as Spir. Salviæ.

Spiritus Mastiches Compositus. Mastic ℥j, myrrh ℥j, olibanum ℥j; rectified spirit Oj; distil.

Spiritus Melissæ Compositus. P. *Eau de Carmes.* Fresh balm in flower ℥xxiv, lemon-peel ℥iv, cinnamon ℥ij, cloves ℥ij, nutmeg ℥ij, coriander seed ℥j, dry angelica root ℥j, rectified spirit ℔viij; macerate for 8 days, and distil in water-bath to dryness.

Spiritus Menthæ Viridis; Spiritus Menthæ Piperitæ; Spiritus Menthæ Pulegii. L. Essential oil ʒiij, proof spirit Cj, water Oj; distil Cj. E. directs Spiritus Menthæ to be prepared from ℔jss of fresh peppermint, as Sp. Carui.

Spiritus Mindereri. See Liquor Ammoniæ Acetatis.

Spiritus Myristicæ. L. & E. (Sp. Nucis Moschatæ, D.) Bruised nutmeg ℥ijss, proof spirit Cj, water Oj; distil Cj. D. directs a previous maceration for 24 hours.

Spiritus Pimentæ. L. Pimento ℥ijss, proof spirit Cj, water Oj; distil Cj. E. as Sp. Carui.

Spiritus Origani. From wild marjoram; as Spir. Salviæ.

Spiritus Pini Turionum. Buds of spruce fir ℔iij, proof spirit ℔vj, water ℔j; distil ℔iv.

Spiritus Pulegii. See Spiritus Menthæ Pulegii.

Spiritus Pyroaceticus. See Naphtha Medicinalis.

Spiritus Rectificatus. The specific gravity of rectified spirit should be 0·838 at 62° [L.]; 0·838 at 60° [E.]; or 0·840 at 60°, or 0·844 at 51° [D.]

Spiritus Rectificatissimus. A stronger spirit, sp. gr. 0·822 to 0·830, is directed in some foreign pharmacopœias.

Spiritus Rosmarini. L. Oil of rosemary ʒij, rectified spirit

Cj, water Oj; mix, and let Cj distil. A superior product is obtained from the fresh herb. L. 1815. Rosemary tops ℔ijss (℔ij to the old gallon), rectified spirit Cj, water q. s.; macerate for 24 hours, and distil a gallon. E. The same, distilling only Ovij. D. ℔jss of the fresh herb, Cj o. m. of proof spirit; distil Ov.

SPIRITUS ROSMARINÆ COMPOSITUS. *Hungary Water*. WIRT. PH. Flowering rosemary ℔iv, sage ℥vj, ginger ℥ij, proof spirit ℔xij, water ℔ij; distil ℔xj. But the original recipe for the Queen of Hungary's water is said to be—Rectified spirit 3 parts, rosemary tops 2 parts; distil.

SPIRITUS RUBI IDÆI. Raspberries ℔iij, rectified spirit ℔ij, distil ℔ij.

SPIRITUS SALIS AMMONIACI. L. 1746. Liquor Ammonia Sesquicarbonatis.

SPIRITUS SALIS AMMONIACI DULCIS. L. 1746. Spiritus Ammoniæ.

SPIRITUS SALIS MARINI. Acidum Hydrochloricum.

SPIRITUS SALVIÆ. Flowering sage ℔j, rectified spirit ℔iij, water ℔j; distil ℔iij.

SPIRITUS SALVIÆ COMPOSITUS. See Sp. Vulnerarius.

SPIRITUS SAPONIS. Spanish soap ℥j, rectified spirit ℥iij, rose water ℥j; digest.

SPIRITUS SASSAFRAS. P. As Spiritus Calami.

SPIRITUS TENUIOR. *Proof Spirit.* L. directs the density to be 0·920 at 62°;—E. (1839) 0·920 at 60°;—D. 0·919 at 60°. It may be made by mixing Ov of rectified spirit with Oiij of distilled water. E. 1841, directs it to be made by mixing Oij of rectified spirit with Oj of water, forming a spirit at 0·912. P. (*alcohol faible*) 0·923.

SPIRITUS TEREBINTHINÆ. See Oleum Terebinthinæ Rectificatum.

SPIRITUS TEREBINTHINÆ ÆTHEREUS. CADET. Alcohol ℔ij, oil of turpentine ℔ss; mix, and add gradually, strong nitric acid ℔ij; distil one half at a gentle heat. VAN MONS substitutes, spirit of nitric æther, with as much rectified oil of turpentine as it will dissolve. [Rectified oil of turpentine is also termed *æthereal spirit of turpentine.*]

Spiritus Terebinthinæ Compositus. See Balsamum Fiovarenti.

Spiritus Thymi. From Thyme, as Spiritus Salviæ.

Spiritus Venalis. *Alcohol du Commerce.* An unrectified spirit of wine is used in many of the compounds of P. The sp. gr. 0·863, or about 41 over proof.

Spiritus Vini Gallici. *Brandy.* Spirit distilled from French wines.

Spiritus Volatilis Aromaticus. See Sp. Ammoniæ Aromaticus.

Spiritus Vulnerarius. P. *Arquebusade.* Fresh leaves of basil, calamint, hyssop, marjoram, balm, mint, origanum, rosemary, sage, mother of thyme, common thyme, wormwood, angelica, fennel, rue, flowering tops of St. John's wort, and of lavender, of each ℥j; proof spirit Oiij. Macerate for 6 days, and distil Oij.

Spongia Cerata. Fine sponge, washed and dried, is dipped into melted bees'-wax, pressed between heated tin plates, and left till cold. It is then cut into suitable pieces, to be used as tents.

Spongia Preparata. Washed sponge, still wet, is bound tightly with string, and placed in a warm room to dry. Sometimes it is previously dipped in white of egg, or mucilage of tragacanth.

Spongia Usta. U. S. Cut sponge into pieces, beat it, and burn it in a close iron vessel until it becomes black and friable. See Pulvis Spongiæ.

Stanni Oxydum. Swediaur. Keep pure tin melted in an open vessel till it is entirely converted into a gray powder; triturate, and sift it.

Stanni Pulvis. See Pulvis Stanni. Tin is also divided by rasping or filing.

Stanni Sulphuretum. *Aurum Musivum.* P. Melt 12 parts of tin with the lowest possible heat in an earthen crucible, add 6 parts of quicksilver, and triturate the amalgam with 7 parts of sulphur and 6 of sal ammoniac. Introduce the mixture into a glass matrass, and heat gradually in a sand-bath till white vapours are disengaged; maintain a gentle heat till these cease, then break the matrass, and remove the golden scales from the darker matter.

STRYCHNIA. L. *Strychnine*, or *Strychnia*. Extract of nux-vomica, made with rectified spirit, is dissolved in cold water, and the filtered solution evaporated to syrup; to this, while yet warm, magnesia is added to saturation. Stir the mixture, set it aside for 2 days, then pour off the supernatant liquor. Press the residue in cloth, boil it in rectified spirit, filter, and distil off the spirit. Digest the residue with a gentle heat, in diluted sulphuric acid mixed with water; set aside for 24 hours, that crystals may form; press, and dissolve them in water, and add ammonia to throw down the strychnia. Dissolve this in boiling spirit, and set aside to crystallize. E. Take ℔j of nux-vomica steam it, slice it, dry it thoroughly, and grind it. Macerate it in Oij of water for 12 hours, boil it, strain, press, and repeat the maceration and decoction twice with Ojss of water. Concentrate the decoctions to the consistence of thin syrup, add ℥jss of lime in the form of milk of lime, dry the precipitate in a vapour-bath, pulverize it, and boil with successive portions of rectified spirit, till the spirit ceases to acquire a bitter taste. Distil off the spirit till the residuum is sufficiently concentrated to crystallize on cooling. Purify the crystals by repeated crystallizations. [Strychnine is more readily obtained, and in greater purity, from St. Ignatius's Bean.] The usual dose of strychnia and its salts to commence with is 1-12th of a grain, or from 1-16th to 1-10th, to be slowly increased, carefully watching its effects. MAGENDIE says the salts are more active than their base.

STRYCHNIÆ ACETAS. Mix one part of powdered strychnine with 5 of boiling distilled water, and add acetic acid till the strychnine is dissolved; filter, concentrate, and crystallize. A slight excess of acid favours the crystallization.

STRYCHNIÆ HYDROCHLORAS. *Muriate* or *Hydrochlorate of Strychnine*. As the acetate, substituting muriatic for acetic acid.

STRYCHNIÆ HYDRIODAS. M. Mix a solution of iodide of potassium with a strong solution of acetate of strychnia; wash the precipitated powder with a little cold water, and dry it carefully.

STRYCHNIÆ IODAS. M. Saturate powdered strychnine with a concentrated solution of iodic acid; treat the mass with boiling alcohol, filter, and let it evaporate spontaneously.

STRYCHNIÆ NITRAS. Saturate warm diluted nitric acid with strychnia, filter, concentrate, and crystallize. A *binitrate* may be obtained by adding to the solution a portion of nitric acid equal to that first employed.

STRYCHNIÆ PHOSPHAS. As the sulphate, substituting phosphoric for sulphuric acid.

STRYCHNIÆ SULPHAS. P. Mix 1 part of powdered strychnine with 5 parts of boiling water, and add sulphuric acid diluted with 5 parts of water, just sufficient to dissolve the strychnine; filter, and crystallize by refrigeration. To form the *bisulphate,* double the quantity of acid.

STYRAX COLATUS. L. Dissolve storax in rectified spirit, strain, and distil off the spirit with a gentle heat till the storax becomes of a proper consistence.

SUBLIMATIS CORROSIVUS. E. See Hydrargyri Bichloridum.

SUCCI ÆTHERIZATI. M. BOUCHARDAT'S *Sucs éthérés.* To the expressed juice of plants, so much æther is added, that after agitating them together, a thin layer of æther rises to the surface. After 24 hours, remove the supernatant æther, by means of a pipette, filter the juice, and return the æther. Preserve the ætherized juice in well-stoppered bottles, and when any of the juice is required, reverse the bottle, that the æther may remain behind. The ætherized juices are said to retain their active properties for an indefinite period. The method is applied with marked advantage to the juice of aconite, anemone, black hellebore, and hemlock. It is probably applicable to many infusions, decoctions, and fluid extracts, as well as to expressed juices.

SUCCI ALCOHOLATI. Juices preserved with spirit. The *Alcoolatures* of M. BERAL. These are prepared from fresh plants, either by adding rectified spirit to the expressed juice, or by digesting the bruised leaves with the spirit before pressing. The latter method, which is adopted in the Paris Codex, is noticed under TINCTURÆ. The *preserved juices* lately introduced into use in this country are prepared according to the following process:—The leaves of the mature plants [when more than half the flowers are fully blown, Mr. SQUIRE,] are bruised in a marble mortar, and placed in a powerful press. The expressed juice is allowed to stand for 24 hours, it is then poured off from the dregs, and rectified spirit added: after standing 24 hours the liquid is filtered. Mr. BENTLEY directs one measure of rectified spirit to be added to four of juice. Mr. SQUIRE, one of spirit to two of juice. The *Homœopathists* usually employ equal parts of spirit and juice, the latter being generally expressed from the *whole* flowering plant, and immediately mixed with the spirit. In some cases they use double or triple the quantity of spirit. GIESKE directs one part by weight of spirit to five of juice. BERAL, and the SAXON PH. direct equal weights. The principal preserved juices used in this country are those of Aconite, Belladonna, Digitalis, Hemlock, Henbane, &c. These are all prepared according to the above directions, from the fresh plants.

SUCCI ANTISCORBUTICI. Succus Cochleariæ Compositus. L. 1788. Juice of scurvy-grass, oranges, water-cresses, each Ojss, spirit of nutmeg f ℥viij. P. Leaves of water-cresses, scurvy-grass, and buck bean, in equal parts. Bruise, express, and filter through paper.

SUCCI EXPRESSI. The juices of fresh plants are obtained by bruising them in a marble mortar, and expressing them in an iron or wooden press. Some plants, having little juice (as the labiate plants) or of a viscous nature (as borage and cabbage), require the addition of an eighth of water. The expressed juices should be filtered cold if practicable; but some (as red cabbage, &c.) require to be previously heated, so as to coagulate their albuminous matter. The acid juices of fruits are allowed to clear themselves by a slight fermentation, in a cool place, before filtering. Buckthorn berries, mulberries, and elder berries, are left for 3 or 4 days, after being crushed between the hands, before pressing. Cherries, barberries, and grapes, are crushed in the hands over a hair sieve, the marc pressed, and the mixed juice allowed to ferment for two days, then filtered, and preserved by Appert's process. Some juices, as those of currants and raspberries, have their clarification remarkably expedited by the addition of the juice of cherries. The expression of quinces, oranges, &c., is facilitated by mixing the crushed fruit with clean chopped rye straw. [APPERT'S mode of preserving vegetable juices is, to bottle them, secure the corks with wire, and place the bottles up to their necks in cold water, with straw between them to prevent breakage; heat to boiling, and when the water has boiled for a few minutes, remove the bottles, and when cool cover the corks with wax or pitch. Juices are also preserved by the addition of alcohol or æther. See Succi Alcoholati; and Succi Ætherizati.]

SUCCI SPISSATI. Inspissated juices are now included among the extracts. See Extracta.

SUCCUS COLCHICI. Mr. BENTLEY directs the cormi, gathered in August, to be bruised and pressed; after the juice has stood for 48 hours, f℥iv of rectified spirit is added to f℥xvj of juice, and afterwards filtered.

SUCCUS GLYCYRRHIZÆ. The foreign extract of liquorice is so named. For a method of purifying it see Extractum Glycyrrhizæ.

SUCCUS HERBARUM COMMIXTARUM. P. Leaves of wild succory, fumitory, borage, and chervil, equal parts. Bruise, express, and filter in a cool place. [A little oil poured on the surface of these juices, in small bottles, will preserve them for a considerable time.]

SUCCUS IRIDIS PALUSTRIS. The fresh juice of the root of yellow flag. Purgative; dose, 80 drops in *Dropsy.*

SUCCUS LIMONIS. GUIBOURT. Peel the lemons, tear with the hand, and place in a cloth with alternate layers of washed rye straw, and press. Strain the juice, leave it in glass or stoneware bottles for five days, then decant, and filter through paper. Unless the seeds are removed, the fruit should be pressed without delay, or the juice will be bitter.

SUCCUS LIMONIS FACTITIUS. Dr. PEREIRA. Citric acid ʒviijss, essence of lemon 4 drops, water f℥xvj.

SUCCUS MALORUM. GUY'S H. *Verjuice.* Bruise crab apples in a mortar, and express the juice. The *Verjus* of the Paris Codex is expressed from grapes. [The other simple juices are prepared according to the general directions above. See Succi Expressi.]

SUCCUS TARAXACI. From the fresh roots, or from the whole flowering plant, as Succus Colchici. For Dr. COLLIER'S mode, see Cremor Taraxaci.

SUFFUMIGATIO. See Fumigatio.

SULPHAS POTASSÆ CUM SULPHURE. See Potassæ Sulphas, &c. See their respective bases for the other sulphates.

SULPHOFORMUM. *Sulphoform.* An oily liquid, obtained by distilling one part of iodoform with three of sulphuret of mercury.

SULPHUR LOTUM. L. 1824. Sublimed sulphur, washed with hot water till all acidity is removed, and dried.

SULPHUR PRECIPITATUM. L. 1824. *Milk of Sulphur.* Boil

together ℔j of sublimed sulphur, ℔ij of quicklime, in Civ of water, filter, and add muriatic acid q. s. to throw down the sulphur. Wash this plentifully with water, until tasteless. [A great part of the commercial *Lac Sulphuris* is precipitated by sulphuric instead of muriatic acid; and consequently contains about half its weight of sulphate of lime.]

SULPHUR SUBLIMATUM. *Flowers of Sulphur.* Sulphur is heated up to 500° or 600° in an earthen vessel, and sublimed into a chamber, or large receiver. Sulphur Sublimatum E. is Sulphur Lotum.

SULPHURIS CARBURETUM. See Carbonis Bisulphuretum.

SULPHURIS HYPOCHLORIDUM. Spread washed sulphur thinly in a proper vessel, or chamber, and pass chlorine gas slowly into it till the sulphur is saturated. Keep it in well-stopped bottles from which the light is excluded.

SULPHURIS IODIDUM. M. and U. S. Mix ℥iv of iodine with ℥j of sulphur in a glass or porcelain mortar; put the mixture into a matrass, close the orifice loosely, and apply a gentle heat sufficient to darken the mass without melting it. When the whole is uniformly darkened, increase the heat so as to melt the iodide, inclining the matrass in different directions. Allow the matrass to cool, break it, and put the iodide into well-stoppered bottles.

SUPPOSITORIUM ANTHELMINTICUM. SWEDIAUR. Aloes ʒiv, muriate of soda ʒiij, flour ʒij, inspissated honey q. s. Divide into suppositories of about 15 grains each. BOERHAAVE. Inspissated honey ℥iv, aloes ℥ss, sulphate of iron ℈ij; mix, and divide into small suppositories.

SUPPOSITORIUM ASTRINGENS. REUSS. Powdered oak-bark ʒij, tormentil ʒij, honey q. s.; make 8 suppositories. See Supp. Rhataniæ.

SUPPOSITORIUM COLOCYNTHIDIS. SPAN. PH. Colocynth ʒss, muriate of soda ʒj, honey ʒj; evaporate to a proper consistence.

SUPPOSITORIUM COMMUNE. Common salt and honey, boiled till sufficiently stiff.

SUPPOSITORIUM COPAIBÆ. COLOMBAT. Solidified copaiva ℈j, butter of cacao ʒj, extract of opium gr. ss.

SUPPOSITORIUM ELATERII. St. B. H. Extract of elaterium gr. ij, hard soap gr. x, flour gr. x, water q. s. Mix.

SUPPOSITORIUM EMOLLIENS. Butter of cacao (oleum concretum cacao) and spermaceti, in equal parts, melted together.

SUPPOSITORIUM HÆMORRHOIDALE. RICHARD. Butter of cacao ʒij, extract of opium gr. j, extract of stramonium gr. j. *For 2 suppositories.*

SUPPOSITORIUM HYDRARGYRI CUM CONIO. Extract of hemlock gr. iv, black oxide of quicksilver gr. iij, suet gr. viij or q. s.; mix.

SUPPOSITORIUM IRRITANS. RICHARD. Butter of cacao ʒij, aloes gr. iv, tartarized antimony gr. j. GAUBIUS. Aloes ℈j, salt ℈j, colocynth gr. v, honey q. s. *To restore the hæmorrhoidal flux.*

SUPPOSITORIUM IODIDI POTASSII. Mr. STAFFORD. Iodide of potassium gr. j to iv, extract of henbane gr. vj, extract of hemlock gr. vj. *In enlarged prostate.*

SUPPOSITORIUM LAXATIVUM. GAUBIUS. Soap ℥j, muriate of soda ʒss, inspissated honey q. s.

SUPPOSITORIUM OPII. St. B. H. Opium gr. ij, hard soap gr. x; mix.

SUPPOSITORIUM QUINÆ. BOUDIN. Sulphate of quinine gr. xv, butter of cacao ʒjss; mix.

SUPPOSITORIUM RHATANIÆ. BRETONNEAU. Butter of cacao ʒij, extract of rhatany gr. xv.

SUPPOSITORIUM SAPONIS. A cone of hard soap is sometimes employed as a laxative suppository.

SUPPOSITORIUM SEDATIVUM. See Supp. Opii, and Supp. Hæmorrhoidale.

SUPPOSITORIUM VAGINALE. GAUDRIOT. Liquid chloride of zinc ♏v, sulphate of morphia gr. ss; mix with ℥ij of the following paste. Thick mucilage of tragacanth 6 parts, white sugar 3, starch 9. Mr. DRUITT prescribes, in *Leucorrhœa*, tannin, gr. x, mucilage of tragacanth q. s.

SYRUPI. Syrups are solutions of sugar in watery liquids. "They should be kept in a place the temperature of which never exceeds 55° F." [L.] Refined sugar is to be used except when otherwise directed. The usual proportions are two parts by weight of sugar to one of liquid, which is nearly the ratio in L. 1824; but the proportion of sugar was increased in 1836.

M. GUIBOURT states that the most perfect syrup consists of 30 parts of sugar to 16 of water. The general directions of D. are to dissolve 29 ounces of refined sugar in fine powder, in 16 fluid ounces of the liquor prescribed, by a gentle heat and frequent agitations; in 24 hours remove the scum, and pour off from the dregs. U. S. & P. direct the specific gravity of syrups to be 1·261 boiling, and 1·319 cold, corresponding with 30° and 35° of Baumé's saccharometer.

SYRUPUS. L. Syrupus Simplex. E. Sugar ℔x, water [boiling, E.] Oiij; dissolve the sugar in the water by a gentle heat. D. directs, powdered sugar ℥xxix, water f℥xvj. U. S. ℔ijss to f℥xvj.

SYRUPUS SIMPLEX ALBUS. P. Very white sugar ℔ij, water ℔j; dissolve without heat, add ℥ij of animal charcoal, and in 12 hours filter through paper.

SYRUPUS ABSINTHII. P. Wormwood ℥ij, boiling water ℥xvj; infuse for 12 hours, strain, and add to the filtered liquor twice its weight of sugar. [Cold water would probably afford a more elegant product.]

SYRUPUS ACETI. E. French vinegar f℥xj, white sugar ℥xiv; boil them together.

SYRUPUS ACETI RUBI IDÆI. P. Raspberry vinegar ℥xvj, sugar ℥xxx; dissolve by a gentle heat in a glass vessel, and strain.

SYRUPUS ACETATIS MORPHIÆ. See Syrupus Morphiæ.

SYRUPUS ACIDI CITRICI. P. Dissolve ʒijss of citric acid in ʒv of water, and add it to ℥xvj (f℥xiij) of boiling syrup.

SYRUPUS CUM ACIDO HYDROCYANICO. P. Medicinal hydrocyanic acid (containing 10 per cent. of real acid) ʒj, syrup ℥xvj. There is no formula for it in this kingdom.

SYRUPUS ACIDI PHOSPHORICI. Phosphoric acid (sp. gr. 1·454) ℥ss, syrup ℥xxxij. [Syrup of raspberries may be substituted for simple syrup.]

SYRUPUS ACIDI TARTARICI. P. As Syrupus Acidi Citrici.

SYRUPUS ACONITI. As Syrupus Belladonnæ. P.

SYRUPUS ADIANTHI. *Capillaire.* P. Maidenhair ℥iv, boiling water Oijss; infuse, strain, add refined sugar ℔v, make a syrup, and clarify with white of egg. Pour the boiling syrup into a water-bath with ℥ij of maidenhair, infuse for two hours, and strain.

SYRUPUS ÆTHERIS. P. *Sirop d'Æther.* Sulphuric æther ℥j, white syrup ℥xvj; mix in a glass vessel having a tap at the lower part, and shake them occasionally for five or six days; when quite clear draw it off into small bottles.

SYRUPUS ALKALINUS. DEVERGIE. Bicarbonate of soda ℥ss, syrup ℥viij. Dose, ʒj three times a day.

SYRUPUS ALLII. D. Garlic sliced ℔j, boiling water f℥xxxij; macerate for 12 hours, strain the infusion, and make a syrup with twice its weight of sugar. U. S. Garlic ℥vj, distilled vinegar f℥xvj; macerate for four days, express, and form a syrup with the clear liquor, and sugar ℔ij.

SYRUPUS ALLII COMPOSITUS. Dr. WILLIS'S Syrup. Garlic cut small ℥ss, bruised aniseed ℥ss, elecampane root ʒiij, liquorice root 3ij, brandy f℥xxiv; digest for two or three days, strain, and form a syrup with ℔jss of sugar.

SYRUPUS ALTHÆÆ. L. Fresh marsh-mallow root ℥viij, water Oiv; boil to Oij, set aside for 24 hours, decant, and make a syrup with ℔ijss of sugar. D. & E. nearly the same.

SYRUP AMYGDALÆ. U. S. (*Sirop d'Orgeat.* P.) Blanch ℔j of sweet, and ℥iv of bitter almonds, and beat them to a paste with f℥iij of water, and ℔j of white sugar; mix the paste thoroughly with f℥xlv of water, strain with strong expression, and dissolve ℔v of sugar in the strained emulsion by the aid of a gentle heat; strain the syrup through fine linen, and keep it in well-closed bottles in a cool place. [P. nearly the same, with the addition of ℥vj of orange-flower water.]

SYRUPUS ANISI. Infuse ʒss of bruised aniseed in ℥iv of hot water; strain, and add 3ij of sugar. For infants.

SYRUPUS ANTHEMIDIS. Chamomile flowers ℔j, boiling water ℔iv; macerate, strain with expression, and form the infusion into a syrup with twice its weight of sugar.

SYRUPUS ANTIMONIATUS. Kermes mineral ℈j, syrup of squills ℥jss, syrup of althæa ℥jss; mix.

SYRUPUS ANTISCORBUTICUS. P. Fresh leaves of scurvy-grass, buck-bean, water-cresses, of each ℔j, horse-radish ℔j, bitter orange-peel ℔j, cinnamon 3iv, white wine ℔iv; macerate two days, distil off ℔j, and add to the distilled liquor half the sugar; strain what remains, decant, and make a syrup with the rest of the sugar; clarify it with white of egg, and when cold add the former syrup.

Syrupus Armoraciæ. Dr. Cullen. Scraped horse-radish ℥j, hot water f℥viij; digest, strain, and dissolve in the liquor twice its weight of sugar. Dose, f℥j frequently, *in hoarseness from relaxation.*

Syrupus Armoraciæ Compositus. See Syrupus Antiscorbuticus.

Syrupus Artemisiæ. From dried mug-wort; as Syr. Absinthii.

Syrupus Artemisiæ Compositus. P. Take of fresh tops of mugwort, pennyroyal, catmint, and savine, each ℥vj, fresh roots of elecampane, lovage, and fennel, each ℨiv, tops of wild marjoram, hyssop, feverfew, rue, and basil, each ℥iijss, aniseed ʒix, cinnamon ℨix, all properly divided; mix ℥xxxij of honey with ℔xxj of water, pour it on the herbs, and let them macerate in a warm place for three days; draw off ʒviij of aromatic liquor, in which dissolve ℥xvj of sugar in a close vessel; strain what remains in the still with expression, and form a syrup with the clear liquor and ℔v ℥iv of sugar; clarify the syrup with white of eggs, and when half cooled add the syrup made with the distilled liquor.

Syrupus Asclepiadis. Dr. Hamilton. Expressed juice of the blood-flower plant (asclepias curassavica), boiled with twice its weight of sugar. Dose, fℨj to fℨiv. *Purgative, emetic,* and *vermifuge.*

Syrupus Asparagi. P. Juice of asparagus ℔j, sugar ℔ij; make a syrup.

Syrupus Aquæ Aurantii. P. Orange-flower water ℔j, very white sugar ℔ij; dissolve and filter. (Similar syrups are made from the distilled waters of Cinnamon, Rose, Peppermint, and Lettuce. P.)

Syrupus Aurantii. L. & E. Fresh orange-peel ℥ijss, boiling water Oj; macerate 12 hours, strain, add sugar ℔iij, and make a syrup.

Syrupus e Succo Aurantiorum. E. 1744. Orange-juice ℔j, sugar ℔ij.

Syrupus Auri. F. H. Powdered gold ℈j, syrup of gum ℥j. *As a local application.*

Syrupus Balsami Peruviani. Prus. Ph. Balsam of Peru ℥j, boiling water ℥xvj; agitate, infuse till cold, and form the filtered liquor into a syrup with ℥xxiv of sugar.

Syrupus Balsami Tolutani. See Syrupus Tolutanus.

SYRUPUS BELLADONNÆ. P. Extract of belladonna gr. xxxij, dissolve in ʒiv of boiling water, and add it to ℥xvj of boiling syrup.

SYRUPUS BERBERIS. As Syrupus Cydoniæ.

SYRUPUS BORAGINIS. P. Dissolve two parts of sugar in one part of the clarified juice of borage, by the heat of a water-bath, and strain.

SYRUPUS BRASSICÆ RUBRÆ. From juice of red cabbage, as Syrupus Boraginis.

SYRUPUS CAHINCÆ. SOUBEIRAN. Alcoholic extract of cahinca gr. lxiv, syrup ℥xvj; dissolve the extract in a little water, and add the solution to the boiling syrup. Dose, ℥j daily.

SYRUPUS CALCIS. TROUSSEAU. Slake ʒijss of quicklime with f℥iij of water, and add it to ℥xxxij of simple syrup; boil 10 minutes, and filter. This is usually diluted with four parts of simple syrup. *In Diarrhœa.*

SYRUPUS CAPRIFOLII. P. From honeysuckle; as Syrupus Violæ.

SYRUPUS CARYOPHYLLI. E. Clove July flowers ℥j, boiling water f℥iv; macerate for 12 hours, strain, and add sugar ℥vij; make a syrup.

SYRUPUS CATECHU. P. Dissolve 128 grains of extract of catechu in ℥ij of water, and add it to ℥xvj of boiling syrup. Contains gr. j of catechu in each ʒj.

SYRUPUS CERASORUM. P. Depurated juice of cherries ℥xvj, sugar ℥xxx; make a syrup.

SYRUPUS CEREFOLII. From the juice of cultivated chervil; as Syrupus Boraginis.

SYRUPUS CHLORIDI CALCIS. Dr. REID. Liquid chloride of lime ʒj, mucilage 3ij, syrup of orange-peel 3x.

SYRUPUS CHONDRI. MOUCHON. Boil ℥viij of carrageen in Oiij of water for half an hour, strain with pressure, and boil the clear liquor with ℔x of syrup till the whole is reduced to ℔x.

SYRUPUS CINCHONÆ. BRANDE. Extract of bark ʒij, syrup of orange-peel f℥ij. P. directs ℥iij of gray bark to be boiled for half an hour in Oj¾ of water, the strained decoction reduced to half, and boiled to a syrup with ℥xvj of white sugar; when cold, filter through paper.

SYRUPUS CINCHONÆ CONCENTRATUS. Mr. DONOVAN. Digest ℥viij of yellow bark in coarse powder in two successive pints of proof spirit, and press strongly; boil the residue for half an hour with a pint of water, strain, and press; repeat this a second and third time; evaporate the mixed decoctions to f℥viij; reduce also the mixed tinctures to f℥viij; mix the concentrated liquors, and boil them with a solution of 55 grains of oxalic acid and 284 grains of dry quinine; add ℥xxj of sugar and ℥iv of gum arabic, and water q. s. to make f℥xxxij of syrup, which strain while hot, through flannel. Mr. D. considers f℥j of this syrup equal to three or four ounces of the decoction.

SYRUPUS CINCHONÆ VINOSUS. P. Soft extract of bark ʒvij, white wine ℥xvj; dissolve, filter, add ℔ij of white sugar, and dissolve in a close vessel.

SYRUPUS CINCHONINÆ. M. Sulphate of cinchonine ℈ij, syrup ℥xvj.

SYRUPUS COCCI ALKALINUS. Cochineal in powder ℈ij, subcarbonate of potash ℈iv; triturate, and add boiling distilled water f℥xvj; strain, add ℥iv of sugar candy. [A popular domestic remedy for hooping cough. Dose, from a tea-spoonful to a table-spoonful, according to the age of the child, 3 or 4 times a day.]

SYRUPUS COCHLEARIÆ. P. Juice of scurvy-grass ℔j, sugar ℔ij. Make a syrup.

SYRUPUS COCHLEARIÆ ARMORACIÆ. See Syr. Armoraciæ.

SYRUPUS CODEIÆ. Codeia gr. xxiv, water f℥iv, sugar ℥viij. Dose, ʒj, in *Hooping Cough.*

SYRUPUS COLCHICI. E. 1817. Fresh colchicum ℥j, vinegar f℥xvj; macerate for 2 days, and strain with gentle expression; add to the clear liquor ℥xxvj of sugar, and boil.

SYRUPUS CONIÆ. *Sirop de Conicine Magistral.* M. VILLE. Simple syrup ʒxiij, conicine 1 drop, alcoholized sulphuric acid 1 drop. Dose, f ʒj.

SYRUPUS COPAIBÆ. PUCHE. Triturate ℥ij of copaiva with ℥ss of powdered gum, and ℥jss water; add 32 drops of essence of peppermint, and ℥xij of simple syrup. Dose, ʒij to ℥j.

SYRUPUS CRESCENTIÆ. Fresh juice of the pulp of calabash (crescentia cujete) boiled with sugar q. s. Prepared in the West Indies. Pectoral, against inward bruises, and in large doses purgative.

Syrupus Croci. L. Saffron ʒx, boiling distilled water Oj; macerate for 12 hours, strain, add ℔iij of refined sugar. [P. Saffron ℥j, malaga wine ℥xvj, sugar ℥xxiv.]

Syrupus Cydoniæ. P. Clarified juice of quinces ℥xvj, sugar ʒxxx, dissolve by a gentle heat. [In the same way syrups are prepared from other fruits.]

Syrupus Cynoglossi. Fuller. Clarified juice of hounds-tongue boiled with its weight of sugar to a syrup. In catarrhous humours.

Syrupus Depurativus. See Syrupus Sarzæ Compositus (Cuisinier's). Some recipes add to each ℔ of the syrup gr. j of corrosive sublimate. See Syrupus Hydrargyri.

Syrupus Dianthi Caryophylli. See Syr. Carophylli.

Syrupus Dictamni. From Dittany of Crete, as Syr. Hyssopi.

Syrupus Digitalis. P. Fox-glove leaves ℈viij, boiling water ℥xvj; infuse for 6 hours, strain the liquor, and make a syrup with twice its weight of sugar. [Guibourt substitutes—Alcoholic extract of digitalis 1 part, dissolved in 8 parts of water, and the filtered solution added to 300 parts of boiling syrup. It is twice the strength of the above. See also Oxysaccharum Digitalis.]

Syrupus Dulcamaræ. P. Infuse ℔j of dulcamara twigs in ℔jss of water for 12 hours, strain, and set aside the liquor, noting its weight. Infuse the residue in ℔iij of water, and strain. Mix this second liquor with ℔viij of syrup, and finish by operating as directed for Syrupus Helminthocorti.

Syrupus Emetinæ. M. Coloured emetine gr. xvj (or *pure* emetine gr. iv), simple syrup ℥vj; mix.

Syrupus Ergotæ. Soubeiran. Powdered ergot ℥jss, white wine ℥xj, macerate for a week, strain, express, filter, and dissolve in the liquor ℥xvj of sugar. [℥j contains ʒss of ergot.]

Syrupus Ergotinæ. Bonjean. Ergotine (Extractum Ergotæ Aquosum) ʒijss, orange-flower water ℥j; dissolve, and add the solution to ℥xvj of boiling syrup. Dose, 2 to 4 spoonfuls in the day.

Syrupus Erysimi. Waller. From the expressed juice of hedge mustard, as Syr. Boraginis; or from a decoction of the dry plant. *In old coughs, and hoarseness.*

SYRUPUS ERYSIMI COMPOSITUS. P. (*Sirop de Vélar.*) Boil ʒij each of pearled barley, raisins, and liquorice root, ℥iij each of dried borage and succory leaves, in ℔xvj of water till reduced to ℔iv; strain with pressure, and pour the boiling decoction on ℔iv of fresh hedge mustard, ℥iv elecampane root, ℥j of maidenhair, ℥ss dried rosemary, ℥ss of French lavender, ʒvj aniseed, all properly divided. Let them infuse for 24 hours, draw off by distillation ℥viij of aromatic liquor, in which dissolve ℥xvj of sugar. Strain the liquor left in the still, let it settle, add to the clear liquor ℔v ℥iv of sugar, and ℥xvj of white honey, boil to a syrup, clarify it, and when half cooled add the syrup prepared from the distilled liquor.

SYRUPUS EXPECTORANS. Dr. NELIGAN. Syrup of hemidesmus f℥iv, tincture of Tolu f℥ss, camphorated tincture of opium fʒj, ipecacuanha wine fʒiij, simple syrup f℥iij. A tablespoonful every 2 hours.

SYRUPUS FERRI. AIKIN. Sulphate of iron ℈iv, tartaric acid ℈ij, water f℥jss; dissolve in a Wedgwood dish, add caustic ammonia in slight excess, evaporate slowly nearly to dryness, redissolve in water with a few drops more ammonia, make it up f℥jss, add ℥ij of sugar, and boil for a minute.

SYRUPUS FERRI ALBUMINATIS. LASSAIGNE. Beat ℥iij of white of egg with ℥iij of distilled water, and filter. Pour into the liquor ʒix of a solution of persulphate of iron, the sp. gr. of which is 1·036. A precipitate falls, on which pour ℥jss of an alcoholic solution of potash, containing 4 per cent. of caustic potash. Agitate till dissolved, and add one and a half times its weight of powdered sugar; dissolve without heat, and filter.

SYRUPUS FERRI PROTOCHLORIDI. Mr. R. PHILLIPS. Mix 800 grains of hydrochloric acid (sp. gr. 1·16) with f℥iij of distilled water, and add 200 grains of iron turnings. Heat till all action has ceased, and filter the solution into f℥xij of thick syrup. Keep it in a stoppered bottle. It contains gr. x of iron in f℥j.

SYRUPUS FERRI PERCHLORIDI. Mr. PHILLIPS. Boil 286 grains of sesquioxide of iron in f℥ij of distilled water, previously mixed with 1200 grains of hydrochloric acid, and filter the solution into f℥xvj of thick syrup. The strength is half that of the tincture. [BERAL prescribes ℈j of dry perchloride of iron to ℥j of syrup.]

SYRUPUS FERRI ET QUINÆ CITRATIS. A syrup is prepared by

Mr. BULLOCK, under this name, but its composition has not been made known. Another form is, citrate of iron and quinine ℥j, syrup of orange-peel Oj.

SYRUPUS FERRI CITRATIS. BERAL. Liquid citrate of iron ℥j, syrup ℥xv, spirit of lemon ʒij. An improved form is, ammonio-citrate of iron gr. xvj, simple syrup ℥j, saccharide of vanilla and cloves (see Saccharum Vanillæ) gr. xvj.

SYRUPUS FERRI CITRATIS ALKALINUS. MIALHE. Syrup ℥xvj, citrate of iron ʒij; dissolve, and add ʒj of bicarbonate of soda.

SYRUPUS FERRI POTASSIO-CITRATIS. Dr. TODD. Solution of potassio-citrate of iron (see Liquor Ferri P. C.) f℥viij, white sugar ℥xvj. Dissolve.

SYRUPUS FERRI IODIDI. E. 1841. (*Substituted for Solutio Ferri Iodidi*, 1839.) Dry iodine 200 grs., clean thin iron wire 100 grs., white sugar in powder ℥ivss, distilled water f℥vj. Boil the iodine, wire, and water together in a glass matrass, at first gently, afterwards briskly, until f℥ij remain. Filter this quickly, while hot, into a matrass containing the sugar. Dissolve the sugar with a gentle heat, and add distilled water to make it up f℥vj. ♏xij contain gr. j of iodide of iron. Dr. A. T. THOMSON prefers a weaker syrup, containing only gr. iij in fʒj. It may be made as the last, using only ʒij of iodine instead of 200 grains. DUPASQUIER's syrup contains but 1 grain in an ounce. [These syrups keep better than the watery solution; they become coloured, however, after a time, but without any deposit taking place if the air is excluded; the colour may in a great measure be removed by boiling them with a little clean iron.]

SYRUPUS FERRI IODIDI COMPOSITUS. RICORD. This may be made by adding f℥j of the E. syrup to ℥ix of compound syrup of sarsaparilla. It contains gr. iv of iodide of iron in ℥j.

SYRUPUS FERRI IODIDI ET FERRI CHLORIDI. Mr. BATTLEY has proposed a syrup containing 3 grains of iodine and 4 of iron in each fʒj; but has not given the quantities of ingredients employed. It may be made as follows:—Diffuse ℥j of iodine in f℥iv of cold distilled water, and add gradually ℥jss of clean iron filings, agitating the mixture constantly till a green solution is obtained. Digest ʒx of iron filings with ℥ivss of muriatic acid (sp. gr. 1·160) till action ceases, and boil for a few minutes. Filter the solution rapidly into a vessel containing

℥xv of white sugar, washing the filters with a little warm water in which a little sugar has been dissolved. Gently heat the whole till the sugar is dissolved. It should measure Oj.

SYRUPUS FERRI ET QUINÆ IODIDI. BOUCHARDAT. Digest ʒj of iodine with ʒss of iron filings and ʒiv of water, with a gentle heat and frequent agitation, till the solution is colourless. Filter it rapidly into a vessel containing ℔ijss of simple syrup. Dissolve also gr. xij of sulphate of quinine in ʒij of water acidulated with sulphuric acid, and add to the former. Taken by spoonfuls, in *scrofulous affections.*

SYRUPUS FERRI LACTATIS. M. CAP. Lactate of iron ʒj, boiling distilled water ℥vj, pure sugar ℥xij. Dose, ℈ij to ʒiv.

SYRUPUS FERRI SUBCARBONATIS. M. MOUCHON. Sulphate of iron ʒjss, subcarbonate of potash ʒjss; powder separately, then triturate together with a little water to form a soft paste, and add this immediately to ℥viij of syrup of gum arabic.

SYRUPUS FERRI SULPHATIS. WILLIS. Sulphate of iron ʒj, water ʒij, syrup of gum ℥xvj.

SYRUPUS FERRI SULPHURETI. CAZENAVE. Sulphuret of iron in fine powder ʒj, syrup of soapwort ℥viij. Dose, f℥ss, twice a day, in *scrofula.*

SYRUPUS FERRI PERSULPHURETI. BOUCHARDAT. Reduce ℥x of syrup by evaporation to ℥ix, and add ℥ij of hydrated persulphuret of iron in a gelatinous state. Mix, and keep it in a close bottle. Give a tea-spoonful 2 or 3 times a day, in *scrofulous and cutaneous affections.* As an antidote for poisoning by the salts of lead, mercury, and copper, give a table-spoonful frequently.

SYRUPUS FERRI TANNATIS. M. BERAL. Simple syrup 375 parts, syrup of vinegar 125 parts, magnetic citrate of iron 10 parts, extract of galls 4 parts.

SYRUPUS FUMARIÆ. P. Clarified juice of fumitory ℔ij; white sugar ℔ij, boil to a syrup.

SYRUPUS GENTIANÆ. P. Gentian ʒxij, boiling water ℥xviij; infuse, strain, and make a syrup with ℥xxxij of sugar. [A more elegant syrup is made by percolating the powdered gentian with cold water.]

SYRUPUS GENTIANINÆ. M. Gentianine gr. xvj, syrup ℥xvj.

SYRUPUS GLECOMÆ. P. From dried ground-ivy, infused in its distilled water; as Syrupus Hyssopi.

Syrupus Geoffrœyæ. Dr. Wright. Decoction of cabbage-tree bark, made into a syrup with twice its weight of sugar. *Vermifuge.* Dose, 1 to 4 table-spoonfuls.

Syrupus Glycyrrhizæ. Liquorice-root ℥iv, boiling water ℥xvj, digest, strain, and make a syrup with sugar q. s.

Syrupus Granati Fructus. P. As Syr. Berberis.

Syrupus [corticis radicis] Granati. Guibourt. Obtain from ℔j of powdered bark of pomegranate root, ℔iv of infusion by percolation. Boil this with ℥xxij of syrup till reduced to ℔ij.

Syrupus Guaiaci. Guibourt. Boil ℔j of guaiacum-wood twice in ℔xij of water to ℔iv. Mix, and strain the decoctions, and mix with ℔iv of syrup, and boil to 30° Baumé boiling.

Syrupus Gummi Ammoniaci. Wurt. Ph. Dissolve ℨij of gum ammoniacum in ℥viij of white wine, by the heat of a water-bath, and add sugar ℥xvj.

Syrupus Gummi Arabici. P. Gum arabic (picked and twice washed for an instant in cold water) ℔j, cold water ℔j; stir them occasionally till the gum is dissolved, strain without expression, and mix it with ℔viij of syrup boiled to 29 degrees (sp. gr. 1·252) boiling.

Syrupus Gummi Tragacanthæ. Mouchon. Gum tragacanth ℥j, water ℥xxxij, macerate for 48 hours, press through linen cloth, and mix the mucilage with ℔viij of syrup heated to 176° F., and strain through coarse cloth. Guibourt directs ℨj of the gum to be macerated with ℥ij of water, strained, mixed with ℨvj of water, and heated with ℨxxxij of syrup. This is much thinner than the former.

Syrupus Hellebori Fœtidi. Sprinkle the fresh leaves of bear's-foot with vinegar, and express the juice. Boil this with twice its weight of sugar. Dose, a teaspoonful at bedtime for 2 or 3 days for children. But its use requires caution.

Syrupus Hemedesmi. Bruised root of hemedesmus Indicus ℔ss, boiling water Oj; digest in a covered vessel with a gentle heat for 3 or 4 hours, strain, add to the liquor twice its weight of refined sugar, and dissolve.

Syrupus Helminthocorti. P. Macerate ℔j of cleansed Corsican moss in ℔ij of warm water; in 24 hours, strain with pressure, filter the liquor, and note its weight. Macerate the residue in ℔ij of warm water, strain, and filter. Mix the last liquor with ℔vj of syrup, and boil it to a thick syrup, the weight of which shall be as much less than ℔vj as the weight of the first liquor; add this rapidly to the syrup, and strain it.

SYRUPUS HYDRARGYRI. There are several forms for mercurial syrups; but they all appear liable to serious objections. PLENK. Quicksilver ʒj, powdered gum acacia ʒiij, syrup ℥ij; triturate, and gradually add ℥j of water. LARREY. Sudorific syrup Oj, bichloride of mercury gr. v, muriate of ammonia gr. v, extract of opium gr. v, Hoffman's anodyne liquor ʒss. Dose, ℥ss to ℥jss. CHERON'S syrup consists of mercurial æther (gr. iv of sublimate to ℈ij of æther) ʒij, syrup ℥viij.

SYRUPUS HYOSCYAMI. P. From the extract; as Syrupus Belladonnæ.

SYRUPUS HYSSOPI. P. Dried tops of hyssop ℥j, hyssop water ℥xxxij; digest in a water-bath for 2 hours, let it cool, filter, dissolve in the infusion twice its weight of sugar, by the heat of a water-bath, and when cold, strain.

SYRUPUS INULÆ. P. As Syrupus Boraginis.

SYRUPUS IODINI. *Sirop Iodique.* FOY. Comp. tincture of iodine ʒiv, mint water ʒiv, syrup ℥xvj. Dose, ʒiv to ℥j.

SYRUPUS IPECACUANHÆ. E. Ipecacuanha in coarse powder ℥iv, rectified spirit f℥xv; digest for 24 hours at a gentle heat, strain, squeeze, and filter; digest the residuum in the same manner first with f℥xiv of proof spirit, then with f℥xiv of water; reduce the mixed fluids to f℥xij, add f℥v of rectified spirit, and mix with Ovij of syrup. It contains about 12 grs. of ipecac. in f℥j, or 10 grs. in ℥j. [The American and French processes will perhaps be considered preferable. P. Extract of ipecacuanha (made with proof spirit) ℥j, syrup ℥144, or Ovj. ℥j represents 16 *French* grains of the root, or 4 of the extract. f℥j will contain the same number of English grains. U. S. Ipecac. coarsely powdered ℥j, proof spirit f℥xvj; macerate for 14 days, and filter. Evaporate to f℥ij, again filter, mix with f℥xxxij of syrup, and heat together in a water-bath. Or it may be made by percolation. The strength is nearly that of P. If reduced to Ojss, each f℥j will represent 16 grains of the root.]

SYRUPUS JALAPINUS. P. Jalap ʒx, coriander ʒss, fennel seed ʒss, water f℥xij; heat to 212° for 20 minutes, let it stand 24 hours, strain, and make a syrup with ℥xxiv of sugar. RIGHINI triturates gr. viij of jalap resin, with ℥j of syrup of rhubarb. Dose, ʒij, or ʒiij for an adult, in water.

Syrupus Juglandis. Extract of walnut leaves gr. viij in simple syrup f℥j.

Syrupus Kermes. Kermes juice ℔j, sugar ℔ij.

Syrupus Krameriæ. U. S. Extract of rhatany ℥ij, water f℥xvj; dissolve, strain, and add sugar ℔ijss.

Syrupus Lactis. Reduce skimmed milk by gentle evaporation to one half, and add twice its weight of sugar.

Syrupus Lactucæ. P. Extract of lettuce gr. viij, syrup ℥j. M. Robinet directs the expressed juice to be boiled with twice its weight of sugar.

Syrupus Levistici. From Loveage; as Syr. Hyssopi.

Syrupus Lichenis. Iceland moss deprived of its bitterness ℥j, syrup ℥xxxij. Make a concentrated decoction of the moss, strain, and add the syrup; boil to a proper consistence.

Syrupus Limonum. L. and E. Juice of lemons (strained L., cleared by subsidence and filtration, E.) Oj, refined sugar ℔ijss; dissolve by a gentle heat, set aside for 24 hours, then remove the scum, and pour off from the dregs. D. directs the juice to be placed in a matrass and subjected to the heat of boiling water; and when cold, strained, and formed into a syrup.

Syrupus Lobeliæ. Mr. Procter. Vinegar of lobelia f℥vj, sugar ℥xij. Dissolve by a gentle heat.

Syrupus Lupulinæ. M. Tincture of lupuline 3j, syrup ʒvij; mix.

Syrupus Magnesiæ. Dorvault. Calcined magnesia ℥j, water ℥iijss; triturate together, put them over the fire in a silver saucepan, and add ℥vj of fine sugar, and ʒij of peppermint water.

Syrupus Malorum. As Syrupus Cydoniæ.

Syrupus Marrubii. P. Dried horehound ℥j, horehound water ℔ij; digest in a water-bath for 2 hours, strain, and add sugar ℔iv.

Syrupi Mellis. See Mellitum Simplex. B.

Syrupus Menthæ. From the herb, as Syrupus Marrubii. Syrupus Aquæ Menthæ, as Syr. Aquæ Aurantii.

SYRUPUS MENYANTHIS. P. As Syr. Boraginis.

SYRUPUS MONESIÆ. DEROSNE. Extract of monesia ʒj, water ʒj, boiling syrup ℥xij; mix.

SYRUPUS MONESIÆ COMPOSITUS. Extract of poppies gr. xvj, orange-flower water ℥ss, hot syrup of monesia ℥xvj.

SYRUPUS MORPHIÆ ACETATIS. P. Dissolve gr. iv of acetate of morphia in a very little water, with a few drops of acetic acid, and mix the solution with ℥xvj of cold syrup.

SYRUPUS MORPHIÆ SULPHATIS. P. With sulphate of morphia, as the last. Each ℥j contains one quarter of a grain of the salt of morphia. [Intended as substitutes for syrup of poppies. Sir C. SCUDAMORE'S syrup is much stronger—acetate of morphia gr. ij, diluted sulphuric acid fʒj; syrup of Tolu fʒxj.]

SYRUPUS MORI. L. Strained mulberry juice Oj, sugar ℔ijss. As Syr. Limonum.

SYRUPUS MUSCI PYXIDATI. Cup-moss ℥j, boiling water Oj; macerate for a few hours, strain, and add sugar ℔iij.

SYRUPUS MYRTI. P. As Syr. Hyssopi.

SYRUPUS NAPHTHALINÆ. DUPASQUIER. Naphthaline gr. xvj; dissolve in the least possible quantity of alcohol heated nearly to boiling, and triturate the solution with ℥iv of syrup.

SYRUPUS NARCISSI. DUFRESNOY. Dried flowers of wild narcissus ℥iv, water ℥xvj; boil for a few minutes, strain, add sugar ℔j, dissolve, clarify the syrup, and boil it down to ℔jss.

SYRUPUS NASTURTII. P. Clarified juice of water-cress ℔j, sugar ℔ij.

SYRUPUS NYMPHÆÆ. P. From the flowers of the white water-lily; as Syr. Violæ.

SYRUPUS OLEI JECORIS ASELLI. DUCLOW. Mix 5 parts of powdered gum with 4 of simple syrup; add 8 parts of cod-liver oil, triturate till perfectly mixed, gradually adding 12 parts of water; lastly, dissolve in the emulsion 24 ounces of sugar by means of a gentle heat. [In the same manner, prepare syrups from oil of skate, castor oil, &c.]

SYRUPUS OPII. D. Extract of opium gr. xviij, boiling water f℥viij; macerate, strain, and add (℥xvj or) q. s. sugar to make a syrup. P. Dissolve gr. xvj of extract of opium in ℥ss of water, add it to ℥xvj of boiling syrup, boil for an instant, and strain.

Syrupus Opii Succinatus. *Sirop de Karabé.* P. Syrup of opium ʒj, succinated spirit of ammonia gr. ij.

Syrupus Ovorum. Fuller. Beat the whites of 3 eggs with ℥vj of plantain water, and work it in a mortar with ℥vj of finely powdered sugar till they form a syrup.

Syrupus Papaveris. L. Syrup of white poppies. *Diacodion.* Poppy heads ℔ij, water Cv; boil to Cij, express, boil to Oiv, set aside for 12 hours, decant, boil to Oij, add sugar ℔v, and make a syrup. [In the preceding editions of the L. and the present E. and D. pharmacopœias, the capsules freed from seeds are ordered; and there is a difference of opinion as to the intention of the college, and a consequent diversity of practice; but we believe the seeds are generally omitted. Dr. Collier says the seeds cause the syrup speedily to ferment. Mr. Southall prepares the syrup by percolating the bruised poppy heads with cold water till exhausted, evaporating, and dissolving the sugar by a sufficient heat.] E. directs ℔jss of sliced poppy-heads (without the seeds) to be infused in Oxv of boiling water for 12 hours, and boiled down to Ov, strained with strong expression through calico, and the liquor boiled to Oijss, and ℔iij of sugar dissolved in it by heat. D. directs f℥xvj of clear concentrated decoction to be obtained from ℥xvij of capsules (without seeds) and ℥xxix of sugar dissolved in it. P. directs ʒiv of alcoholic extract of poppies to be dissolved in ʒiv of water, and the solution added to ℔iv (3 French pounds) of boiling syrup, continuing the boiling till it attains the proper consistence. [This is weaker than the L. syrup, but probably of more uniform strength.]

Syrupus Paulliniæ *vel* Guaranæ. Dr. Gavrelle. Extract of paullinia ℈ijss, syrup ℥xxxij.

Syrupus Pectoralis. L. 1746. Black maidenhair ʒv, liquorice root ʒiv, boiling water Oiv; macerate for some hours, strain, add to the infusion twice its weight of sugar, and make a syrup.

Syrupus Persicarum Florum. P. Depurated juice of peach flowers ℔j; refined sugar ℔ij; dissolve the sugar in the juice by the heat of a water-bath.

Syrupus Persimmonis. Unripe persimmons (fruit of the Diospyros Virginiana) slightly crushed ℥viij, boiling water Oj;

infuse till cold and strain. Boil with ℥viij of sugar to the consistence of syrup. *Astringent.*

SYRUPUS PŒONIÆ. P. From the flowers; as Syrupus Violæ.

SYRUPUS POTASSII CYANIDI. M. *Sirop d'hydrocyanate de potasse.* Clarified syrup ℥xvj, medicinal hydrocyanate of potash (a solution of one part of cyanide of potassium in 8 of water) ʒj.

SYRUPUS POTASSII IODIDI. CAZENAVE. Iodide of potassium ʒij, syrup ℥vj. A spoonful 3 or 4 times in 24 hours.

SYRUPUS POTASSII SULPHURETI. P. Liver of sulphur gr. viij, water gr. xvj, syrup ℥j.

SYRUPUS IODHYDRARGYRATIS POTASSII. PUCHE. Iodhydrargyrate of potassium gr. xvj, tincture of saffron ℈ijss, syrup ℥xvj. [PUCHE'S Compound Antisyphilitic Syrup consists of Iodhydrargyrate of potassium gr. xvj, iodine gr. xvj, iodide of potassium ʒv, syrup of red poppies ℥xvj.]

SYRUPUS PRUNI VIRGINIANÆ. Mr. PROCTER. Macerate ℥iv of powdered bark of wild cherry with f℥xij of water, and put it into a percolator, adding water till f℥xij of liquid are obtained, returning the first portions if not clear. Dissolve in this liquor ℔ij of white sugar. Dose about ℥j. *Tonic and calmative.*

SYRUPUS QUINÆ CITRATIS. M. Acid citrate of quinine ℈ss, clarified syrup ℥xvj. Dissolve. f℥ss to f℥j in 24 hours.

SYRUPUS QUINÆ SULPHATIS. P. Dissolve gr. xxxij of sulphate of quinine dissolved in ʒij of water with a few drops of alcoholized sulphuric acid, and mix the solution with ℥xvj of white syrup, without heat.

SYRUPUS QUINÆ SULPHO-TARTRATIS. Sulpho-tartrate of quinine 1 part, water 3, hot syrup 20 parts.

SYRUPUS QUINÆ CUM CAFFÆO. Prepare Ojss of clear infusion from ℥iv of roasted coffee: dissolve in it ℔v of refined sugar, and add to the syrup ʒjss of sulphate of quinine dissolved in a little water, with the addition of a few drops of sulphuric acid.

SYRUPUS QUINÆ DIKINATIS. See Syr. Cinchonæ Concentratus.

SYRUPUS QUINQUE RADICUM. E. 1744. Of each of the 5 roots

(see Species Diureticæ) ʒij, water Ov; boil to Oiij, strain, and boil to a syrup with ℔iv of sugar.

SYRUPUS RAPI. GUIBERT. Juice of raw turnips boiled with sugar q. s. *For Hooping-cough.*

SYRUPUS RHAMNI. L. & E. *Syr. Spinæ Cervinæ.* Juice of buckthorn berries (cleared by subsidence) Oiv, ginger sliced ʒvj, bruised pimento ʒvj, sugar ℔iv; macerate the ginger and pimento with Oj of the juice for 4 hours with a gentle heat, and strain; boil the rest to Ojss, and dissolve the sugar in the mixed liquors. D., the same proportions.

SYRUPUS RHATANIÆ. See Syrupus Krameriæ.

SYRUPUS RHEI. U. S. Rhubarb sliced ℥ij, boiling water f℥xvj; macerate for 24 hours, strain, and add sugar ℔ij. Dissolve, and boil to a proper consistence. [ZWELFER'S syrup was made with ℥vj of rhubarb, ʒvj of cream of tartar, ʒij of sulphate of potash, boiling water ℔ijss (Oij), white sugar ℔iijss.]

SYRUPUS RHEI AROMATICUS. U. S. Rhubarb ℥ijss, cloves ℥ss, cinnamon ℥ss, nutmeg ʒij, proof spirit f℥xxxij; macerate for 14 days, strain, evaporate by water-bath to f℥xvj, filter while hot, and mix with Oiv f℥xvj of syrup previously heated.

SYRUPUS RHEI ET SENNÆ. E. 1744. Rhubarb ℥j, senna ℥ij, fennel seed ʒij, cinnamon ʒij, boiling water Oijss; macerate for 12 hours, strain, and boil with ℔iij of sugar to a syrup.

SYRUPUS RHŒADOS. L. & E. To Oj of water, heated in a water-bath, gradually add ℔j of red poppy petals; then remove from the fire, macerate for 12 hours, strain, and make a syrup with ℔ijss of sugar.

SYRUPUS RIBIS; SYRUPUS RUBI IDÆI; and other fruits. As Syrupus Mori [P.], or Syrupus Limonis.

SYRUPUS ROSÆ. L. *Syrupus Rosæ Solutivus.* Dried petals of the 100-leaved rose ℥vij, boiling water Oiij; macerate for 12 hours, and strain. Evaporate the strained liquor to Oij, strain, and dissolve in it ℔vj of white sugar. E. directs ℔j of fresh petals to be infused for 12 hours in Oiij of boiling water, and ℔iij of sugar dissolved in the strained liquor by heat.

SYRUPUS ROSÆ GALLICÆ. E. Dried petals of red rose ℥ij, boiling water Oj, pure sugar ℥xx; infuse for 12 hours, strain, and dissolve the sugar by heat.

SYRUPUS RUTÆ. It is not in the British pharmacopœias, though generally kept in the shops. It may be made by infusing ℥j of rue in Oj of boiling water, and adding to the strained liquor twice its weight of sugar. But it is often prepared, as Dr. PEREIRA observes, by triturating about 8 drops of the oil with Oj of simple syrup. Dr. ROYLE directs ♏xij of the oil to be dissolved in f℥ss of spirit, and mixed with Oj of syrup. BERAL prepares it with the alcoholized juice, of which 24 drops may be added to each ounce of syrup. DORVAULT directs it to be prepared as Syr. Hyssopi.

SYRUPUS SALICINÆ. Salicine ʒj, boiling water ℥j, sugar ℥ij.

SYRUPUS SAMBUCI. Boil the juice of elder berries for an instant with twice its weight of sugar.

SYRUPUS SAPONARIÆ. M. GUIBOURT. Infuse ℥ij of dried soapwort in ℥xvj of boiling water for 12 hours, strain with expression, and form the infusion into a syrup with twice its weight of sugar. M. COSSERAN directs ℥ij of the alcoholic extract to be mixed with ℥iv of water, and added to ℥xxxij of syrup previously reduced by boiling to ℥xxvj.

SYRUPUS SARZÆ. L. E. & D. Sarsaparilla ℥xv, boiling water Cj; macerate for 24 hours, boil to Oiv, strain, add ℥xv of sugar, and boil to a syrup.

SYRUPUS CUM EXTRACTO SARSAPARILLÆ. P. Alcoholic extract of sarsaparilla ℥vj (which, to correspond with Troy pounds, must be reduced to ℥ivss: otherwise avoird. weight may be used), water ℔iv, dissolve by heat of water-bath, filter while hot, add ℔viij of sugar, and dissolve without boiling. [Each ʒj corresponds with gr. xv of extract, or ℈ij of the root.]

SYRUPUS SARSAPARILLÆ COMPOSITUS. U. S. Powdered sarsaparilla ℔ij, rasped guaiacum ℥iij, red roses, senna, and liquorice root, of each (bruised) ℥ij, proof spirit Oviij (Ox o.m.) Macerate for 14 days, then express and filter; evaporate the tincture by water-bath to Oiij f℥iv (Oiv o.m.); add ℔viij of white sugar, and dissolve it to form a syrup. To this, when cold, add oil of anise ♏v, oil of sassafras ♏v, oil of partridgeberry ♏iij, previously triturated with a little of the syrup. It may also be made by the following process: Reduce the first 5 ingredients to a coarse powder, mix them with f℥48 of water, and after 24 hours transfer the whole to an apparatus for displacement, and gradually add more water till Ovj f℥viij (Oviij o.m.) of filtered liquid are obtained. Evaporate, and proceed as before. [These are regarded as improved forms of the

Sirop de Cuisinier of the French Codex; which is prepared by infusion from 2 ℔ of sarsaparilla, 2 ounces of dried borage flowers, 2 ounces of pale roses, 2 ounces of senna, 2 ounces of aniseed, 2 ℔s of sugar, and 2 ℔s of honey; the syrup being clarified by white of egg. Avoirdupois weights are here intended. For a process for a more concentrated syrup or sweet fluid-extract by Mr. HODGSON, see Extractum Sarzæ Compositum.]

SYRUPUS SARZÆ IODURETUS. M. RICORD. Syrup of sarsaparilla 50 parts, iodide of potassium 1 part.

SYRUPUS SASSAFRAS. FULLER, *altered.* Digest ℥ij of sassafras shavings in Ojss of boiling water, in a close vessel, for a few hours: strain, and dissolve in the clear infusion twice its weight of sugar. [It is also made from the vinous infusion.]

SYRUPUS SCILLÆ. E. Vinegar of squill Oiij, sugar ℔vij; dissolve by a gentle heat, and agitation. [U. S. f℥xvj to ℥xxiv.]

SYRUPUS SCILLÆ COMPOSITUS. U. S. *Hive Syrup.* Squill and seneka, bruised, each ℥v, water Oiv; boil to Oij, add sugar ℔iv ℥vj, evaporate to Oiij, and while hot dissolve in it 60 grains of tartarized antimony. It may also be made by displacement. [The weights are adjusted to imperial measure.] Mr. ECKY directs ℔j of his Extr. Senegæ et Scillæ to be mixed with ℔vj of clarified honey at 160° F. and gr. xvj of tartar emetic to be added to each f℥xvj of the syrup.]

SYRUPUS SENNÆ. L. Senna ℥ijss, fennel seed ℨx, boiling water Oj; digest for an hour, strain, add manna ℥iij, sugar ℨxv and boil to a syrup. E. Senna ℥iv, boiling water f℥xxiv; infuse for 12 hours, strain with strong expression so as to obtain f℥xxij of liquid. Concentrate ℔iv of treacle as far as possible in a vapour-bath, add to it the infusion, stirring carefully, and removing the vessel from the bath as soon as the mixture is complete. If Alexandria senna be used, it should be carefully freed from cynanchum leaves.

SYRUPUS SENNÆ CONCENTRATUS. See Extractum Sennæ Fluidum.—Another method of preparing it is that of Mr. DUHAMEL. Macerate ℥viij of coarsely-powdered senna with f℥xvj of proof spirit for 12 hours, put it into a displacement apparatus, and pour in water till f℥xlviij have passed. Evaporate to f℥v, and dissolve in it ℥v of sugar. Strain, and when cold, add for each f℥j two drops of oil of fennel dissolved in a little comp. spirit of sulphuric æther.

SYRUPUS SENEGÆ. U. S. Seneka root ℥iv, water f℥xvj; boil to f℥viij, strain, and add sugar ℔j; make a syrup.

SYRUPUS SIMPLEX. Syrupus Sacchari. See Syrupus.

SYRUPUS SODÆ HYPOSULPHITIS. MOUCHON. Hyposulphite of soda ℥j, water ℥xij, sugar ℥xxiij. Dissolve with a gentle heat, and filter. Dose, ℥j to ℥ij.

SYRUPUS SORBI. SAUVAN. Boil Oj of juice of unripe service with ℔iij of sugar. *Astringent.*

SYRUPUS STRAMONII. From the extract, as Syr. Belladonnæ.

SYRUPUS SUDORIFICUS. Comp. Syrup of Sarsaparilla.

SYRUPUS SULPHURETI POTASSÆ. See Syr. Pot. Sulphureti.

SYRUPUS SYMPHITI. E. 1744. Mr. BOYLE'S Syrup. Fresh comfrey root ℔ss, plantain leaves ℔ss; bruise, express the juice, boil to half, and make a syrup with an equal weight of sugar.

SYRUPUS TANNINI. FOY. Tannin ℥ij, water ℥xvj, sugar ℥xxxij.

SYRUPUS TARTARICUS. See Syrupus Acidi Tartarici.

SYRUPUS TOLUTANUS. L. *Syrupus Balsamicus.* Balsam of Tolu ℨx, boiling water Oj; boil in a covered vessel for half an hour, stirring occasionally, filter the liquor when cool, and dissolve in it ℔ijss of refined sugar. P. directs ℥iv of the balsam to be digested in a covered water-bath with ℥xvj of water for 12 hours, stirring it now and then; the liquor is then filtered, and twice its weight of very white sugar dissolved in it by a gentle heat in a close vessel. The syrup is then filtered through paper. A less elegant syrup is prepared by adding gradually ℥j of tincture of Tolu to ℔ij (E.) or ℔jss (D.) of recently prepared simple syrup, shaking the mixture after each addition. M. MARCHAND proposes the following formula:—Balsam of Tolu 16 parts, white sugar 32, cold water 60, syrup 1000. Powder the balsam with the sugar, place it in an earthen or tin pot, mix the water with it, and pour over them the syrup, boiling. Leave it covered up for 12 hours, stirring now and then, and filter through paper. The balsam is economized by this process, but the flavour of the product is not equal to that of P., though much finer than that of E. and D.

SYRUPUS TRAGACANTHÆ. GUIBOURT. Make a mucilage with ℨj of tragacanth, and ℥ij of water; add ℥vj more water, heat in a water-bath for half an hour, mix with it ℥xxxij of syrup, boil to a due consistence, and strain through flannel.

SYRUPUS TUSSILAGINIS. P. Coltsfoot flowers ℔j, boiling water ℔ij; macerate for 12 hours, strain, press, and add sugar ℔iv. [℥ij of dried flowers may be substituted for ℔j of fresh.]

SYRUPUS ULMI. SOUBEIRAN. Alcoholic extract of elm bark ℈iij, syrup ℥xijss. Dose, ʒiv, frequently, in *skin diseases.*

SYRUPUS URTICARIÆ. Clarified nettle juice boiled with an equal weight of sugar to a due consistence. *Diuretic.*

SYRUPUS VALERIANÆ. P. Bruise ℔j of valerian root, and put it into a still with ℔viij of water. In 12 hours distil off ℔jss; strain and filter what remains, mix the liquor with ℔viij of simple syrup, evaporate to ℔vjss, and add the distilled water.

SYRUPUS VANILLÆ. Vanilla ℥ij, white sugar ℥xviij, water ℥ix. Beat the vanilla with a few drops of spirit, then with part of the sugar, and water q. s. to form a soft paste; add the rest of the sugar and water, and digest for 18 or 20 hours in a glass vessel placed in a water-bath. Strain, and clarify with white of egg if required.

SYRUPUS VIOLÆ. E. Fresh violets ℔j, boiling water Oijss, pure sugar ℔vijss. Infuse the flowers for 24 hours in water in a covered glass or earthenware vessel; strain, without squeezing, and dissolve the sugar in the filtered liquor. P. directs the violets to be agitated with 3 times their weight of warm water (at 113° F.), then to be infused in twice their weight of boiling water for 12 hours, strained with expression through well-rinsed linen, and the clear infusion made into a syrup with twice its weight of sugar. [Care should be taken in the selection of the sugar, as some samples have an alkaline reaction. The washing of the flowers is intended to remove a yellow colouring matter which renders the syrup very liable to change.]

SYRUPUS VIOLÆ SOLUTIVUS. WIRTEM. PH. Violets ℥iv, senna ℥ij, boiling water ℔j; digest, strain, and add sugar ℥xvj.

SYRUPUS VIOLÆ TRICOLORIS. GUIBOURT. Wild pansy (the dried herb) ℥j, boiling water ℥viij; infuse for 12 hours, strain, and dissolve in the clear infusion twice its weight of sugar.

SYRUPUS ZINCI IODIDI. DR. A. T. THOMSON. Iodine ʒiv, zinc (finely divided) ʒij, water f℥iv; agitate till the liquor is colourless, and filter the solution into f℥xij of simple syrup previously reduced by boiling to f℥viij.

SYRUPUS ZINGIBERIS. L. & E. Ginger sliced ℥ijss, boiling

water Oj; macerate for 4 hours, and add sugar ℔ijss, and dissolve. U. S. Tincture of ginger f ℥iv, syrup Ovj f ℥viij (one *old* gallon). Mix, and by means of a water-bath evaporate to a proper consistence.

TABELLÆ. *Tablettes.* See TROCHISCI.

TARAXACINE. M. POLEX. Boil the milky juice of dandelion root with water, concentrate and filter the liquid, and let it evaporate spontaneously in a warm place. Purify the crystalline matter by redissolving, filtering, and crystallizing.

TARTARUM BORAXATUM. KAEPELER. Dissolve 250 parts of borax and 75 of cream of tartar in boiling water; filter, evaporate till a portion dropped on a cold slab solidifies. Powder it in a warm mortar, and keep it in well-stopped bottles. CAMBORNAC'S Soluble Cream of Tartar is, Bitartrate of potash ℥xij, borate of soda ℥vj, tartaric acid ʒiij. Dissolve in water, clarify the solution by white of egg, and proceed as for Potassæ Boro-tartras, P., which see.

TELA VESICATORIA. *Blistering Tissue.* See Sparadrapum Vesicans, P. The same composition may be spread on waxed paper, oiled silk, adhesive or isinglass plaster, sarcenet, or other convenient material. OETTHINGER directs the following composition to be spread with a brush on stretched sarcenet:—Powdered cantharides ʒiij, æther ℥j; digest for 24 hours, strain, add sandarach ʒiv, mastic ʒij, turpentine ℈j, oil of lavender 12 drops. Another method is to use the Extractum Cantharidis Aceticum, which may be spread on paper, waxed cloth, adhesive plaster, &c.

THEINA. THEIN, or CAFFEIN. To a decoction of tea, or of raw coffee (for both yield the same principle), add solution of diacetate of lead so long as it occasions a precipitate. Filter the liquid, and pass sulphuretted hydrogen through it to free it from lead; again filter, and concentrate that crystals may form; or it may be evaporated to dryness, and the residue carefully sublimed.

TESTÆ PREPARATÆ. L. Wash oyster-shells with boiling water, and prepare them in the same way as chalk.

THERIACA ANDROMACHI. L. 1746. *Venice Treacle.* Consists of 61 ingredients, and contains 1 grain of opium in 75. The Theriaca of P. consists of 72 ingredients, and contains gr. j of opium in 72. Electuarium Theriaca, PRUS. PH., contains gr. v of opium in ℥j. For these polypharmic electuaries (which are rarely prescribed in this country, and probably never made according to the authorized formulæ) may be substituted the following:—

THERIACA EDINENSIS. E. 1744. Serpentary, valerian, contrayerva, each ℥iv; aromatic powder ℥iij, guaiacum resin ℥ij, castor ℥ij, nutmeg ℥ij, saffron ℥j, opium ℥j, clarified honey ℥75. Dissolve the opium in a little wine, and mix it with the other dry ingredients in powder, and the honey. It contains 1 gr. of opium in 100.

TINCTURÆ. *Spirituous and Æthereal Tinctures.* The dry ingredients, divided by cutting or bruising, are macerated in the spirit for the time prescribed, in well-closed vessels, shaking occasionally. The liquor is then strained off, the residuum pressed, and the tincture cleared by subsidence or filtration. Another method of preparing tinctures is by *percolation.* The dry materials, reduced to a coarse, or moderately fine powder, are moistened with enough spirit to form a thick pulp; after 12 hours (or sometimes without delay) the mass is put into a cylinder (the lower end of which is furnished with a pierced diaphragm, or obstructed by cotton, or tied over with cloth), and the solvent poured into the upper part of the cylinder. The degree of fineness to which the materials are to be reduced, and the firmness with which the mass is to be packed in the cylinder, vary with the different articles, and can only be learned by experiment. Dr. BURTON proposes to inclose the dry ingredients in a calico bag, and suspend it in the spirit contained in a cylindrical vessel; a plan which in many cases is very convenient, and shortens the time required for maceration. M. PERSONNE found that most substances required 5 times their weight of spirit to extract their active principles. M. HŒNLE'S method of making his *concentrated tinctures* is this: Digest 8 parts of the vegetable powder with 16 of the spirit of wine (0·857 sp. gr.) for 4 days at 72° F., stirring occasionally. Express, and filter; add to the residue as much spirit as it has absorbed, and again express and filter. Mix the liquors, the weight of which should be 16 parts. In this way are prepared concentrated tinctures of the leaves of aconite, belladonna, conium, hyoscyamus, &c.; the flowers of arnica and chamomile; the roots of ipecacuanha, valerian, &c. For the methods of preparing tinctures from *fresh* plants, see Tinctura Aconiti, and Succi Alcoholati. The tinctures of the French Codex are generally stronger than those of the British Pharmacopœias.

TINCTURA ABSINTHII. E. 1783. Dried tops of wormwood ℥iv,

rectified spirit ℔ij; macerate for 2 days, strain, macerate for 4 days with ℥ij more of the herb, and strain. P. one part of the herb to 4 of proof spirit.

TINCTURA ABSINTHII ALKALINA. See Essentia Absinthii.

TINCTURA ABSINTHII COMPOSITA. DAN. PH. Wormwood ℥ij, gentian ʒiv, holy thistle ʒiv, orange-peel ʒiv, aniseed ʒj, proof spirit ℔iij.

TINCTURA ACONITI. U. S. Aconite (dried leaves) ℥iv, diluted alcohol (proof spirit) f℥xxxij; macerate for 14 days, express, and filter through paper. It may also be prepared by moistening the aconite in powder, with diluted alcohol, allowing it to stand for 24 hours, then transferring it to an apparatus for displacement; and gradually pouring upon it diluted alcohol until f℥xxxij of liquor are obtained. Dose, 20 to 30 drops. [P. directs the dried leaves to be macerated 15 days with 4 times their weight of proof spirit.]

TINCTURA ACONITI CUM FOLIIS RECENTIBUS. P. Fresh aconite is bruised, and macerated for 15 days, with an equal weight of rectified spirit, then strained with expression, and the liquor filtered. [Tinctures are directed to be made from several fresh plants in the same way. They are stronger than the ordinary tinctures, and not to be substituted for them except when expressly ordered. See Succi Alcoholati.] Dose, 2 to 12 drops.

TINCTURA ACONITI ÆTHEREA. P. Powdered aconite ℥iv, sulphuric æther ℥xvj, (nearly f℥xxiv.) It is best prepared by *percolation* in a cylindrical glass vessel, furnished with a stopper, and terminating at the lower end in a funnel, which is to be obstructed with a little cotton. The powder being introduced over the cotton, pour on it enough æther to moisten it, put in the stopper, fix the tube into the neck of a bottle, and leave it for 48 hours. Then add gradually the rest of the æther, and lastly, enough water to displace the æther absorbed.

TINCTURA RADICIS ACONITI CONCENTRATA. Dr. TURNBULL. Powdered aconite root ℔j, rectified spirit ℔ij; digest for 7 days, express the tincture, and filter. *For outward use.* [Dr. FLEMING directs ℥xvj of the root, dried and powdered, to be macerated with f℥xvj of rectified spirit for 4 days, and the tincture strained. The root is then treated by percolation with more spirit, till the tincture obtained amounts to f℥xxiv. As an anodyne, antineuralgic, and calmative, he gives ♏v 3 times a day, increasing the dose one ♏ daily if required; an antiphlogistic ♏v, repeated in 4 hours, and afterwards half the dose if required. Its effects must be carefully watched. These stronger tinctures should not be dispensed unless specially ordered.]

TINCTURA ACONITINÆ. See Solutio Aconitinæ.

TINCTURA ALÖES. L. Aloes ℥j, extract of liquorice ℥iij, distilled water Ojss, rectified spirit Oss; macerate for 14 days, and strain. E. directs f℥xij of spirit, and f℥xxviij of water; 7 days. D. ℥ss of aloes, ℥jss of liquorice, f℥viij of water, and f℥viij of proof spirit.

TINCTURA ALÖES COMPOSITA. L. (Tinct. Aloes et Myrrhæ. E. and U. S.) *Elixir Proprietatis.* Aloes ℥iv, saffron ℥ij, tincture of myrrh Oij; macerate for 14 days, and strain. D. omits the saffron.

TINCTURA ALÖES ALKALINA. SWEDIAUR. Aloes ℥ss, extract of liquorice ʒjss, cinnamon water f℥viij, proof spirit f℥viij, subcarbonate of soda ℥j; digest in a sand-bath, and strain.

TINCTURA ALÖES ÆTHEREA. E. 1817. Aloes ʒjss, myrrh ʒjss, saffron ʒj, spirit of sulphuric æther ℔j; digest for eight days.

TINCTURA AMARA. See Tinct. Absinthii Comp.

TINCTURA AMBERGRISEÆ. P. One part of ambergris to four (by weight) of spirit at ·863.

TINCTURA AMBERGRISEÆ ALKALINA. Ambergris ℈ij, carbonate of potash ʒij; triturate, and add spirit of roses (made with alcohol) ℥viij; dissolve by heat.

TINCTURA AMBERGRISEÆ ÆTHEREA. P. Ambergris ℥j, sulphuric æther ʒiv (fʒvj); macerate in a stoppered bottle for four days, and filter.

TINCTURA AMMONIÆ COMPOSITA. L. Spiritus Ammonia Succinnatus. Mastic ℈ij, rectified spirit fʒix; digest until dissolved, decant, add oil of lavender ♏xiv, oil of amber ♏iv, stronger solution of ammonia Oj, and mix. [Without the oil of amber this forms the *Eau de Luce* of the shops.]

TINCTURA GUMMI AMMONIACI. P. Gum ammoniac ʒiv, rectified spirit Oj; digest 15 days, and strain.

TINCTURA ANGELICÆ. AUSTR. PH. Dried angelica root ℥j, proof spirit ʒvj; digest and filter.

TINCTURA ANGUSTURÆ. D. Angustura (cusparia) bark ʒij, rectified spirit f℥xxxij; macerate seven days, and filter.

TINCTURA ANISODI. Dried leaves of anisodus luridus ʒj, proof spirit ʒviij; digest and filter. Maximum dose, 20 drops. It causes dilatation of the pupils.

TINCTURA ANTHEMIDIS. AUSTR. PH. Dried chamomile flowers ʒij, proof spirit ℔j.

TINCTURA ANTISCORBUTICA. P. Tinctura Armoraciæ Composita. Horse-radish root ʒviij, black mustard-seed ℥iv, muriate of ammonia ʒij, proof spirit ʒxvj, compound spirit of scurvy-grass ʒxvj; macerate for a week.

TINCTURA ANTIARTHRITICA. Dr. GRAVES'S *Gout Tincture.* Orange-peel ℥ij, rhubarb ʒj, powder of aloes and canella ʒij, brandy Oij; digest for a week. A spoonful night and morning with water.

TINCTURA ANTI-PHTHISICA. E. 1744. Acetate of lead ʒjss, sulphate of iron ʒj, rectified spirit fʒxvj; digest without heat. Dose, 20 to 40 drops.

TINCTURA ANTIMONII. L. 1745. Crude antimony ℔ss, subcarbonate of potash ℔j; mix, and fuse together in a strong fire for an hour, and digest the powdered mass in f℥xxxij of rectified spirit.

TINCTURA ARNICÆ. PRUS. PH. Arnica flowers ℥jss, spirit of wine (at 0·900) ℔j; digest and filter.

TINCTURA ARNICÆ ÆTHEREA. P. From the flowers; as Tinct. Aconiti Ætherea.

TINCTURA AROMATICA. Tinct. Cinnamomi Composita.

TINCTURA ASARI. P. One part of dried asarum to four of spirit at 0·863.

TINCTURA ASSAFŒTIDA. L. & E. Assafœtida ℥v, rectified spirit Oij; macerate for 14 days. D. Triturate ℥iv of assafœtida with fʒviij of water, and add fʒxxxij of rectified spirit; digest 14 days, and filter.

TINCTURA ASSAFŒTIDÆ ÆTHEREA. P. As Tinct. Castorei Ætherea.

TINCTURA ASTRINGENS. Dr. COPLAND, *for sponginess of the*

gums. Catechu ℥ss, myrrh ℥ss, cinchona ʒij, balsam of Peru ʒjss, spirit of horse-radish ℥jss, rectified spirit of wine ℥jss; digest.

TINCTURA AURANTII. L. E. & D. Dried orange-peel ℥iijss, proof spirit Oij; macerate 14 [7 E.; 3 D.] days, and strain.

TINCTURA BALSAMICA. E. 1744. Copaiva ℥j, balsam of Peru ʒiij, balsam of Tolu 3ij, benzoin ʒss, saffron ℈j, rectified spirit f℥xvj; digest four days in a sand-bath and strain.

TINCTURA BALSAMI COPAIBÆ. One part of copaiva, to eight of alcohol.

TINCTURA BALSAMI PERUVIANI. L. 1788. Balsam of Peru ℥iv, rectified spirit f℥xvj; digest until dissolved.

TINCTURA BALSAMI TOLUTANI. L. Balsam of Tolu ℥ij, rectified spirit Oij; macerate till dissolved, and filter. [E. ℥iijss of balsam to Oij of rectified spirit. D. ℥j of balsam to f℥xvj of spirit.]

TINCTURA BALSAMI GILEADENSIS. GUIBOURT. One part of balsam to eight of rectified spirit.

TINCTURA BELLADONNÆ. U. S. Belladonna leaves (dried) ℥iv, proof spirit f℥xxxij; macerate for 14 days, express, and filter. It may also be made by displacement. BAILEY'S and that of GUY'S H. are of the same strength. Dose, ♏v to xxx. Mr. BLACKETT'S *saturated* tincture is made by macerating ʒx of the extract in ℔j of proof spirit. Dose, ♏ij to iij. Care must be taken not to confound these different preparations. P. directs it to be made both from the dry and fresh plant, as Tinctura Aconiti.

TINCTURA BELLADONNA ÆTHEREA. P. As Tincture Aconiti Ætherea.

TINCTURA BENZOINI. P. Benzoin ℥iv, rectified spirit Oj; digest for 6 days.

TINCTURA BENZOINI COMPOSITA. L. & D. *Balsamum Traumaticum*, or FRYAR'S *Balsam*. Benzoin ℥iijss, strained storax ℥ijss, balsam of Tolu 3x, aloes 3v, rectified spirit Oij; macerate for 14 days. E. Benzoin ℥iv, balsam of Peru ℥ijss, E. I. aloes ℥ss, rectified spirit Oij. Seven days.

TINCTURA BONPLANDIÆ. Tinctura Angusturæ.

TINCTURÆ BRUCINÆ. M. Brucine gr. xvj, rectified spirit ℥j.

TINCTURA BUKU. E. & D. Buku (or Buchu) leaves ℥v, proof spirit Oij; digest for seven days; [or prepare it by percolation, E.]

TINCTURA CAINCÆ. Cahinca root ℥j, proof spirit Oss; macerate 15 days. A tincture is also prepared from 1 part of alcoholic extract, and 11 of brandy. Dose, ʒj to ʒij daily.

TINCTURA CALAMI. AUST. PH. Dried root of sweet flag ℥ij, proof spirit ℔j; digest and strain.

TINCTURA CALAMI COMPOSITA. POL. PH. Calamus ℥iij, zedoary ℥j, ginger ℥j, green oranges ℥ij, proof spirit Oij.

TINCTURA CALUMBÆ. L. and E. Calumba root ℥iij, proof spirit Oij; macerate for 14 days. [E. 7 days; or more conveniently by percolation; allowing the powdered root to soak in a little of the spirit for 6 hours before putting it into the percolator. E. and U. S.]

TINCTURA CAMBOGIÆ ALKALINA. Gamboge ℥ss, subcarbonate of potash ℥j, proof spirit or brandy ℥xij. Dose, ʒss to ʒj.

TINCTURA CAMBOGIÆ AMMONIATA. SWEDIAUR. Gamboge ʒss, spirit of ammonia ℥iv.

TINCTURA CAMPHORÆ. L. E. and D. *Spirit of Camphor.* Camphor ℥v [E. ℥ijss], rectified spirit Oij. Dissolve. [P. directs 1 part camphor to 7 of spirit, and a weaker solution, 1 part of camphor to 40 of proof spirit.]

TINCTURE CAMPHORÆ COMPOSITA. L. (Tinct. Opii Camphorata, L. 1787.) *Paregoric Elixir.* Camphor ℈ijss, opium gr. 72, benzoic acid gr. 72, oil of aniseed fʒj, proof spirit Oij; macerate for 14 days and filter. [The oil of aniseed was rejected in 1809, and the name at the same time altered, after which time two preparations were usually kept, under the old and new names. In 1836 the college readmitted the oil.] For E. see Tinct. Opii Camphorata. D. (Tinct. Opii Camphorata) as L.

TINCTURA CANNABIS INDICÆ. BENGAL PH. Resinous extract of Indian hemp gr. xxiv, proof spirit f℥j. Dose, from 5 to 10 drops in neuralgia, cholera, &c. In tetanus much larger doses are given.

TINCTURA CANTHARIDIS. L. and E. (*Tinctura Lyttæ.* L. 1809.) Powdered Spanish flies ʒiv, proof spirit Oij; macerate for 14 days. E. directs 7 days' maceration; or by percolation. D. ʒij of flies to f℥xxiv of proof spirit, 7 days. [P. One part of flies to 8 of spirit.]

TINCTURA CANTHARIDIS ÆTHEREA. P. Powdered cantharides ℨiv, acetic æther ℨxxxij; macerate for 8 days in a stoppered bottle, express, and filter.

TINCTURA CANTHARIDIS ACETICA (EPISPASTICA). Dr. FEHR. Bruised cantharides ℨiv, strong acetic acid ℨiv, rectified spirit ℨiv; digest for some days, express, and filter. It is probably more active than the Acetum Cantharidis. L.

TINCTURA CANTHARIDIS NITRICA. M. RIGHINI. Cantharides in fine powder 64 parts, nitric acid 32 parts; pour the acid on the flies, and when the action has ceased, pour on it by little and little, 750 parts of rectified spirit. Macerate for 8 hours, frequently stirring; then express, and filter. It should contain no free acid.

TINCTURA CAPSICI. L. D. and E. Capsicum ℥x, proof spirit Oij; macerate for 14 days. [It is best prepared by percolation, which may be commenced as soon as the capsicum (in moderately fine powder) is made into a pulp with a little of the spirit. E.]

TINCTURA CAPSICI ACETICA. VAN MONS. Capsicum ℨij, vinegar ℨxij, proof spirit ℨxij; digest.

TINCTURA CAPSICI CONCENTRATA. Dr. TURNBULL, *for external use.* Capsicum ℨiv, rectified spirit ℨxij; macerate for 7 days; or rather prepare it by percolation. [It is also used instead of the pepper in cookery, under the name of Essence of Cayenne.]

TINCTURA CAPSICI CUM VERATRIA. Dr. TURNBULL. Dissolve gr. iv of veratria in ℨj of the last tincture. *For external use.*

TINCTURA CAPSICI ET CANTHARIDIS. Cantharides ℥x, capsicum ℥j, proof spirit Oj; macerate for 10 days.

TINCTURA CARDAMOMI. L. & E. Cardamom seeds (without the capsules) ℨiijss, proof spirit Oij; macerate 14 days. E. directs ℨivss of the seeds, and to be prepared in preference by percolation, as Tinct. Capsici, the seeds being ground in a coffee-mill.

TINCTURA CARDAMOMI COMPOSITA. L. & E. Cardamom seeds ℥ijss, caraway seed ℥ijss, cochineal ℥j, cinnamon ℥v, raisins stoned ℨv, proof spirit Oij; macerate for 14 days, [7 days, or by percolation, E.] D. omits the raisins and cochineal. Dr. PEREIRA remarks that some druggists improperly weigh the capsules with the seeds. It may be added that some omit to remove the seeds from the raisins, the tannin of which precipitates quina and other alkaloids when the tincture is added to mixtures containing them. Some employ Sultana raisins, which are devoid of seeds.

TINCTURA CARUI COMPOSITA. GUY'S H. Caraway seed ʒiij, pimento ʒiij, cinnamon ℥ss, raisins ℥iv, proof spirit Ojss; macerate for 14 days, and strain.

TINCTURA CARYOPHYLLI. BRUNS. PH. Cloves ℥ij, rectified spirit ℥xij. [P. Digest bruised cloves with 4 times their weight of unrectified spirit at ·863 (41 over proof) for 15 days.]

TINCTURA CASCARILLA. L. E. D. Cascarilla ℥v, proof spirit Oij; macerate for 14 days. [17 days E. & D.; or by percolation as Tinct. Cinchonæ, E.]

TINCTURA CASSIÆ. E. Cassia in moderately fine powder ℥iijss, proof spirit Oij. Proceed by percolation, the cassia being first macerated with a little of the spirit for 12 hours. Or digest 7 days.

TINCTURA CASTOREI. L. & E. Castor ℥ijss, rectified spirit Oij; macerate 14 days [or prepare it by percolation, E.] D. orders proof spirit. P. as Tinct. Caryophylli.

TINCTURA CASTOREI AMMONIATA. E. Castor ℥ijss, assafœtida ʒx, spirit of ammonia Oij; digest for 7 days. [This is the Elixir Fœtidum of foreign pharm.; and, with the addition of ʒv of opium, it forms the Elixir Uterinum, or Elixir Castorei Thebaicum.]

TINCTURA CASTOREI ÆTHEREA. P. Castor ℥iv, sulphuric æther ℥xvj [nearly f℥xxiv]. Let them macerate for 4 days in a stoppered bottle, and filter.

TINCTURA CATECHU. L. E. & D. *Tinctura Japonica.* Catechu ℥iijss, cinnamon ℥ijss, proof spirit Oij; macerate for 14 [7 E. & D.] days [or by percolation, E.]

TINCTURA CATECHU COMPOSITA. POL. PH. Catechu ʒiv, myrrh ʒiv, balsam of Peru ʒj, spirit of scurvy-grass ℥viij. An excellent mouth tincture.

TINCTURA CENTAURII MINORIS. As Tinctura Absinthii.

TINCTURA CEPHALICA. E. 1744. [Simplified.] Valerian ℥iv, serpentary ℥j, tops of rosemary ʒiv, white wine Ov; digest 3 days.

TINCTURA CEPHALICA PURGANS. Add to the last—senna ℥ij, black hellebore ℥j, wine ℔ij.

TINCTURA CHENOPODII. SWEDIAUR. Mexican tea 1 part, proof spirit [or spirit of sulphuric æther, VAN MONS] 4 parts. Macerate 15 days.

TINCTURA CHIRAYTÆ. Dr. SIGMOND. Chirayta herb ℥j, proof spirit f℥viij; digest for 7 days.

TINCTURA CHIRAYTÆ COMPOSITA. Dr. REECE. Chirayta ℥ij, sassafras ℨiij, red santal wood ℨij, proof spirit f℥xxiv. Macerate 14 days.

TINCTURA CIMICIFUGA. Dr. HILDRETH. Bruised root of cimicifuga racemosa (black snake root) ℥iv, proof spirit Oj. Dose, fʒj to fʒij.

TINCTURA CINARÆ. Mr. COPEMAN. Fresh artichoke leaves, bruised, ℔ij, rectified spirit ℔j; digest for 7 days, express, and filter.

TINCTURA CINCHONÆ. L. E. & D. Yellow Peruvian bark (or other species prescribed) ℥viij, proof spirit Oij; macerate 14 days, and filter. E. and U. S. direct it to be made by percolation; the bark in fine powder to be moistened with a little of the spirit, left thus for 10 or 12 hours [48 U. S.], then firmly packed in the cylinder, and the rest of the spirit poured on it. D. orders ℥iv of pale bark to f℥xxxij of proof spirit, by maceration, 7 days.

TINCTURA CINCHONÆ COMPOSITA. L. & E. Pale bark [yellow, E., in fine powder if by percolation] ℥iv, dry orange peel ℥iij, serpentary root ʒvj, saffron ʒij, cochineal ℨj, proof spirit Oij; macerate 14 days. [E. 7 days, or by percolation.] HUXHAM'S Tincture of Bark was exactly that of L., except that French brandy was used. D. Pale bark ℥ij, orange peel ℥ss, cochineal ℈ij, serpentary ʒiij, saffron ʒj, proof spirit f℥xx.

TINCTURA CINCHONÆ AMMONIATA. L. 1824. Peruvian bark ℥iv, aromatic spirit of ammonia f℥xxxij; macerate for 10 days.

TINCTURA CINCHONINÆ. *Alcohol de Cinchonine.* M. Sulphate of cinchonine gr. xij, rectified spirit f℥jss.

TINCTURA CINNAMOMI. L. D. and E. Cinnamon ℥iijss, proof spirit Oij; macerate 14 days. [E. as Tinct. Cassiæ.]

TINCTURA CINNAMOMI COMPOSITA. L. Cinnamon ʒj, cardamom ʒiv, long pepper ʒijss, ginger ʒijss, proof spirit Oij. 14 days. E. directs cinnamon ℥j, cardamom ℥j, long pepper ʒiij, proof spirit Oij; by digestion 7 days, or rather by percolation, the spices being finely powdered.

Tinctura Cnici Benedicti. Bruns. Ph. Blessed thistle ℥vj, rectified spirit Oij.

Tinctura Coccinellæ Septempunctatæ. Niemann. Digest 60 or 80 common lady-birds in ℥j of rectified spirit for 8 days, and strain. *Antiodontalgic.*

Tinctura Cocci. Ams. Ph. Cochineal (bruised) 1 part, proof spirit 8 parts. Digest for 8 days and strain. Sauter directs a *saturated* tincture as an *antispasmodic.*

Tinctura Cocci Ilicis. Ellis. Kermes ℥ij, brandy f℥vij; digest in a stoppered bottle.

Tinctura Cocci Ammoniata. Dr. Eberle. Cochineal ℥ss, water of ammonia ℥ss, rectified spirit f℥viij. Dose, 5 drops, *in Hooping-cough.*

Tinctura Cochleariæ Composita. See Tinct. Antiscorbutica.

Tinctura Colchici. L. and E. (Tinct. Seminum Colchici, D.) Colchicum seeds (bruised, L. ground in a coffee-mill, E.) ℥v, proof spirit Oij. Macerate for 14 days. E. by percolation, as Tinct. Cinchonæ. Dose, ♏xxx to fʒj. [P. from the dried cormi, one part to four of proof spirit.]

Tinctura Florum Colchici. Dr. Wilson's *Eau Medicinale.* Mix two parts of fresh juice of colchicum flowers with one of brandy; after a few days filter or decant.

Tinctura Extracti Colchici. Bateman. Extract of colchicum gr. viij, proof spirit fʒj.

Tinctura Colchici Composita. L. (Spiritus Colchici Ammoniatus, L. 1824.) Colchicum seeds ℥v, aromatic spirit of ammonia Oij. Macerate for 14 days. Dose, ♏xv to fʒj.

Tinctura Colocynthidis Dahlbergi. Colocynth pulp ʒiv, spirit of aniseed ℥vj; digest for three days, express, and filter. [Prus. Ph. Colocynth ℥j, star-aniseed ʒj, proof spirit ℔j.] Dose, xv or xx drops.

Tinctura Colombæ. D. See Tinctura Calumbæ. U. S. ℥iv colombo to f℥xxxij of proof spirit.

Tinctura Conii. L. and D. Dried hemlock ℥v, cardamom

seed ℥j, proof spirit Oij. Macerate for 14 days. E. directs fresh hemlock ℥xij, tincture of cardamoms f℥x, rectified spirit f℥xxx. Bruise and press the hemlock, and transmit first the tincture, and then the spirit through the pressed residuum, into the juice, gently adding water q. s. to push through the spirit remaining in the percolator. [Dr. PEREIRA suggests a tincture of the *fruit;* but does not give the proportions.] P. directs tinctures to be prepared from the dried leaves, with four times their weight of proof spirit, and with æther in the same proportion; and also a tincture from the fresh leaves, as Tinct. Aconiti.

TINCTURA CONII ÆTHEREA. P. As Tinctura Aconiti Ætherea.

TINCTURA CONTRAYERVÆ. P. Contrayerva root ℥iv, spirit of wine (0·863) Oj.

TINCTURA CORNUS CIRCINATÆ. Dr. REECE. Extract of round-leaved cornel (dog-wood) ℥j, brandy Oj.

TINCTURA CROCI. E. Saffron ℥ij, proof spirit Oij. Prepare by digestion or percolation.

TINCTURA CROTONIS. SOUBEIRAN. Croton oil 16 drops, rectified spirit ℥j. POPE. Croton seed ʒj, rectified spirit ℥jss. BATEMAN. Croton oil four drops, tincture of myrrh f℥j. NIMMO. Eight drops of oil to f℥j of rectified spirit.

TINCTURA CUBEBÆ. L. Cubebs ℥v, rectified spirit [D. & U. S., proof spirit] Oij; macerate for 14 days. A concentrated tincture (sold as essence of cubebs) may be conveniently made by percolation of any desired strength. Mix the ground berries with sufficient rectified spirit to moisten them; after 12 hours put the pulp into a percolator, and pour more spirit till the tincture equals the weight of the cubebs, or more according to strength required.

TINCTURA CULLILAWAN. WIRT. PH. Culilawan bark ʒiv, rectified spirit ℔jss; digest for four days, and filter.

TINCTURA CURCUMÆ. VAN MONS. Turmeric ℥j, rectified spirit ℥vj.

TINCTURA CUSPARIÆ. E. Cusparia bark ℥ivss, proof spirit Oij; by digestion, or percolation.

TINCTURA DELPHINII. AUGUSTIN. Larkspur seed ℥j, rectified spirit ℔ss; digest. Dose, ♏x to xx, in *Asthma.*

TINCTURA DELPHINIÆ. See Solutio Delphiniæ.

TINCTURA DIGITALIS. L. & E. Dried foxglove ℥iv, proof spirit Oij; macerate for 14 days. E. By percolation, as Tinct. Capsici. L. 1824 and D. direct ℥iv of dried digitalis to f ℥xxxij of spirit. Dose, from ♏x, sometimes gradually increased to ♏xl.

TINCTURA DIGITALIS ÆTHEREA. P. As Tinctura Aconiti Ætherea.

TINCTURA DIGITALIS COMPOSITA. VAN MONS. Digitalis ℥ij, spirit of bitter almonds ℥xvj.

TINCTURA ELATERII. Extract of elaterium gr. viij, rectified spirit f ℥viij. Dose, f ʒss to f ʒij.

TINCTURA ERGOTÆ. GUY'S H. Ergot of rye ℥jss, proof spirit Oj; macerate for 14 days, and strain. Dose, from ♏xx to f ʒij. [A stronger tincture is used by Dr. BLUNDEL; see Essentia Secalis Cornuti.]

TINCTURA ERGOTÆ ÆTHEREA. Powdered ergot ℥ij, white sand ℥ij; mix, and place them in an apparatus for displacement, and pouring on them ℥ix of sulphuric æther, to produce ℥viij of tincture. Dose ♏xxx to f ʒj. PHARM. JOURNAL. For a stronger preparation see Essentia Secalis Cornuti Ætherea.

TINCTURA ERGOTÆ AMMONIATA. Mr. GORE. Bruised ergot ℥iv, aromatic spirit of ammonia Oss; macerate for a month, express, and filter. Dose, 30 drops every 10 minutes till it excites *uterine contractions.*

TINCTURA EUPHORBII. PRUS. PH. Euphorbium ʒj, rectified spirit ℔j.

TINCTURA FEBRIFUGA. Dr. CLUTTON. Febrifuge spirit Oss, angelica root 3jss, serpentary ʒjss, cardamom seed ʒjss; digest, and filter.

TINCTURA FELLIS. Inspissated ox-gall ℥ij, proof spirit Oj; digest until dissolved.

TINCTURA FERRI ACETATIS. D. Acetate of potash 2 parts, sulphate of iron 1 part; rub them together, dry with a moderate heat, triturate with 26 parts of rectified spirit, digest for 7 days in a stoppered bottle, shaking frequently, and decant. Dose ♏xx to ʒj.

TINCTURA FERRI ACETATIS CUM ALCOHOLE. D. Acetate of potash ℥j, sulphate of iron ℥j, rub together, dry, digest in a well-stoppered bottle for 24 hours with f ℥xxxij of alcohol (sp. gr. ·810), shaking frequently and decant. Dose, ♏xx to f ʒj.

TINCTURA FERRI ACETATIS ÆTHEREA. PRUS. PH. To 9 parts of strong acetic acid add moist oxide of iron (see Ferrugo) in excess; digest, filter, and add 1 part of acetic æther, and 2 of rectified spirit.

TINCTURA FERRI AMMONIO-CHLORIDI. L. *Tinct. Ferri Ammoniati.* Ammonio-chloride of iron ℥iv, proof spirit Oj; dissolve. Dose, ♏x to xl.

TINCTURA FERRI AURANTIACA. WIRTEMB. PH. Iron filings ℥iv, Seville oranges, deprived of their seed, No. 4; beat them together, leave them for 2 days, then add Madeira wine ℥x, spirit of orange-peel ℥ij; digest, express, and filter.

TINCTURA FERRI PROTO-IODIDI. CALLOUD. Sulphate of iron ℥j, iodide of potassium ʒx; powder separately, triturate together, and add rectified spirit Oj. Filter, and keep in well-closed bottles quite filled; f ʒj contains about 4 grains of dry iodide of iron.

TINCTURA FERRI MALATIS. See Tinctura Martis Cydoniatum.

TINCTURA FERRI SESQUICHLORIDI. L. *Tinctura Ferri Muriatis.* E. Sesquioxide of iron [red oxide, E.] ℥vj, hydrochloric acid Oj; digest for 3 days, add Oiij of rectified spirit, and filter. [Tinct. Ferri Muriatis, E. 1817, was made with the black oxide.]

TINCTURA FERRI CHLORIDI ÆTHEREA. P. *Teinture de Bestuchef.* Dry perchloride of iron ʒj, spirit of sulphuric æther 3vij; mix in a stoppered bottle, and keep it from the light. [It was formerly made with 3j of proto-chloride of iron, and ʒix of spirit of æther.]

TINCTURA FERRI TARTARIZATA. *Tinct. Martis Tartarizata.* Pure iron filings 100 parts, cream of tartar 250, rectified spirit 50 parts; put the filings and tartar into an iron kettle with sufficient water to form a soft paste; leave them for 24 hours, add 3000 parts of soft water, and boil for 2 hours, stirring constantly, and supplying the waste of water. Decant and filter the liquor, and evaporate it till it marks 32° (1·286), and add the spirit. Dose, 3 to 6 drops.

TINCTURA FEVILLÆ CORDIFOLIÆ. DR. HAMILTON. Macerate 8 or 10 bruised cocoons (seeds of the plant) in Oj of spirit for 2 or 3 days; and diluting the tincture with Oj of water. Dose f ℥ss. Stomachic; in larger doses, *purgative and emetic.*

TINCTURA FILICIS ÆTHEREA. PESCHIER. Buds of male fern 1 part, sulphuric æther 8 parts; by percolation and digestion.

TINCTURA FULIGINIS. L. 1746. Wood-soot (the most compact and shining pieces) ℥ij, assafœtida ℥j, proof spirit Oij; digest for a few days, and filter.

TINCTURA GALANGÆ. AMST. PH. Galangal root ℥j, proof spirit ℥vj.

TINCTURA GALBANI. D. Galbanum ℥ij, proof spirit f ℥xxxij; digest for 7 days, and filter.

TINCTURA GALLÆ. L. E. & D. Gall nuts ℥v, proof spirit Oij; macerate for 14 days. [E., by digestion 7 days, or percolation.]

TINCTURA GAMBOGIÆ AMMONIATA. SWEDIAUR. Gamboge gr. xxxvj, spirit of ammonia ℥iv.

TINCTURA GENTIANÆ COMPOSITA. L. *Tinctura Amara.* Gentian ℥ijss, dried orange-peel ʒx, cardamom seed ʒv, proof spirit Oij; macerate for 14 days [7 days, D.], and filter. E. omits the cardamom, and adds canella ʒvj, cochineal ʒss. By digestion 7 days, or percolation.

TINCTURA GENTIANÆ AMMONIATA. *Elixir Antiscrofuleux.* P. Gentian ℥j, carbonate of ammonia ʒij, proof spirit ℥xxxij. [Dr. PERHYLE's Elixir differs in substituting ʒiij of crystallized subcarbonate of soda for the ammonia.]

TINCTURA GENTIANINÆ. M. Gentianine gr. v, proof spirit f ʒx.

TINCTURA GERANII. Dried roots of geranium maculatum ℥v, proof spirit Oij. *Astringent.* Chiefly used in gargles, &c.

TINCTURA GINGIVALIS. PORT. PH. Myrrh ℥j, catechu ℥j, tincture of Peruvian balsam 3j, spirit of scurvy-grass ℥iv, rectified spirit ℥iv; 4 days.

TINCTURA GRANI PARADISI. Grains of paradise ℥j, proof spirit Oj; macerate for 10 days.

TINCTURA GRATIOLÆ. Dr. REECE. Dried hedge-hyssop ℥iv, proof spirit f ℥xxxij.

TINCTURA GUAIACI. L. & E. Guaiacum resin ℥vij, rectified

spirit Oij; macerate for 14 days. [D., ℥iv to f℥xxxij.] Dose, fℨj to fℨij.

TINCTURA GUAIACI ALKALINA. Dr. DEWEES. Guaiacum ℥v, carbonate of potash (or of soda) ℨiij, pimento ℥ij, proof spirit Oij. A teaspoonful 3 times a day, in *dysmenorrhœa*, &c.

TINCTURA GUAIACI COMPOSITA. L. *Tinct. Guaiaci Ammoniata.* E. Guaiacum resin ℥vij, aromatic spirit of ammonia Oij; macerate for 14 days. [E. directs simple spirit of ammonia, and 7 days' digestion.] Dose, fℨj to fℨij, in *chronic rheumatism*, &c.

TINCTURA GUAIACI FŒNICULATA. SWED. PH. Guaiacum resin ℥j, oil of fennel ℨss; digest with a gentle heat for 24 hours, and add ℔j of spirit of wine of 0·900 sp. gr.

TINCTURA LIGNI GUAIACI. P. One part of the wood to 4 parts, by weight, of proof spirit.

TINCTURA LIGNI GUAIACI COMPOSITA. PRUS. PH. *Essentia Lignorum.* Rasped guaiacum ℥iij, sassafras ℥ij, rhodium wood ℥ss, red santal ℥j, yellow santal ℥j, rectified spirit ℔ij.

TINCTURA HELLEBORI [NIGRI]. L. & D. Black hellebore root ℥v, proof spirit Oij; macerate for 14 days, and filter. Dose, ♏xxx to fℨj, with caution.

TINCTURA HELLEBORI ALBI. See Tinctura Veratri.

TINCTURA HIPPOCASTANEI. M. JOBERT. Horse-chestnut bark ℥iv, proof spirit Oj; macerate for 15 days, and filter. *Tonic.*

TINCTURA HUMULI. D. See Tinctura Lupuli.

TINCTURA HIBISCI ABELMOSCHI. Dr. REECE. Musk seed ℥ij, proof spirit f℥xvj.

TINCTURA HYOSCYAMI. L. E. & D. Dried henbane leaves ℥v, proof spirit Oij; macerate for 14 days, [7 days, or by percolation, E.] Dose, fℨss to fℨjss.

TINCTURA HYPERICI. Flowering tops of St. John's-wort ℥v, rectified spirit Oj; digest for 3 days.

TINCTURA IMPERATORIÆ. Masterwort root ℥ij, proof spirit f℥xvj. Digest and strain. (Pharm. Journ.)

TINCTURA INULÆ. P. Powdered elecampane ℥iv, proof spirit Oj; digest for 15 days.

TINCTURA IODINII. M. P. D. & Dr. COINDET. One part of

iodine, to 12 parts by weight of rectified spirit. E. & U. S. are virtually the same—℥j of iodine to f ℥xvj of rectified spirit. [It alters spontaneously, and is decomposed by water.] Dose, 4 to 8 drops (COINDET); others extend the dose to 20 drops, or more.

TINCTURA IODINII COMPOSITA. L. Iodine ℥j, iodide of potassium ℥ij, rectified spirit Oij; dissolve. Dose, from ♏v to xxx. GUIBOURT recommends iodine 5 parts, iodide of potassium 6 parts, rectified spirit 50, distilled water 100 parts.

TINCTURA IODINII ÆTHEREA. M. Iodine ℈ij, sulphuric æther ℥j (f ℥jss.)

TINCTURA IPECACUANHÆ. P. Ipecac. ℥iv, proof spirit ℥xvj, (nearly Oj). [The Vinum Ipecac. is so named in E. 1744.]

TINCTURA IPECACUANHÆ ANISATA. ALIBERT. Ipecacuanha ℥j, spirit of aniseed ℥iv, sugar ʒiv; digest.

TINCTURA IRIDIS. Fresh powdered orris root 1 part, rectified spirit 8 parts. (Sold as *Esprit de Violettes.*)

TINCTURA JALAPÆ. L. E. and D. Jalap (in powder) ℥x, (℥vij E.) proof spirit Oij; digest for 14 days.

TINCTURA JALAPÆ COMPOSITA. E. 1744. Jalap root ʒvj, black hellebore root ʒiij, juniper berries ℥ss, guaiacum shavings ℥ss, French brandy f ℥xxiv; digest for 3 days, and strain. [P. Jalap ℥viij, turpeth root ℥j, scammony ℥ij, proof spirit ℔viij.]

TINCTURA JALAPÆ COMFORTANS. AMST. PH. Jalap ℥ij, lemon-peel ℥j, cinnamon ʒss, aniseed ʒij, rectified spirit ℥viij, proof spirit ℥viij. Macerate for 8 days.

TINCTURA JAPONICA. See Tinctura Catechu.

TINCTURA JUGLANDIS. DAM. PH. Green shells of walnut ℥vj, proof spirit f ℥xxiv; digest 6 days.

TINCTURA JUSTICIÆ. Dr. AINSLIE. Root of panicled justicia ℥iij, proof spirit Oij. Used as Tinct. Calumbæ.

TINCTURA KALINA. See Solutio Potassæ Alcoholica.

TINCTURA KALMIÆ. Dr. STABLER. Leaves of mountain laurel (Kalmia latifolia) ℥ij, rectified spirit f ℥xvj. Dose, 30 drops, 4 or 6 times a day; as an arterial sedative.

TINCTURA KINO. L. and E. Kino ℥ijss, rectified spirit Oij;

macerate for 14 [7, E.] days. D. Kino ℥iij, proof spirit f ℥xxiv.

TINCTURA KRAMERIÆ. See Tinctura Rhataniæ.

TINCTURA LACCÆ. E. 1744. Gum lac ℥j, myrrh ℥ss, solution of subcarbonate of potash q. s.; rub together to a soft paste, dry it, and digest in spirit of scurvy-grass Ojss.

TINCTURA LACTUCARII. E. Powdered lactucarium ℥iv, proof spirit Oij; digest, or percolate.

TINCTURA LACTUCÆ VIROSÆ. P. From the fresh leaves, as Tinctura Aconiti recentis.

TINCTURA LAVANDULÆ COMPOSITA. L. Spirit of lavender Ojss, spirit of rosemary Oss, cinnamon ʒijss, nutmeg ʒijss, red saunders wood ʒv; macerate for 14 days, and strain. [For E. and D. see Spiritus Lavandulæ Compositus.]

TINCTURA CORTICIS LIMONUM. SOUBEIRAN. Dried lemon-peel ℥iv, proof spirit ℥xvj. Digest 15 days. [When intended for aromatizing syrups, &c., the *fresh* peel should be used.]

TINCTURA LIRIODENDRI. Digest ℥iv of bruised tulip-tree bark in Oj of proof spirit for 7 days. Tonic and diaphoretic. Dose, f ʒj.

TINCTURA LOBELIÆ. E. Dried lobelia (inflata) in moderately fine powder ℥v, proof spirit Oij; prepare by digestion or percolation. Dose, 20 to 40 drops.

TINCTURA LOBELIÆ ÆTHEREA. E. As the last, substituting spirit of sulphuric æther for proof spirit. [WHITLAW'S Æthereal Tincture is—dried lobelia ℔j, rectified spirit Oiv, spirit of nitric æther Oiv, spirit of sulphuric æther ℥iv; macerate for 14 days in a dark place, and filter. Dose, ♏v to xx.]

TINCTURA LUPULI. L. *Tinctura Humuli.* D. Hops ℥vj, proof spirit Oij; macerate for 14 days and strain. [E. is the same as Tinctura Lupulinæ.]

TINCTURA LUPULINÆ. U. S. (Tinct. Lupuli, E.) Lupuline ℥v, rectified spirit Oij, macerate for 14 days, and filter. [Or by percolation, E.]

TINCTURA LUPULI COMPOSITA. F. H. *Liqueur des teigneux.* Hops ℥j, smaller centaury ℥j, orange-peel ʒij, carbonate of potash ℈j, proof spirit Oj.

TINCTURA MACIDIS. Mace ℥j, rectified spirit Oss; macerate for 8 days.

TINCTURA MAGNOLIÆ. Recently dried bark, or cones of Magnolia glauca ℥iv, proof spirit or brandy Oj. *In chronic rheumatism.*

TINCTURA MARTIS CYDONIATUM. PRUS. PH. Impure malate of iron (extractum martis cydoniatum) ℥j, spirit of cinnamon ℥vj.

TINCTURA MARTIS TARTARIZATA. See Tinct. Ferri Tartarizata.

TINCTURA MASTICHES. Mastic ℥ij, rectified spirit f℥ix. [Used in making Eau de Luce, or Tinctura Ammoniæ Composita.]

TINCTURA MATTICONIS. Dr. H. LANE. Matico leaves ℥ijss (℥iij Dr. JEFFREYS), proof spirit Oj; macerate for 14 days, and strain. Dose, fℨss to fℨij. *Styptic.*

TINCTURA OLEI MENTHÆ PIPERITÆ, PULEGII, ET VIRIDIS. U. S. ℥ij of the oil to f℥xvj of rectified spirit. [The *Infusion* of mint was termed *Tincture* in E. 1744.]

TINCTURA MONESIÆ. ST. ANGE. Monesia (extract) ℨss, proof spirit ℥viij. Mr. DONOVAN. Monesia ℥j, proof spirit f℥ixss, water f℥ij; macerate, and decant. DEROSNE. Monesia ℥ss, water ℥vijss, spirit ℥ij.

TINCTURA MOSCHI. D. Musk ℨij, rectified spirit f℥xvj; macerate for 7 days. P. ℥iv to Oj.

TINCTURA MOSCHI ARTIFICIALIS. VAN MONS. Artificial musk ℨj, rectified spirit f℥ij [ℨx, BERZELIUS.]

TINCTURA MYRISTICÆ COMPOSITA. *Essence Cephalique.* P. Nutmeg ℥ij, cloves ℥ij, cinnamon ℥jss, pomegranate flowers ℥jss, rectified spirit Oij; macerate for 15 days, and strain.

TINCTURA MYRRHÆ. L. and E. Myrrh ℥iij [℥iijss, E.], rectified spirit Oij; macerate for 14 days [7 days or by percolation, E.] D. Myrrh ℥iij, rectified spirit f℥viij, proof spirit f℥xxiv.

TINCTURA MYRRHÆ ÆTHEREA. P. As Tinct. Castorei Ætherea.

TINCTURA MYRRHÆ ET ALÖES. E. 1744. Myrrh ℥ij, aloes ℥j, rectified spirit Ojss; digest for 8 days.

TINCTURA MYRRHÆ ALKALIZATA. E. 1744. Powdered myrrh ℥jss, solution of subcarbonate of potash q. s.; mix into a soft paste, dry it, and add rectified spirit Oj; digest for 6 days, and strain.

TINCTURA NERVOSA RIEMERII. Volatile liquor of hartshorn ʒiv, rectified spirit ℥ij, oil of juniper ʒj.

TINCTURA NICOTIANÆ ÆTHEREA. P. Powdered tobacco leaves ℥iv, sulphuric æther ℥xvj (nearly f℥xxiv). By percolation.

TINCTURA NUCIS VOMICÆ. D. Rasped nux vomica ℥ij, rectified spirit f℥viij; macerate for 7 days, and filter. [M. Extract of nux vomica gr. x, rectified spirit ℥iij.]

TINCTURA ODONTALGICA. Tincture of opium ʒj, sulphuric æther ʒiij, oil of cloves 3 drops. See Tinct. Pyrethri, and Guttæ Odontalgicæ.

TINCTURA OPII. L. Powdered opium ℥iij, proof spirit Oij; macerate for 14 days. D. ʒx of opium to f℥xvj of spirit. E. Opium sliced ℥iij, rectified spirit f℥xxvij, water f℥xiijss. Digest the opium in the water near the boiling temperature for 2 hours, break it down with the hand, strain, and express; macerate the residuum in the rectified spirit for 24 hours, then strain, and express strongly; mix the watery and spirituous infusions, and filter.

TINCTURA CUM EXTRACTO OPII. P. Extract of opium ℥j, proof spirit ℥xij; dissolve, and filter.

TINCTURA OPII ACETATA. U. S. Opium ℥ij, vinegar f℥xij, rectified spirit f℥viij; rub the opium with the vinegar, then add the spirit; and, having macerated for 14 days, express, and filter. [*Vinaigre d'opium*, P. is identical except that the liquids are by weight. ♏x, U. S., or gr. x, P. represent gr. j of opium.]

TINCTURA OPII AMMONIATA. E. *Scotch Paregoric.* Benzoic acid ʒvj, saffron ʒvj, opium ℥ss, oil of aniseed ʒj, spirit of ammonia Oij; digest 7 days. [The spirit of ammonia must be that of E. which contains caustic ammonia. That of L. does not hold the morphia in solution.]

TINCTURA OPII CROCATA. See Vinum Opii.

TINCTURA OPII CAMPHORATA. E. *Paregoric Elixir.* Camphor ℈ijss, opium sliced ℈iv, benzoic acid ℈iv, oil of anise fʒj, proof spirit Oij. Digest for 7 days, and filter. D. Opium in powder ʒj, benzoic acid ʒj, oil of anise ʒj, camphor ℈ij, proof spirit f℥xxxij. U. S. the same, with ℥ij of clarified honey. Dose, from fʒj to fʒij. For L. see Tinctura Camphoræ Composita.

TINCTURA OREOSELINI. VAN MONS. Fresh spignel leaves ℥ij, spignel seeds ʒj, proof spirit ℥xiv; macerate for some days.

TINCTURA PAREIRÆ. Sir B. BRODIE. Pareira brava root ℥ij, French brandy Oj; digest for 7 days.

TINCTURA PAULLINIÆ. Dr. GAVRELLE. Extract of paullinia ℥j, proof spirit ℥xvj; dissolve.

TINCTURA PHELLANDRII. NIEMANN. Seeds of water-fennel (phellandrium aquaticum) ℥ss, rectified spirit ℥vj; digest for 24 hours, and add burgundy wine ℥vj; digest, and filter.

TINCTURA PHOSPHORI ÆTHEREA. P. Sliced phosphorus ʒj, sulphuric æther ℥vj ʒij; macerate for a month in the dark, and decant.

TINCTURA PIMPINELLÆ. PRUS. PH. Burnet saxifrage root ℥v, rectified spirit Oij.

TINCTURA PINI. AUSTR. PH. Buds of spruce fir ℥ij, proof spirit ℔j.

TINCTURA PINI COMPOSITA. SAX. PH. Buds of spruce fir ℥iij, rasped guaiacum ℥ij, sassafras ʒj, juniper berries ℥jss, rectified spirit ℔j; digest, and filter.

TINCTURA PIPERIS STOMACHICA. *Essentia Stomachica Polychresta.* SPIELMAN. Capsicum ʒj, black pepper ʒij, long pepper ʒij, white pepper ʒij, solution of acetate of potash ℥vj, spirit of ammonia ℥j; digest, and filter.

TINCTURA PIPERIS ANGUSTIFOLIÆ. See Tinct. Matticonis.

TINCTURA PISCIDIÆ ERYTHRINÆ. Dr. HAMILTON. Jamaica dogwood ʒj, rectified spirit f℥iv; digest for 7 days. Full dose, as a narcotic, fʒj.

TINCTURA POPULI. VAN MONS. Poplar buds ʒiv, rectified spirit ℥xxiv; macerate and filter.

TINCTURA POTASSÆ. See Solutio Potassæ Alcoholica.

TINCTURA POTASSÆ HYDRIODATIS. Dr. COINDET. Iodide of potassium ʒss, proof spirit ℥j.

TINCTURA POTASSII SULPHURETI. *Tinctura Sulphuris.* QUINCY. Sulphuret of potash ℥iv, spirit of wine ℥xvj, digest 24 hours, and strain.

TINCTURA PYRETHRI. CADET. Pellitory of Spain root ℥j, spirit of rosemary ℥viij. P. Pellitory ℥iv, spirit of wine (0·863 sp. gr.) Oj; or spirit of sulphuric æther Oj.

TINCTURA PYRETHRI COMPOSITA. BRANDE. Pellitory root ʒiv, camphor ʒiij, opium ʒj, oil of cloves ʒij, rectified spirit ℥vj; digest for 8 days, and filter. [Another Comp. Tincture of Pellitory, called *Paraguay-Roux*, is thus prepared—Pellitory root ℥j, Para cress (flowers of Spilanthus oleraceus) ℥iv, leaves of Italian elecampane (Inula bifrons) ℥j, rectified spirit f℥viij. Macerate for 15 days, express and filter.]

TINCTURA PURGANS. P. See Tinctura Jalapæ Comp. Dr. FULLER prescribes—Senna ℥iij, rhubarb ℥j, scammony ℈iv, brandy Oiv.

TINCTURA QUASSIÆ. E. & D. Quassia chips ʒx, proof spirit Oij. [U. S. ℥ij to f℥xxxij.]

TINCTURA QUASSIÆ COMPOSITA. E. Cardamom seed ʒiv, cochineal ʒiv, cinnamon ʒvj, quassia ʒvj, raisins ℥vij, proof spirit Oij. Digest for 7 days.

TINCTURA QUINÆ. M. Sulphate of quinine gr. vj, rectified spirit ℥j, (or gr. v to fʒx.) Dr. COPLAND—gr. viij to ℥j.

TINCTURA QUINÆ IMPURÆ. PIORRY. *Teinture de Quinine brute.* Crude quinine ℥j, rectified spirit ℥xij, distilled water ℥xij.

TINCTURA QUINÆ SULPHATIS ACIDA. Dr. COPLAND. Sulphate of quinine gr. xlviij, compound tincture of orange-peel f℥vss, dilute sulphuric acid f3ij, (or elixir of vitriol ♏xlv.) Dose, fʒss to fʒij.

TINCTURA QUINÆ HYDROCYANOFERRATIS. Mr. DONOVAN. Ferroprussiate of quinine gr. xxxij, rectified spirit f℥j. Dose, fʒj.

TINCTURA RHATANIÆ. *Tinctura Krameriæ.* U. S. Powdered rhatany root ℥vj, proof spirit f℥xxxij; digest, or percolate.

TINCTURA RHATANIÆ AROMATICA *vel* COMPOSITA. PAREIRA. Rhatany root ℥iij, dried orange-peel ℥ij, proof spirit Oj. REECE. Rhatany ℥ij, orange-peel ℥ss, canella (or cinnamon) 3jss, proof spirit f℥xxxij. NIEMANN. Rhatany ℥iij, orange-peel ℥ij, serpentary ʒiv, saffron ʒj, proof spirit ℔ij. Digest for 12 days.

TINCTURA RHEI COMPOSITA. L. Rhubarb ℥ijss, liquorice root ʒvj, ginger ʒiij, saffron ʒiij, proof spirit Oij; macerate for 14 days, and strain. [The two following tinctures of rhubarb were ordered before 1836, for which this was then substituted.

Tinctura Rhei. L. 1824. Rhubarb ℥ij, cardamom seed ℥ss, saffron ℈ij, proof spirit f℥xxxij. Tinctura Rhei Composita. L. 1824. Rhubarb ℥ij, liquorice root ℥ss, ginger ℈ij, saffron ʒij, proof spirit f℥xvj, water f℥xij.]

TINCTURA RHEI. E. Rhubarb ℥iijss, cardamom seed ℥ss, proof spirit Oij. By percolation (the rhubarb in moderately fine powder) or digestion. D. (Tinct. Rhei Comp.) Rhubarb ℥ij, ginger ʒss, cardamom ℥ss, saffron ℈ij, proof spirit f℥xxxij.

TINCTURA RHEI ET ALOES. E. *Elixir Sacrum.* Rhubarb in moderately fine powder ℥jss, aloes (E. I. or Soc.) ʒvj, cardamom seed bruised ʒv, proof spirit Oij. By percolation.

TINCTURA RHEI ANISATA. Dr. COPLAND. Rhubarb ℥ij, liquorice root ℥ij, aniseed ʒj, sugar ʒj, proof spirit Oij; macerate for 14 days.

TINCTURA RHEI AQUOSA [ALKALINA]. PRUS. PH. Rhubarb ℥jss, carbonate of potash ʒiij, boiling water ℥xij; macerate for 12 hours, and strain, and add spirit of cinnamon ℥ij.

TINCTURA RHEI ET GENTIANÆ. E. Rhubarb (in moderately fine powder, if by percolation) ℥ij, gentian (coarsely powdered) ℥ss, proof spirit Oij. By percolation or digestion.

TINCTURA RHEI ET SENNÆ. U. S. *Warner's Gout Cordial.* Rhubarb ℥j, senna ʒij, coriander seed ʒj, fennel seed ʒj, red saunders ʒij, saffron ℈ss, liquorice (ext.) ʒss, raisins (stoned) ℥vj, proof spirit f℥xlviij; macerate for 14 days, and filter.

TINCTURA RHODII. GRAY. Rhodium wood ℥iv, rectified spirit f℥xvj; digest for 14 days.

TINCTURA RHODODENDRI. NIEMANN. Leaves of rhododendron chrysanthum ℥ij, French brandy ℔ss, sherry wine ℔ss; digest for 15 days.

TINCTURA RHOIS [TOXICODENDRI *vel* RADICANTIS]. P. From the fresh leaves, as Tinct. Aconiti cum fol. rec. Dose, 5 to 10 drops, gradually increased to 25. It may also be made from the dried leaves, as Tinct. Aconiti. P.

TINCTURA RICINI. PAROLA. An alcoholic and an æthereal tincture are directed to be made by digesting bruised castor-oil seeds in five times their weight of rectified spirit or of sulphuric æther. These tinctures are stated to be four times the strength of the oil.

TINCTURA ROSMARINÆ. BRUNS. PH. Flowering tops of rosemary ℥jss, spirit of rosemary ℥vj; digest, express, and filter.

TINCTURA ROSÆ. Mr. SQUIRE. Dried red rose ℥v, rectified spirit f℥ij; rose water f℥viij; digest for three or four days, express, and filter; digest the mass with Oss of proof spirit for three days, press off, and mix the liquors. [Tinct. Rosarum, L. 1846. Inf. Rosæ.]

TINCTURA SABADILLÆ. Dr. TURNBULL. Digest the seeds of cevadilla (freed from their capsules, [as directed in preparing veratria, E.] and bruised) for 10 days in as much rectified spirit as will cover them. *For external use only, in rheumatism,* &c.

TINCTURA SABINÆ COMPOSITA. L. 1788. *Elixir Myrrhæ Comp.* Extract of savin ℥j, tincture of castor f℥xvj, tincture of myrrh f℥viij; digest until dissolved.

TINCTURA SACRA. See Vinum Alöes.

TINCTURA SALUTIFERA. E. 1744. Angelica root, calamus aromaticus, galangal, gentian, zedoary, bay berries, cardamom seed, cinnamon, long pepper, of each ʒj, French brandy Oij.

TINCTURA SANGUINARIÆ. U. S. Blood root ℥iv, proof spirit f℥xxxij; macerate for 14 days, or prepare by percolation. Dose, as a stimulant and alterative, 30 to 60 drops; as an emetic fʒiij—iv.

TINCTURA SAPONIS. P. White soap ℥iij, subcarbonate of potash ʒj, proof spirit ℥xij: dissolve.

TINCTURA SAPONIS CAMPHORATA. U. S. Soap shavings ℥iv, camphor ℥ij, oil of rosemary fʒiv, rectified spirit f℥xxxij.

TINCTURA SAPONIS TEREBINTHINATA. *Baume de vie externe.* White soap ℥iij, oil of turpentine ℥iij, spirit of wild thyme ℔ij, water of ammonia ℥ij.

TINCTURA SARCOCOLLÆ. SARD. PH. Sarcocol ℥ij, rectified spirit ℥xvj; digest for 7 days, and strain.

TINCTURA SARZÆ. SOUBEIRAN. Cut sarsaparilla ℥iv, proof spirit Oj. Macerate 15 days.

TINCTURA SARZÆ COMPOSITA. *Liqueur depurative.* FRANCOIS. Sarsap., guaiacum, China root, sassafras, of each ℥j, proof spirit f℥xvj. A table-spoonful every morning.

TINCTURA SATURNINA. E. 1783. Acetate of lead ℈iv, sulphate of iron ʒj, rectified spirit ℔j; macerate without heat, and filter.

Tinctura Scammonii. P. Scammony ℥iv, rectified spirit Oj.

Tinctura Scillæ. L. E. and D. Dried squill ℥v, proof spirit Oij; macerate for 14 days, and filter. [7 days, or by percolation, E.]

Tinctura Scillæ Alkalina. Sobernheim. Squill ℥ij, solution of potash fʒij, rectified spirit ℥xij.

Tinctura Scillæ cum Elaterio. St. B. H. Tincture of squills fʒij, vinegar of colchicum fʒij, spirit of nitric æther f℥j, extract of elaterium gr. j. Dose, ♏xv to fʒj.

Tinctura Secalis Cornuti. See Tinctura Ergotæ.

Tinctura Senegæ. Hann. Ph. Seneka root ℥j, proof spirit ℥vj.

Tinctura Sennæ Composita. L. and D. Senna ℥iijss, caraway seed ʒiijss, cardamom ʒj, raisins ℥v, proof spirit Oij; macerate for 14 days, and strain. [The old Elixir Salutis contained guaiacum wood, which is said to increase the activity of senna.]

Tinctura Sennæ Composita. E. *Tinctura Sennæ et Jalapæ.* U. S. Sugar ℥ijss, coriander seed bruised ℥j, jalap in moderately fine powder ʒvj, senna ℥iv, caraway seed ʒv, cardamom seed ʒv, raisins bruised ℥iv, proof spirit Oij; digest for 7 days, or percolate. [U. S. is very similar, but weaker.]

Tinctura Sennæ Aromatica. See Tinctura Rhei et Sennæ.

Tinctura Serpentariæ. L. and D. Serpentary root ℥iijss, proof spirit Oij; macerate for 14 days. [E. 7 days, or by percolation; and adds ʒj of cochineal.]

Tinctura Solani Ætherea. P. Powdered leaves of garden nightshade ℥iv, sulphuric æther ℥xvj; by percolation.

Tinctura Spartii. Dr. Pearson. Spanish broom seeds ℥ij, proof spirit f℥viij; macerate for 10 days. Dose, from fʒj to fʒij or fʒiij daily.

Tinctura Staphisagriæ Concentrata. Dr. Turnbull. Digest stavesacre seeds in twice their weight of rectified spirit. *For external use only, in neuralgic and rheumatic affections,* as a substitute for Solutio Delphiniæ.

Tinctura Stramonii. U. S. Bruised stramonium seeds ℥iv, proof spirit f℥xxxij; macerate for 14 days, or percolate. Dose, ♏x to xxx. [P. From the dried leaves; also from the fresh leaves; and an æthereal tincture; as Tinct. Aconiti.]

TINCTURA STRYCHNIÆ. M. Strychnine gr. iij, rectified spirit f ʒxij. Sir J. WYLIE, gr. iij to ℥j of spirit.

TINCTURA STYPTICA. L. 1746. Calcined sulphate of iron ʒj, French brandy, coloured by the cask, ℔ij.

TINCTURA SUCCINI. P. Amber in fine powder ℥j, rectified spirit ℥xvj; digest for 6 days, and filter. [The *Æthereal* tincture, as Tinct. Castorei Ætherea.]

TINCTURA SUCCINI ALKALINA. E. 1744. Rub ℥ij of amber with q. s. solution of subcarbonate of potash to form a soft paste; dry this, and digest it in f℥xvj of rectified spirit for 8 days. See also Potestates Succini.

TINCTURA SUDORIFICA. E. 1744. Serpentary root ʒv, cochineal ʒiv, castor ʒj, saffron ℈ij, opium ℈j, spirit of mindererus f℥xvj; digest for three days, and strain.

TINCTURA TABACI. AUGUSTIN. Tobacco leaves ℥j, proof spirit ℔j; digest for three days.

TINCTURA TEREBINTHINÆ. P. Venice turpentine ℥iv, rectified spirit Oj.

TINCTURA TOLUTANA. E. See Tinct. Balsami Tolutani.

TINCTURA TOXICODENDRI. See Tinctura Rhois Toxicodendri.

TINCTURA VALERIANÆ. L. and D. Valerian root ℥v, proof spirit Oij; macerate for 14 days, [7 days, D.; by percolation or digestion, E.]

TINCTURA VALERIANÆ COMPOSITA. L. *Tinct. Val. Ammoniata.* E. and D. Valerian root ℥v, aromatic (simple, E. and D.) spirit of ammonia Oij; macerate for 14 days, [7 days, D. Proceed by percolation or digestion, E.]

TINCTURA VALERIANÆ ÆTHEREA. P. Valerian ℥iv, æther ℥xvj; by percolation.

TINCTURA VANILLÆ. P. Vanilla pods ℥j, spirit of wine (at 0·863 sp. gr.) ℥iv. Other pharm. order from ℥vj to ℥xij of spirit.

TINCTURA VERATRI. E. *Tinct. Hellebori Albi.* White hellebore ℥iv, proof spirit Oj. Dose, from ♏x.

TINCTURA VERATRIÆ. M. Veratria gr. iv, rectified spirit ℥j. Dose 10 to 25 drops. [*For external use,* Dr. TURNBULL employs veratria from ℈j to ʒj, rectified spirit ℥ij.]

TINCTURA VULNERARIA. P. The ingredients for spiritus vulnerarius are digested for 15 days with Oij of rectified spirit, and the liquor expressed and filtered.

TINCTURA ZEDOARIÆ. AMST. PH. Zedoary root 1 part, rectified spirit 8; digest, and filter.

TINCTURA ZINCI ACETATIS. D. Sulphate of zinc 1 part, acetate of potash 1 part, rub together, and add 16 parts of rectified spirit; macerate for a week, agitating occasionally, and filter.

TINCTURA ZINGIBERIS. L. Ginger sliced [in coarse powder, E.] ℥ijss, rectified spirit Oij; macerate for 14 days [or proceed by percolation, E.] D. directs proof spirit. A stronger tincture is directed by U. S. Ginger ℥viij, rectified spirit f ʒxxxij. Macerate for 14 days, and express. This is the *Essence of Ginger* of the shops.

TROCHISCI, *Troches* or *Lozenges*. These are small dry masses of confectionary of a determinate form; such as the flat *lozenges* (Tabellæ, *Tablettes*, P.); the hemispherical *drops* (Pastilli, *Pastilles*, P.); pipes, comfits, *grains*, &c. Double refined sugar should be used, and (except for *drops*) should be reduced to a fine powder, as should also the other dry ingredients. Some French pharmaciens apply the term *Pastilles* as a general name for these compounds. Another form of lozenge will be found under PASTA. Only those lozenges which are *medicated* require notice in this work.

Several compounds, not containing sugar, were formerly prepared in a similar form, but are now obsolete; except a few which are used as external applications (to which alone the term is now applied in the French Codex), and which are here placed after the rest.

TROCHISCI ACACIÆ. E. *Troch. Amyli vel Gummosi.* Gum arabic ℥iv, white starch ℥j, pure sugar ℔j; pulverize them, and make them into a proper mass with rose water for forming lozenges. P. Powdered gum ℔j; sugar ℔iij, orange-flower water ℥ij. Make a mucilage with the orange-flower water and part of the gum; add the rest of the gum previously mixed with the sugar, and make into lozenges. For another form of gum lozenge, see Pasta Gummi. The *transparent* gum paste or lozenges may be thus made: Dissolve ℔vj of picked gum arabic without heat in ℔viij of water, and add the solution to ℔vij of simple syrup. Evaporate by a gentle heat to a very thick syrup, adding towards the end f ℥iv of orange-flower water. Finish as directed for Pasta Jujubæ.

TROCHISCI ACIDI CITRICI. P. Citric acid ʒiij, sugar ℥xvj, essence of lemon 16 drops, mucilage of tragacanth q. s. Mix, and divide into 10-grain lozenges.

TROCHISCI ACIDI LACTICI. M. Lactic acid ʒij, sugar ℥j, oil of vanilla 4 drops, mucilage of tragacanth q. s.

TROCHISCI ACIDI OXALICI. SOUBEIRAN. Oxalic acid in fine powder ʒj, sugar ℥viij, oil of lemon 8 drops, mucilage of tragacanth q. s. In 10-grain lozenges.

TROCHISCI ACIDI TARTARICI. D. Tartaric acid ʒij, sugar ℥viij, oil of lemon ♏x, mucilage q. s.

TROCHISCI ALTHÆÆ. *Tablettes de Guimauve.* P. Powdered decorticated marsh-mallow root ℥ij, sugar ℥xiv, mucilage of tragacanth (made with orange-flower water) q. s. Divide into lozenges of 13 grains each. (See Pasta Althææ.)

TROCHISCI AMYLI. L. 1788. *Troch. Bechici Albii.* Starch ℥jss, liquorice powder ʒvj, orris ℈iv, sugar ℔jss, mucilage of tragacanth q. s.

TROCHISCI ANTHELMINTICI. PIDERIT. Sulphate of iron ʒss, worm-seed ʒjss, sugar ʒvj, mucilage q. s. For 32 lozenges. PHŒBUS. Worm-seed ℈j, chocolate ℈j, sugar ℈ij, mucilage of tragacanth q. s. See Troch. Santoninæ. [Lozenges containing calomel are also employed to destroy worms. The following are said to be the formulæ for CHING'S Worm Lozenges. *Yellow.* Calomel 1 part, sugar 28 parts, mucilage of tragacanth (made with infusion of saffron) q. s. Each lozenge to contain 1 grain of calomel. *Brown.* Calomel ʒj, resinous extract of jalap ℈j, white sugar ℈ijss, mucilage of tragacanth q. s. For 120 lozenges.]

TROCHISCI ANISI. DORVAULT directs them to be prepared from the oil as orange drops. See Tro. Aurantii. They are more frequently sold in the form of pipes, for which Mr. BARTLETT gives the following form :—Sugar ℔iij, umber (to colour) ʒiij, oil of aniseed 50 drops, mucilage q. s.

TROCHISCI ANTIMONII. P. *Tablettes de Kunkel.* Levigated black antimony ℈j, sweet almonds ℈ij, sugar ℈xiij, cardamom ℈j, cinnamon ʒiv; beat the blanched almonds with the sugar, add the other powders, mix intimately, and make a mass, with mucilage of tragacanth. Divide into lozenges of 15 grains each.

TROCHISCI ANTI-CATARRHALES. *Tablettes de Tronchin.* Gum

acacia ℥viij, oil of aniseed 6 drops, extract of opium gr. xij, mineral kermes ʒj, extract of liquorice ℥ij, sugar ℥xxxij, mucilage of tragacanth q. s. In 10-grain lozenges. VANDAMME'S *Tablettes Anticatarrhales.* Benzoic acid ʒij, sugar ℥xxxij, orris ʒiv, gum acacia ℥ij, starch ℥iv, water ℥iv. Divide into lozenges of 15 grains each.

TROCHISCI AURANTII. Orange lozenges may be made as Troch. Limonis, flavouring with oil of orange-peel, and colouring with a little infusion of saffron. The Drops (Pastilli, P.) are thus made: Sugar in coarse powder (prepared by first passing it through a hair sieve, and then removing the finer powder by a lawn sieve,) ℥xij, oil of orange flowers ʒj, orange-flower water q. s. Make a paste with part of the sugar and the water; heat it to boiling, stir in the rest of the sugar, and, lastly, the oil; then drop it from a metal rod in small portions on a tinned plate.

TROCHISCI AURI. CHRESTIEN. Auro-chloride of soda gr. iv, sugar ℥j, mucilage of tragacanth q. s. For 60 lozenges, 2 daily.

TROCHISCI AURI CYANIDI. CHRESTIEN. Cyanide of gold gr. ij, chocolate paste ℥j. Make into 24 lozenges. From 1 to 4 in the day.

TROCHISCI BALSAMICÆ. See Troch. Tolutani.

TROCHISCI BECHICI. (Albi et nigri.) See Troch. Amyli, and Troch. Glycyrrhizæ.

TROCHISCI BISMUTHI. TROUSSEAU. Trisnitrate of bismuth ℥ij, sugar ʒxx, mucilage q. s. In 120 lozenges.

TROCHISCI BORACIS. Borax ʒij, sugar ʒiv, mucilage of tragacanth q. s. In 30 lozenges.

TROCHISCI BUTYRI CACAO. Concrete oil of cacao ℥ij, sugar ℥ivss, mucilage of tragacanth, made with rose water, q. s.

TROCHISCI CÆRULEI. RODRIGUEZ. Pure Prussian blue ʒj, p. gum acacia ʒj, sugar ʒij, cinnamon ℈j, syrup of lemon-peel q. s. Divide into 20 pastilles.

TROCHISCI CALCIS CHLORINATÆ. Chloride of lime ʒss, sugar ʒxx, mucilage q. s. For 120 lozenges.

TROCHISCI CALOMELANOS. P. Calomel ʒj, sugar ʒxj, mucilage of tragacanth q. s.; into 60 lozenges.

TROCHISCI CAMPHORÆ. Powdered camphor ʒj, sugar ℥j, mucilage of tragacanth q. s.; for 60 lozenges. They should be kept in a stoppered bottle. They are frequently made with a less proportion of camphor.

TROCHISCI CANNABIS. M. EBRIARD. Extract of Indian hemp gr. xij, sugar ℥iij, mucilage of tragacanth q. s.; divide into 144 lozenges.

TROCHISCI CARBONATIS CALCIS. See Tro. Cretæ.

TROCHISCI CARBONIS. P. Prepared charcoal ℥iv, sugar ℥xij, mucilage of tragacanth q. s.; in lozenges of 16 grs. each.

TROCHISCI CARBONIS CUM CHOCOLATA. M. CHEVALLIER. Prepared charcoal ℥j, sugar ℥j, chocolate ℥iij, mucilage of tragacanth q. s.

TROCHISCI CARDIALGICI. See Tro. Cretæ.

TROCHISCI CATECHU. E. 1744. Catechu ℥ij, sugar ℔ss, tragacanth ℥ss, rose water q. s. P. *Tablettes de Cachou.* Extract of catechu ℥iv, sugar ℥xvj, mucilage of tragacanth q. s.; make into 10 or 12 gr. lozenges. *Grains de Cachou* are the same mass variously aromatized with essential oil, and tincture of ambergris and musk, and formed into small globules or pills; they are frequently silvered.

TROCHISCI CATECHU ET MAGNESIÆ. Pure magnesia ℥ij, powdered catechu ℥j, p. sugar ℥xiij, mucilage of tragacanth made with cinnamon water q. s.; make 480 lozenges.

TROCHISCI CHOCOLATE ET IPECACUANHÆ. P. Ipecacuanha ℥j, vanilla chocolate ℥xij; liquefy the chocolate by a gentle heat, incorporate with it the ipecac.; roll it into small balls of gr. xiij each, and flatten them on a warm tinned plate.

TROCHISCI CHOCOLATE ET FERRI. BOUCHARDAT. Fine chocolate ℥xiv, iron reduced by hydrogen ℥j. Soften the chocolate by heat, mix with the iron, and divide into lozenges of 15 grains each. Levigated iron filings are sometimes substituted for reduced iron. Others the sesquioxide. See Chocolata Martis.

TROCHISCI CINCHONÆ. P. Powdered bark ℥ij, cinnamon ʒij, sugar ℥xiv, mucilage of tragacanth q. s.; into 15 gr. lozenges.

TROCHISCI CRETÆ. E. *Heartburn Lozenges.* Prepared chalk ℥iv, gum acacia ℥j, nutmeg ʒj, sugar ℥vj, water q. s. [These are substituted for the old Tabeliæ Cardialgicæ (Heartburn

Lozenges), L. 1745. Prepared chalk ℥iv, prepared crab's claws ℥ij, bole ℥ss, nutmeg ℈j, sugar ℥iij, water q. s.]

TROCHISCI CROTONIS. SOUBEIRAN. Croton oil ♏v, starch ℈j, sugar ʒj, chocolate ʒij; divide into 30 lozenges.

TROCHISCI EMETINÆ PECTORALES. M. Sugar ℥iv, coloured emetine gr. xxxij (or pure emetine gr. viij), mucilage q. s.; divide into 256 lozenges. They may be coloured with carmine. One every hour.

TROCHISCI EMETINÆ EMETICI. M. Coloured emetine gr. xxxij, sugar ℥ij, mucilage q. s.; in 64 lozenges. Dose, 1 for children, 3 or 4 for adults.

TROCHISCI FERRI. P. Levigated iron filings ℥j, sugar ℥x, cinnamon ʒij, mucilage of tragacanth q. s.; in 480 lozenges. See Troch. Chocolata et Ferri.

TROCHISCI FERRI CITRATIS. BERAL. Liquid citrate of iron ʒj, sugar ʒvjss; mix, dry, pulverize and form a mass with mucilage of tragacanth q. s.; divide into lozenges of 15 gr. each. A later formula directs—Ammonia citrate of iron gr. xv, sugar ʒiv, sugar of vanilla and cloves (see Saccharum Vanilla) gr. xv. Mix, and divide into 12-grain lozenges.

TROCHISCI FERRI IODIDI. Syrup of iodide of iron (E.) f℥iij, gum ℥j, sugar ℥ixss; in 240 lozenges, each containing gr. ss of iodide of iron.

TROCHISCI FERRI LACTATIS. M. CAP. Lactate of iron 3ss, sugar ʒvj, mucilage q. s.; in 30 lozenges.

TROCHISCI GLYCYRRHIZÆ. E. *Tro. Bechici Nigri.* Extract of liquorice ℥vj, gum acacia ℥vj, sugar ℔j; dissolve them in hot water, and evaporate to a paste. See Pasta Glycyrrhizæ Alba, Fusca, Opiata, and Nigra.

TROCHISCI GLYCYRRHIZÆ ET OPII. This was the name of Tro. Opii in E. 1817. [A different formula is given in U. S. Powdered opium ℥ss, liquorice powder (the extract, or juice) ℥x, gum acacia ℥x, sugar ℥x, oil of anise fʒij, water to form a mass; divide into lozenges of 6 grains each.] See Trochisci Opii.

TROCHISCI GUMMI ARABICI. See Tro. Acaciæ, and Pasta Althææ.

TROCHISCI GUMMI TRAGACANTHI. E. 1744. Sugar ℔j, compound powder of tragacanth ℥iij, rose water ℥iv.

TROCHISCI IPECACUANHÆ. U. S. Ipecacuanha in fine powder ℥ss, sugar ℥xiv, arrow root ℥iv, mucilage of tragacanth q. s. Divide into lozenges of 10 grains each. P. Ipecac. ℥j, sugar ℥xlvij, mucilage of tragacanth q. s.; into 1920 lozenges (¼ of a gr. of ipec. in each). See Tro. Chocolatæ et Ipecac.

TROCHISCI IPECACUANHA ET CAMPHORÆ. Ipecac. gr. xv, camphor ʒj, sugar ℥j mucilage of tragacanth q. s. Make 60 lozenges. [Each contains 1 grain of camphor, and ¼ of a grain of ipecac.]

TROCHISCI IRIDIS. Orris powder ʒj, sugar ℥ij, mucilage of tragacanth q. s.

TROCHISCI JUJUBÆ. See Pasta Jujubæ.

TROCHISCI KERMETIS. P. Kermes mineral ʒij, sugar ℥xvij, gum acacia ℥j; orange-flower water ℥j; mix, and divide into lozenges of 12 grains each.

TROCHISCI LACTUCÆ. SPRAGUE. Concentrated extract of lettuce, extract of liquorice, gum acacia, of each equal parts. Mix, and divide into lozenges.

TROCHISCI LACTUCARII. Dr. DUNCAN. Prepared as Tro. Opii, substituting lactucarium for opium.

TROCHISCI LICHENIS. P. Dried jelley of Iceland moss ℥ij, sugar ℥iv, gum acacia 3jss; mix with water q. s. See Pasta Lichenis.

TROCHISCI LIMONIS. Oil of lemon ʒj, sugar ℥xij; mix, and form into lozenges with mucilage of tragacanth; or into drops, as those of orange. See Troch. (Pastilli) Aurantii.

TROCHISCI MAGNESIÆ [Carbonatis]. E. Carbonate of magnesia ℥vj, sugar ℥iij, nutmeg ℈j; form a mass with mucilage of tragacanth.

TROCHISCI MAGNESIÆ [CALCINATÆ]. U. S. Magnesia ℥iv, sugar ℔j, nutmeg ʒj, mucilage of tragacanth q. s. Mix, and divide into 10-gr. lozenges.

TROCHISCI MANNÆ. VAN MONS. Tragacanth ʒj, sugar ℥xij, manna ℥iij, orange-flower water q. s. Mannite may be substituted for manna.

TROCHISCI MENTHÆ PIPERITÆ. U. S. Sugar ℔j, oil of peppermint f 3j, mucilage of tragacanth q. s. Make into lozenges of 10 grains each. P. Sugar ℥xvj, oil of peppermint ʒj, mucilage of tragacanth q. s. [The drops (pastilli) are made with sugar ℥xij, oil ʒj, peppermint water q. s.; as those of orange.]

TROCHISCI MORPHIÆ. E. Muriate of morphia ℈j, tincture of Tolu f℥ss, sugar ℥xxv; dissolve the muriate in a little hot water, mix it and the tincture with the sugar, beat into a mass with mucilage, and divide into lozenges of 15 grains each. Each lozenge contains 1-40th of a grain of muriate of morphia.

TROCHISCI MORPHIÆ ET IPECACUANHÆ. E. As the last, adding ʒj of ipecacuanha.

TROCHISCI NAPHTHALINÆ. DUPASQUIER. Naphthaline ℈v, sugar ℥xx, oil of aniseed to flavour; form a mass with mucilage of tragacanth, and divide into lozenges of gr. xv each. [Expectorant: may be taken to the extent of 20 in the day.]

TROCHISCI E NITRO. E. 1783. Nitre ℥iij, sugar ℥ix, mucilage of tragacanth q. s.

TROCHISCI NITRI CAMPHORATI. CHAUSSIER. Opium gr. vj, camphor gr. xxiv, nitre gr. xlviij, sugar ʒiij, mucilage q. s.; mix, and divide into 48 lozenges.

TROCHISCI OCULORUM CANCRORUM. Crabs' eyes ʒj, sugar ʒvij, mucilage of tragacanth with orange-flower water q. s.

TROCHISCI OPII. E. Opium ʒij, tincture of Tolu f℥ss, pure sugar ℥vj, extract of liquorice ℥v, gum acacia ℥v. Reduce the opium to a fluid extract (as in making Extractum Opii), mix it intimately with the liquorice reduced to the consistence of treacle; add the tincture, sprinkle in the powdered gum and sugar, and beat the whole into a proper mass, which is to be divided into 10-grain lozenges. One grain of opium is contained in 6 or 7 lozenges. [Dr. DUNCAN recommends reducing the opium and extract of liquorice to powder, mixing them with the powdered gum, beating them first with the tincture, then with f℥viij of syrup (and water if required), using ℥vijss of the extract and ℥ijss of gum, instead of ℥v of each.]

TROCHISCI PAPAVERIS. Extract of poppies ℥ij, sugar ℥viij, tragacanth powder ℥iv, water q. s.

TROCHISCI PAULLINIÆ. Dr. GAVRELLE. Extract of paullinia (guarana) ℥j, sugar with vanilla ℥xxiv, mucilage of tragacanth q. s. Divide into lozenges of gr. xij each. 16 to 20 daily.

TROCHISCI PECTORALES. Dr. GRUNN. Sugar ℥viij, manna ℥iv, extract of lettuce ℥ij, ipecacuanha ʒivss, squill ℥j, mucilage of tragacanth q. s. Divide into lozenges of 15 grains each.

TROCHISCI POTASSÆ CHLORATIS. Chlorate of potash ʒij, sugar ʒxij, mucilage of tragacanth q. s. Reduce the chlorate to powder by itself, then triturate it with a little of the mucilage, and lastly beat it with the sugar. Divide into 60 lozenges. (There would probably be danger of an explosion in making these on a large scale.) Mr. MURRAY recommends them for the cure of *Consumption*. They are sometimes useful in *Sore Throat*. 4 to 8 daily.

TROCHISCI POTASSÆ SUPEROXALATIS. P. Superoxalate of potash ʒiij, sugar ℥xvj, oil of lemon ♏xvj, mucilage of tragacanth q. s. Divide into lozenges of 10 grains each.

TROCHISCI QUINÆ SULPHATIS. SOUBEIRAN. Sulphate of quinine gr. xxxij, sugar ℥xvj, mucilage of tragacanth q. s. Divide into lozenges of 15 grains each.

TROCHISCI RHEI. P. Rhubarb ℥j, sugar ℥xj, mucilage of tragacanth q. s. Divide into lozenges of gr. xv each.

TROCHISCI RHEI AROMATICI. Turkey rhubarb ℥ij, cinnamon ʒj, sugar ℥xj, mucilage of tragacanth q. s. In 480 lozenges.

TROCHISCI SANTONINÆ. M. CALLOUD. Santonine ʒj, sugar ℥ivss, mucilage of tragacanth q. s. For 144 lozenges. Dose, from 5 to 10 in the day.

TROCHISCI SCILLÆ. Squill in powder ʒj, extract of liquorice ℥j, sugar ℥x, mucilage of tragacanth q. s. For 480 lozenges.

TROCHISCI SCILLÆ ET IPECACUANHÆ. As the last, adding ℈iv of ipecacuanha.

TROCHISCI SODÆ BICARBONATIS. E. Bicarbonate of soda ℥j, sugar ℥iij, powdered acacia ℥ss, mucilage q. s. The *Pastilles de Vichy*, P., contain bicarbonate of soda ℥j, sugar ℥xix, mucilage of tragacanth q. s. In ℈j lozenges. Mr. DARCET'S formula is that of P., with the addition of oil of peppermint or other flavouring ingredient.

TROCHISCI SODÆ CHLORINATÆ. Solution of chloride of soda ʒj, sugar ʒx, gum arabic ʒij, mucilage of tragacanth q. s. [ʒss of camphor may be added.] To be held in the mouth when exposed to infection.

TROCHISCI SODÆ CUM ZINGIBERE. Bicarbonate of soda ℥ij to ℥iv, ginger ℥j, sugar ℥x, mucilage of tragacanth q. s. For 480 lozenges.

TROCHISCI SPONGIÆ. P. Burnt sponge ℥iv, sugar ℥xij, mucilage of tragacanth (made with cinnamon water) to form a mass. Divide into 12-grain lozenges.

TROCHISCI E SULPHURE. L. 1788. Washed sulphur ℥ij, sugar ℥iv, mucilage q. s. P. Sulphur ℥ij, sugar ℥xvj, mucilage of tragacanth with rose water q. s. [Tro. Diasulphuris. E. 1744. Sulphur ℥j, flowers of benzoin ʒj, sugar ℥iv, mucilage of tragacanth q. s.]

TROCHISCI TARTARI SOLUBILIS. GUIBOURT. Borotartrate of potash ℥j, sugar ℥vij, mucilage of tragacanth q. s.; flavoured with lemon.

TROCHISCI TOLUTANI. P. Balsam of Tolu ℥j; dissolve in ℥j of rectified spirit, add ℥ij of water, heat in a water-bath, and filter; make a mucilage with the filtered liquor and ℈iv gum tragacanth, add sugar ℥xvj, and form a paste for lozenges.

TROCHISCI VANILLÆ. GUIBOURT. Vanilla ℥j, sugar ℥vij, mucilage of tragacanth q. s. The vanilla must be powdered with the sugar.

TROCHISCI VIOLARUM. SARD. PH. Sugar ℔viij, juice of violets ℥iij, orris powder ℥j.

TROCHISCI ZINCI. Dr. COPLAND. Sulphate of zinc ʒiv, sugar ℥xvj, mucilage of tragacanth q. s. Mix, and divide into 480 lozenges.

TROCHISCI ZINGIBERIS. SOUBEIRAN. Ginger ℥j, sugar ℥vij, mucilage of tragacanth q. s. Form into lozenges of 15 gr. each.

The following are for outward use:—

TROCHISCI ALBI RHASIS. E. 1744. White lead ℥x, sarcocol ℥iij, tragacanth ʒij, starch ʒij, camphor ʒss, rose water q. s. Make them into troches, S. A.

TROCHISCI ESCHAROTICI. P. Bichloride of mercury ʒij, starch ʒiv, mucilage of tragacanth q. s. Porphyrize the sublimate, add the rest, and form the paste into 3-gr. troches of the form of a grain of oat.

TROCHISCI MINII. E. 1744, and P. 1837. Bichloride of mercury ℥ij, red lead ʒj, crumb of bread ℥j, distilled water (rose water, E.) q. s. As the last.

TROCHISCI ESCHAROTICI ZINCI. See Causticum Zinci.

UNGUENTA. *Ointments.* As a general rule, the fats, resins, and wax should be melted by the heat of a water-bath, then the powders, liquids, &c. added, and the whole stirred with a wooden spatula till cool. Note—by *lard* is here intended hog's lard properly prepared and washed; by *suet,* prepared mutton suet; and by wax, yellow bees'-wax. Both the *Pommades* and the *Onguents* of the Paris Codex are placed under this division of the work.

UNGUENTUM ACETI. Dr. CHESTON. White wax ℥iv, olive oil ℔j; melt together, add ℥ij of vinegar, and stir till cold.

UNGUENTUM ACIDI MURIATICI. Dr. CORRIGAN. Muriatic acid ʒj, spermaceti ointment ℥j. Mix. For *scalled heads,* night and morning, after the scabs have been removed by a poultice.

UNGUENTUM ACIDI NITROSI. E. 1817. Lard ℔j; melt in an earthen vessel, add gradually nitrous acid ʒvj, and stir diligently as it cools. D. Olive oil ℔j, lard ʒiv, nitric acid fʒvss. See also Unguentum Oxygenatum.

UNGUENTUM ACIDI NITRICI OPIATUM. Dr. EBERLE. Beef suet ℥j, nitric acid fʒj, powdered opium ʒj.

UNGUENTUM ACIDI PHOSPHORICI. SOUBEIRAN. Phosphoric acid (sp. gr. 1·454) ʒj, lard ℥j. *In frictions on osseous tumours.*

UNGUENTUM ACIDI SULPHURICI. D. Sulphuric acid ʒj (fʒss), lard ℥j; mix. Dr. DUNCAN says 1 part of acid to 16 of lard, in *scabies.* GUY'S H. Sulphuric acid fʒj, lard ℥j; oil of turpentine fʒj is sometimes added.

UNGUENTUM ACONITI. Dr. TURNBULL. Alcoholic extract of aconite ʒj, lard ʒij. *In neuralgia,* as a substitute for Ung. Aconitinæ.

UNGUENTUM ACONITI AMMONIATUM. Dr. TURNBULL. Ammoniated extract of aconite ʒj, lard ʒiij. *In old rheumatic cases and paralysis.* As efficacious as Ung. Aconitinæ.

UNGUENTUM ACONITI ANTIMONIATUM. Tartar emetic ointment ℥j, extract of aconite ʒj.

UNGUENTUM ACONITINÆ. Dr. TURNBULL. Aconitine gr. ij, triturate with 6 drops of alcohol, and add ʒj of lard. It must not be used where there is the slightest abrasion of the skin. It is sometimes necessary gradually to increase the proportion of aconitine to 4 or 5 grains.

Unguentum Adipis. L. 1788. Beat ℔ij of prepared lard with f℥iij of rose water; melt with a gentle heat, set aside, pour off the lard from the water, and stir it till cold.

Unguentum Æruginis. E. Resinous ointment ℥xv, verdigris in fine powder ℥j. D. Ointment of white resin ℔j, prepared verdigris ℥ss.

Unguentum Album. That of L. 1746, is Unguentum Cetacei; that of E. 1744, Ung. Plumbi Carbonatis.

Unguentum Album Camphoratum. L. 1746. Spermaceti ointment ℔ij, camphor (rubbed with a little oil) ʒjss. E. White lead ointment ℔vjss, powdered camphor ℥j.

Unguentum Alkalinum. Cazenave. Subcarbonate of potash ʒij, lard ℥ij. Cullerier. Subcarbonate of soda ʒij, wine of opium ʒj, lard ℥j. Devergie uses from 9 to 15 grains of carbonate of soda with ℥j of lard in *Lichen;* 15 to 30 in *Lepra, Ichthyosis,* and *Psoriasis;* and 30 to 60 in *Porrigo favosa.*

Unguentum Alkalinum Camphoratum. Cazenave. Subcarbonate of potash ℈j, lard ʒvij, camphor gr. iij. *In Sycosis.*

Unguentum Allii. Equal parts of fresh garlic and lard beaten together. It is applied to the feet in *hooping-cough.*

Unguentum Alöes. Dupuytren. Aloes ℥j, lard ℥iv.

Unguentum Alöes Compositum. Bat. Ph. Aloes ʒij, ox-gall ʒiij, petroleum ʒiij, lard ℥iij. Germ. H. Aloes ℥j, inspissated gall ʒij, althæa ointment ℥j. *Vermifuge.* Applied over the abdomen of children.

Unguentum Althææ. L. 1746. *Dialthæa.* Oil of mucilages ℔ij, yellow wax ℔ss, resin ℥iij, Venice turpentine ℥ss.

Unguentum Aluminis. Sundelin. Alum ʒj, fresh butter washed ℥ij; mix. *For Hæmorrhoids.*

Unguentum Aluminis Compositum. Banyer's *Ointment.* Powdered litharge ℔ss, burnt alum ℥ij, calomel ℥jss, Venice turpentine ℔ss, lard ℔ij. To be ground together till perfectly smooth, and diluted with more lard at the time of using.

Unguentum Ammoniacale. P. *Pommade de Gondret.* Suet ℥j, lard ℥j; melt together in a wide-mouthed bottle, add ℥ij of solution of ammonia (sp. gr. 0·923), close the bottle, and shake till cold. Gondret's formula is, lard ʒvj, suet ʒiv, almond oil ʒij, strong water of ammonia 3xij. In winter he puts 3ij less suet, and ʒij more lard. They are mixed as above. Rubefacient, and if covered with a compress vesicant, in from 3 to 5 minutes.

UNGUENTUM AMMONIÆ CARBONATIS. Sesquicarbonate of ammonia ʒj, lard ℥j; mix.

UNGUENTUM AMMONIÆ HYDRIODATIS. ELLIS. Hydriodate of ammonia (iodide of ammonium) ℈j, lard ℥j. [GIBERT: ʒj to ℥j.]

UNGUENTUM ANTHRAKOKALI. Dr. POYLA. Anthrakokali 1 part, lard 30 parts.

UNGUENTUM ANTIMONII POTASSIO-TARTRATIS. L. (*Ung. Antimoniale*, E.) Potassio-tartrate of antimony ℥j, lard ℥iv. Mix. [Triturate them carefully together into a smooth and uniform mass, E.] D. (*Ung. Tartari Emetici*) directs ʒj of tartar emetic to ℥j of lard.

UNGUENTUM ANTIMONII CUM SACCHARO. Dr. JENNER. Tartarized antimony 3ij, spermaceti ointment ʒix, sugar ʒj, red sulphuret of mercury gr. v.

UNGUENTUM ANTIMONIALE CAMPHORATUM. Dr. FABRE'S *Ointment for chronic affections of the liver.* Muriate of ammonia ʒj, tartarized antimony 3ss, camphor gr. xxv, musk gr. x, lard ℥j..

UNGUENTUM ANTIHÆMORRHOIDALE. See Ung. Hæmorrhoidale.

UNGUENTUM ANTIHERPETICUM. CHEVALLIER. Chloride of lime 3iij, subsulphate of mercury 3ij, oil of almonds ʒvj, lard ℥ij. ALIBERT. Red sulphuret of quicksilver 3jss, camphor ʒss. cerate ℥ij.

UNGUENTUM ANTIPSORICUM. E. 1744. Elecampane root ℥iij, sharp-leaved dock ℥iij; bruise, and boil with water Oijss, vinegar f℥xvj, till reduced to half; add to the liquor ℥x of water-cress and ℔iv of lard; boil till the moisture is exhaled, express, and add ℥iv of wax and ℥iv of oil of bay. [With ℥viij of strong mercurial ointment, it forms Unguentum Antipsoricum Compositum.] The Ung. Sulphuris was substituted in E. 1792.

UNGUENTUM AQUÆ ROSÆ. U. S. Oil of almonds f℥ij, spermaceti ℥ss, white wax ʒj; melt together, add f℥ij of rose water, and stir constantly till cold.

UNGUENTUM ARCÆI. Ung. Elemi Compositum.

UNGUENTUM ARGENTI NITRATIS. GUY'S H. Nitrate of silver ℈j, lard ℥j; mix. M. JOBERT'S Ointments (for white swellings), Nos. 1, 2, and 3, contain respectively 4, 8, and 12 parts of nitrate of silver to 30 of lard. Mr. MACDONALD prescribes 1 part of the nitrate with 7 and a half of lard to smear bougies in gonorrhœa. Mr. GUTHRIE'S ophthalmic ointment consists of nitrate of silver gr. x, liquid diacetate of lead ♏xv, lard ʒj. VELPEAU'S, gr. j of the nitrate to ℥j of lard. MACKENZIE'S, gr. v to ℥j.

UNGUENTUM ARGENTI OXYDI. SERRE. Oxide of silver gr. xvj, lard ℥j.

UNGUENTUM ARSENICI. GUY'S H. Levigated white arsenic ℈ij, lard ℥j; mix. [A weaker ointment, gr. ij of arsenic to ℥j of lard, is used by Mr. LUKE in *Onychia Maligna.*]

UNGUENTUM ARSENICI CUM SULPHURE. GUY'S H. Levigated white arsenic ℈ij, sulphur ʒj, lard ℥j. Sir A. COOPER. White arsenic ʒj, sulphur ʒj, spermaceti cerate ℥j. Mr. MARSHALL. Arsenic and sulphur each ℈j to ℥j of cerate.

UNGUENTUM ARSENICI IODIDI. BIETT. Iodide of arsenic gr. ijss, lard ℥j.

UNGUENTUM ARSENIATIS SODÆ. F. H. Arseniate of soda 3j, lard ℥ij.

UNGUENTUM ARSENICALE. CARMICHAEL. Arseniate of iron ʒss, phosphate of iron ʒij, spermaceti cerate ʒvj.

UNGUENTUM ARTHANITÆ. From sow-bread leaves as Ung. Conii. *Used externally as a Vermifuge.*

UNGUENTUM ASTRINGENS. GUIBOURT. Cypress and gall-nuts, pomegranate-peel, sumach, and mastic, of each ℥j, rose ointment ℥xix. *For Hernia.*

UNGUENTUM AURI. M. LEGRAND. Powdered gold gr. xij, lard ℥j. M., *for endermic use.* Gold divided by mercury 3j, lard ℥j; when the blisters become dry, substitute auro-chloride of gold gr. viij, lard 3ss. The latter form is used to relieve *rheumatic pains.*

UNGUENTUM ATROPIÆ. Dr. BROOKES. Atropia gr. v, lard ʒiij.

UNGUENTUM BALSAMI PERUVIANI. Balsam of Peru ʒj, lard ℥j.

UNGUENTUM BALSAMI PERUVIANI COMPOSITUM. Dr. COPLAND. Lard ℥ij, white wax ʒiv; melt in a water-bath, and add balsam of Peru ʒij, oil of lavender ♏xij. *To restore the hair.*

UNGUENTUM BARII IODIDI. M. BIETT. Iodide of barium gr. iij to iv, lard ℥j.

UNGUENTUM BASILICUM. See Unguentum Resinæ.

UNGUENTUM BASILICUM NIGRUM. See Ung. Picis Nigræ.

UNGUENTUM BASILICUM VIRIDE. L. 1746. Prepared verdigris ℥j, olive oil ℥iij, resin ointment ℥viij.

UNGUENTUM BELLADONNÆ. SOUBEIRAN. Fresh belladonna leaves 1 part, lard 2 parts; bruise the leaves, mix them with the lard, and boil them gently together till the leaves become crisp; digest, and strain with pressure. [PEREIRA. Extract of belladonna ʒj to ʒij, lard ℥j; mix. CHAUSSIER. Extract ʒij, simple cerate ℥j.]

UNGUENTUM BELLADONNÆ ANTIMONIATUM. M. ROLLOT. Antimonial ointment ℥j, extract of belladonna ʒj.

UNGUENTUM BENZOINI. M. DESCHAMPS. Benzoin coarsely powdered 1 part, fresh lard 25 parts; heat for 2 or 3 hours in a water-bath and strain. [M. D. recommends this as a basis for ointments, as benzoin resists rancidity and the decomposition of metallic salts and oxides. Poplar buds have the same effect. See Ung. Populeum.]

UNGUENTUM BISMUTHI. PEREIRA. Trisnitrate of bismuth ʒj; spermaceti cerate ʒiv. Mix. FULLER. Oil of almonds ℥ij, spermaceti ʒiij, magistery of bismuth ʒj.

UNGUENTUM BORACIS. Powdered borax ʒj to ʒij, lard ℥j. Mix.

UNGUENTUM BORACIS COMPOSITUM. HARLESS. Borax ʒj, balsam of Peru ʒjss, oil of almonds ℥j, yolk of egg ʒij, white of egg ʒij. Mix.

UNGUENTUM BROMINII COMPOSITUM. M. Hydrobromate of potash ℈j, bromine 10 drops, lard ℥j. Mix.

UNGUENTUM CADMII. RADIUS. Sulphate of cadmium gr. j to ij, lard ʒj.

UNGUENTUM CÆRULEUM. Mercurial ointment is so termed; so also is Ung. Cobalti Oxydi.

UNGUENTUM CALAMINÆ. D. Ointment of yellow wax ℔v, prepared calamine ℔j. Mix. [The calamine should be examined, as it is often adulterated.]

UNGUENTUM CALCIS OPIATUM. GUIBOURT. Cucumber ointment ℥ij, slaked lime ʒij, wine of opium ʒij. Mix. *For Piles.*

UNGUENTUM CALCIS CHLORIDI. Chlorinated lime ℈j to ʒj, lard or fresh butter ℥j. Mix.

UNGUENTUM CALCIS MURIATIS. SUNDELIN. Muriate of lime 3j, digitalis powder ʒij, concentrated vinegar ℈ij, lard ℥j. *For chronic glandular swellings.*

UNGUENTUM CALOMELANOS. GUY'S H. Calomel ʒj, wax ointment ℥j. Dr. UNDERWOOD. Calomel ʒj to ʒij, elder-flower ointment ℥j. Dr. PEREIRA. ʒj of calomel to ℥j of lard.

UNGUENTUM CALOMELANOS COMPOSITUM. BANYER'S *Ointment for Milk Scall.* Calomel 3ij, burnt alum ʒiv, carbonate of lead ʒiv, Venice turpentine ʒvj, spermaceti ointment ℥jss. Dr. A. T. THOMSON in *Lepra,* Calomel ʒj, tar ointment ʒiv, spermaceti ointment ℥j.

UNGUENTUM CAMPHORÆ. RASPAIL. Powdered camphor ℥j, lard ℥iij.

UNGUENTUM CANTHARIDIS. L. & D. (Ung. Infusi Cantharidis, E.) Powdered cantharides ℥j water f℥iv; boil to half, strain, add to the liquor ℥iv of resin cerate, and evaporate to a proper consistence. E. Infuse ℥j of powdered cantharides in f℥v of boiling water for a night, express, and filter. Add ℥ij of lard, and boil till the water is dispersed; then add ℥j each of wax and resin, and when these are liquefied, remove the vessel from the fire, and add ℥ij of Venice turpentine. D. & U. S. as L., but twice the quantities.

UNGUENTUM CANTHARIDIS. E. Cantharides in fine powder ℥j, resinous ointment ℥vij. Add the flies to the melted ointment, and stir briskly, as it concretes on cooling.

UNGUENTUM CUM EXTRACTO CANTHARIDIS. M. CAP. Alcoholic extract of cantharides gr. viij, oil of roses ʒj, beef marrow ℥ij, oil of lemon ♏xl. *To promote the growth of the hair.*

UNGUENTUM TINCTURÆ CANTHARIDIS. DUPUYTREN. Tincture of cantharides [P.] ʒj, lard ʒix. It may be coloured and perfumed at pleasure.

UNGUENTUM CANTHARIDIS CUM HYDRARGYRO. Lard 65 parts, powdered flies 29, strong mercurial ointment 6 parts. Mix. Used in Normandy to *indolent tumours*.

UNGUENTUM CANTHARIDINÆ. SOUBEIRAN. Cantharidine gr. j, lard ℈vij, white wax ʒj. Mix accurately.

UNGUENTUM CARBONIS. RADIUS. Charcoal ℥j, lard ℥ij.

UNGUENTUM CATECHU. Catechu ℥iv, alum ℈ix, resin ℥iv, olive oil ℥x, water q. s. Used in India to *Ulcers*.

UNGUENTUM CERÆ ALBÆ. D. White wax ℔j, lard ℔iv.

UNGUENTUM CERÆ FLAVÆ. D. Purified yellow wax ℔j, lard ℔iv. GUY'S H. Yellow wax ℥vijss, olive oil Oj.

UNGUENTUM CERÆ CUM ACETO. Dr. CHESTON. Wax ointment ℔j, vinegar ℥ij, melt, and stir until cold.

UNGUENTUM CERUSSÆ ACETATIS. Ceratum Plumbi Acetatis.

UNGUENTUM CETACEI. L. Spermaceti ʒvj, white wax ℈ij, olive oil f℥iij; melt, and stir till cold. D. White wax ℔ss, spermaceti ℔j, lard ℔iij.

UNGUENTUM CHLORINII. Solution of chlorine ʒij, lard ℥j.

UNGUENTUM CITRINUM. E. Ung. Hydrargyri Nitratis.

UNGUENTUM CINCHONÆ. BIETT. Red bark ʒij, almond oil ʒij, beef marrow ʒvj. *In Porrigo Decalvans.*

UNGUENTUM COBALTI OXYDI. AMST. PH. Simple cerate ℥xvj, liquid diacetate of lead ℥iv, powdered smalts ℥iv.

UNGUENTUM COCCULI. E. Beat the kernels of Cocculus Indicus in a mortar, first alone, and then with five times their weight of lard, gradually added.

UNGUENTUM COLOCYNTHIDIS. Powdered colocynth ℥j, lard ℈viij; mix. *In frictions on the abdomen as a purgative.*

UNGUENTUM CONII. D. Fresh hemlock ℔j, lard ℔j; boil the leaves in the lard until they begin to become crisp, and strain through linen.

UNGUENTUM COSMETICUM. QUINCY. Oil of almonds ℥ij, spermaceti ℈iij, trisnitrate of bismuth ʒj, oil of rhodium 6 drops. See also Ceratum Cosmeticum.

UNGUENTUM CREASOTI. L. & U. S. Creasote fʒss, lard ℥j; mix. [E. ʒj to ℥iij.]

UNGUENTUM CREASOTI CUM HYDRARGYRO. Dr. HILDRETH. Strong mercurial ointment ʒiv, creasote ♏x to xxx. *In Scrofulous Ophthalmia with Opacity of the Cornea.*

UNGUENTUM CRETÆ COMPOSITUM. St. GEO. H. As Ung. Plumbi Comp., but with f ℥xxxij of olive oil.

UNGUENTUM CRINISCUM. QUINCY. Labdanum ʒvj, bears' grease ℈ij, powdered southernwood ʒiij, oil of mace ʒj, balsam of Peru ʒij.

UNGUENTUM CROTONIS. AINSLEY. Croton oil ♏x, cerate or lard ℥ss; mix. CAVENTOU'S *Rubefacient Pommade:* Lard 2½, wax ½; melt together, and when cool scrape it, and mix without heat with 1 part of croton oil.

UNGUENTUM CUCUMIS. GUIBOURT. Melt together 4 parts of lard and 1 of veal suet; strain, and mix it well with 3 parts of juice of cucumber; in 24 hours pour off the juice, and add fresh juice; repeat this process 10 times. Melt, and to each ℔ add ʒiij powdered starch; let it settle, pour off the ointment from the sediment, strain through a cloth, and stir till cold.

UNGUENTUM CUPRI SUB-ACETATIS. D. Prepared verdigris ℥ss, triturate with olive oil ℥j, and mix with ℔j of ointment of white resin, previously melted. See Ung. Æruginis for E.

UNGUENTUM CUPRI AMMONIATI. SWEDIAUR. Solution of ammonio sulphate of copper ℈j, simple cerate ℥j.

UNGUENTUM CUPRI CARBONATIS. M. DEVERGIE. Carbonate of copper ʒij, lard ℥j. *In Impetigo and Eczema of the Scalp.*

UNGUENTUM DELPHINIÆ. Dr. TURNBULL. Delphine gr. x to xxx, olive oil ʒj; rub together, and add ℈j of lard.

UNGUENTUM DEOBSTRUENS. Dr. HUNEFIELD. Muriate of ammonia in fine powder ℈j, strong mercurial ointment ℥j, extract of hemlock ℈jss.

UNGUENTUM DEPILATORIUM. CAZENAVE. Subcarbonate of soda 6, slaked lime 4, lard 30.

UNGUENTUM DIALTHÆÆ. See Ung. Althææ.

UNGUENTUM DIGESTIVUM. P. Venice turpentine ℥ij, yolk of 2 eggs; mix, and add ℈ss of oil of St. John's-wort. With an equal weight of mercurial ointment it forms *Digestif Mercuriel;* or with an equal weight of liquid styrax, *Digestif Animé.* ℥iv of simple digestive with ℈j of vinum opii, form *Digestif Opiacê* of F. H.

UNGUENTUM DIGESTIVUM VIRIDE. Dr. KIRKLAND. Yellow resin ℥j, elemi ℥j, wax ℥j, green oil ℥vj; melt together, and when nearly cool, add ʒij of oil of turpentine.

UNGUENTUM DIGITALIS. As Ung. Conii. L. 1746 directs it to be prepared with fresh butter, and several successive quantities of the plant boiled in it. M. RUDEMACHER. Extract of digitalis ʒij, lard ℥j; spread on lint, and the throat covered with it, in *Croup*.

UNGUENTUM ECTROTICUM. F. H. Mercurial ointment 12 parts, wax 5, black pitch 3. *To prevent the pitting of small-pox pustules.*

UNGUENTUM ELEMI. L. *Ung. Arcæi.* Elemi ℔j, prepared suet ℔ij; melt together, remove from the fire, and add ℥x of common turpentine, and ℥ij of olive oil, and strain through linen. D. Elemi ℔j, white wax ℔ss, lard ℔iv. Strain while hot.

UNGUENTUM ELEMI CUM ÆRUGINE. Ointment of elemi ℔ss, prepared verdigris ʒj; mix.

UNGUENTUM EMETINÆ. Dr. TURNBULL. Emetime gr. xv, rectified spirit q. s., lard ℥ss. *As a rubefacient.*

UNGUENTUM EMOLLIENS. CHEVALLIER. Concrete oil of cacao ℥iv, oil of almonds 3ij, mucilage of quince seeds 3ij.

UNGUENTUM EPISPASTICUM, FORTIUS ET MITIUS. E. 1817. As Ung. Cantharidis, and Ung. Infusi Cantharidis, E.

UNGUENTUM EPISPASTICUM FLAVUM. P. Bruised cantharides ℥iv, lard ℥liv; digest for 3 hours in a water-bath, strain, and express; add ʒij of turmeric, digest, strain, melt the product with ℥viij of wax, stir the mixture, and when nearly cool add ʒij of oil of lemon.

UNGUENTUM EPISPASTICUM VIRIDE. P. Powdered cantharides ℥j, poplar ointment ℥xxviij, white wax ℥iv. Melt the wax with the ointment, add the flies, and stir till cold.

UNGUENTUM ESCHAROTICUM. Sir B. BRODIE. Prepared verdigris ʒij, sulphate of copper ʒij, nitric oxide of mercury ʒij, bichloride of mercury ʒj, lard q. s. LANDOLPHI—Arsenical caustic (pulvis escharoticus arsenicalis) ʒss, acetate of morphia gr. iij, white cerate 3vijss.

UNGUENTUM EUPHORBII. Dr. NELIGAN. Powdered euphorbium

gr. xxv to xxx, lard ℥j; mix. To keep up a discharge from issues.

Unguentum Ferri Arseniatis. Arseniate of iron ʒj, spermaceti ointment ʒxij.

Unguentum Ferri Iodidi. Pierquin. Iodide of iron ʒj, lard ℥j.

Unguentum Oxydi Ferri. Germ. H. Red oxide of iron ʒss, lard ʒiv. Mix. *In Chronic Ophthalmia.*

Unguentum Ferri Phosphatis. Phosphate of iron ʒiij, spermaceti ointment ℥j.

Unguentum Ferri Prussiatis. U. C. H. Levigated Prussian blue ʒij, potash-tartrate of antimony gr. iv, spermaceti ointment ℥j. [Dr. Thomson, ʒj Prussian blue to ℥j of lard.]

Unguentum Ferri Sulphatis. M. Velpeau. Sulphate of iron from ʒj to ℈ij, lard ℥j. *In Erysipelas.*

Unguentum Flavum. Prus. Ph. Lard ℔viij, powdered turmeric ℈ij, water q. s. Boil together till the moisture is consumed, and add wax ℔ss, resin ℔ss. Melt and strain.

Unguentum dictum Flos Unguentorum. Resin, frankincense, wax, suet, each ℔ss; olibanum ℥ijss, common turpentine ℥ijss, camphor ℈ij, myrrh ℥j, wine Oss; boil together.

Unguentum Fuliginis. M. Blaud. Wood soot ℥ss, lard ℥ij; mix. *In cutaneous diseases.*

Unguentum Fuliginis Compositum. Acetic extract of wood soot ʒiv, dried salt ʒx, lard ℥xiv. *For Tinea.*

Unguentum Fuligokali. Deschamps. Fuligokali ʒj to ℈ij, lard ℥iv.

Unguentum Fuligokali Sulphureti. Sulphuretted fuligokali ℈ij, water ʒij; mix, and add lard ℥iv. Mix.

Unguentum Fuscum. P. Levigated nitric oxide of mercury ʒj, resin ointment ℥ij; mix.

Unguentum Gallarum. D. Galls ℥j, lard ℥iij; mix. [In this and the following ointments, the nut-galls should be reduced to a very fine powder.]

Unguentum Gallæ Compositum. L. Galls ʒij, opium ʒss, lard ℥ij.

UNGUENTUM GALLÆ CUM CAMPHORA. Galls ʒij, camphor ʒss, lard ℥j.

UNGUENTUM GALLÆ CUM CUPRI SULPHATE. Galls ʒj, sulphate of copper ℈j, lard ℥j. *An Indian remedy for Ringworm of the Scalp.*

UNGUENTUM GALLÆ CUM MORPHIA. Dr. PARIS. Morphia gr. ij, olive oil fʒij; rub together, and add zinc ointment ℥j, galls ʒj. Mix.

UNGUENTUM GALLÆ ET OPII. E. Galls ʒij, opium ʒj, lard ℥j. GUY'S H. (Ung. Gallæ Opiatum.) Galls ʒij, opium (softened with water) ʒj, liquid diacetate of lead fʒij, lard ℥j. Mix.

UNGUENTUM GRAPHITIS. VAN MONS. Black lead ℥j, lard ℥ij. [Dr. PEREIRA says ʒj or ʒij to ℥j of lard.]

UNGUENTUM HÆMORRHOIDALE. (See Ung. Gallæ, &c. above.) Dr. GEDDING'S. Carbonate of lead ʒiv, sulphate of morphia gr. xv, stramonium ointment ℥j, olive oil q. s. VALLEZ. Extract of elder leaves gr. xvj, burnt alum gr. viij, poplar ointment ʒiv, 4 times a day. See Linimentum Hydrargyri Nitratis; Ung. Calcis Opiatum, &c.

UNGUENTUM HELLEBORI COMPOSITUM. RAYER. White hellebore ℥j, muriate of ammonia ʒiv, lard ℥viij. See Ung. Veratri, and Ung. Sulph. Comp.

UNGUENTUM HYDRARGYRI FORTIUS. L. (Ung. Hydrargyri, E. & D.) Mercury ℔ij, lard ℥xxiij, suet ℥j. Rub the mercury with the suet and a little of the lard until the globules disappear; then add the rest of the lard, and mix. [This ointment is not well prepared so long as metallic globules may be seen in it with a magnifier of 4 powers, E.] D. & P. omit the suet. [The extinction of the quicksilver may be greatly facilitated by triturating it with a portion of *old* mercurial ointment, as recommended by Mr. HIGGINBOTTOM of Northampton in 1814; or of lard, which has been long exposed, in a divided state, to the action of the air. See Adeps Oxygenatus. Many other modes of abridging the time and labour required in accomplishing this object have been proposed; but none of them are more effectual, or freer from objection, than these.]

UNGUENTUM HYDRARGYRI MITIUS. L. Stronger mercurial ointment ℔j, lard ℔ij; mix. D. orders ℔j of quicksilver to ℔ij of lard. E. directs the strong ointment to be diluted with twice or thrice its weight of lard.

Unguentum Hydrargyri Camphoratum. Guy's H. Camphor (rubbed with 30 drops of olive oil) ʒj, stronger mercurial ointment ʒj; mix.

Unguentum Hydrargyri cum Ammoniæ Muriate. Dupuytren. Stronger mercurial ointment ℥ij, muriate of ammonia in fine powder ʒj. *Applied to chronic glandular enlargements.*

Unguentum Hydrargyri Opiatum. Guy's H. Opium (softened with 30 drops of water) ʒj, milder mercurial ointment ʒj.

Unguentum Hydrargyri cum Pice. Barthez, *to prevent the scars from Small Pox.* Mercurial ointment 24 parts, wax 10, black pitch 6.

Unguentum Hydrargyri cum Soda. F. H. *Savon Mercuriel.* Mercurial ointment ʒiijss, solution of caustic soda ℥iij; triturate until they combine.

Unguentum Hydrargyri Ioduretum. Hanke. Weak mercurial ointment ʒj, iodine gr. vj, iodide of potassium ʒjss.

Unguentum Hydrargyri Ammonio-chloridi. L. [Ung. Precipitati Albi, E.; Ung. Submuriatis Hydr. Ammoniati, D.] White precipitate ʒj, lard ℥jss; mix.

Unguentum Hydrargyri Chloridi. See Ung. Calomelanos.

Unguentum Hydrargyri Chloridi cum Sapone. Jadelot. Calomel ʒj, soap ʒj, olive oil ʒij, water ʒj.

Unguentum Hydrargyri Bichloridi. Guy's H. Bichloride of mercury gr. iij, spermaceti ointment ℥j. The powdered sublimate should be rubbed perfectly smooth with a little of the ointment, and the rest added, and well mixed. [The *Pommade de Cirillo*, P., is made with ʒj of sublimate to ℥j of lard, well ground together. Dr. Corrigan uses an ointment containing gr. v of sublimate to ʒj of lard, in the treatment of *Porrigo.*]

Unguentum Hydrargyri Chloro-iodidi. M. Recamier. Chloro-iodide of mercury gr. iij, lard or cerate ʒv; mix accurately.

Unguentum Hydrargyri Cyanidi. Cazenave. Cyanide of mercury gr. viij, lard ʒj. A few drops of essence of lemon or bergamot are sometimes added.

Unguentum Hydrargyri Iodidi. L. Iodide of mercury ℥j, white wax ℥ij, lard ℥vj; melt the wax and lard together, and add the iodide in fine powder. [M. directs only gr. xx of the iodide to ℥jss of lard; CAZENAVE, ℈j to ℥j of lard.]

UNGUENTUM HYDRARGYRI BINIODIDI. L. As the last, substituting the *red* iodide.

UNGUENTUM HYDRARGYRI ET AMMONIÆ MURIATIS. BIETT. Sal Alembroth ℈j, lard ℥j; mix.

UNGUENTUM HYDRARGYRI PROTO-NITRATIS. BIETT. Proto-nitrate of mercury ℈j, lard ℥j; mix.

UNGUENTUM HYDRARGYRI NITRATIS. L. (*Ung. Citrinum*, E.) Quicksilver ℥j, nitric acid f ʒxj, lard ℥vj, olive oil f ℥iv; dissolve the mercury in the acid, and mix the warm solution with the lard and oil, previously melted together. [If the acid should not be of the full strength, the quantity should be proportionally increased. The density of the acid ordered by the College being 1500, if a weaker acid is used, one 24th more must be added for every 10 less density. Thus, if the density of the acid employed in the above ointment has a density of only 1490, ♏27 (the 24th of f ʒxj) must be added, making f ʒxj ♏xxvij. This rule applies pretty exactly down to 1420. The principal causes of failure in making this ointment are, an insufficient quantity of acid, and too low a temperature. (See Mr. SCHACT's paper, Pharm. Journal, vol. iv.) The heat, however, should not exceed 212° F.] E. (*Ung. Citrinum*) directs ℥iv of quicksilver to be dissolved, with a gentle heat, in f ℥viij f ʒvj of pure nitric acid, and the solution to be added, whilst hot, to ℥xv of lard, melted with f ℥xxxij of olive oil, and still hot, in a vessel capable of holding 6 times the quantity, and thoroughly mixed. If the mixture do not froth up, increase the heat a little till this takes place. [This formula is founded on that of Messrs. DUNCAN & Co., of Edinburgh. U. S. substitutes neatsfoot oil for olive oil. Mercury ℥j, nitric acid f ʒxj, neatsfoot oil f ℥x, lard ℥iij. This is said to retain its soft consistence better than the preceding.]

UNGUENTUM HYDRARGYRI NITRATIS MITIUS. E. 1817. As Ung. Hydr. Nit., with 3 times the quantity of oil and lard. [See Linimentum Hydrargyri Nitratis. It is often reduced extemporaneously with spermaceti ointment. The following is the Linimentum Hydr. Nitratis of the Manchester Pharmacopœia:—Ointment of nitrated quicksilver ℥ijss, simple cerate ʒvijss, olive oil f ʒvss. In using these ointments, a bone or wooden spatula must be employed.]

UNGUENTUM HYDRARGYRI NITRICO-OXYDI. L. & D. White wax ℥ij, lard ℥vj; melt together, add nitric oxide of mercury in very fine powder ℥j, and mix.

UNGUENTUM OXYDI HYDRARGYRI. E. Red oxide of mercury ℥j, lard ℥viij.

UNGUENTUM HYDRARGYRI OXYDI CINEREI. E. 1817. Gray oxide of quicksilver 1 part, lard 3 parts; mix. [Mr. DONOVAN'S Ointment, proposed as a substitute for Ung. Hydrargyri, is made by mixing 1 part of black oxide of mercury (procured by decomposing calomel with solution of pure potash, or by pouring a solution of nitrate of mercury into caustic alkaline solution) with 16 parts of lard, and maintaining the mixture at a heat of between 300° and 320° for at least an hour, stirring them continually; then remove, and stir until cold. Not more than 21 or 24 grains of the oxide enter into combination with ℥j of lard.]

UNGUENTUM HYDRARGYRI SUBSULPHATIS. ALIBERT. Turbith mineral ʒij, lard ℥iv. BIETT. Turbith mineral ʒj, sulphur ʒij, lard ℥iij, oil of lemon 15 drops.

UNGUENTUM HYDRARGYRI BIPHOSPHATIS. ALBANO. Biphosphate of mercury ʒj, lard ʒxj. Mix accurately.

UNGUENTUM HYDRARGYRI SULPHURETI RUBRI. ALIBERT. Red sulphuret of mercury ℥j, lard ℥xvj.

UNGUENTUM HYDRIODATIS POTASSÆ. See Ung. Potassii Iodidi.

UNGUENTUM HYDROBROMATIS POTASSÆ. See Ung. Potassii Bromidi.

UNGUENTUM HYOSCYAMI. GAUGER. Fresh henbane leaves bruised ℔ij, olive oil ℔iv ℥ix, wax ℔j ℥iij. Digest for some hours, boil for a ¼ of an hour, and strain.

UNGUENTUM HYPOCHLORIDIS SULPHURIS. See Ung. Sulph. Hypochloridis.

UNGUENTUM IMPERATORIÆ. *Pommade Anticancéreuse de Milius.* Powdered masterwort ʒjss, tincture of masterwort ℥j, lard ℥ij; mix.

UNGUENTUM INULÆ. Fresh elecampane root (boiled till soft and pulped) ℥jss, lard ℥j; mix. *In Itch.*

UNGUENTUM IODINII. U. S. Iodine ℈j, rectified spirit ♏xx; rub together, and add ʒj of lard. [D. ℈j, GUY'S H. gr. xv of iodine, to ℥j of lard.] For E. see the next.

UNGUENTUM IODINII COMPOSITUM. L. & U. S. (Ung. Iodinei, E.) Iodine ʒss, iodide of potassium ʒj, rectified spirit fʒj; rub together, and add ℥ij of lard; mix perfectly. [P. Iodine ℈ij, iodide of potassium ʒij, lard ℥ij.] LUGOL'S *Ointments*, Nos. 1, 2, 3, and 4 contain respectively gr. x–xv–xvij–xx of iodine, with ℈j, ʒij, ʒijss of iodide of potassium, and ℥ij of lard. Triturate the iodine and iodide with a little water, and mix with lard.

UNGUENTUM IODINII CUM OLEO NICOTIANÆ. Dr. DOVER. Iodine gr. xij, iodide of potassium ℈iv, oil of tobacco 50 drops, lard ʒij. *To relax rigid muscles.*

UNGUENTUM IODHYDRARGYRATIS POTASSII. LAMOTHE. Iodhydrargyrate of potassium ℈j, lard ℥j.

UNGUENTUM IODO-NARCOTICUM. F. H. Iodide of potassium ℈iv, extract of henbane ʒj, extract of hemlock ʒj, camphor ℈iv, lard ʒx.

UNGUENTUM IPECACUANHÆ. Dr. TURNBULL. Powdered ipecac. ʒij, olive oil ʒij, lard ℥ss. Rubbed on the skin for a few minutes once or twice a day, it produces an eruption.

UNGUENTUM JATROPHÆ. Dr. HAMILTON. The milky juice of the English physic nut (Jatropha Curcas) with half its weight of lard. *In Piles.*

UNGUENTUM JUNIPERI. Juniper leaves 1 part, resinous ointment 6 parts, boil gently, and strain.

UNGUENTUM LAURO-CERASI. JAMES. Oil of cherry-laurel ʒj, lard ℥j.

UNGUENTUM LAURINUM. P. Fresh bay-leaves ℔j, bay-berries ℔j, lard ℔ij; digest the bruised leaves and berries with the lard till the moisture is consumed, and express.

UNGUENTUM LAVANDULÆ. BAUME. Lard ℔ijss, lavender flowers ℔x, white wax ℥iij; melt the lard, digest with ℔ij of the flowers for 2 hours, and strain; repeat this with fresh flowers till all are used; melt the ointment, and leave it at rest to cool; separate the moisture and dregs, and melt the ointment with the wax.

UNGUENTUM LINARIÆ. Fresh toad-flax (in flower) ℔j, lard ℔ij. As Ung. Sambuci.

UNGUENTUM LITHARGYRI ACETATIS. CH. Wax ointment ℥j, Goulard's extract of lead ʒss; mix.

Unguentum Lupuli. Van Mons. Dried hops ℥ij, lard ℥x; as Ung. Conii.

Unguentum Lupulinæ. Freake. Lupulin ℈j, lard ʒiij.

Unguentum Manganesii Oxydi. Virey. Oxide of manganese ʒij, lard ℥j.

Unguentum Manganesii Oxydi cum Sulphure. Oxide of manganese ℥j, sulphur ℥j, white soap ℥j, lard ʒiij. *In Porrigo.*

Unguentum Manganesii Sulphatis. Augustin. Equal parts of sulphate of manganese and lard.

Unguentum Maticonis. Mr. Young. Powdered matico ʒiij, opium gr. iij, lard ℥j. Mix.

Unguentum Mezerei. U. S. & P. Mezereon bark dried ℥iv, lard ℥xiv, white wax ℥ij. Moisten the mezereon with rectified spirit, and beat it to a smooth paste; digest in a water-bath with the lard for 12 hours, strain with strong pressure, and allow the ointment to cool slowly. Separate from the dregs, and melt it with the wax. M. Guibourt proposes to mix ʒij of alcoholic extract of mezereon with ℥ix of lard, and ℥j of wax. *To keep up a discharge from blistered surfaces.*

Unguentum Monesiæ. Dr. St. Ange. Monesia ʒj, lard ℈j; mix. Derosne. Oil of almonds 4 parts, white wax 2, extract of monesia 1, water 1.

Unguentum Naphthalinæ. M. Emery. Naphthaline ʒss, lard ʒvijss; mix. *In Psoriasis, Lepra,* &c.

Unguentum Nervinum. E. 1744. Male southern-wood, marjoram, mint, pennyroyal, rue, rosemary (all fresh), each ℥vj; boil with Oiv of neats-foot oil and ℔iij of beef-suet, till the moisture is exhaled. Then press, and strain out the liquor, add Oss of oil of bays and make an ointment.

Unguentum Nicotianæ. See Ung. Tabaci.

Unguentum Nutritum. P. Litharge ℈iij, vinegar ℈iv, olive oil ℈ix; heat gently, and stir constantly until they combine.

Unguentum Olei Aselli. This may be made with cod-liver oil, white wax, and spermaceti, in the same proportions as Ung. Cetacei. If the *stearine* of cod-liver oil can be obtained, it may be melted with a fourth of its weight of wax. A little camphor may be added. [M. Deschamps employs a *soap* of cod-liver oil as a plaster or ointment, and as the basis of other preparations. Dissolve ʒj of caustic soda in ℥ijss of water, and mix it with f ℥viij of the oil.] BREFELD. Oil 10, extract of lead 5, lard 10.

UNGUENTUM OLEI ASELLI CUM FULIGINE. M. CARRON. Cod-liver oil ℥ij, extract of wood-soot ℥ij, citrine ointment ʒj, beef marrow ℥vj.

UNGUENTUM OPHIOGLOSSI. From the green leaves and spikes of adderstongue; as Ung. Sambuci.

UNGUENTUM OPII. GUY'S H. Opium (softened with 30 drops of water) ʒj, wax ointment ℥ij.

UNGUENTUM OPIATUM CUM FELLE. AUGUSTIN. Opium ʒij, calves' gall ℥ij; digest for 2 days, add lard ℥ij, oil of bergamot 10 drops.

UNGUENTUM OPIATUM CUM SUCCO GASTRICO. BRERA. Opium ʒj, gastric juice of a calf q. s. Digest for 24 hours, and add lard ℥j, or q. s.

UNGUENTUM OPHTHALMICUM. The following are selected from the many magistral and hospital formulæ bearing this name. [N.B. The dry ingredients should be very finely powdered, and triturated with the fatty matters till perfectly smooth.]

1. ACKERMANN'S. Nitric-oxide of mercury ℈j, camphor gr. vj, fresh butter ℥ij.

2. DESSAULT'S. Red oxide of mercury ʒj, tutty ℥j, acetate of lead ʒj, burnt alum ʒj, corrosive sublimate ℈ss, rose ointment ℥j. Grind for a long time on porphyry.

3. DUPUYTREN'S. Red oxide of mercury gr. x, sulphate of zinc ℈j, lard ℥ij.

4. FRICKE'S. Nitrate of silver gr. x, balsam of Peru ʒss, zinc ointment ℥ij.

5. HUFELAND'S. Black oxide of mercury gr. ij, oil of walnut ʒij.

6. JANIN'S. Tutty ʒij, bole ʒij, white precipitate ℥j, lard ℥ss.

7. LOHSSE'S. Iodine gr. jss, iodide of potassium ℈j, lard ℥ss. *In Opacity of the Cornea.*

8. PELLIER'S. Nitric oxide of mercury ʒjss, calamine ℥jss, tutty ℥ss, vermilion ℈j, balsam of Peru 15 drops, lard ℥ij.

9. REGENT'S. Red oxide of mercury ℥j, acetate of lead ʒj, camphor gr. v, washed butter ʒxviij.

10. Rust's. Liquid diacetate of lead ʒss, wine of opium ʒss, washed fresh butter ʒij.

11. Spielmann's. Acetate of lead ℈j, spermaceti cerate ʒv, compound tincture of benzoin ℈ij.

12. St. Yves'. Nitric oxide of mercury ℈j–℈ij, oxide of zinc ℈j, fresh butter ℥j, wax ℈iv, camphor gr. xv.

13. H. des Enfans. Oxide of zinc gr. xv, calomel gr. xij, camphor gr. viij, fresh butter ʒij, tincture of catechu ʒss. *In Scrofulous Ophthalmia.*

14. Scarpa. Tutty ʒj, aloes gr. ij, calomel gr. ij, butter ʒiijss. See also Ung. Argenti Nitratis; Ung. Hydr. Nitratis Mitius; Ung. Zinci, &c.

Unguentum Ovorum. Soubeiran. Yolk of 1 egg, wax ʒiv, oil of almonds ℥jss. Behrends. Yolk of egg, honey, fresh linseed oil, of each q. p. Mix.

Unguentum Oxygenatum. Alyon. Lard ℥xvj, nitric acid ℥ij; heat together in a glass or porcelain vessel till the mixture begins to boil; then remove from the fire and stir till cold.

Unguentum Paulliniæ. Extract of paullinia (guarana) ʒij, lard ℥ij.

Unguentum ad Perniones. *Chilblain ointment.* Kapeler. Oil of almonds ℥ij, white wax ʒj, spermaceti ʒij, hydrochloric acid ʒij, Peruvian balsam ʒj. Devergie. Lard ʒvijss, creasote 10 drops, solution of diacetate of lead 10 drops, extract of opium gr. j. Mix.

Unguentum Phosphoratum. P. Phosphorus 1 part, lard 50 parts, put them into a bottle loosely corked, and heat it gradually by means of a water-bath: when the water boils, take out the bottle, stop it close, and shake it briskly till the ointment is cooled.

Unguentum Phytolaccæ. Dr. Wood. Powdered leaves or root of Phytolacca decandra (American Poke) ʒj, lard ℥j. *In psora, tinea capitis,* &c.

Unguentum Olei Picis. Giraud. Distilled oil of tar ʒj, lard ℥j.

Unguentum Picis Liquidæ. L. & D. Tar ℔j, suet ℔j; melt together, strain, and stir till cold. E. Tar ℥v, bees'-wax ℥ij.

UNGUENTUM PICIS NIGRÆ. L. *Black Basilicon.* Black pitch ℥ix, wax ℥ix, resin ℥ix, olive oil f℥xvj; melt together, and strain.

UNGUENTUM PICIS COMPOSITUM. St. B. H. Tar ointment ℔ss, cerate of acetate of lead ℔ss. GUY'S H. Equal weights of sulphur ointment and tar ointment.

UNGUENTUM PICROTOXINÆ. JAEGER. Picrotoxine gr. x, lard ℥j; mix.

UNGUENTUM PIPERIS NIGRI. D. Lard ℔j, black pepper ℥iv; mix.

UNGUENTUM PIPERIS COMPOSITUM. BATE. Elecampane ℥ij, sulphur ℥ij, black pepper ℥jss, rose water ointment ℥xvj, oil of rhodium (or other scent) ℈ij. *For the cure of Itch.*

UNGUENTUM PLATINI. HOEFER. Perchloride of platinum ʒj, extract of belladonna ʒij, lard ℥iv; mix.

UNGUENTUM PLUMBI ACETATIS. E. Simple ointment ℥xx, acetate of lead ℥j; mix.

UNGUENTUM PLUMBI CARBONATIS. E. *Ung. Album.* Simple ointment ℥v, carbonate of lead ℥j; mix.

UNGUENTUM PLUMBI CAMPHORATUM. *Ung. Album Camphoratum.* E. 1744. Add to the last ℈ij of camphor, ground with a little oil.

UNGUENTUM PLUMBI COMPOSITUM. L. KIRKLAND'S *Neutral Ointment.* Melt ℔iij of lead plaster with Oj of olive oil. Mix ℥viij of prepared chalk with f℥vj of distilled vinegar: add the warm solution to the plaster and oil, also warm, and stir till cold.

UNGUENTUM PLUMBI CUM AQUA LAURO-CERASI. GIACOCOMINI'S *Pommade,* for chilblains, &c. Lard ℥j, cherry-laurel water ʒij, acetate of lead 3ij. COTTERAU adds—camphor ʒj, tar ʒjss.

UNGUENTUM PLUMBI CUM ACIDO HYDROCYANICO. Dr. A. T. THOMSON. Acetate of lead ʒss, diluted hydrocyanic acid fʒiij, spermaceti ointment ℥iij.

UNGUENTUM PLUMBI CHLORIDI. Mr. TUSON. Chloride of lead ʒj, simple cerate ℥j.

UNGUENTUM PLUMBI IODIDI. L. Iodide of lead ℥j, lard ℥viij; rub together.

UNGUENTUM PLUMBI TANNATIS. SUNDELIN. Decoction of oak bark (from ℥j of bark) ℥vj, liquid diacetate of lead ℥jss; mix, set aside for an hour, collect the precipitate on a filter, and mix it, still moist, with ℥j of lard; gr. x. of camphor may be added. Dr. TOTT, for *bed-sores.* Fresh tannate of lead 12 parts, lard 30.

UNGUENTUM PLUMBAGINIS. Black lead ʒj to ʒij, lard ℥j.

UNGUENTUM POMATUM. L. 1746. See Ung. Simplex.

UNGUENTUM POPULEUM. M. DESCHAMPS. Buds of poplar 2 parts, water 1 part, fresh lard 12 parts; boil in a tinned vessel till the moisture is evaporated, strain through linen, and stir now and then whilst cooling. See Ung. Benzoini.

UNGUENTUM POPULEUM COMPOSITUM. To ℔vss of the last ointment add fresh leaves (bruised) of poppy, belladonna, henbane, common nightshade, each ℥viij; boil gently, till they become crisp, strain, and press.

UNGUENTUM POTASSII BROMIDI (*vel* POTASSÆ HYDROBROMATIS). M. Hydrobromate of potash ʒss, lard ℥j. GUIBOURT directs 1 part to 12. See also Ung. Brominii Compositum.

UNGUENTUM POTASSII CYANIDI. LOMBARD. Cyanide of potassium gr. ij to iv, lard ℥j. CAZENAVE. Cyanide of potassium gr. xij, oil of almonds ʒij, cold cream ℥ij. [Rubbed on the sound skin to relieve neuralgic and rheumatic pains.]

UNGUENTUM POTASSII IODIDI. *Ung. Potassæ Hydriodatis.* D. Hydriodate of potash (Iodide of potassium) ℈j, lard ℥j. It is frequently made stronger: GUY'S H. and Dr. MANSON direct ʒss, P. ʒj, and M. ℈ij of the iodide to ℥j of lard. Dr. COINDET. Iodide of potassium ʒss, solution of potash 2 drops, lard ℥jss, white wax ʒiij. M. GRAS prescribes 3ss of iodide of potassium to ℥j of lard as an *Itch Ointment.* [The iodide of potassium should be first rubbed with a few drops of spirit or oil, or a little of the lard, till perfectly smooth; or it may be dissolved in its weight of water. But this latter expedient must not be adopted when the salt is to be mixed with mercurial ointment, unless a reaction between them is desired.]

UNGUENTUM POTASSII IODIDI IODURETUM. M. See Ung. Iodidi Compositum.

UNGUENTUM POTASSII IODIDI OPIATUM. Dr. A. T. THOMSON. Iodide of potassium ʒjss, lard ℥jss, tincture of opium fʒj.

UNGUENTUM POTASSII SULPHURETI. ALIBERT. Sulphuret of potassium ʒiij, carbonate of soda ʒiij, lard ℥iij. *For Ringworm.*

UNGUENTUM POTASSII IODIDI CUM HYDRARGYRO. SCHONLEIN. Ointment of iodide of potassium, mercurial ointment, oil of henbane by infusion, each ℥ij, oil of juniper ʒj.

UNGUENTUM PURGATIVUM. See Ung. Colocynthidis. BOERHAAVE'S Ung. Purgans contains aloes ʒj, ox-gall ʒj, althea ointment ℥j. To be applied about the navel.

UNGUENTUM QUINÆ CITRATIS. Citrate of quinine ℈ss, lard ʒj.

UNGUENTUM QUINÆ FORTIUS. Sulphate of quinine ʒj, lard ʒij. Used in frictions for the cure of intermittents.

UNGUENTUM QUINÆ HYDRIODATIS IODURETUM. RIGHINI. Ioduretted hydriodate of quinine ʒss, spermaceti ʒv, oil of almonds ʒx; melt the spermaceti with the oil, and add the salt of quinine.

UNGUENTUM RESINÆ ALBÆ. D. Lard ℔iv, white resin ℔ij, yellow wax ℔j; melt together, and strain.

UNGUENTUM RESINOSUM. E. Resin ℥v, lard ℥viij, wax ℥ij; melt together.

UNGUENTUM RESOLVENS. HUFELAND. Marsh-mallow ointment ℥j, fresh ox-gall ℥ss, soap ℥ss, oil of petroleum ʒj, camphor ʒj; mix.

UNGUENTUM RHATANIÆ. M. TROUSSEAU. Extract of rhatany ʒjss, butter of cacao ʒv; mix.

UNGUENTUM ROSATUM. P. *Pommade Rosat.* Washed lard ℔ij, petals of 100-leaved rose ℔iv: bruise half the flowers, mix with the lard, and in 2 days melt, strain, and express: add the rest of the flowers; and in 24 hours melt, strain, and express; colour with alkanet root. [That of E. 1744, is Ung. Pomatum; see also Ung. Aquæ Rosæ.]

UNGUENTUM RUBEFACIENS. RICHARD. Cantharides ʒj, camphor ʒj, lard ℥j.

UNGUENTUM RUTÆ. SPAN. H. Fresh rue ℥ij, wormwood ℥ij, mint ℥ij, lard ℥xvj; boil till the moisture is expelled.

UNGUENTUM SABADILLINÆ. Dr. TURNBULL. Sabadilline gr. xv to xx, lard ℥j; used as Ung. Veratriæ, but less efficient.

UNGUENTUM SABINÆ. D. Fresh sabine ℔ss, lard ℔ij; boil

till the leaves are crisp, strain, and add ℔ss of yellow wax. [A heat below boiling is preferable.]

UNGUENTUM SAMBUCI VIRIDE. D. Fresh elder leaves bruised ℔iij, lard ℔iv, suet ℔ij. Boil the leaves in the lard till they become crisp, then strain with expression; lastly add the suet, and melt them together.

UNGUENTUM SAMBUCI. L. Elder flowers ℔ij, lard ℔ij; boil together till the flowers become crisp, and express. [Care must be taken to keep the heat moderate towards the end of the process.]

UNGUENTUM SATURNINUM. See Ung. Plumbi Acetatis.

UNGUENTUM SCILLÆ. Powdered squills ʒss, lard (mercurial ointment, BRERA) ℥j; mix.

UNGUENTUM SCROPHULARIÆ. D. Fresh leaves of knotty figwort ℔ij, lard ℔ij, suet ℔j; boil together till the leaves become crisp and strain, with expression. A specific in *Pemphigus gangrenosus*. Dr. W. STOKES.

UNGUENTUM SIMPLEX. E. Olive oil f℥vss, white wax ℥ij; melt together. U. S. White wax ℔j, lard ℔iv; melt together with a moderate heat, and stir until cold. [Ung. Simplex, E. 1746, was lard washed with rose water.]

UNGUENTUM SINAPIS COMPOSITUM. Dr. FERRIAR. Resin ointment ℥j, soap ℥ss, mustard-flour ℈j, camphor ℈ij.

UNGUENTUM SODÆ MURIATIS. TAVIGNOT. Common salt from ʒj gradually increased to ʒiv, lard ℥j. Rub together till perfectly smooth. *To inflamed eyelids.*

UNGUENTUM STANNI CHLORIDI. M. NAUCHE. Perchloride of tin gr. jss, lard ℥j; mix ʒj to be rubbed in daily.

UNGUENTUM STANNI OXYDI. BATE. Oxide of tin rubbed with oil of St. John's-wort was formerly applied for the cure of blindness; with Locatelle's balsam and honey, for indolent ulcers.

UNGUENTUM STAPHISAGRIÆ. SWEDIAUR. Powdered stavesacre ℥j, lard ℥iij; digest for 3 hours and strain.

UNGUENTUM STRAMONII. U. S. Fresh stramonium (cut) ℔j, lard ℔iij; boil until the leaves become friable, strain, add yellow wax (previously melted) ℔ss, and stir till cold. [It is also made with ℥j of the powdered leaves, and ʒiv of lard. Dr. PEREIRA.]

UNGUENTUM STRYCHNIÆ NITRATIS. WENDT. Nitrate of strychnia gr. jss, lard ʒij.

UNGUENTUM STYRACIS. CH. Wax ointment ℥j, strained storax ʒj. P. Oil of nuts ℥xij, liquid storax ℥viij, resin ℥xvj, elemi ℥viij, yellow wax ℥viij; melt together and strain.

UNGUENTUM SUBERIS USTI. Burnt cork gr. iv, acetate of lead gr. xv, fresh butter q. s. *For Piles.*

UNGUENTUM SULPHURIS. L. Sublimed sulphur ℥iij, lard ℥vj, oil of bergamot ♏xx; mix. E. and D. direct 1 part of sulphur to 4 of lard.

UNGUENTUM SULPHURIS COMPOSITUM. L. *Itch Ointment.* Sulphur ℥vj, white hellebore ℥ij, nitre ʒj, soft soap ℔ss, lard ℔jss, oil of bergamot ♏xxx. U. S. Sulphur ℥j, ammoniated mercury (white precipitate) ʒj, benzoic acid ʒj, oil of bergamot f ʒj, sulphuric acid f ʒj, powdered nitre ʒij, lard ℔ss. To the melted lard add the other ingredients, and stir constantly until cold. P. Lard ℥xvj, washed sulphur ℥viij, muriate of ammonia ℥ss, alum ℥ss; mix carefully.

UNGUENTUM SULPHURIS ALKALINUM. BATEMAN. Subcarbonate of potash ʒiv, rose water ℥j, vermilion ʒj, oil of bergamot ʒss, sulphur ℥xj, lard ℥vj.

UNGUENTUM SULPHURIS SAPONACEUM. F. H. Saponis ℥j, water q. s. Dissolve, and add ℥j of sulphur.

UNGUENTUM SULPHURIS CUM CARBONE. RICHARD. Charcoal ℥j, sulphur ℥j, lard ℥v.

UNGUENTUM SULPHURIS CUM ZINCO. SAX. PH. JASSER'S *Ointment for Tinea Capitis.* Sulphur ℥ij, sulphate of zinc ℥j, bay ointment ℥j, lard ℥vj.

UNGUENTUM SULPHURIS HYPOCHLORIDI. Dr. COPLAND. Hypochloride of sulphur ʒj, spermaceti ointment ℥j; mix.

UNGUENTUM SULPHURIS IODIDI. M. One part of ioduret of sulphur to 18 or 19 parts of lard. CAZENAVE, 1 part to 30. Dr. DAVIDSON, ℈j to ℈ij of ioduret of sulphur to ℥j of lard. PEREIRA, gr. x to xxx to ℥j of lard.

UNGUENTUM TABACI. U. S. Fresh leaves of tobacco ℥j, lard ℥xij. As Ung. Stramonii. [Mr. CHIPPENDALE recommends the following to be used every night, or night and morning, in frictions, to relieve *Neuralgia.* Extract of tobacco ʒj, simple cerate ʒvij. A little neroli or other mild scent may be added.]

UNGUENTUM OLEI TABACI. Empyreumatic oil of tobacco 20 drops, simple ointment ℥j. *It must be used with caution.*

UNGUENTUM TANNINI. RICHARD. Tannin ʒij, water ʒij, lard ℥jss; mix. CAZENAVE: Tannin ℈j, lard ʒxxx.

UNGUENTUM TARTARI EMETICI. See Ung. Antimonii Potassio-tartratis.

UNGUENTUM TEREBINTHINÆ COMPOSITUM. GUY'S H. Oil of turpentine f℈j, camphor ʒj, resin cerate ℥j.

UNGUENTUM TEREBINTHINÆ AMMONIATUM. DEBREYNE. Oil of turpentine ℥j, liquid ammonia ʒj, spirit of camphor ʒiv, lard ℥x: mix. *In Sciatica.*

UNGUENTUM AD TINEAM. F. H. Ointment of nitrate of quicksilver ʒiv, tar ointment ℥j. H. OF ST. LOUIS. Caustic soda ʒij, sulphuret of potash ʒij, lard ℥iij. HENKE. Hydrochloric acid ʒiv, althæa ointment ʒiv, juniper ointment ℥ij; mix.

UNGUENTUM TRIPHARMACUM. L. 1746. Lead plaster ℥iv, olive oil f℥ij, vinegar f℥j; melt, and stir till they combine.

UNGUENTUM TUTIÆ. D. *Ung. Zinci Oxydi impuri.* Prepared tutty ℥ij, white wax ointment ℥x; mix.

UNGUENTUM VERATRI. L. White hellebore powder ℥ij, lard ℥viij, oil of lemon ♏xx; mix. D. ℥iij of hellebore to ℔j of lard.

UNGUENTUM VERATRIÆ. M. Veratria gr. iv, lard ℥j; mix. Dr. TURNBULL directs from gr. x to xx grains of veratria to ℥j of lard; the veratria to be first rubbed with a little oil till perfectly smooth. M. SAUVAN prefers the acetate of veratria; from 4 to 12 grs. to ℥j of lard. Dr. T. directs about the size of a nut of the ointment to be rubbed from 5 to 15 minutes, night and morning, over the seat of the disease, taking care that the skin is perfectly sound. But when applied over a large surface, as in dropsical effusions, the quantity used should contain from 2 to 4 grains of veratria.

UNGUENTUM VERMIFUGUM. BATAVIAN PH. Aloes ℈j, inspissated ox-gall ℈jss, lard ℥jss.

UNGUENTUM VIRIDE. L. 1746. Green oil ℔iij, yellow wax ℥x; melt together, and stir till cool.

UNGUENTUM ZINCI. L. & E. Oxide of zinc ℥j, lard (simple liniment, E. Ointment of white wax, D.) ℥iij; mix.

Unguentum Zinci cum Myrrha. Knachstedt. Oxide of zinc 3ij, calamine ʒij, lycopodium ʒij, acetate of lead ʒss, myrrh ʒss, lard ℥jss.

Unguentum Zinci cum Opio. Henke. Fresh butter ℥j, oxide of zinc ʒss, opium in powder gr. j. *In Chronic Impetigo.*

Unguentum Zinci Cyanidi. Cuvier. Cyanide of zinc gr. xij, lard 3v, butter of cacao 3v; mix.

Unguentum Zinci Iodidi. Dr. Ure. Iodide of zinc 3j, lard ℥j.

Unguentum Zinci Sulphatis. Scarpa. Sulphate of zinc 3j, lard ℥j. Klein. Sulphate of zinc ℈j, fresh butter ʒij.

Unguentum Zinci et Lycopodii. Rosenstein. Lycopodium ʒj, oxide of zinc ʒj, lard ℥ss. See Cerates and Liniments for other formulæ.

Urea Factitia. Mix 28 parts of well-dried ferrocyanate of potash with 14 of black oxide of manganese (both in fine powder), and heat them to dull redness on an iron plate. Lixiviate with cold water; add 20½ parts of dry sulphate of ammonia, concentrate by evaporation with a heat not exceeding 212° F., decant the concentrated liquid, treat it with rectified spirit, and crystallize. *Diuretic*—dose, from gr. x to ℈j.

Ureæ Nitras. Nitric acid throws down this salt from a concentrated solution of urea. Dose, gr. jss 3 times a day, in *Anasarca.*

Usquebagh. L. 1677. French brandy ℔xxiv, liquorice root ℔j, stoned raisins ℔ss, cloves ℥ss, mace 3ij, ginger ʒij. Macerate for 14 days. [Replaced by Tinct. Cardamomi Composita.]

Vegetabilium Preparatio. The following is the substance of the directions of the pharmacopœia for the collection, preservation, and preparation of vegetable simples. A few additions from other authorities are included in brackets.

Vegetables should be collected in dry weather, when neither wet with dew nor rain. They should not be kept longer than a year. To dry them, spread them lightly, shortly after they are gathered, and dry them with a gentle heat. [The temperature should be between 100° and 212°. Brande.] Preserve them, in convenient vessels, from the access of damp or light.

Most *Roots* should be dug up before the leaves and stalks

shoot forth. [*Annual* roots, just before the time of flowering; *biennial* after the vegetation of the first year has ceased; *perennial* in the spring before vegetation has commenced. Dr. WOOD.] Lay up the roots that are to be kept fresh in sand. Cut the cormi of meadow-saffron, and the bulbs of squill, before drying them, into thin transverse slices, after removing their dry coats. [Fleshy roots may be sliced, and after drying in the air, exposed to a heat of 100°; the sliced bulbs should be dried at the same temperature. Dr. WOOD. Dr. HOULTON says that colchicum may be dried by placing the cormi, without slicing them, in a dry situation after removing the loose coats, and carefully extracting the eye or bud, the rudiment of the future plant.]

Barks are to be collected at the season in which they are most readily separated from the wood. [This, with few exceptions, is late in the spring, or early in the summer. BRANDE.]

Leaves are to be gathered after the flowers are fully blown, and before the seeds ripen. *Seeds* when fully ripe, and kept in their seed-vessels. *Flowers* when recently blown.

Pulps. See Pulpæ, page 276.

Gum-Resins. Opium should be kept carefully freed from extraneous substances; and kept *soft* for pills, and *hard* (dried by water-bath) for powders. Those Gum-Resins should be preferred which require no purification. If less pure, boil them in water until they become soft; press through hempen cloth, and set by, that the resinous part may subside. Evaporate the supernatant liquor, and towards the end add the resin, and mix. The easily fusible gum-resins may be inclosed in an ox-bladder. and kept in boiling water till soft enough to be pressed through hempen cloth. [See Extractum Styracis, and Extractum Scammonii. Mr. BRANDE recommends reducing ammoniacum, assafœtida, and galbanum to powder in cold weather, and passing the powder through a sieve.]

VERATRIA. L. Boil ℔ij of bruised sabadilla in 3 successive gallons of rectified spirit, in a retort with a receiver fitted to it. Press the sabadilla, distil off the spirit from the mixed and filtered liquors, and evaporate the residue to the consistence of an extract. Boil this 3 times or oftener in water, acidulated with a little diluted sulphuric acid, and evaporate the clear liquor to the consistence of syrup. To this, when cold, add magnesia to saturation, stir it, squeeze, and wash it twice or thrice; then dry it, and digest it twice or thrice in spirit, filtering the solutions; distil off the spirit, boil what remains in water, to which a little sulphuric acid and animal charcoal have been added, for a quarter of an hour, and strain. Lastly, the charcoal being well washed, evaporate the liquors to the consistence of syrup, and add as much solution of ammonia as will suffice to precipitate the veratria. Wash and dry it. E. directs the sabadilla seeds to be infused in boiling water, and in 24 hours squeezed and dried; then beaten in a mortar, and the seeds separated from the capsules by agitation in a deep vessel. The seeds are then ground, and exhausted by percolation with rectified spirit, the spirituous solutions concentrated by distillation so long as no deposit forms, and the residuum poured while hot into 12 volumes of cold water. To the filtered liquor and washings of the residuum add excess of ammonia, wash the precipitate slightly with cold water, and dry it, first by imbibition with filtering paper, and then in a vapour-bath. [The sulphate, tartrate, and other salts of veratria, are obtained in the same manner as the corresponding salts of morphia.]

VINA. The medicated wines are prepared in the same manner as tinctures: they should be made in well-closed vessels, and macerated without heat. The L. College in the pharmacopœia of 1824, substituted a *diluted spirit* for wine still retaining the name; but the wine (*sherry*) was restored in that of 1836.

VINUM ABSINTHII. P. Dried wormwood ℥j, white wine ℥xxxij, rectified spirit ℥j; macerate the leaves in the spirit; in 24 hours add the wine, macerate for 2 days and strain.

VINUM ALKALINUM DIURETICUM. SYDENHAM. Ashes of broom ℥xij, Rhenish wine Oiv.

VINUM ALÖES. L. *Tinct. Sacra. Tinct. Hieræ Picræ.* Aloes ℥ij, canella ʒiv, sherry Oij; macerate for 14 days, occasionally shaking, and strain. E. Aloes ℥jss, cardamom ʒjss, ginger ʒjss, sherry Oij. Digest for 7 days and strain. D. Aloes ℥iv, canella ℥j, sherry f℥xlviij, proof spirit f℥xvj.

VINUM ALOETICUM ALKALINUM. L. 1746. Subcarbonate of potash ℥viij, aloes ℥j, myrrh ℥j, saffron ℥j, muriate of ammonia ʒvj, white wine f℥xxxij; macerate for a week, and filter. [Dr. A. T. THOMSON proposes the following modification:—Carbonate of soda ℥iij, carbonate of ammonia ʒivss, myrrh ʒvj, aloes ʒvj, sherry f℥xxiv.] Dose, fʒj.

VINUM ANTIMONII POTASSIO-TARTRATIS. L. *Vinum Antimoniale.*

E. Potassio-tartrate of antimony ℈ij, sherry Oj; dissolve. For D., see Liquor Tartari Emetici.

VINUM ANTISCORBUTICUM. P. Horse-radish root ℥j, scurvy-grass ʒiv, water-cress leaves ʒiv, buck-bean ʒiv, mustard seed ℥iv, muriate of ammonia ʒij, wine ℥xxxij, compound spirit of scurvy-grass ʒiv.

VINUM AROMATICUM. P. Aromatic species ℥iv, vulnerary spirit ℥ij, red wine ℥xxxij. For outward use M. RICORD sometimes adds from 1 to 6 per cent. of tannin.

VINUM BUCHU. BRANDES. Buchu leaves ℥ijss, white wine Oj.

VINUM CAINCÆ. Cahinca (bruised) ℥j, Malaga wine ʒxvj; macerate for 6 days, and strain.

VINUM CENTAURII COMPOSITUM. HOFFMANN'S *Elixir Viscerale.* Centaury, orange-peel, extract of blessed thistle, gentian, myrrh, cascarilla, each ʒj, sherry Oij.

VINUM CEPÆ. SOUBEIRAN. Two onions sliced, white wine Ojss; digest and strain. *For Gravel.*

VINUM CHALYBEATUM. See Vinum Ferri.

VINUM CINCHONINÆ. M. Cinchonine ℈j, wine f ʒxxxvj.

VINUM CINCHONÆ. P. Peruvian bark ℥ij, proof spirit ℥iv, macerate for 24 hours, and add red wine ℥xxxij. Macerate the bruised bark with the spirit for 24 hours, and add the wine. Macerate for 8 days, shaking it occasionally, strain with expression, and filter.

VINUM CINCHONÆ ET VALERIANÆ. PRINCE L. L. BONAPARTE. Yellow Peruvian bark ℥ij, valerian ℥j, rectified spirit ℥iv, acidulous white wine Oj. Macerate for 8 days, and decant. Dose, f ℥iij in 24 hours.

VINUM COLCHICI. L. & E. Dried colchicum cormus ℥viij, sherry wine Oj: macerate for 14 days, and filter. [U. S. Dried colchicum ℥xij, sherry f ℥xxxij. 14 days.] Dose, ♏xxx to f ʒj.

VINUM COLCHICI SEMINIS. U. S. Colchicum seeds bruised ℥iv, white wine f ℥xxxij; macerate for 14 days, occasionally shaking, and filter. [Dr. WILLIAMS says it is unnecessary to bruise the seeds, and that British wines will not answer.] Dose, f ʒss to f ʒj.

VINUM COLCHICI OPIATUM. EISENMANN. Wine of colchicum

seed ʒiij, tincture of opium ℈ss. Dose, 20 to 30 drops. *In Gout.*

VINUM COLOCYNTHIDIS. VAN MONS. Colocynth ℥ij, white wine ℥xxiv; macerate for 8 days, and filter.

VINUM CORNUS CIRCINATÆ. REECE. Extract of round-leaved dogwood (by cold water) ʒiij, white wine Ojss.

VINUM CROCEUM. L. 1746. Saffron ℥j, Canary wine f℥xvj.

VINUM CYNARÆ. LEWIS. Equal parts of unclarified juice of artichoke leaves and white wine. A wineglassful twice a day, in *Dropsies.*

VINUM DIGITALIS. PORT. PH. Dried fox-glove ℥j, good white wine ℔ij. Macerate for 4 days, and strain.

VINUM DIURETICUM MITIUS. M. DEBREYNE. Nitre ʒiij, juniper berries ℥jss, white wine Oij.

VINUM DIURETICUM FORTIUS. Jalap ʒij, squill ʒij, nitre ʒiv, white wine Oij.

VINUM DULCAMARÆ. Dr. CURRIE. Dulcamara stalks and leaves ℔j, sherry Oij; macerate for 14 days.

VINUM ERGOTÆ. U. S. Bruised ergot ℥ij, white wine f℥xvj; macerate for 14 days, and filter. Dose, from ʒj to ʒiij.

VINUM FERRI. L. 1809 and P. Iron filings ℥ij, sherry f℥xxxij; mix, set aside for a month, and filter. [In 1824 the following was substituted: in 1836 it was omitted. Iron filings ℥j, supertartrate of potash ʒvj, water f℥j; mix, keep them exposed in an open vessel, and daily moistened and stirred, for 6 weeks. Then dry it with a gentle heat, powder, and mix with water Ojss, proof spirit Oj.] Mr. DONOVAN recommends ℥ij of rust of iron to be added to Oj of hock, and digested in a water-bath at about 100° F. for an hour, shaking it frequently. Then remove it from the bath, and the next day filter it. M. SOUBEIRAN recommends proto-tartrate of iron gr. xvj, tartaric acid gr. xvj; triturate in a glass mortar, add Ojss of white wine, and filter. GUY'S H. directs the washed and still moist precipitate from ℈j of sulphate of iron and ℈j gr. v of carbonate of soda, to be mixed with ʒj gr. xij of bitartrate of potash, and the mixture digested for 3 days, in a close vessel, with Oss of sherry.

VINUM FERRI ACETATIS. M. SOUBEIRAN. Acetate of iron gr. xxxij, white wine ℥xvj.

VINUM FERRI CITRATIS. Liquid citrate of iron ℥j, Malaga wine ʒxxxij. [For another form, see Tinctura Ferri Aurantiaca.]

VINUM FERRI IODIDI. PIERQUIN. Iodide of iron ʒiv, Bourdeaux wine Oj. CALLOUD. Sulphate of iron gr. xij, iodide of potassium gr. xvj, white wine ℥j; dose, fʒss to fʒj.

VINUM GENTIANÆ. E. Gentian ℥ss, yellow bark ℥j, canella ʒj (each in coarse powder), dried orange-peel sliced ʒij, proof spirit f℥ivss; digest for 24 hours, add f℥xxxvj of sherry, digest for 7 days, express, and filter.

VINUM GLYCYRRHIZÆ. FULLER'S *Sweet Tincture.* Liquorice (Italian juice) ℥j, cochineal ℈ij, canary wine Oij. Sometimes ʒj of saffron is added.

VINUM GRATIOLÆ. NIEMANN. Hedge hyssop ʒij, white wine ℥xvj. Digest at a gentle heat for 4 hours, and strain. Dose, f℥j, frequently, in *Hypochondria.*

VINUM ILICIS. M. ROUSSEAU. Powdered holly leaves ʒij, white wine ℥vj; infuse for twelve hours.

VINUM INULÆ. P. Elecampane root ℥j, rectified spirit ℥j, white wine ℥xxxij.

VINUM IPECACUANHÆ. L. E. & D. Ipecacuanha bruised [in moderately fine powder, E.] ℥ijss, sherry wine Oij; macerate for 14 days [7 E. and D.], and filter.

VINUM LIRIODENDRI. Fresh bark of tulip-wood ℥ij, rectified spirit ℥ij, white wine Oj. Macerate for 8 days.

VINUM OPII. L. & E. SYDENHAM'S *Liquid Laudanum.* Purified extract of opium ℥ijss [E. opium ℥iij], cloves ʒijss, cinnamon ʒijss, sherry Oij; digest for 14 days [7 E.], and filter. D. Opium ℥j, cinnamon ʒj, cloves ʒj, sherry wine f℥xvj. U. S. Powdered opium ℥ij, cinnamon ʒj, cloves ʒj, wine f℥xvj. SYDENHAM'S was the same, with the addition of ℥j of saffron, and he directed it to be digested in a water-bath for 2 or 3 days, until it acquired a due consistence. P., as Sydenham's, macerated 15 days.

VINUM OPII FERMENTATIONE PARATUM. ROUSSEAU'S *Laudanum. Black Drop.* Choice opium ℥iv, honey ℥xij, hot water ℔v, yeast ʒij. Dissolve the opium and honey separately in hot water, mix, and add the yeast. Keep it at about 86° F. for a month, express, filter, distil off ℥xvj, and evaporate the residuum to ℥x; add to it ℥ivss of strong spirit (obtained by rectifying the product of distillation), mix, and filter; 4 drops are considered equivalent to ½ grain of extract of opium, or nearly one grain of crude opium.

VINUM PERSIMMONIS. Crushed persimmons (green fruit of the *Dyospyros Virginiana*) ℔j, port wine Ojss; place it daily in the sun for 14 days, strain, and filter. Dose, f ʒij to f ʒiv; *astringent.*

VINUM PIMPINELLÆ. SOBERNHEIM. Burnet saxifrage ℥jss, white wine Oj.

VINUM PURGANS ET TONICUM. PIERQUIN. Senna ℥j, rhubarb ℈vj, cloves ʒj, saffron ʒj, sherry Oij; macerate for 5 or 6 days, often shaking, and decant.

VINUM QUINÆ. M. Sulphate of quinine gr. xij, white wine f ℥xxxvj.

VINUM QUINÆ AROMATICUM. Dr. GOLLIER'S *Aromatic Quinine Wine.* Disulphate of quinine gr. xviij, citric acid gr. xv, sound orange wine one bottle (or f ℥xxiv.)

VINUM RHEI. L. 1788. Rhubarb ℥ijss, cardamom seed ℈iv, saffron ʒij, sherry f ℥xxxij, proof spirit f ℥viij; digest for 10 days. E. Rhubarb in coarse powder ℥v, canella ʒij, proof spirit f ℥v, sherry Oj, f℥xv; digest for 7 days, express strongly, and filter.

VINUM SARSAPARILLÆ. BERAL. Alcoholic extract of sarsaparilla ℥j, white wine ℥xvj.

VINUM SARSAPARILLÆ COMPOSITUM. Comp. extract of sarsa. ℥j, Madeira wine f ℥vij.

VINUM SENNÆ. SWED. PH. Senna ℥iv, coriander seed ʒij, fennel seed ʒij, sherry ℔ijss; digest for 3 days, add stoned raisins ℥iij; macerate for 24 hours, and strain with expression.

VINUM SCILLÆ. P. Dried squill ℥j, Malaga wine ℥xvj; macerate for 12 days.

VINUM SCILLÆ COMPOSITUM. RICHTER. Dried squill ℥j, orange-peel ʒiij, sweet flag ʒiij, juniper berries ʒij, white wine ℔iv; digest for 3 days, filter, and add ℥ij of oxymel of squills.

VINUM SCILLITICUM AMARUM. P. Peruvian bark ℥ij, winter's bark ℥ij, lemon-peel ℥ij, swallow-wort ʒiv, angelica root ʒiv, squill ʒiv, wormwood ℥j, balm ℥j, juniper berries ʒiv, mace ʒiv, white wine Ovij.

VINUM STRAMONII. BATAV. PH. Stramonium seeds ℥ij, Malaga wine ℥viij, rectified spirit ℥j; digest, and filter.

VINUM SUDORIFICUM. As Vin. Sarsap. Comp.

VINUM TABACI. E. Tobacco leaves ℥iijss, sherry wine Oij; digest for seven days, express strongly, and filter. U. S. directs ℥j of tobacco, f℥xvj of wine, which is the original form of Dr. Fowler. Dose, from ♏x to xl.

VINUM VERATRI. L. White hellebore root ℥viij, white wine (sherry) Oij; macerate for 14 days, and strain.

VINUM VERATRI OPIATUM. Mr. MOORE's substitute for *Eau Medicinale:* Wine of white hellebore ʒiij, tincture of opium ʒj.

VINUM VIPERINUM. L. 1746. Dried vipers ʒij, white wine ℔iij; macerate for 7 days.

VITRIOLUM CAMPHORATUM. PORT. PH. Nearly identical with Lapis Divinus, P.

VITRUM ANTIMONII. See Antimonii Vitrum.

ZINCI ACETAS. U. S. Acetate of lead ℔j; dissolve it in Oiij of distilled water, add ℥ix of granulated zinc, and agitate them in a stoppered bottle for 5 or 6 hours, till the liquid yields no precipitate with iodide of potassium. Filter, evaporate to 1-5th, and set aside to crystallize. If coloured, redissolve the crystals in water, and drop in a filtered solution of chloride of lime until it ceases to let fall oxide of iron; then filter, add a few drops of acetic acid, and crystallize.

ZINCI CARBONAS [IMPURA] PREPARATA. See Calamina Præparata.

ZINCI CARBONAS. To a solution of pure sulphate of zinc add a solution of carbonate of soda; wash the precipitate, and dry it.

ZINCI CHLORIDUM. P. and U. S. Dissolve ℥xx of zinc in muriatic acid q. s.; add ℥j of nitric acid, evaporate to dryness in an earthen vessel, dissolve in water, add ℥j of chalk, leave it for 24 hours in the cold, then filter, and evaporate to dryness. M. RIGHINI has proposed another method:—Dissolve separately in f℥xxiv of water, ℥iij ℈ij of pure sulphate of zinc, and ʒijss of pure crystallized chloride of barium; heat the mixed solution gently for a few minutes, filter, evaporate to f℥ij, digest with animal charcoal and a few grains of chloride of barium; filter, and concentrate by evaporation, so that, when left to itself, flaky crystals may form, which must be kept in well-stoppered bottles.

ZINCI CYANIDUM. P. *Cyanuret of Zinc.* To a solution of

pure sulphate of zinc, gradually add a solution of cyanide of potassium; collect the precipitate, and carefully wash and dry it. Dose, from a quarter of a grain.

Zinci Ferrocyanidum. To a strong solution of sulphate of zinc, add a solution of ferro-prussiate of potash, or of ferrocyanic acid; collect the precipitate, wash it, and dry it. The solutions should be hot. Dose, gr. j to iv.

Zinci Iodidum. Digest iodine with half its weight of finely-divided zinc, with a little water, and agitate frequently till the solution is colourless. Evaporate with a gentle heat. M. directs it to be prepared by sublimation, from 170 parts of iodine, and 20 of zinc. It must be kept from the air.

Zinci Lactas. Woehler. To ℔ij of sour milk add ℥j of sugar of milk in fine powder, and ℥j of clean zinc filings. Digest with a gentle heat for several days, adding more sugar of milk as it dissolves. Heat the mixture to boiling, filter whilst hot, and let it cool gradually in a close vessel. If not sufficiently pure, recrystallize it. It may also be made by decomposing lactate of lead by sulphate of zinc.

Zinci Oxydum. L. Sulphate of zinc ℔j, sesquicarbonate of ammonia ℥vjss; dissolve them separately in Oxij of water, filter, mix the solutions, wash the precipitate, and burn it for two hours in a strong fire. E. directs sulphate of zinc ℥xij, carbonate of ammonia ℨvj, water Oiv; proceed as L., squeezing the precipitate in a cloth, and drying it before burning it. D. orders it to be prepared by putting the metal in small pieces into a large crucible heated to whiteness, and placed with its mouth inclined to that of the furnace. After each piece of zinc is thrown in, the crucible is loosely covered by inverting another crucible over it. [The *hydrated* oxide is obtained by precipitating a solution of pure sulphate of zinc by solution of potash, avoiding excess.]

Zinci Sulphas. L. Dissolve ℥v of fragments of zinc in Oij of diluted sulphuric acid; filter, evaporate until a pellicle appears, and set aside to crystallize. E. directs it to be made by a similar process, or by recrystallizing the commercial sulphate. [Commercial sulphate of zinc contains sulphate of copper and iron. The former metal may be separated by boiling the solution with metallic zinc, but not the iron. The latter may be precipitated by chloride of lime.] D. as L., from 13 parts of zinc, 20 of sulphuric acid, and 120 of water. U. S. as L.

ZINCI VALERIANAS. PRINCE L. L. BONAPARTE. To valerianic acid, in a retort, add hydrated oxide of zinc to saturation, and slowly evaporate the solution; remove the pellicle as it forms on the surface, dry it, and preserve in a well-corked bottle. M. BRUN BUISSON directs ℥xxxij of valerian with ℔viij of water, and ℥iij of sulphuric acid, to be macerated for 2 days, and distilled as long as the product reddens litmus paper. The distilled water is exposed to the air for a month, after which it is put into a matrass with 225 grains of recently precipitated oxide of zinc, digested on a sand-bath for 8 or 10 hours at 176° F., agitating occasionally, filtered hot, evaporated to 3-4ths, and the remainder dried on earthen plates. M. LEFORT procures the acid by distilling 2⅔℔ of valerian root, 13$\frac{1}{7}$ ℔ of water, sulphuric acid ℥iij, bichromate of potash ℥ij, after 24 hours' maceration. Proceed as above. M. MURATORI obtains it by the mutual decomposition of sulphate of zinc and valerianate of lime. Dose, gr. ½ to 1½.

ADDITIONAL AND CORRECTED FORMULÆ.

ATROPIA. Digest 80 parts of powdered belladonna root with 60 of alcohol (sp. gr. ·830) for some days: express the tincture, and digest the root with more alcohol. Express, mix, and filter the tinctures, and add one part of slaked lime. In 24 hours filter, add sulphuric acid in slight excess, and again filter. Distil off half the spirit, add 6 parts of distilled water, draw off the rest of the spirit, and concentrate the solution to one-third. When cold, drop into a solution of carbonate of potash as long as it occasions a precipitate; collect this, press it between bibulous paper, and dry it. Dissolve it in 5 parts of alcohol, filter the solution, dilute it with 6 parts of water, evaporate the spirit, and set the solution aside that crystals may form. [A powerful poison, only employed externally.]

EXTRACTUM CUBEBÆ FLUIDUM. By evaporating, with a very gentle heat, a tincture prepared by digestion or percolation, with rectified spirit. PUCHE directs the cubebs to be treated by percolation with proof spirit, so as to obtain a liquid equal in weight with the cubebs. See Ext. Cubebæ Oleo-resinosum, Essentia Cubebæ, and Tinctura Cubebæ.

HYDRARGYRI BROMIDUM. When a solution of bromide of potassium is added to a solution of proto-nitrate of mercury, an insoluble white precipitate falls, which is a bromide or sub-bromide of mercury. Dose, one grain twice a day. By the direct action of bromine on mercury, or its peroxide, a soluble salt is obtained, the dose of which is from 1-16th to 1-4th of a grain.

INFUSUM ANTHEMIDIS ET AURANTII. Dr. PERCIVAL. Chamomile flowers ℥j, dried orange-peel ℥ss, cold water ℔iij. Macerate for 24 hours.

INFUSUM CARNIS BUBULÆ. *Beef Tea.* Having given Dr. SEYMOUR's formula for this preparation (see Jusculum cum Carne bovis) we add that of Professor LIEBIG. Let ℔j of beef, free from fat, be minced very small, as for sausage-meat; mix it with an equal weight of cold water, and heat it slowly to boiling; let it boil for a minute or two, and strain it through a cloth. It may be coloured with roasted onion or burnt sugar, and salted to the taste.

INFUSUM SARZÆ ACIDUM. Dr. HANCOCK. Sarsaparilla 3x, boiling water Oj, muriatic acid ♏xxx to xl. Infuse in a glass vessel for some hours, and strain. Dr. H. says the efficacy of the infusion is greatly increased by the acid.

PILULÆ ACIDI CARBONICI. Mr. MORSON. Mix ʒss of bicarbonate of soda, and gr. xxv of tartaric acid, coarsely powdered, with the smallest possible quantity of syrup and mucilage to form a mass. Divide into 12 pills.

PILULÆ RHEI ET ZINGIBERIS. Rhubarb ʒijss, ginger ʒjss, thin syrup q. s. In 5-grain pills.

SOLUTIO FERRI BROMIDI. This solution (referred to p. 52) is described under Ferri Bromidum. It must be kept on excess of iron until filtered for use.

SOLUTIO POTASSÆ CHLORATIS. To the formula, p. 318, add—This name is also given to the following solution of chlorine. CHARING CROSS H. Chlorate of potash ʒss, hydrochloric acid f℥ss, distilled water f℥iv. Dose, ♏xx in f℥j of water.

SYRUPUS RUBI FRUTICOSI. Mr. SALTER recommends the following as a cheap and pleasant colouring syrup:—Squeeze ripe blackberries in a flannel bag, and to the pressed fruit add cold water equal in measure to the juice obtained, and press again; mix the liquors, add to every pint ℔jss of sugar, and boil for a minute or two. [We have seen syrup of blackberries which retained its agreeable colour and flavour more than twelve months; but it was made from the undiluted juice, with about twice its weight of sugar.]

UNGUENTUM FERRI OXYDI NIGRI. BREFELD. Beef suet ℥xvj, lard ℥xvj, black oxide of iron ℥ij; heat them together in an iron vessel, constantly stirring them with an iron rod till the mixture becomes black; let the sediment subside, pour off the liquid ointment, and add to it Venice turpentine ℥ij, oil of bergamot ʒj, bole (rubbed with a little olive oil) ℥j; mix thoroughly. (A modification of WAHLER's *Ointment for Chilblains.*)

PREPARATIONS AND COMPOUNDS EMPLOYED AS COUNTER-POISONS.

ANTIDOTE FOR PRUSSIC ACID. Messrs. SMITH, Edinburgh. Prepare persulphate of iron (see Ferrugo, and Ferri Persulphas) from 4 parts of crystallized sulphate of iron; dissolve the dry salt, with 3 parts of cryst. sulphate, in 32 parts of water. Dissolve separately, in the same quantity of water, 5 parts of pure subcarbonate of potash. Label the alkaline solution No. 1, and the iron solution No. 2. 35 ♏ of each are sufficient to decompose 100 ♏ of the London acid; but it is safer to give it in excess. f ʒij of No. 1 should be given in a little water, and the same of No. 2 immediately after. These solutions should be kept in readiness, as a short delay renders them unavailing. As a more ready mode of preparing the antidote, Messrs. Smith recommend the following. Dissolve 10 grains of sulphate of iron in f ℥j of water, and add f ʒj of tincture of muriate (sesquichloride) of iron. In another vial dissolve ℈j of subcarbonate of potash with an ounce or two of water. Give the latter as quickly as possible, followed immediately by the former.

MAGNESIA as an *Antidote* to White Arsenic (Arsenious Acid). The necessity of using magnesia, which has not been over-calcined, has been stated before. (See Magnesia, page 202.) But it may be well to give more particular directions for preparing it. M. BUSSY directs an earthen crucible to be half filled with carbonate of magnesia, and heated till the bottom becomes obscurely red. The magnesia is to be constantly stirred as long as there is an evident escape of gas and vapour. When this ceases, a small quantity is diffused in water, and muriatic acid added. If there is only a trifling disengagement of gas, the operation may be considered as finished. It may also be made in the moist way. Dissolve sulphate of magnesia in 25 times its weight of water. Dissolve also caustic potash (potassæ hydras), equal to half the weight of the salt, in 20 times its weight of water. Mix the solutions, collect the precipitate on a linen cloth, wash it, and press it strongly; or, if wanted for immediate use, the washing may be dispensed with. Either kind should be given diffused in water, half or three-quarters of an ounce to a pint. [This antidote has been regarded as preferable to the hydrated oxide of iron (see Ferrugo); but the recent investigations of M. Personne seem to show that the arsenite of iron is less soluble in the secretions of the stomach than arsenite of magnesia. In either case vomiting should be promoted. This form of magnesia is also one of the best antidotes in poisoning by *acids*.]

Antidotes to Metallic Poisons. The salts of mercury, copper, and lead, are decomposed by the hydrated protosulphuret and persulphuret of iron (see Ferri Protosulphuretum, and Ferri Persulphuretum Hydratum, page 135), and the compounds produced are comparatively inert. Duflos proposes the following mixture as an antidote to the metallic poisons, including white arsenic. Saturate 32 ounces of water of ammonia (·970) with sulphuretted hydrogen gas; mix the liquor with 48 ounces of distilled water, and add a solution of 2 and a half ounces of protosulphate of iron, in 16 ounces of water. Close the bottle with bladder, and allow the precipitate to subside; pour off the liquid, and wash the precipitate. Lastly, 2 and a half ounces of protosulphate of iron dissolved in 16 ounces of water, and 1 ounce of calcined magnesia (as above), diffused in a little water, are added to the former precipitate.

Antidotes to Vegetable Alkaloids, and substances containing them. M. Bouchardat has much confidence in the following solution in poisoning by opium, salts of morphia, hemlock, aconite, belladonna, strychnine, colchicum, &c. In the case of digitalis, he regards it as useless. Iodine gr. iij, iodide of potassium gr. vj, water 16 ounces. The stomach having been emptied, the mixture is to be given by glassfuls, still encouraging the vomiting; and to be followed (in the case of narcotics) by strong infusion of coffee. Dr. Garrod states that *purified animal charcoal* (see Carbo Animalis Purificatus) absorbs and renders inert the active principles of many vegetable poisons. He prescribes it in doses of an ounce or more diffused in warm water, in poisoning by opium or morphia, nux-vomica or strychnia, belladonna, &c.

APPENDIX.

I.

WEIGHTS AND MEASURES.

THE weights and measures now employed in compounding medicines in Great Britain are derived from the *Troy Pound* and the *Imperial Gallon*, and are thus divided:—

APOTHECARIES' WEIGHT.

℔ Pound.		℥ Ounces.		ʒ Drachms.		℈ Scruples.		Gr. Grains.		Minims of water.
1	=	12	=	96	=	288	=	5760	=	6319·54
		1	=	8	=	24	=	480	=	526·62
				1	=	3	=	60	=	65·82
						1	=	20	=	21·94
								1	=	1·09

The Troy Pennyweight, 24 grains, is not used in compounding medicines.

APOTHECARIES' MEASURE.

C. Congius. Gallon.		O. Octarii. Pints.		f℥ Fluid Ounces.		fʒ Fluid Drachms.		♏. Minims.		Grains of water.
1	=	8	=	160	=	1280	=	76800	=	70000
		1	=	20	=	160	=	9600	=	8750
				1	=	8	=	480	=	437·5
						1	=	60	=	54·7
								1	=	0·9

The above weights and measures are those exclusively intended in this Work, except where otherwise stated.

AVOIRDUPOIS WEIGHT.

℔ Pound.		oz. Ounces.		dr. Drachms.		gr. Grains.		French Grammes.
1	=	16	=	256	=	7000	=	453·544
		1	=	16	=	437·50	=	28·346
				1	=	27·34	=	1·771

Avoirdupois weight is used in the sale of drugs, but its use in compounding medicines is not sanctioned by any Pharmacopœia. But as it is not usual to keep Troy weights of any large size, their place is supplied by their equivalent Avoirdupois weights, in compounding officinal preparations. The following table, from Dr. Duncan's Edinburgh Dispensatory, will facilitate the required computation.

TABLE FOR CONVERTING TROY INTO AVOIRDUPOIS WEIGHTS.

Troy ounces.		Avoirdupois ounces.	Avoirdupois grains.	Troy ounces.		Avoirdupois ounces.	Avoirdupois grains.
1	=	1	42½	7	=	7	297½
2	=	2	85	8	=	8	340
3	=	3	127½	9	=	9	382½
4	=	4	170	10	=	10	425
5	=	5	212½	11	=	11	30
6	=	6	255	12	=	12	72½

175 Troy ounces are equal to 192 Avoirdupois.

Troy ℔.		Avoirdupois. ℔.	oz.	gr.	Troy ℔		Avoirdupois. ℔.	oz.	gr.
1	=	0	13	72½	18	=	14	12	430
2	=	1	10	145	19	=	15	10	65
3	=	2	7	217½	20	=	16	7	137½
4	=	3	4	290	30	=	24	10	425
5	=	4	1	362½	40	=	32	14	275
6	=	4	14	435	50	=	41	2	125
7	=	5	12	70	60	=	49	5	412½
8	=	6	9	142½	70	=	57	9	262½
9	=	7	6	215	80	=	65	13	112½
10	=	8	3	287½	90	=	74	0	400
11	=	8	0	360	100	=	82	4	250
12	=	9	13	432½	175	=	144	0	0
13	=	10	11	67½	200	=	164	9	62½
14	=	11	8	140	300	=	246	13	312½
15	=	12	5	212½	400	=	293	2	125
16	=	13	2	285	500	=	411	6	375
17	=	13	15	359½	1000	=	822	13	312½

A more copious table will be found in Professor Redwood's improved edition of Gray's Supplement.

The following are the divisions of the *old wine gallon*, adopted in the editions of the London Pharmacopœia previous to 1836; and in the last edition of the Dublin, and United States Pharmacopœias. Its use is no longer legal.

C.		O.		f℥.		fʒ.		f℈		Minims.
1	=	8	=	128	=	1024	=	3072	=	61440
		1	=	16	=	128	=	384	=	7680
				1	=	8	=	24	=	480
						1	=	3	=	60
								1	=	20

COMPARISON BETWEEN THE OLD AND NEW MEASURES.

	Grains of distilled Water.		Cubic Inches.	
	OLD.	NEW.	OLD.	NEW.
Gallon - -	58317·8	70000	231	277·274
Pint - -	7289·7	8750	28·875	34·659
f℥j - - -	455·6	437·5	1·804	1·733
fʒj - - -	56·9	54·7	·225	·216

[In the Dublin Ph., 1807, the weight of a gallon (old measure) of water is stated to be 58443 grains; in that of 1826, 58327·5 grains. U. S. estimates it at 58328·8 grains.]

The old gallon is very nearly $\frac{5}{6}$ths of the new; the new $\frac{6}{5}$ths of the old. 115500 imperial gallons are exactly equal to 138637 old. The exact factor for converting the old measure into new is ·83311; and for converting new into old 1·20032.

RELATIVE VALUE OF [THE FORMER] APOTHECARIES' MEASURE, AND THE PRESENT IMPERIAL MEASURE, FROM THE AMERICAN DISPENSATORY.

OLD.		NEW.				NEW.		OLD.				
		O.	f℥	fʒ	♏			C.	O.	f℥	fʒ	♏
Cong.	=	6	13	2	23	Cong.	=	1	1	9	5	8
O.	=		16	5	18	O.	=		1	3	1	38
f℥	=		1	0	20	f℥j	=				7	41
fʒ	=			1	2½	fʒj	=					58

To find the weight of any given measure of a liquid, multiply the weight of water it will contain by the specific gravity, water being 1·000. The weight of a gallon of any liquid, in avoird. ℔s and decimal parts, is at once seen from its density, merely removing the decimal point one place to the right. Thus a gallon of æther at ·750 weighs 7·50 (7½) lbs.

The medical weights of France were formerly the *grain*, the *scrupule* of 24 *grains*, the *gros* of 3 *scrupule*, the *once* of 8 *gros*, the *livre* of 16 *onces*. After the introduction of the decimal or metrical system, the value of these weights was modified. The *livre*, formerly equal to 489·5 grammes, was made to correspond with 500 grammes. In 1840 the old weights altogether ceased to be legal. The present weights of France, and their equivalents in English grains, are :—

		Troy Grains.			Troy Grains.
Milligramme	=	·0154	Décagramme	=	154·34
Centigramme	=	·1543	Hectogramme	=	1543·40
Décigramme	=	1·5435	Kilogramme	=	15434·00
Gramme	=	15·4340	Myriagramme	=	154340·00

The measures of capacity in France are multiples and divisions of the LITRE, which is the measure occupied by a kilogramme (15434 Troy grains) of distilled water at its greatest density. It is equal to rather more than 35 fluid ounces, or 1·7608 imperial pints. 4½ litres make an imperial gallon, within f ℥x.

The unit of the British India ponderary system is the tola, equal to 180 Troy grains. 32 tolas are equal to ℔j Troy. The maund is equal to 100 Troy ounces.

In the United States of America, the old wine gallon and its divisions are adopted by the Pharmacopœia. The apothecaries' weights are the same as in this country.

COMPARISON OF THERMOMETRIC SCALES.

To convert the degrees of Centigrade into those of Fahrenheit, multiply by 9, divide by 5, and add 32.

To convert degrees of Centigrade into those of Reaumur, multiply by 4 and divide by 5.

To convert degrees of Fahrenheit into those of Centigrade, deduct 32, multiply by 5, and divide by 9.

To convert degrees of Fahrenheit into those of Reaumur, deduct 32, divide by 9, and multiply by 4.

To convert degrees of Reaumur into those of Centigrade, multiply by 5 and divide by 4.

To convert degrees of Reaumur into those of Fahrenheit, multiply by 9, divide by 4, and add 32.

TABLE SHOWING THE RELATIONS OF THE WEIGHTS AND MEASURES OF VARIOUS LIQUIDS.

	Specific Gravity.	A Fluid ounce weighs	Imperial Pint weighs	Troy ounce measures		Avoirdupois ounce measures		A Gallon weighs in Avoirdupois	
		Grains.	Grains.	f℥	♏	f℥	♏	℔s	oz
Water (distilled)	1·000	437½	8750	8	46	8	0	10	0
Alcohol. L.	·815	356½	7131	10	46	9	49	8	2½
Alcohol. E.	·796	348	6964	11	2	10	3	7	15⅜
Rectified Spirit	·838	366½	7332½	10	28	9	33	8	6
Proof Spirit. L.	·920	402½	8050	9	31	8	42	9	3 3/16
Proof Spirit. E. 1841. . .	·912	399	7980	9	37	8	46	9	1⅞
Æther	·750	328⅛	6562½	11	42	10	40	7	8
Spirit of Nitric Æther. L. .	·834	365	7297½	10	31	9	35	8	5 7/16
Olive Oil	·9153	400½	8009	9	35	8	44	9	2 7/16
Syrup. (*Normal.* GUIBOURT.)	1·320	577½	11550	6	39	6	4	13	3¼
Syrup. BRANDE (*thick.*) . .	1·450	634½	12687½	6	4	5	30	14	8
Sulphuric Acid. L.	1·845	807	16144	4	45	4	20	18	7 3/16
Nitric Acid	1·500	656¼	13125	5	51	5	20	15	0
Muriatic Acid	1·160	507½	10150	7	35	6	54	11	9 9/16

II.

TABLE OF PROPORTIONATE DOSES FOR DIFFERENT AGES, FROM GAUBIUS, ETC.

				EXAMPLES.		
Under ½	year	1-15th of a full dose.	Gr.	¾	1¼	2
" 1	"	1-12th "	"	1	1¾	2½
" 2	"	1-8th "	"	1½	2½	4
" 3	"	1-6th "	"	2	3½	5
" 4	"	1-5th "	"	2½	4	6
" 7	"	1-3d "	"	4	7	10
" 14	"	1-half "	"	6	10	15
" 20	"	2-3ds "	"	8	13	20
Above 21	"	the full dose	"	12	20	30
At 63	"	11-12ths "	"	11	18	27
" 77	"	5-6ths "	"	10	16	25
" 100	"	2-3ds "	"	8	13	20

Dr. Pereira quotes from Hufeland a table of doses differing from the above, of which the following is an abridgment:—

Years,	25	20	15	12	10	8	6	4	3	2	1
Doses,	40	35	30	27	25	23	21	18	16	13	10

Months,	11	9	7	5	3	2	1	½
Doses,	9	8	7	6	5	4	2	1

The dose being 40 grains for an adult, the doses for the different ages will be the number of grains placed under the years and months; and in the same proportion for other doses.

Dr. Young gives the following simple formula:—

For children under 12 years the doses of most medicines must be diminished in the proportion of the age to the age increased by 12. Thus, at 2 years, the dose will be 1-7th of that for an adult, viz.:—

$$\frac{2}{2 + 12} = \text{1-7th.}$$

Sex, temperament, constitutional strength, and the habits and idiosyncrasies of individuals must be taken into account. Nor does the same rule apply to all medicines. *Calomel*, for instance, is generally borne better by children than by adults; while *Opium* affects them more powerfully, and requires the dose to be diminished considerably below that indicated in the Table.

III.

TABLE SHOWING THE PROPORTION OF ACTIVE INGREDIENTS IN CERTAIN COMPOUND MEDICINES.

POTASSIO-TARTRATE OF ANTIMONY.

One grain in f ʒiv of the *Wine:* and in gr. v of the *Ointment.*

ARSENIOUS ACID.

One grain of arsenious acid is contained in f ʒij (110 grains) of *Solution of Arsenite of Potash;* in f ℥ss of DE VALLENGER'S Mineral Solution; in 100 grains *Liqueur Arsenicale,* P.; in 5000 grains of DEVERGIE'S Solution; in 15 *Asiatic Pills;* in gr. xxv of the *Cerate* (U. S.); in gr. xiij of the ointment (GUY'S H.); and in gr. x of Sir A. COOPER'S [or gr. xiv of GUY'S H.] *Ointment of Arsenic with Sulphur.*

IODIDE OF ARSENIC.

One grain is contained in 96 grains or 105 ♏ of DONOVAN'S Solution (*Liq. Hydriodatis Arsenici et Hydrargyri*); in 100 grains of SOUBEIRAN'S; in ℥j of WACKENRODER'S (*Liq. Arsenici Periodidi*); and in 192 grains of BIETT'S *Ointment.*

ARSENIATES.

One grain of Arseniate of Ammonia is contained in ℥j of BIETT'S *Solution;* and one of Arseniate of Soda in f ℥j of PEARSON'S.

CHLORIDE OF BARIUM, OR MURIATE OF BARYTES.

One grain is contained in ♏ viij of the L. & E. *Solution,* and in ♏ iv of D.

CANTHARIDES.

One grain makes f ℈iv of the L., f ʒij of the E., and gr. viij of the P. *Tincture.* One grain in ♏ x of *Acetum Cantharidis,* in gr. vj of the *Cerate* (E.), and gr. iij of the *Plaster.*

COLCHICUM.

One grain of the *seed* makes ♏ viij of the simple *Tincture* (L. E. & D.); ♏ viij of the *Compound Tincture;* ♏ viij of the *Wine.* (U. S.)

One grain of the dried cormus makes ♏ v of the *Wine* (L. & E.); one grain of fresh cormus, ♏ xvj of *Vinegar of Colchicum.*

CONIUM.

One grain of dried hemlock makes ♏ viij of the *L. Tincture;* one grain of *fresh* ♏ iijss of the *E. Tincture.*

DIGITALIS.

One grain of the dried leaves makes f ℈viij of the *Infusion,* L. 1836, but only f ʒj of that of L. 1824; f ʒj of the D. *Infusion;* and ℈iv of the E. Also ♏ x of the *Tincture.*

IODINE.

One grain of iodine is contained in ♏ xvj of the E. *Tincture;* in gr. xiij (about ♏ xvj) of that of D. M., &c.

One grain, with 2 of iodide of potassium, in ♏ xl of the *Compound Tincture;* in f ℥iv *Liq. Iodidi Potassii Comp.;* and (with gr. iv of the iodide) in f ʒj of *Liq. Iodinei Comp.* E.

MERCURY AND ITS SALTS.

One grain of quicksilver is contained in gr. iij of the *Mercurial Pill;* in gr. ij and 2-3ds of *Quicksilver with Chalk,* L.; and in gr. jss of *Quicksilver with Chalk* and Q. with *Magnesia,* D.

One grain is also contained in gr. ij of the *stronger,* and gr. vj of the *weaker, Ointment;* in gr. vj of *Mercurial Liniment,* and gr. v. of *Mercurial Plaster.*

One grain of Calomel is contained in gr. v. of *Comp. Calomel Pills;* the *Pills of Calomel and Opium,* E., contain gr. ij of Calomel, and 2-3ds of a grain of Opium in each pill.

One grain of Bichloride of Mercury is contained in f ℥ij (or 876 grains) of the Solution (*Liq. Hydr. Bichloridi*), L.; and in 1000 grains of that of P.

One grain of Nitric Oxide of Mercury is contained in gr. ix of the L. & E. Ointment.

One grain of Ammonio-chloride of Mercury is contained in gr. iij of the *Ointment.*

One grain of Iodide of Mercury is contained in gr. v of the *Pills* (L.); and in 8 pills of Magendie's Form.

One grain of the Iodide and Biniodide of Mercury is contained in gr. ix of their Ointments. (L.)

MORPHIA.

One grain of Muriate of Morphia is contained in 106 ♏ or 94 grains of the E. *Solution;* in 100 grains of Dr. Christison's. A solution, containing gr. j in ℥ss, is used at Apoth. Hall, &c. But the solutions of Morphia used in different establishments vary considerably in strength. See Liquor Morphiæ, &c.

OPIUM (CRUDE).

One grain of opium is used in making ♏ iv of the E. & D., and ♏ vjss of the U. S. *Vinegar of Opium;* ♏ x of the U. S. and gr. x of P. *Acetated Tincture of Opium;* ♏ xiv of the *Tincture* (L. & E.); ♏ 240 (450 drops, CHRISTISON) of the *Camphorated Tincture of Opium,* E.; ♏ 267 (500 drops, CHRISTISON) of the D., and the same of the *Compound Tincture of Camphor,* L.; ♏ 80 [equal to 150 drops, CHRISTISON] of the *Ammoniated Tincture of Opium,* E.; ♏ 13½ of *Wine of Opium,* E.; and ♏ 16 of D. [It is probable that the whole of the active principles of the Opium are not taken up in either the Tincture, Wine, or Vinegar of Opium; and that, consequently, the above quantities do not exactly represent one grain of Crude Opium. Dr. CHRISTISON says, that f ℥j of good Tincture of Opium should leave, on evaporation, from 17 to 22 grains of extract.]

One grain of Opium is contained in 36 grains of the L. *Confection,* in 43 of the E. and 25 of the D. *Electuary* of Opium; in 5 grains of *Storax Pill,* L. & D.; in 2 *Pills* of *Lead of Opium,* E.; in 5 grains of the new or 10 grains of the old *Thebaic Pills,* E.; and in from 6 to 8 Opium Lozenges. Each Pill of Calomel and Opium, E., contains 2-3ds of a grain of Opium. One grain is contained in ℈ij of the L., and 37 grains of the E. *Powder of Chalk with Opium;* in ℈ss of *Compound Powder of Ipecacuanha;* in ℈j of *Compound Powder of Kino;* and in ℈ss of Powder of Hartshorn Opium, L., 1824, and Pulvis Opiatus, E., 1813.

PURIFIED EXTRACT OF OPIUM.

One grain of Purified Extract of Opium is contained in ♏ xvj of *Wine of Opium,* L.; in f ℥j of *Syrup of Opium* [D. 1807]; and in gr. xiij of the P. *Tincture.*

PRUSSIC ACID (HYDROCYANIC ACID).

One grain of (anhydrous) Prussic Acid is contained in 50 grains (about 55 ♏) of *Hydrocyanic Acid*, L.; in about 30 grains of *Hydrocyanic Acid*, E.; and in about 63 grains of *Prussic Acid*, D. [Dr. BARKER states that the Dublin contains 1·5 or 1·6 per cent. of real acid; and Dr. KANE says it is prepared of this strength at the Apothecaries' Hall of Ireland. Dr. CHRISTISON, however, asserts that it contains 3·3 per cent. of acid. Mr. DONOVAN says, 2·5 or 2·8 per cent.; Mr. LAMING, 1·75 to 1·25 per cent. In the Annals of Pharmacy it is said to contain 2 per cent.; and the Editor of the "Pharmaceutical Journal" has shown that the ingredients are capable of yielding an acid of 2·66 per cent.] SCHEELE'S process yields an acid of variable strength, and there is no fixed standard to which it should be adjusted; as sent out by different makers it contains from 3 to 6 per cent. of real acid, or from 1 grain in 33 to 1 in 17. The acid of the UNITED STATES, AUSTRIAN, BADEN, HAMBURGH (?), and PRUSSIAN Pharmacopœias is of the same strength as the London. The Medicinal Prussic Acid of MAGENDIE and the PARIS CODEX contains 1 grain of acid in 9½ grains, or 10½ per cent. Mr. LAMING'S Acid contains 1 grain in f ʒj.

Bitter Almond Water is made of various strengths, there being no standard formula in this country. In Germany, where it is prescribed medicinally, the avarage, in 18 examples, was about 4-5ths of a grain of Prussic acid in an ounce, equivalent to ♏ 44 of the Acidum Hydrocyanicum dilutum, L.

IV.

TABLE OF CERTAIN ENGLISH AND FRENCH SYNONYMES, SHOWING UNDER WHAT LATIN NAMES THEY ARE PLACED IN THIS WORK.

The alphabetical arrangement of the Pocket Formulary renders a general Index unnecessary. The following list is chiefly intended to facilitate reference in a few instances in which the Latin names attached to the compounds in the body of the work do not exactly represent the English or French names by which they are generally known. The French names are printed in *Italics*. This table also includes an Index to the additional formulæ, and to others not placed in their proper alphabetical order.

Alcool Sulphurique. Acidum Sulphuricum Alcoholisatum.
Alcoolats. Distilled Spirits. Spiritus.
Alcoolatures. See Succi Alcoholati.
Antidotes, preparations of. See pages 424 and 425.
Arquebusade. Spiritus Vulnerarius.
Atropia. Atropine. See page 422.
Battley's Sedative Solution. See Liquor Opii.
Beef Tea. See Infusum Carnis, page 423.
Black Drops. See Guttæ Nigræ; and Vinum Opii fermentatione paratum.
Blistering Tissue. See Sparadrap. Vesicans; and Tela Vesicatoria.
Bromide and Perbromide of Mercury. See page 422.
Canquoin's Caustic. Causticum Zinci.
Cachou Aromatique. See Trochisci Catechu.
Capillaire. Syrupus Adianthi.
Caustiques de Filhos. See Pasta Viennensis.
Cephalic Snuff. Pulvis Asari Compositus; and Pulvis Sternutatorius.
Cold Cream. Ceratum Galeni.
Corn Plaster. Emplastrum Æruginis.
Court Plaster. Emplastrum Icthyocollæ.
Cream of Taraxacum. See Succus Taraxaci.
Crême de Tronchin. Linctus Cacao.
Dalby's Carminative. Mistura Carminativa Infantilis.
Dupuytren's Pommade. Unguentum Tincturæ Cantharidis.
Eau d'Arquebusade. Spiritus Vulnerarius.
Eau de Carmes. Spiritus Melissæ Compositus.
Eau de Cologne. Aqua Coloniensis.
Eau de Javelle. Liquor Potassæ Chlorinatæ.
Eau de Luce. Tinctura Ammoniæ Composita.
Eau Magnesienne. See Liquor Magnesia Carbonatis.
Eau Phagedenique. Lotio Hydrargyri Flava.
Eau de Rabel. Acidum Sulphuricum Alcoholicum.
Eau de Travez. Apozema Emeto-catharticum.
Eau de Vichy. Aqua Vicensis.
Electuary of Clinkers. See Electuarium Anticachecticum.
Elixir of Vitriol. Acidum Sulphuricum Aromaticum.
Elixir, Haller's Acid. Acidum Sulphuricum Alcoholisatum.
Essential Salt of Bark. Extractum Cinchonæ Siccum.
Essence of Mustard. Linimentum Sinapis.
Farines Emollientes. See Species Emollientes.
Farines Résolutives. See Species Resolventes.
Fluid Magnesia. Liquor Magnesia Carbonatis.
Fluid Extract of Cubebs. See page 422.
Gall, Inspissated. Extractum Fellis.
Gelée pour le Goître. Linimentum Gelatinosum Ioduretum.
Granville's (Dr.) Counter Irritants. Linimentum Ammoniæ Compositum.
Grains de Cachou. See Trochisci Catechu.
Grains de Santé. Pilulæ Aloës Rosatæ.
Grains de Vie. Pilulæ Aloës cum Mastiche.
Granules de Digitaline. See Pilulæ Digitalinæ.
Goat's Milk, Artificial. Decoctum Sevi.
Gout Cordial. Tinctura Rhei et Sennæ.

Gowland's Lotion. Lotio Hydrargyri Amygdalina.
Gregory's Powder. Pulvis Rhei Compositus, E.
Gregory's Mixture. Mistura Rhei Composita.
Haller's Acid Elixir. Acidum Sulphuricum Alcoholisatum.
Hahnemann's Soluble Mercury. Hydrargyri Precipitatum Nigrum.
Hahnemann's Prophylactic Solution. Solutio Belladonnæ.
Heberden's Ink. Mistura Ferri Aromatica.
Hive Syrup. Syrupus Scillæ Compositus.
Huile de Morue. Oleum Morrhuæ.
Infusion of Sarsaparilla (Dr. Hancock's Acid). See page 423.
Ioduretted Dog's-grass. Mistura Iodinii cum Dec. Graminis.
Ioduretted Sarsaparilla. Mistura Iodinii cum Sarzâ.
Jesuit's Drops. See Elixir Antivenereum.
Juices (preserved). See Succi Alcoholati.
Jujubes. See Pasta Jujubæ.
Justamond's Caustic. Arsenicum Antimoniatum.
Kentish's Liniment. Linimentum Terebinthinatum.
Kimbel's Anticroupal Mixture. Mistura Scillæ et Valerianæ.
Kirkland's Cerate. Ceratum Neutrale.
Kitchener's Peristaltic Persuaders. Pil Rhei et Carui.
Labarraque's Solution. Liquor Sodæ Chlorinatæ.
Lady Hesketh's, or Lady Webster's Pills. See Pilulæ Alöes et Masticbes.
Lausanne Compound. See Pulvis Sulphuris Compositum.
Lip Salve. Ceratum Rosatum, P.
Liqueur Depurative. Tinct. Sarzæ Composita.
Liquid Blister. Acetum Cantharidis.
Liston's Plaster. See Emplastrum Icthyocollæ.
Marmalade dè Zanetti. Lohoc Expectorans.
Oil of Flints. Liquor Potassæ Silicatis.
Paraguay-Roux. See Tinct. Pyrethri Comp.
Pilules Gaziferes. See Pil. Acidi Carbonici, page 423.
Plummer's Pills. Pil. Hydrargyri Chloridi Compositæ.
Pommades. See Unguenta.
Pommade de Dupuytren. Ung. Tincturæ Cantharidis.
Pommade de Gondret. Unguentum Ammoniacale.
Pommade de Jadelot. See Linimentum Sulphuro-Saponaceum.
Pommade d'Autenrieth. Unguentum Antimonii.
Poudre de Gutette. See Pulvis Antiepilepticus.
Poudre de Pihorel. Pulvis Antipsoricus.
Purple of Cassius. Aurum Stanno Paratum.
Pyro-acetic Spirit. See Naphtha.
Roche's Embrocation. Linimentum Succini.
Rousseau's Drops. Vinum Opii ferment. paratum.
Saccharures and Saccharoles. See Sacchara.
Sachets. Sacculi.
Scott's Pills. Pilulæ Andersonis.
Sel de Guindre. Pulvis Sodæ Sulphatis Compositus.
Sirop d'Orgeat. Syrupus Amygdalæ.
Sirop de Cuisinier. Syrupus Sarsaparillæ Compositus.
Solutions. See Liquor and Solutio.
Solution of Bromide of Iron (Mohr.) See page 423.

Solution of Chlorate of Potash. See page 423.
Soluble Cream of Tartar. Potassæ Boro-tartras.
Sucre Ferrugineux. Ferri Carbonis Saccharatum.
Syrup of Blackberries. Syrupus Rubi Fruticosi. See page 423.
Tablettes. Trochisci.
Taffetas Vesicant. Sparadrapum Vesicans; and Tela Vesicatoria.
Tanjore, or Asiatic Pills. Pilulæ Arsenici.
Tisanes. See Ptisanæ.
Tisane de Feltz. Decoctum Sarzæ cum Icthyocollâ.
Tisane de Vinache. Decoctum Sarzæ cum Sennâ.
Traitement Arabique. See Electuarium Arabicum.
Trousseau's Tonic. Electuarium Nigrum.
Vallet's Pills. Pilulæ Ferri Carbonatis.
Vesicatoire Volant. Sparadrapum Vesicans.
Wahler's Chilblain Ointment. See Ung. Ferri Oxydi Nigri, page 424.
Ward's White Drops. Liquor Hydrargyri et Ammoniæ Nitratis.
Ward's Paste. Confectio Piperis Nigri.
Whitlaw's Tincture. See Tinctura Lobeliæ Ætherea.
Young's Purging Mixture. Liquor Sodæ Tartarizatæ effervescens.

V.

:ONS AND CONTRACTIONS MORE OR LESS FREQUENTLY MET WITH IN PRESCRIPTIONS.

(Copied by permission, with slight abridgment, from the last edition of "Selecta e Præscriptis.")

A., *aa.*, *ana*, of each ingredient. In the Pharmacopœia the term *singulorum* is employed instead of ana.
Abdom., *Abdomen*, the belly; *abdominis*, of the belly; *abdomini*, to the belly.
Abs. febr., *Absente febre*, in the absence of the fever.
Ad 2 vic., *Ad duas vices*, at twice taking.
Ad 3tiam vicem, *Ad tertiam vicem*, for three times.
Ad gr. acid, *Ad gratam aciditatem*, to an agreeable sourness.
Ad def. animi, *Ad defectionem animi*, to fainting.
Ad libit., *Ad libitum*, at pleasure.
Add., *Adde* or *addantur*, add, or let be added.
Adjac., *Adjacens*, adjacent.
Admov., *Admove*, or *admoveatur*, or *admoveantur*, apply, or let be applied.
Ads. febre, *Adstante febre*, when the fever is on.
Adv., *Adversum*, against.
Aggred. febre, *Aggrediente febre*, while the fever is coming on.
Altern. horis, *Alternis horis*, every other hour.
Alvo adst., *Alvo adstricta*, when the belly is bound.
Aq. astr., *Aqua astricta*, frozen water. *Aq. bull.*, *Aqua bulliens*, boiling water. *Aq. com.*, *Aqua communis*, common water. *Aq. fluv.*, *Aqua*

fluviatalis, river water. *Aq. mar.*, *Aqua marina*, sea water. *Aq. niv.*, *Aqua nivalis*, snow water. *Aq. pluv.*, *Aqua pluviatilis*, or *Aqua pluvialis*, rain water. *Aq. ferv.*, *Aqua fervens*, hot water. *Aq. font.*, *Aqua fontana*, or *Aqua fontis*, or *Aqua fontalis*, spring water.

Bis ind., *Bis indies*, twice a day.
Bib., *Bibe*, drink (thou).
BB., *Bbds.*, *Barbadensis*, Barbadoes; as *Aloe Barbadensis.*
B. M., *Balneum Mariæ*, or *Balneum Maris*, a warm water bath.
Bull., *Bulliat*, or *bulliant*, let boil.
Bui., *Butyrum*, butter.
B. V., *Balneum vaporosum*, or *Balneum vaporis*, a vapour bath.
C. Cum, with.
Cærul. Cæruleus, blue.
Cap., *Capiat*, let the patient take.
Calom., *Calomelas*, calomel, or chloride of mercury.
C. C., *Cornu cervi*, hartshorn. *Cucurbitula cruenta*, a cupping glass with the scarificator.
C. C. U., *Cornu cervi ustum*, burnt hartshorn.
Coch., a spoonful, a table-spoonful. *Cochleat.*, *Cochleatim*, by spoonfuls. *Coch. ampl.*, *Cochleare amplum*, a large (or table) spoonful. *Coch. infant.*, *Cochleare infantis*, a child's spoonful. *Coch. magn.*, *Cochleare magnum*, a large spoonful. *Coch. med.*, *Cochleare medium*, *Coch. mod.*, *Cochleare modicum*, a middling spoonful; i. e. a child's or dessert spoonful; about f℥ij. *Coch. parv.*, *Cochleare parvum*, a small (or tea) spoonful; about f ʒj.
Col., *Cola*, strain. *Colatus*, strained.
Colet., *Colat.*, *Coletur*, let it be strained; *Colaturæ*, to the strained liquor.
Colent., *Colentur*, let them be strained.
Color., *Coloretur*, let it be coloured.
Comp., *Compositus*, compounded.
Con., *Concisus*, cut.
Cong., *Congius.*
Cons., *Conserva*, a conserve; also, keep thou.
Cont. rem., *Continuentur remedia*, let the remedies be continued.
Coq., *Coque*, boil; *Coquantur*, let them be boiled. *Coq. ad med. consumpt.*, *Coque ad medietatis consumptionem*, boil to the consumption of half. *Coq. in S. A.*, *Coque in sufficiente quantitate aquæ*, boil in a sufficient quantity of water.
Cort., *Cortex*, bark.
C. v., *Cras vespere*, to-morrow evening.
C. m. s., *Cras mane sumendus*, to be taken to-morrow morning.
C. n., *Cras nocte*, to-morrow night.
Crast., *Crastinus*, for to-morrow.
Cuj., *Cujus*, of which
Cujusl., *Cujuslibet*, of any.
Cyath. theæ, *Cyatho theæ*, in a cup of tea.
Cyath., *Cyathus*, *vel*, *C. vinar.*, *Cyathus vinarias*, } a wineglass: from f℥jss to f℥ij.
Deaur. pil., *Deaurentur pilulæ*, let the pill be gilt.
Deb. spiss., *Debita spissitudo*, a proper consistence.
Dec., *Decanta*, pour off.
Dec., *Decubitus*, of lying down.

De d. in d., *De die in diem*, from day to day.
Deglut., *Deglutiatur*, may be (or let be) swallowed.
Dej. alvi, *Dejectiones Alvi*, stools.
Det., *Detur*, let it be given.
Dieb. alt., *Diebus alternis*, every other day.
Dil., *Dilue.*, *dilutus*, dilute (thou), diluted.
Diluc., *Diluculo*, at break of day.
Dim., *Dimidius*, one-half.
D. in 2plo, *Detur in duplo*, let twice as much be given.
D. in p. æq., *Dividatur in partes æquales*, let it be divided into equal parts.
D. P., *Dir. prop.*, *Directione propria*, with a proper direction.
Donec alv. bis dej., *Donec alvus bis dejiciatur*, until the bowels have been twice evacuated.
Donec alv. solv. fuer., *Donec alvus soluta fuerit*, until the bowels shall be opened.
Donec dol. neph. exulav., *Donec dolor nephriticus exulaverit*, until the nephritic pain be removed.
D., *Dosis*, a dose.
Eburn., *Eburneus*, made of ivory.
Ed., *Edulcorata*, edulcorated.
Ejusd., *ejusdem*, of the same.
Elect., *Electuarium*, an electuary.
Enem., *Enema*, a clyster; *enemata*, clysters.
Exhib., *Exhibeatur*, let it be exhibited.
Ext. sup. alut. moll., *Extende super alutam mollem*, spread (thou) upon soft leather.
F., *Fac*, make; *fiat*, *fiant*, let it be made.
F. pil. xij, *Fac pilulas duodecim*, make 12 pills.
Fasc., *Fasiculus*, a bundle which can be carried under the arm.
Feb. dur., *Febre durante*, during the fever.
Fem. intern., *Femoribus internis*, to the inner part of the thighs.
F. venæs., *Fiat venæsectio*, bleed.
F. H., *Fiat haustus*, let a draught be made.
Fict., *Fictilis*, earthen.
Fil., *Filtrum*, a filter; *Filtra*, filter (thou),
Fist. arm., *Fistula aramata*, a clyster pipe and bladder fitted for use.
Fl., *Fluidus*, liquid; also, by measure.
F. L. A., *Fiat lege artis*, let it be made by the rules of art.
F. M., *Fiat mistura*, let a mixture be made.
Frust., *Frustillatim*, in little pieces.
F. S. A., *Fiat secundum artem*, let it be made according to art.
F. S. A. R., *Fiat secundum artis regulas*, let it be made according to the rules of art.
Gel quâv., *Gelatinâ quâvis*, in any kind of jelly.
G. G. G., *Gummi guttæ Gambiæ*, gamboge.
Gr., *Granum*, grain; *grana*, grains.
Gr. vj. *pond.*, *Grana sex pondere*, six grains by weight.
Gtt., *Gutta*, a drop; *guttæ*, drops.
Gutt. quibusd., *Guttis quibusdam*, with a few drops.
Guttat., *Guttatim*, by drops.
Har. pil. sum. iij., *Harum pilularum sumantur tres*, let 3 of these pills be taken.

Hb., *Herba*, a herb,
H. D., or *Hor. decub. Hora decubitûs*, at the hour of going to bed.
H. p. n., *Haustus purgans noster*, a formula of purging draught made according to a practitioner's private pharmacopœia.
H. S., or *Hor. som.*, *Hora somni*, just before going to sleep.
Hor. un. spatio, *Horæ unius spatio*, at the expiration of an hour.
Hor. interm., *Horis intermediis*, in the intermediate hours.
Hora 11*mâ. mat.*, *Horâ undecimâ matutinâ*, at the eleventh hour in the morning.
Ind., *Indies*, from day to day, or daily.
In pulm., *In pulmento*, in gruel.
Inc., *Incide*, cut (thou); *incisus*, being cut.
Inf., *Infunde*, pour in.
Jul., *Julepus*, *Julepum*, *Julapium*, a julep.
Inj. enem., *Injiciatur enema*, let a glyster be given.
Kal. ppt., *Kali præparatum* (*Potassæ carbonas*, Ph. L.), prepared kali, or carbonate or subcarbonate of potash.
Lat. dol., *Lateri dolenti*, to the side that is painful.
M., *Misce*, mix; *mensurâ*, by measure; *manipulus*, a handful; *minimum*, a minim.
Mane pr., *Mane primo*, very early in the morning.
Man., *Manipulus*, a handful.
Min., *Minimum*, a minim; *minutum*, a minute.
M. P., *Massa pilularum*, a pill mass.
M. R., *Mistura*, a mixture.
Mic. pan., *Mica panis*, crumb of bread.
Mitt., *Mitte*, send; *mittatur*, or *mittantur*, let be sent.
Mitt. sang. ad ℥xij *saltem*, *Mitte sanguinem ad uncias duas saltem*, take away blood to 12 ounces at least.
Mod. præsc., *Modo præscripto*, in the manner prescribed.
More dict., *More dicto*, in the manner directed.
Mor. sol., *More solito*, in the usual manner.
Ne tr. s. num., *Ne tradas sine nummo*, do not deliver it unless paid.
N. M., *Nux Moschata*, a nutmeg.
No., *Numero*, in number.
O., *Octarius*, a pint.
Ol. lini s. i., *Oleum lini sine igne*, cold-drawn linseed oil.
Omn. hor., *Omni horâ*, every hour. *Omn. bid.*, *Omni biduo*, every two days. *Omn. bih.*, *Omni bihorio*, every two hours.
O. M., or *Omn. man.*, *Omni mane*, every morning.
O. N., or *Omn. noct.*, *Omni nocte*, every night.
Omn. quad. hor., *Omni quadrante horæ*, every quarter of an hour.
O. O. O., *Oleum olivæ optimum*, best olive oil.
Ov., *Ovum*, an egg.
Oz., the ounce avoirdupois, or common weight.
P. e., *Part. æqual.*, *Partes æquales*, equal parts.
P. d., *Per deliquum*, by deliquescence.
Past., *Pastillus*, *Pastillum*, a little ball of paste, to take like a lozenge, &c.
P., *Pondere*, by weight.
P. C., *Pondus civilis*, civil weight (avoirdupois weight).
P. M., *Pondus medicinale*, medicinal (apothecaries') weight.
Ph. D., *Pharmacopœia Dublinensis*. *Ph. E.*, *Pharmacopœia Edinensis*.

Ph. L., *Pharmacopœia Londinensis.* *Ph. U. S.*, *Pharmacopœia of the United States.*
Part. vic., *Partitis vicibus*, in divided doses.
Per op. emet., *Peractâ operatione emetici*, when the operation of the emetic is finished.
Pocul., *Poculum*, a cup; *Pocill.*, *Pocillum*, a little cup.
Post sing. sed. liq., *Post singulas sedes liquidas*, after every loose stool.
Ppt., *Præparata*, prepared.
P. r. n., *Pro re nata*, according as circumstances arise (i. e., occasionally).
P. rat. æt., *Pro ratione ætatis*, according to the age of the patient.
Pug., *Pugillus*, a pinch; a gripe between the thumb and two first fingers.
Pulv., *Pulvis: pulverizatus*, a powder,—powdered.
Q. l., *Quantum lubet*, } as much as you please.
Q. p., *Quantum placet*, } as much as you please.
Q. s., *Quantum sufficiat*, or *Quantum satis*, as much as is sufficient.
Quor., *Quorum*, of which.
Q. v., *Quantum vis*, *Quantum volueris*, as much as you will.
℞, *Recipe*, take.
Red. in pulv., *Redactus in pulverem*, powdered.
Redig. in pulv., *Redigatur in pulverem*, let it be reduced to powder.
Reg. umb., *Regio umbilici*, the umbilical region.
Repet., *Repetatur*, *Repetantur*, let it be continued.
S. A., *Secundum artem*, according to art.
Scat., *Scatula*, a box.
S. N., *Secundum naturam*, according to nature.
Semidr., *Semidrachma*, half a drachm.
Semih., *Semihora*, half an hour.
Sesunc., *Sesuncia*, an ounce and a half.
Sesquih., *Sesquihora*, an hour and a half.
Si n. val., *Si non valeat*, if it does not answer.
Si op. sit., *Si opus sit*, if there be occasion.
Si vir. perm., *Si vires permittant*, if the strength will bear it.
Signatura, a label.
Sign. n. pr., *Signetur nomine proprio*, let it be written upon with the proper name (not the trade name).
Sing., *Singulorum*, of each.
S. S. S., *Stratum super stratum*, layer upon layer.
Ss., *semi*, a half.
St., *Stet*, let it stand; *Stent*, let them stand.
Sub. fin. coct., *Sub finem coctionis*, when the boiling is nearly finished.
Sum. tal., *Sumat talem*, let the patient take one like this.
Sum., *Summitates*, the summits, or tops.
Sum. Sume, *sumat*, *sumatur*, *sumantur*, *sumendus*, take thou, let him take, to be taken.
S. V., *Spiritus Vinosus*, ardent spirit of any strength.
S. V. R., *Spiritus Vini rectificatus*, rectified spirit of wine.
S. V. T., *Spiritus Vini tenuis*, proof spirit.
Tabel., *Tabella*, (dim. of *tabula*, a table) a lozenge.
Temp. dext., *Tempori dextro*, to the right temple.
T. O., *Tinctura Opii*, tincture of opium.

T. O. C., *Tinctura Opii camphorata*, paregoric elixir. It is now called *Tinct. camphoræ composita.*
Trit., *Tritura*, triturate.
Tra., *Tinctura*, tincture.
Troch., *Trochisci*, troches or lozenges.
Ult. præscr., *Ultimo præscriptus*, the last ordered.
V. O. S., *Vitello ovi solutus*, dissolved in the yolk of an egg.
Vom. urg., *Vomitione urgente*, the vomiting being troublesome.
V. S. B., *Venæsectio brachii*, bleeding in the arm.
Zz., *Zingiber*, ginger.

To the above comprehensive list we subjoin a few abbreviations used by Continental physicians :—

F. S. L. or *F. S. A.*, *Faites selon l'art*, made according to art.
M. S. L., *Melez selon l'art*, mix according to art.
M. D. S., *Misce, detur, signetur*, let it be mixed, delivered, labelled.
P. ég., *Parties égales*, equal parts.
Pinc., *Pincée*, a pinch.
Poig., *Poignee*, a handful.
Pr., *Prenez*, take.
Q. q., *Quantité quelconque*, any quantity.
Rec. or *Rp.*, *Recipe*, take.
T., *Transcrivez; I.*, *Instruction; S.*, *Signature;* placed before the directions for taking or using the medicine.

THE END.

ADDITIONS.

Absinthina. Dr. Luck. Treat dried wormwood with alcohol of sp. gr. ·863, until exhausted of bitterness. Having distilled the clear liquid to a syrup, transfer it to a stoppered bottle, and shake it up with ether. When the ether has separated, remove it with a syringe. Repeat this several times, and distil the mixed ethereal solutions. From the dry remainder some brown resin is to be removed by means of water rendered alkaline by ammonia. The Absinthine is left.

Acetum Digitalis. Prus. Ph. Dried foxglove ℥j, vinegar ℥viij. Macerate for 6 days, press, filter. Dose, to ♏xxx.

Acidum Aceticum Glaciale. D. Acetate of lead, dried in an oven at about 300° till it ceases to lose weight, is exposed to an atmosphere of *dry* muriatic acid gas, in a flask or retort, until the whole of the salt appears damp. A Liebig's condenser being adapted, heat is applied by means of a chloride of zinc bath, until the whole of the acetic acid has passed over. The muriatic acid gas should be slowly disengaged from the materials directed for Acidum Muriaticum, using 8 ounces of salt for every 16 ounces of dry acetate of lead; and before being conducted into the vessel containing the latter, should be made to bubble through oil of vitriol, and then passed through a long tube packed with fragments of fused chloride of calcium. The sp. gr. is 1·065.

Acidum Aceticum Forte. D. Glacial acetic acid f℥vj, distilled water f℥iv. Mix.

Acidum Aceticum e Ligno Venale. D. Acetic acid of commerce. Purified pyroligueous acid. The sp. gr. should be 1·044.

Acidum Arseniosum Purum. D. Commercial white arsenic is directed to be placed in a Florence flask, the neck of which is inserted into a larger flask, and a regulated heat applied to the former by suspending it beneath a semi-cylindrical hood of sheet iron, a few inches above a small charcoal fire, under a flue with a good draught, to protect the operator from inhaling any vapors that may escape. Dose, from $\frac{1}{16}$ of a grain to $\frac{1}{8}$.

ACIDUM ARSENIOSUM PRÆPARATUM. White arsenic levigated as Creta præparata.

ACIDUM HYDROCYANICUM SCHEELII. The original process of Scheele does not yield an acid of uniform strength, and is probably never followed. It is therefore impossible to state precisely what is intended when Scheele's acid is prescribed, or to discover the ground on which it is preferred by certain physicians to the preparation of the Pharmacopœia, which is of a known and definite strength. As prepared by different makers it has been found to contain from 3 to 5 per cent. of real acid. The following is Scheele's process: Mix ℥ij of Prussian blue with ℥vj of red precipitate of mercury, and add ℥vj of water. Boil for some minutes, constantly agitating; pour the whole on a filter, and wash the residuum on the filter with ℥ij of hot water, which is to be added to the filtered liquor. Add to this ℥jss of clean iron filings, and ʒiij of sulphuric acid, shake well, and let it settle; then pour the clear liquor into a retort, and distil a fourth part into a receiver well luted and kept cold.

ACIDUM MURIATICUM PURUM. E. Take equal weights of pure muriate of soda (see Sodæ murias purum) well dried, of pure sulphuric acid, and of water. Put the salt into a glass retort, and add the sulphuric acid, previously mixed with a third of the water, and cooled. Fit on a receiver containing the rest of the water. Distil with a gentle heat as long as any acid passes over, keeping the receiver constantly cool by cold water or snow. Density, 1·170. Dilute f℥xliv of oil of vitriol with f℥xxxij of water; and when the mixture has cooled, pour it upon ℥xlviij of dried chloride of sodium previously introduced into a gallon globular flask. A gentle heat being applied, let the gas be conducted into a bottle containing f℥xliv of distilled water, by means of a tube dipping about half an inch beneath its surface, and let the process be continued until the product measures Oiij, keeping the receiver cold. Sp. gr. 1·176.

ACIDUM NITRICUM FUMANS. PRUS. PH. Distilled from ℔iv of nitre and ℔ij of oil of vitriol.

ACIDUM SULPHURICUM. *Oil of Vitriol.* It is made on the large scale by conveying the vapors produced by the combustion of sulphur mixed with an eighth part of nitre, into leaden chambers containing a little water: or sulphur is burned alone, and the vapors from nitre and sulphuric acid also conveyed into the chamber. The weak acid thus obtained is concentrated first in leaden boilers, then in platinum or glass retorts, till its density is not less than 1·840. It is also obtained from iron pyrites. The commercial acid is liable to be contaminated with various impurities. The London College does not direct its purification, but requires its density to be 1·843, that it be free from color and smell, and give no vapors of nitrous acid when mixed with an equal measure of water. Diluted with 12 parts of water, sulphuretted hydrogen should not throw down a yellow precipitate. 100 grains require for saturation 285 grains of cr. carbonate of soda.

ÆTHER CANTHARIDALIS. ŒTTINGER. Powdered cantharides 1 part, æther 2 parts; digest for 3 days, and express.

ALCOHOL AMYLICUM. D. *Fusel Oil.* Take of the light liquid, which may be obtained at any large distillery by continuing the distillation for some time after the pure spirit has been all drawn off, q. p. Introduce it into a small still or retort, connected with a condenser, and apply heat so as to cause distillation. As soon as the oil begins to come over unmixed with water, the receiver should be changed, and the distillation being resumed and carried nearly to dryness, the desired product will be obtained. The liquid drawn over during the first part of the distillation will consist of an aqueous fluid surmounted by a stratum of fusel oil: the latter should be separated and preserved for use. [Used in preparing Valerianic Acid.]

ALOIN. Mix powdered Barbadoes aloes with clean sand, and lixiviate it with cold water in a percolator. Evaporate the solution *in vacuo* to the consistency of syrup, and set it aside for two or three days. Press the crystalline mass between folds of blotting paper, and purify by repeated crystallization from hot water. Dose, gr. i to ij.

ALUMINÆ TANNAS. An article has been sold under this name which does not appear to be a definite compound, and contains but little tannin.

AMMONIÆ BITARTRAS. To a solution of a given quantity of tartaric acid, add q. s. of ammonia or its carbonate to neutralize it; then add to it a solution of the same quantity of tartaric acid. The bitartrate precipitates.

AMMONIÆ CARBONAS PYRO-OLEOSUM. See Sal Cornu Cervi.

AMMONIÆ CITRAS. See Liquor Ammoniæ Citratis.

AMMONIÆ SESQUICARBONAS. L. Sesquicarbonate (formerly carbonate or subcarbonate) of ammonia. *Volatile Salts.* Mix ℔j of powdered sal ammoniac (ammoniæ hydrochloras) with ℔iss of prepared chalk, and sublime with a gradually increased heat. Dose, gr. v to xv.

AMMONIÆ TARTRAS. See Liquor Ammoniæ Tartratis.

AMMONIA TARTARIZATA. Saturate a solution of 150 grains of cream of tartar with 118 grains, or q. s., of sesquicarbonate of ammonia. Evaporate to dryness, with a very gentle heat. *Diuretic;* in doses of a few grains.

AMMONIÆ SUCCINAS. Mix one part of pure succinic acid with four parts of water, and add ammonia in slight excess; filter, evaporate, and crystallize. This compound is also prepared in a liquid form by saturating spirit of hartshorn with succinic acid. *Antispasmodic* and *sudorific.*

AMMONIO-CITRAS FERRI. See Ferri Ammonio-citras.

AMMONIACUM PRÆPARATUM. L. Boil lump ammoniacum in sufficient water to cover it, strain through a hair sieve, and evaporate it so far that it shall be hard when it is cold.

ANTIHECTICUM POTERII. Fuse together 4 parts of regulus of antimony and 5½ of fine tin; pour it on a metal plate, reduce it to powder, and deflagrate it in a red-hot crucible with 15 parts of nitre: keep it hot for some time, then wash it, and dry with a gentle heat. Dose, gr. ij to x, in hectic fevers, &c.

ANTIMONII TARTARIZATI LIQUOR. See Vinum Antimonii Potassio-tartratis.

ANTIMONII ET SODII SULPHURETUM. SCHLIPPE'S *Antimonial Salt.* M. VANDEN CORPUT. Mix 8 parts of effloresced sulphate of soda, 6 of sulphuret of antimony, and 3 of charcoal, and expose to a red-heat in a covered Hessian crucible till the fused mass ceases to throw up a scum. Boil the residue in a porcelain vessel with 1 part of sulphur, and sufficient distilled water, and set the filtered liquor aside for crystallization.

ANTIMONII TANNAS. Add to a decoction of cinchona bark a solution of potassio-tartrate of antimony as long as a precipitate is thrown down; collect and dry the precipitate. It may also be made with a solution of tannin instead of the decoction. Dose, iij to viij grs. in some mucilaginous liquid, as a contra-stimulant.

ANTIMONIUM TARTARIZATUM. E. & D. See Antimonii Potassio-tartras.

AQUA AMYGDALE AMARÆ. U. S. Oil of bitter almonds ♏xvj, carbonate of magnesia ʒj; rub together, then with f℥xxxij of distilled water gradually added, and filter. [This is weaker than the P. & PRUS. PH.]

AQUA CERASORUM AMYGDALATA. PRUS. PH. Sour cherries dried and bruised with their stones ℔j, bruised bitter almonds ℔j, water q. s. Distil ℔xxiv.

AQUA CINNAMOMI SPIRITUOSA. PRUS. PH. (*Aqua Cinnamomi Vinosa.*) Bruised cinnamon ℔ij, proof spirit ℔ij, water q. s. Distil ℔ix.

AQUA MAGNESIÆ CITRATIS. M. MAURY. Mix ʒij of calcined magnesia, ʒj of carbonate of magnesia, ℥iss of sugar (with a drop or two of oil of orange or lemon-peel), citric acid ʒviss, in a Oj bottle of water. Cork immediately; in half an hour it will be ready to drink. *Laxative.*

AQUA PARIETARIÆ. P. From wall pellitory; as Aq. Lactucæ.

AQUA PHAGEDÆNICA. See Lotio Hydrargyri flava.

AQUA VULNERARIA ACIDA. See Mistura Vulneraria.

ARNICINA. From arnica montana, as Lobelina. Dose scarcely determined.

ARSENIAS AMMONIÆ, &c. See Ammoniæ Arsenias, &c.

ARSENICI ET HYDRARGYRI HYDRIODAS. See Liquor Arsenici et Hydr. Hydriodatis.

ARSENICUM PURUM. D. Place ʒij of white oxide of arsenic at the sealed end of a hard German glass tube, of ½ inch diameter, and 18 inches long; and having covered it with 8 inches of dry and coarsely-powdered charcoal, and heated the portion containing the charcoal to redness, place a few ignited coals beneath the oxide so as to effect its slow sublimation. The metallic arsenic will be found attached to the cool end.

ASSAFŒTIDA PRÆPARATA. L. As Ammoniacum Præparatum.

ATROPIA. *Atropine*, or *Belladonnin.* Exhaust fresh powdered belladonna root with alcohol (822°); add to the tincture 1 part of slaked lime for 24 of root, and digest for 24 hours, frequently shaking; add sulphuric acid by drops until in slight excess; filter, distil off rather more than half the spirit; add water to the residuum, and evaporate the remainder of the spirit rapidly with a moderate heat; again filter, and evaporate the liquid to $\frac{1}{12}$th the weight of root used; add to the cold liquid a strong solution of carbonate of potash, drop by drop, taking care not to render the liquid alkaline. In a few hours filter again, add carbonate of potash as long as a precipitate falls, and in 12 or 24 hours collect the atropine on a filter, press it between folds of blotting paper, and dry it. Moisten it with water, and again press and dry it; dissolve it in five times its weight of alcohol; decolorize by shaking it with animal charcoal; filter, distil off the spirit, and evaporate so that the atropia may crystallize. M. RABOURDIN prepares it from the expressed juice of the plant, coagulated by heat, and filtered. To each quart add ʒj of caustic potash and ℥j of chloroform; agitate for a minute and let it rest; in half an hour pour off the supernatant liquor from the colored chloroform, and wash the latter with water as long as this becomes colored. Distil off all the chloroform in a small retort by means of a water-bath, and dissolve the residuum in a little water acidulated with sulphuric acid. To the filtered solution add carbonate of potash in slight excess; collect the precipitate, and dissolve it in alcohol. The solution, by spontaneous evaporation, yields crystals of atropine. M. MEIN obtained 3 grains from 1000 grains of the root. A powerful poison. Dose, from $\frac{1}{30}$ gradually increased to $\frac{1}{5}$th of a grain; or *endermically* from $\frac{1}{30}$ to $\frac{1}{10}$th of a grain; to the sound skin, 8 or 10 grains to ℥j of ointment.

ATROPIÆ SULPHAS. L. Mix fʒij of diluted sulphuric acid with f℥ss of distilled water, and gradually add ℈viiss of atropia, or sufficient to saturate it. Let the solution be filtered, and evaporated with a gentle heat, that crystals may form. *Intended for outward use only.*

BALNEUM ALUMINIS. Dr. ASHWELL. Dissolve 1℔ of alum in each gallon of water. To be used at 98° F.

BALNEUM CREASOTI. CUT. H. Creasote ʒij, glycerine ℥ij, boiling water Cj. Mix. To be added to Cxxix of water.

BALNEUM GLYCERINII COMPOSITUM. CUT. H. Tragacanth ℔j, glycerine ℔ij, water Cij; boil till dissolved. Oj to Cxxx of water.

BALNEUM IODINII. CUT. H. Iodine ʒij, solution of potash ℥ij, water Oj. Dissolve. Oij to be added to Cxxx of water.

BALNEUM MARINUM. CUT. H. Common salt ℔viij, sulphate of magnesia ℔ij, solution of chloride of calcium ℔j, water Cij. Dissolve. Add Oj to Cxxx of water. See also Aqua Marina. A common substitute is 1 part of salt to 30 of water. As a pediluvium, add a handful of salt to a pailful of water; to which a little mustard is sometimes added.

BALNEUM MERCURIALE. CUT. H. Corrosive sublimate ℥iij, hydrochloric acid ℥j, water Cij. Oj to be added to Cxxx of water.

BALNEUM MURIATICUM. RICHARD. Muriatic acid ℥ij-iv, water 16 pails. *In prurigo and lichen.*

BALNEUM OLEOSUM. Cold baths of olive or other oils, to which aromatic plants may be added, are used in the East as a preservative from the plague: the patient remains in them about half an hour.

BALNEUM QUERCI. DR. ELAESSER. Boil 3 handfuls of oak-bark (tied up in linen) in 3 quarts of water for half an hour, and add to a bath for a child.

BALNEUM SULPHURIS COMPOSITUM. CUT. H. Precipitated sulphur ℔iv, hyposulphite of soda, ℔j, sulphuric acid ʒij, water Cij. Mix. A pint to be added to 30 gallons of water.

BALNEUM TEREBINTHINATUM. Dr. T. SMITH. Camphine from ¼ to ½ pint, common soda ℔ij, oil of rosemary ℥ss, water q. s. "It calms the pulse, softens the skin, and renders respiration freer." For children and delicate women, f℥ij of camphine may be sufficient.

BETEL. A masticatory compound, consisting of the leaves of Piper betel, Areka nuts, and lime. *Sialagogue.*

BIBIRINA. Dr. RODIE. The bark of the Bebeeru or greenheart tree is first boiled with a solution of carbonate of soda, then exhausted with water acidulated with sulphuric acid, and ammonia added as long as it occasions a precipitate. To purify it, Dr. MACLAGAN directs the impure alkali to be washed and mixed with an equal weight of moist oxide of lead (Plumbi oxydum hydratum), and the mass dried and exhausted with alcohol. The clear solution decanted and evaporated, leaves the alkaloid, which may be further purified by dissolving it in pure ether. Tonic and anti-periodic. Dose, gr. ij—xij.

BIBIRINÆ SULPHAS. By dissolving bebeerine in diluted sulphuric acid, till the acid is neutralized, and evaporating the solution. Or from the bark, as Quinæ Sulphas, E. Dose, gr. j—iij, *as a tonic;* or gr. v—xx, *as an antiperiodic.*

BISMUTHI NITRAS. L. [*B. Trisnitras*, L. 1836; *B. Subnitras*, D., *Bismuthum Album*, E.] To f℥iss of nitric acid, mixed with f℥j of distilled water, add ℥j of bismuth, and apply heat till it is dissolved. Pour the solution into Oiij of distilled water, and strain the mixture through linen to separate the powder: wash this with distilled water, and dry it with a gentle heat. E. directs the metal to be gradually added to the nitric acid gently heated, and a very little water to be added as soon as crystals or a white powder begin to form; the solution to be then poured into the water, the precipitate collected on a calico filter, washed quickly with cold water, and dried in a dark place. D. directs ℥ij of the metal to be dissolved in f℥iij of pure nitric acid diluted with f℥iij of water, and the clear solution evaporated to f℥ij before pouring it into Cj of distilled water. [Dose, from 5 grs., sometimes increased to 15 or 20, as a tonic and antispasmodic, particularly in pyrosis and gastrodynia.]

BOLUS STANNI. GUY'S H. Tin-filings ℥ss, comp. tragacanth powder ʒss, syrup q. s. In 3 boluses. Dose 1 to 3.

CADMII SULPHAS. Dr. PEREIRA. Dissolve 7 parts of cadmium in 6½ parts of sulphuric acid with 15 of water and a little nitric acid. Evaporate to dryness, redissolve in water, filter, and evaporate by a gentle heat, that crystals may form. Uses, as sulphate of zinc.

CAFFEINA. *Caffeine*, or *Theine*. Boil pulverized unroasted coffee in distilled water, strain, and add acetate of lead to the decoction as long as it throws down a precipitate; pass sulphuretted hydrogen through the filtered solution, refilter, and evaporate so that crystals may form on cooling. The salts of caffein may be made by adding to a diluted acid sufficient caffeine to neutralize it, and exposing the solution to a heat of 104° F. Dose, gr. j. every hour or two, in hemicrania, &c.

CARBO LIGNI. Obtained by burning wood, without access of air. *Antiseptic*. Dose, gr. x to ʒij.

CASSIA PRÆPARATA. L. Macerate broken cassia pods, in sufficient distilled water to cover them, for 6 hours, constantly stirring; strain the washed pulp through a hair sieve, and evaporate in a water-bath to the consistence of a confection. Dose, ʒij—vj.

CATAPLASMA CEPÆ. Onions roasted and mashed.

CATAPLASMA AD DECUBITUM. PRUS. PH. Boil ℥ij of oak bark in q. s. water, to yield ℥viij of strained decoction; add to this ℥ij of liquid diacetate of lead, collect the precipitate on a filter, and put it into a bottle with ʒij of rectified spirit.

CATAPLASMA FICI. A dried fig, roasted, or boiled (sometimes in milk), and split, is sometimes applied to gum-boils, &c.

CATAPLASMA GALVANICUM. RECAMIER. It consists of cotton wadding containing a layer of very thin zinc plates and another layer of copper ones. This pad, conveniently quilted, is inclosed in a bag one face of which is of quilted calico, the other of impermeable tissue. The natural perspiration, confined by the impermeable tissue, excites galvanic action between the metals.

Cataplasma Hyoscyami. Gl. H. As Cataplasma Papaveris.

Cataplasma Oryzæ. Rice flour, with boiling water q. s.

Cataplasma Vini Rubri. Gl. H. Linseed meal ℥iss, boiling water ℥v; stir it over a slow fire for a minute, remove, and add ℥ij of red wine.

Causticum Acidum Hydrargyri Nitratis. Cut. H. Dissolve ℥j of quicksilver in ℥ij of nitric acid (sp. gr. 1·50).

Causticum Arseniosum Compositum. Cut. H. Calomel ℥iiss, vermilion ℈ij, arsenious acid ℈j to ʒij. Mix.

Causticum Cantharidis Compositum. Cut. H. Powdered cantharides ℥ij, strong pyroligneous acid ℥viij, tannin ʒj. Macerate for a week, and strain.

Causticum Depilatorium. Cut. H. Quick-lime ʒj, yellow sulphuret of arsenic ℈ij, starch powder ʒvj. Mix.

Causticum Hydrargyri cum Arsenico. Cut. H. Quicksilver ℥ss, arsenious acid ʒss, nitric acid ℥j. Dissolve.

Causticum Iodinii. Lugol. Iodine ℥ss, iodide of potassium ℥ss, distilled water ℥j. Mix.

Causticum Nitricum. Dr. Rivallie's *Solidified Nitric Acid.* On a piece of lint placed in an earthen vessel, gradually drop concentrated nitric acid; press the gelatinous mass into a suitable shape, and apply it, with the forceps, on the part. Remove it carefully in 15 or 20 minutes. *For Cancerous Tumors*, &c.

Causticum Potassæ Bichromatis. A saturated solution of bichromate of potash.

Causticum Potassæ Compositum. Cut. H. Hydrate of potash ℥ss, quick-lime ℥ss, glycerine q. s. Mix.

Causticum Potentiale. See Potassæ Hydras.

Causticum Sabinæ Compositum. Cut. H. Powdered savin ℥ss, burnt alum ℥j, levigated nitric oxide of mercury ʒj. Mix.

Causticum Suphuricum. Saffron, triturated with oil of vitriol to a plastic paste.

Causticum Zinci Chloridi Compositum. Cut. H. Chloride of zinc ʒiv, chloride of antimony ʒij, powdered starch ʒj, glycerine q. s. Mix.

Cera Alba. *Bleached or White Wax.* Melted bees'-wax is allowed to run through a perforated vessel upon a cylinder revolving in water; the ribands thus formed are exposed to the weather till their color is removed, and are then melted into cakes.

Ceratum Cacao. Butter of cacao, and oil of almonds, equal parts. *Cosmetic.*

Ceratum Cretæ Compositum. Manch. H. Lead plaster ℥viij, olive oil f℥iv, prepared chalk ℥iv, distilled vinegar f℥iv, diacetate of lead fʒiv.

Ceratum Lauro-cerasi. See Ceratum Calmans.

Cerevisia Sarsæ. *Spanish Jarave.* Pour 4 gallons of boiling water on ℔ij Rio Negro sarsaparilla, ℥viij powdered guaiacum bark, ℥iv each of rasped guaiacum wood, anise seed, and liquorice root; ℥ij of bark of mezereon root, ℔ij of treacle, and 12 bruised cloves. Shake it thrice a day, and keep it in a warm place. When fermentation has set in it is fit for use. Dose, a small tumblerful.

Charta Exploratoria. Prus. Ph. Infuse 1 part of litmus in 4 of water, and dip white paper into it, and dry. If the infusion be slightly reddened by the smallest quantity of sulphuric acid, it forms red litmus paper. Used to detect acids, the latter for alkalies.

Charta Resinosa. Prus. Ph. Paper thinly spread with common pitch.

Chlorinii Liquor. D. Put ℥ss of powdered peroxide of manganese into a gas bottle, add f℥iij of muriatic acid diluted with f℥ij of water; apply a gentle heat, and cause the gas to pass through f℥ij of water, and then into a Oiij bottle containing f℥xx of distilled water, and whose mouth is loosely plugged with tow. When the air has been entirely displaced by the chlorine, cork the bottle loosely, and shake it till the chlorine is absorbed. It should now be transferred to a pint stoppered bottle, and preserved in a dark cool place. L. (Liquor Chlorinii) directs the gas from f℥j of hydrochloric acid and ʒij of binoxide of manganese to be passed into Oss of distilled water. E. (Chlorinei Aqua) directs 60 grs. of common salt, and 350 grs. of red oxide of lead, to be triturated together; put into a stoppered bottle with f℥viij of water, and fʒij of oil of vitriol, and agitated till the oxide becomes almost white. The clear liquid to be used. [Dose, fʒss to fʒij, largely diluted. See also Solutio Chlorinii.]

CHLOROFORMYL. (*Chloroform.*) L. Put ℔iv of chlorinated lime, mixed with Ox of water, into a retort, and add Oss of rectified spirit. The mixture must not occupy more than a third part of the retort. Heat by a sand-bath, and as soon as boiling commences instantly withdraw the fire, lest the retort should be broken by the sudden and increased heat. Let the liquor distil as long as anything subsides from it, renewing the heat if required. Add to the distilled liquor 4 times as much water, and stir the mixture well. Carefully separate the heavier liquid which shall have subsided, and agitate it now and then during an hour with ʒj of bruised chloride of calcium. Then again distil the liquid from a glass retort into a glass receiver. [Free from color; of a grateful smell; sp. gr. not less than 1·48; hardly at all soluble in water; does not redden litmus; rubbed on the skin it quickly disappears, leaving scarcely any smell. L.] D. Chloroformum. Slake 5℔ av. of fresh lime with Oij of boiling water; put it into a sheet-iron or copper still, with 10℔ of chlorinated lime, and add 3¾ gallons of water previously mixed with ℥xxv of rectified spirit, and raised to 100°. Connect the still with the condenser and apply heat, which must be withdrawn the moment distillation commences. Let the lower stratum of the distilled product, which need not exceed Oij, be agitated twice in succession with an equal volume of distilled water, and then in a separate bottle with half its volume of pure sulphuric acid. Lastly, let it be shaken in a matrass with ʒij of finely powdered peroxide of manganese, and rectified from this at a very gentle heat. Sp. gr. 1·496. The lighter liquid and washings should be reserved, to be put into the still with the next charge. Dose, 2 to 10 drops, as an antispasmodic; but chiefly used by inhalation to produce insensibility.

CIGARETTÆ BALSAMICÆ. Soak a piece of thick blotting paper in a solution of nitre, and dry it; then brush it over with compound tincture of benzoin. A piece 3 inches long and 1¼ wide is rolled into a Cigarette. *In aphonia*, &c.

CINNABARIS. E. See Hydrargyri Bisulphuretum.

COLLODION. MIALHE. Dissolve ℥j of gun-cotton in ℥xvj of

rectified æther, and add f℥j of alcohol. It may be strained through coarse muslin; and thinned with more æther if too thick. [The gun-cotton for this purpose may be made by mixing ℥x of powdered nitre with ℥xv or ℥xx of strong sulphuric acid in a porcelain vessel, and stirring into it ℥¼ of carded cotton wool, moving it constantly with glass rods for a few minutes (Mr. DAVENPORT says half an hour); then washing it thoroughly in a large quantity of cold water, squeezing, and again opening it under a stream of water. Press it strongly in a dry cloth, then open it, and dry it gradually in a warm place free from danger.] U. S. To ℥x of nitrate of potassa in powder add f℥viiiss of sulphuric acid in a Wedgewood mortar, and triturate them until uniformly mixed; then add ℥ss of fine carded cotton freed from impurities, and, by means of the pestle and a glass rod, imbue it thoroughly with the mixture for 4 minutes. Transfer the cotton to a vessel containing water, and wash it in successive portions by agitation and pressure, until the washings cease to have an acid taste, or to be precipitated by chloride of barium. Having separated the fibres, dry the cotton with a gentle heat, dissolve it by agitation in Oiiss (Oij imp.) of æther, previously mixed with f℥j of rectified spirit.

COLLODION CANTHARIDALE. Dr. ILISCH. Treat ℥xvj of coarsely powdered cantharides with ℥xvj of æther, and ℥iij of acetic æther. In ℥ij of the percolated liquid dissolve ℈j of gun-cotton. Or dissolve gr. xv of pure cantharidine and ℈j of gun-cotton in ℥iss of sulphuric æther and ℥ss of acetic æther. M. ŒTTINGER prefers a mixture of cantharidal æther (see Æther Cantharidalis), and collodion; and applies 2 coats of the mixture. For children 1 part of cantharidal æther to 2 of collodion.

COLLODION TINCTUM. CUT. H. Collodion ℥j, palm oil ʒss, alkanet root q. s. to color it. Mix, and strain. The color of this compound renders its appearance less disagreeable, as an application to the skin, and the oil gives it a degree of flexibility.

COLLUTORIUM CREASOTI. Dr. FAULCON. Creasote ʒss, infusion of sage Oj. *In mercurial salivation.*

COLLUTORIUM DISINFECTANS. F. H. Chloride of lime gr. xv, mucilage fʒj, water f℥j, syrup of orange-peel fʒiv. Mix.

COLLUTORIUM SODÆ POTASSIO-TARTRATIS. MIALHE. Rochelle salts ℥j, water ℥iij, syrup of currants ℥j. *For reducing tur-*

gescence of the mucous membrane. [See also Gargarisma, for other mouth washes.]

COLLYRIUM ATROPIÆ. Atropine gr. j, distilled water ℥j. A few drops only to be used. BOUCHARDAT, for his *stronger* solution for dilating the pupil, prescribes one grain of atropine to ʒv of water; one or two drops to be used. His *weaker* solution consists of one grain to 1000 grains of water. *In hernia of the iris, and ulcerations of the cornea.*

COLLYRIUM PLUMBI CUM OPIO. MAN. H. Goulard water f℥xij, tincture of opium fʒij. [Wine of opium is often used.]

COLOCYNTHIS PRÆPARATA. *Trochisci Alhandal.* PRUS. PH. Colocynth pulp (without seeds) ℥v, powdered gum Arabic ℥j; form them into a paste with water q. s.; dry, and reduce to powder.

COLUMBINA. WITTSTOCK. Exhaust columbo root by rectified spirit, evaporate to dryness, dissolve the extract in water, and agitate with an equal bulk of æther. Remove the æther with a syphon, distil off the greater part, and set it aside. Wash the crystals with cold æther, and press them in bibulous paper. Dose, 1 to 3 grains daily, in *Dyspepsia.*

CONFECTIO CATECHU COMPOSITUM. D. Compound powder of catechu ℥v, simple syrup f℥v. Mix.

CONFECTIO SULPHURIS. D. Sublimed sulphur ℥ij, bitartrate of potash ℥j, clarified honey ℥j, syrup of ginger and syrup of saffron, of each f℥ss.

CONFECTIO TEREBINTHINÆ. D. Oil of turpentine f℥j, p. liquorice root ℥j, clarified honey ℥ij; rub the oil with the powder, then add the honey, and beat them together. Dose, ʒij, or more. [For other Confections, see *Conserva* and *Electuarium.*]

CONSERVA SABINÆ. HAN. PH. Fresh savine 1 part, sugar 2 parts.

CUPRI AMMONIATI SOLUTIO. E. As Liquor Cupri Ammoniosulphatis, L.

CUPRI SUBACETAS PRÆPARATUM. D. Reduce verdigris to powder by careful trituration in a porcelain mortar, and separate the finer parts for use by a sieve.

DECOCTUM ADANSONIÆ. DUCHASSAING. Bark of the Baobab

tree (Ad. digitata) ʒvj, water Oiss; boil to Oj, and strain. Used as a substitute for Decoct. Cinchonæ.

Decoctum Aloes Concentratum. Mr. Westall. Extract of liquorice ʒxiv, carbonate of potash ʒij, myrrh and aloes of each ʒiij, water Oj. Boil gently to f℥xiij, strain, and put the liquid into a bottle with ʒiij of saffron, and f℥xiv of comp. tinc. of cardamoms. Macerate for 10 days, and strain through linen. [With an equal quantity of water it forms the decoction of the L. Pharmacopœia.]

Decoctum Araliæ Spinosæ. From the bark of the Angelica tree; as Dec. Cinchonæ.

Decoctum Arundinis. Root of the Province-reed (Arundo Donax) ℥j, water Oj; boil and strain. *To prevent the secretion of milk.* A wine-glassful frequently.

Decoctum Bael. Dried unripe fruit of bael (Ægle Marmelos) ℥ij, water Oj; boil to O¼, and strain. Dose, f℥iss, twice or thrice a day, *in dysentery, diarrhœa,* &c.

Decoctum Baptisiæ Tinctoriæ. Dr. Thacker. Root of wild indigo ℥j, water Oj; boil and strain. Dose f℥ss every 4 or 8 hours, *in threatened mortification;* also applied externally.

Decoctum Caffei. M. Dauvin. Boil ʒx of raw coffee berries in f℥viij of water to f℥v. To be given in 3 doses during the intermissions of intermittent fevers.

Decoctum Cannabis. See Cerevisia Cannabis.

Decoctum Ceanothi. Dr. Wood. Root of Ceanothus Americanus (red-root) ʒij, water f℥xvj; boil gently, and strain. *In syphilis.*

Decoctum Cinchonæ Pallidæ, and Dec. Cinchonæ Rubræ. L. From the yellow and red bark, as above.

Decoctum Cinchonæ Factitium. Pruss. Ph. Willow bark ℥ss, horse-chestnut bark ℥ss, calamus root ʒij, cloves ʒij; boil in f℥xvj of water to f℥viij. [As a substitute for D. Cinchonæ, when it cannot be obtained.]

Decoctum Corticis Peruviani. See D. Cinchonæ.

Decoctum Corticis Brasiliensis. Bark of the Acacia astringens ℥j, water f℥xvj; boil to f℥viij. Dose, ℥j—ij. Chiefly *in gonorrhœa.*

Decoctum Curcumæ. Turmeric root ℥j, distilled water Oss;

boil a few minutes and strain. Chiefly used as a test for alkalies.

DECOCTUM COPALCHI. Copalchi bark ℥ss, water Oj; boil for 10 or 15 minutes, and strain. Dose, ℥ss to ℥j, 2 or 3 times a day.

DECOCTUM ELATERII RADICIS. LAVAGNA. Dried root of elaterium ʒiv, water f℥xlviij; boil to f℥xxiv. A wine-glassful daily in 3 doses. *Diuretic and purgative in dropsies.*

DECOCTUM EUPATORII PERFOLIATI. Dr. WOOD. Boil ℥j of the dried herb in Oiiss of water to Oj. Dose f℥iv—viij. *Emetic and cathartic.*

DECOCTUM GALEOPSIS. LEJEUNE. Boil ℥ss of the tops of Galeopsis grandiflora in Oj of water to Oss, and sweeten. Milk is sometimes substituted for water. The whole to be taken in 24 hours. *In phthisis.*

DECOCTUM LICHENIS ISLANDICI. D. Iceland moss ℥j, water Oiss; wash the moss with cold water, then boil it for 10 minutes in a covered vessel, and strain while hot. For L. see Dec. Cetrariæ.

DECOCTUM LINI COMPOSITUM. D. *Infusum Lini Compositum.* Linseed ℥j, liquorice root ʒiv, water Oiss; boil for 10 minutes in a covered vessel, and strain while hot.

DECOCTUM LYCOPODII. RADIUS. Herb lycopodium, cut small, 2 heaped spoonfuls; water Oj; boil to Oss. A teacupful warm every 10 minutes, in *retention of urine.*

DECOCTUM MILLEFOLII. Dried tops of yarrow ℥j, water Oj; boil for a quarter of an hour in a covered vessel, and strain. Dose, f℥iss 3 times a day: and as a *fomentation to bruises,* &c.

DECOCTUM MYRRHÆ. D. Myrrh ʒij, water f℥viiiss; triturate the myrrh, with the water gradually added; then boil for 10 minutes in a covered vessel, and strain.

DECOCTUM PINI TURIONUM. Buds of the Norway spruce fir, or the silver fir, ʒvj, water Oj; boil gently, and strain. *Diuretic.*

DECOCTUM QUASSIÆ COMPOSITUM. CUT. H. Quassia ℥j, ginger ℥j, boiling water Cj; macerate for 4 hours, and strain. More properly an *infusion.*

DECOCTUM SCOPARII. D. Broom tops (dried) ℥ss, water Oss; boil for 10 minutes, and strain.

DECOCTUM SPIRÆÆ TOMENTOSÆ. Dr. WOOD. Boil ℥j of the

dried plant (hardhack) in Oj of water, and strain. *Tonic astringent.* Dose, f℥iss—ij.

DECOCTUM STATICIS ARMERIÆ. Dr. EBERS. Boil ℥j of the dried herb (common thrift) in Oj of water, and strain. *Diuretic.* By glassfuls. Some other species, Statice Caroliniana, and S. Limonium, are used in the same form, as *astringents.*

DECOCTUM THLASPI BURSÆ PASTORIS. Boil half a handful of the herb (shepherd's purse) with f℥xvj of water to f℥xij. To be taken at twice, in the day; in *uterine hæmorrhage.*

ELATERIUM. D. See Extractum Elaterii.

ELECTUARIUM AROMATICUM. E. Aromatic powder one part, syrup of orange-peel two parts. Mix.

ELECTUARIUM PIPERIS. E. See Confectio Piperis.

ELECTUARIUM RESINÆ. See Confectio Resinæ.

ELIXIR AURANTIORUM COMPOSITUM. PRUS. PH. Thin orange peel ℥vj, cassia ℥ij, carbonate of potash ℥j, Madeira wine ℔iv. Macerate for 6 days, express, and dissolve in the tincture ℥j each of the extracts of gentian, wormwood, buckbean, and cascarilla. Filter.

ELIXIR WORONEJE. Rectified spirit ℔viiss, sal ammoniac ʒj, nitre and pepper, each ℈iiiss, nitromuriatic acid ʒss, vinegar ℔iss, petroleum (native white or rose naphtha) ʒss, olive oil ℥ss, oil of peppermint ℥vij. Digest for 12 hours, and strain. Dose, 2 teaspoonfuls every quarter of an hour. *In Cholera.*

[For other Elixirs, see TINCTURÆ.]

EMBROCATIO COMMUNIS. GUY'S H. Sesquicarbonate of ammonia ℥iv, vinegar Ov, or q. s., proof spirit Oiiss. Mix.

EMBROCATIO IODINII. Dr. TODD'S *Iodine paint.* Iodine gr. lxiv, iodide of potassium ʒss, alcohol ℥j. The part to be painted over with a camel-hair pencil. [It produces smarting, and frequently vesication or an eruption.]

EMPLASTRUM ADHÆSIVUM NIGRUM. *Court Plaster.* See Empl. Ichthyocollæ.

EMPLASTRUM PLUMBI CARBONATIS. See Empl. Cerussæ. A similar compound is used in America under the name of MAHY'S plaster.

EMPLASTRUM PLUMBI COMPOSITUM. GUY'S H. Lead plaster ℥viij, frankincense ℥ij, oxide of iron ℥j; mix.

EMPLASTRUM POTASSII IODIDI. L. Strained frankincense ℥vj, wax ʒvj; melt together, and add ℥j of iodide of potassium rubbed smooth with fʒij of olive oil, and stir till cold. To be spread on linen, rather than on leather.

EMPLASTRUM SEVI COMPOSITUM. GUY'S H. Equal parts of suet, wax, and resin, melted together and strained.

EMPLASTRUM SINAPIS. Flour of mustard mixed with warm water or vinegar, to form a stiff paste. As a counter-irritant. It should not be left on too long.

EMPLASTRUM STIBIATUM. *Empl. Antimonii Tartarizati.*

EMPLASTRUM ZINGIBERIS. Powdered ginger, mixed with sufficient boiling water to form a paste, and spread on cloth or paper.

ENEMATA. The following are the usual quantities used:—

Age.		*Laxative.*		*If to be retained.*
For Adults	..	8 to 12 oz.	..	3 to 4 oz.
8 to 16 years	..	6 to 8 "	..	2 to 3 "
3 to 8 "	..	3 to 6 "	..	1½ to 2 "
Younger	..	2 "	..	1 "

ENEMA ALBUMINIS. RICORD. Infusion of linseed ℥xij, whites of 2 or 3 eggs. Mix. *In chronic diarrhœa.*

ENEMA ANTHELMINTICUM. Decoction of male fern, or of Corsican moss, is used, sometimes with the addition of ℥j of castor oil. For *Ascarides*, Enema aloes and En. Ferri muriatis are employed. See also Enema Vermifugum.

ENEMA CAMPHORÆ. Simple camphor liniment ʒiv, gruel q. s.

ENEMA FERRI MURIATIS. Dr. DARWALL. A few drops of the tincture in warm water or gruel is recommended as a remedy for *ascarides*, in children.

ENEMA FERRI PERCYANIDI. Triturate gr. v of Prussian blue with f℥ij of water; to be used daily, increasing the dose if necessary. [An American remedy for *ascarides.*]

ENEMA PLUMBI. Dr. NEWBOLD. Acetate of lead gr. vj, tepid water f℥vj; to be repeated in 2 hours. *In strangulated hernia.*

ENEMA SIMPLEX. GUY'S H. Gruel, or decoction of barley, or of linseed, f℥xvj.

EPITHEMA GLYCERINÆ. Mr. STARTIN. Gum tragacanth ʒij—iv, lime water f℥iv, glycerine ℥j, rose water f℥iij. Form a jelly. Applied to superficial burns, scalds, and excoriations.

ESSENTIA ABIETIS. See Extractum Abietis Fluidum.

ESSENTIA ANISI. D. Essential oil of anise f℥j, rectified spirit f℥ix; mix with agitation. [For making Aqua Anisi.]

ESSENTIA ANTHEMIDIS. See Liquor Anthemidis. The name is also given to a tincture of quassia, flavored with oil of chamomile. [GRAY.]

ESSENTIA CALUMBÆ. See Liquor Calumbæ.

ESSENTIA CAMPHORÆ. See Liquor Camphoræ.

ESSENTIA CARUI. D. As Essentia Anisi.

ESSENTIA CINCHONÆ. See Infusum Cinchonæ Spissatum, and Liquor Cinchonæ.

ESSENTIA CINNAMONII. D. As Essentia Anisi.

ESSENTIA FŒNICULI. D. As Essentia Anisi.

ESSENTIA GENTIANÆ. See Liquor Gentianæ.

ESSENTIA GUAIACI. See Extractum Guaiaci Fluidum.

ESSENTIA MENTHÆ PULEGII. D. As Essentia Anisi. [It is also prepared by the other formulæ directed for Essentia Menthæ Pip.]

ESSENTIA MYRISTICÆ MOSCHATÆ. D. As Essentia Anisi.

ESSENTIA PIMENTÆ. D. As Essentia Anisi.

ESSENTIA PHELLANDRII AQUATICI. COTTEREAU. Digest ℥j of bruised water-fennel seeds in f℥iv of proof spirit. Dose, 4 to 30 drops.

ESSENTIA RHEI. See Liquor Rhei.

ESSENTIA ROSÆ. See Liquor Rosæ, and Tinctura Rosæ.

ESSENTIA ROSMARINI. D. As Essentia Anisi.

EXTRACTUM ABIETIS FLUIDUM. Evaporate a decoction of the young tops of the black spruce fir to the consistence of treacle.

EXTRACTUM ABRI PRECATORII. As Ext. Glycyrrhizæ; which it resembles.

EXTRACTUM ACONITI SICCUM SEU PULVERATUM. PRUS. PH.

Mix ℥iv of extract of aconite carefully with ℥j of powdered sugar of milk, and dry the mass in a warm place, adding so much powdered sugar of milk as will make the weight ℥iv. The other narcotic extracts are treated in the same way. Dose, as the Extracts.

Extractum Alconorcæ. By evaporating a decoction of the American Alconorque bark. *Astringent,* 10 grs. to ℈j.

Extractum Aloes Barbadensis. L. From Barbadoes aloes; as Ext. Aloes.

Extractum Apocyni. From the root of apocynum cannabinum, as Extractum Anthemidis. Dose, gr. iij—iv.

Extractum Aurantii [corticis fructûs]. By digesting the dried peel with proof spirit, afterwards with proof spirit with an equal quantity of water, evaporating the mixed tinctures.

Extractum Calisayacum. Ellis. Bruised yellow (Calisaya) bark ℔ij; boil in Cj of distilled water acidulated with f℥ss of hydrochloric acid; strain, and boil the residue with two successive portions of acidulated water. Filter the mixed decoctions, add ℥ij or q. s. of lime previously slaked; stir the mixture well, let the precipitate subside, wash it well, dry it, exhaust it with hot alcohol, evaporate the solution by water-bath to a pilular consistence. Dose, 1 to 4 grains; medium dose, 2 grains. Sulphuric acid renders it more soluble and active.

Extractum Cannabis Indicæ Purificatum. D. Dissolve ℥j of extract of Indian hemp of commerce in f℥iv of rectified spirit, and when the dregs have subsided, decant the clear liquid, and evaporate by water-bath. [See Resina Cannabis Indicæ.]

Extractum Carnis. Treat 6 pounds (av.) meat as directed for Infusum Carnis (Liebig's), and evaporate it by a gentle heat to ℥iij. Keep it from the air.

Extractum Colchici Alcoholicum. P. As Ext. Ipecacuanhæ.

Extractum Conii Siccum. As Ext. Aconiti Siccum.

Extractum Copalchi. From copalchi bark, as Ext. Rhei. Dose, 1 to 2 grains.

Extractum Erigeronis. From Canadian Fleabane; by evaporating an aqueous infusion. Dose, 5 to 10 grains.

Extractum Ferri Pomatum. Pruss. Ph. Peel ℔vj of unripe crab-apples, and beat them to a pulp; add ℔j of coils of iron wire; digest in a vapor bath for 8 days, take out the wire and express. Evaporate the liquor, when clear, in porcelain vessels, with constant stirring to a soft extract. Dissolve it in 4 parts of water, filter, and evaporate with constant stirring. Dose, gr. v—x, daily.

EXTRACTUM FILICIS. Dr. EBERS. Digest dried root of male fern (Aspidium Filix mas) in rectified spirit, strain, distil off most of the spirit, and evaporate what remains to an extract. Dose, ℈j to ℈ij (?) in *tapeworm*. See the next.

EXTRACTUM FILICIS ETHEREUM. See Oleum Filicis.

EXTRACTUM GRANATI [Fructûs Corticis]. From the decoction.

EXTRACTUM HYOSCYAMI ALCOHOLICUM. U. S. & P. As Extractum Aconiti Alcoholicum. Dose, ¼ gr. to ij.

EXTRACTUM LINI CATHARTICI. Dr. B. LANE. Macerate the dried herb in 8 or 10 times its weight of boiling water for a few hours, strain with pressure, and evaporate the clear liquor by a gentle heat. Dose, 5 to 10 grains twice a day, as a laxative and diuretic. It yields one-sixth of extract.

EXTRACTUM MALTI. Pour over ground malt sufficient hot water (between 170 and 200°) to cover it; leave it for 24 hours, strain without pressure, and evaporate the clear liquor immediately, to the thickness of treacle.

EXTRACTUM NUCIS VOMICÆ AQUOSUM. PRUS. PH. Macerate the coarsely powdered nuts in four parts of boiling water for 24 hours, express; macerate the residuum in three parts of boiling water, and express. Evaporate the mixed and clear liquor to a soft extract by a gentle heat, and dry it in a warm place.

EXTRACTUM PARIETARIÆ. From fresh pellitory of the wall, as Extractum Aconiti.

EXTRACTUM PIPERIS FLUIDUM. U. S. From black pepper, as EXT. CUBEBÆ FLUIDUM, separating the piperine by expression through a cloth, and keeping the liquid portion for use.

EXTRACTUM RHEI FLUIDUM. U. S. Mix ℥viij of coarsely powdered rhubarb with the same weight of sand; add f℥xij of proof spirit, and let the mixture stand for 24 hours. Transfer the mass to a percolator, and gradually pour upon it proof spirit until the liquid which passes has little of the odor or taste of rhubarb. Evaporate the tincture by water-bath to f℥v, then add ℥v of sugar; dissolve, and mix the fluid extract with f℥iv of tincture of ginger, in which are dissolved ♏iv each of oil of fennel and oil of anise.

EXTRACTUM RUMICIS AQUATICI. From the root of water-dock, as Extractum Gentianæ, or Extractum Glycyrrhizæ. Dose, ℈j to ʒj, in *cutaneous diseases.* Rumex Hydrolapathum (*great water-dock*), and R. Obtusifolius are also used.

EXTRACTUM SARSÆ LIQUIDUM. L. Boil ℔iijss of sarsaparilla in Ciij of distilled water to Oxij; pour off the liquid, and strain it while hot. Boil the root again in Cij of water, to Cj, and strain. Evaporate the mixed decoctions to f℥xviij, and when cold, add f℥ij of rectified spirit. [Each f℥j represents ℥ij of the root, and f℥xvj of the decoction.]

EXTRACTUM SARSÆ COMPOSITUM FLUIDUM. See Liquor Sarsæ Compositum.

EXTRACTUM SARSAPARILLÆ FLUIDUM. U. S. Sarsaparilla ℥xvj, liquorice root, sassafras root bark, each ℥ij (all bruised), mezereon sliced ʒvj, proof spirit Oiij o. m. (Ovj f℥viij imp.): macerate for 14 days, then express, and filter. Evaporate the liquid by water-bath to f℥xij, add to it, while still hot, ℥xij of sugar, and remove from the bath as soon as the sugar is dissolved.

EXTRACTUM SCILLÆ ACETICUM. Mr. NIBLETT. Digest powdered squills ℔j in acetic acid ℥iij, and distilled water Oj, with a gentle heat, for 48 hours. Express strongly, and, without straining, evaporate to a proper consistence. [One grain of this is said to equal three of the powder.]

EXTRACTUM SPIGELIÆ ET SENNÆ FLUIDUM. U. S. Mix ℔j of pink root, and ℥vj of senna, each in coarse powder, with f℥xxxij of proof spirit; in 2 days transfer it to a percolator, and gradually pour upon it proof spirit until f℥lxiv are obtained. Evaporate by water-bath to f℥xvj, add ʒvj of carbonate of potash, and lastly (after the sediment has dissolved), ℥xviij of sugar, previously triturated with fʒss each of oil of caraway and oil of anise, and dissolve by a gentle heat.

EXTRACTUM SPIGELIÆ MARILANDICÆ. M. THELU. Exhaust dried Carolina pink by proof spirit, by percolation; distil off most of the spirit, evaporate the residuum by water-bath. Dose, gr. viij to ʒss.

EXTRACTUM ULMI. SOUBEIRAN. By percolation with proof spirit.

EXTRACTUM VALERIANÆ FLUIDUM. U. S. Valerian in coarse powder ℥viij, ether f℥iv, rectified spirit f℥xij. Mix the valerian with half the ether and spirit, previously mixed: put it into a percolator, and add the rest gradually, then add proof spirit until f℥xvj of liquid have passed. Let it evaporate spontaneously in a shallow vessel to f℥v. Pour more proof spirit into the percolator until f℥x have passed, to which add the former f℥v, taking care to dissolve in rectified spirit any oleo-resinous deposit. Let the mixture stand 4 hours, with occasional agitation, then filter, and add rectified spirit to make up f℥xvj. [fʒj contains ʒss of valerian.]

EXTRACTA SICCA *vel* PULVERATA. PRUS. PH. These are made by mixing 4 parts of the extract with 1 of powdered sugar of milk, setting the mixture in a warm place until dry. Triturate the mass to powder, adding more of the sugar if necessary, to make the weight the same as that of the extract used. These are consequently of the same strength as the extract.

FARINA TRITICI TOSTA. Wheat flour slightly baked, so as to acquire a pale buff tint; as a food for infants and invalids, particularly in diarrhœa.

FARINI HORDEI PRÆPARATA. PRUS. PH. Into a tin cylinder compress barley-flour till the vessel is two-thirds full. Suspend it in the body of a still two-thirds filled with water; fit on an alembic, and let the water be kept boiling for 2 days, 15 hours each. Remove the upper layer, powder the rest, and keep it in a dry place.

FERRI CHLORIDUM HYDRATUM. *Ferri Proto-murias.* Digest sulphuret of iron in excess, with diluted muriatic acid; filter, and evaporate, that crystals may form. Keep them from the air.

FERRI PER-CHLORIDUM. P. Dissolve red oxide of iron (Ferri Peroxydum) in hydrochloric acid, evaporate the solution to dryness by a water-bath; and preserve it in well-closed bottles.

FERRI ET MAGNESIÆ CITRAS. VANDEN CORPUT. Dissolve hydrated peroxide of iron in citric acid, as for Ferri Citras, and neutralize the solution with carbonate of magnesia. Filter, evaporate, and dry as Ferri Ammonio-citras. Dose, gr. iij to viij, in solution or in pills.

Ferri et Potassæ Citras. Mr. Hemingway. Dissolve a known quantity of citric acid in water, neutralize it with carbonate of potash; add to this as much acid as before used; digest with hydrated oxide of iron, gradually added till a portion remains undissolved. Evaporate the filtered solution as directed for Ferri Ammonio-citras.

Ferri et Sodæ Citras. As the last; substituting carbonate of soda for carbonate of potash. The doses and uses of the last three are the same as for Ferri Ammonio-citras.

Ferri Iodidi Syrupus. See Syrupus Ferri Iodidi.

Ferri Limatura Lævigata. P. Ferrum Pulveratum. Prepared iron filings ground by means of a slab and muller of porphyry to a fine powder, without moisture. See Ferri Pulvis.

Ferri Oxydum Magneticum. D. See Ferri Oxydum Nigrum.

Ferri Peroxydum. D. (*Ferri Oxydum Rubrum*, 1826.) Place hydrated peroxide of iron in an oven, in a few folds of filtering paper, and when it has become dry to the touch, transfer it to a covered crucible, and expose it for a few minutes to an obscure red heat.

Ferri Peroxydum Hydratum. D. (Ferrugo, E.) To f℥x of water add fʒvj of pure sulphuric acid, and with the aid of heat dissolve in it 8 ounces of sulphate of iron. Mix fʒiv of pure nitric acid with f℥ij of water, add it to the solution, and concentrate by boiling, until, upon the sudden disengagement of much gas, the liquid passes from a dark to a red color. Let this now be poured into Oij of solution of caustic potash, and when the mixture has been well stirred, place it on a calico filter, and let it be washed with distilled water until the liquid which passes through ceases to give a precipitate when dropped into a solution of barium. Inclose the precipitate, in its pasty state, in a porcelain pot, the lid of which is rendered air-tight by lard. See Ferrugo for E.

Ferri Biphosphas. (?) Dr. Routh. To metaphosphoric acid, boiling in a platina capsule, add as much phosphate of iron as it will dissolve, and let the solution solidify by cooling and exposure to the air. Dose, gr. j to ij, twice or thrice a day. *In debility, with nervous depression and anæmia.* [Whether the above is a definite chemical compound may be questioned. Until its composition is ascertained, the above name, under which it is prescribed by Dr. Routh, may be provisionally retained.]

Ferri Bitartras cum Potassæ Sulphate. Mr. Tyson. Triturate ℨiij of sulphate of iron with ℨiss of nitric acid, and add f℥vj. of water, and ℨvj of bitartrate of potash. Boil, filter while warm, and evaporate to dryness. Dose, gr. v—xx.

Ferri Pulvis. D. (Ferrum Reductum.) *Iron reduced by hydrogen.* Introduce into a gun-barrel as much peroxide of iron as will occupy about 10 inches, confining it to the middle portion of the barrel by plugs of asbestos. Heat the part containing the oxide to redness, and pass through it hydrogen gas (procured from zinc and diluted sulphuric acid, and dried by passing through oil of vitriol, and afterwards through a tube containing caustic potash), till the gas escapes without loss. Remove the fire, a slow current of the gas still being continued; and when cool, remove the metallic contents of the barrel, and preserve in an accurately stopped vessel. [Particular directions are given for conducting the process, for which we must refer to the D. Pharmacopœia.] Dose, gr. v, frequently repeated.

Ferri Sulphas Granulatum. D. Dissolve the iron as in Ferri Sulphas, page 135, receive the filtered solution into f℥viij of rectified spirit, and stir the mixture as it cools. Let the granular crystals be drained, washed on a funnel or small percolator with ℥ij of spirit, pressed repeatedly between blotting-paper, dried beneath a glass bell over a dinner-plate half filled with oil of vitriol, and preserved in a well-stopped vessel. Dose, gr. ss to gr. v.

Ferri et Aluminæ Bisulphas. Sir James Murray. 10 parts of well-washed alumina, 3 of soft iron filings, 5 of carbonate of potash or of soda, with water and carbonic acid, under strong pressure, yield a solution, to which sulphuric acid is added in excess. The salt is obtained in crystals. Dose, from 5 to 10 grains.

Ferri Proto-sulphuretum Hydratum. Add a solution of byhydrosulphuret of soda to one of proto-sulphate of iron: wash the precipitate quickly on a cloth filter, squeeze out most of the water, and keep the paste from the air. In this state it is used as an antidote for poisoning by corrosive sublimate. It may be safely taken in considerable doses. [For the anhydrous proto-sulphuret, see Ferri Sulphuretum.]

Ferri Per-sulphuretum Hydratum. Into a dilute solution of liver of sulphur, drop *very gradually* a neutral solution of persulphate of iron, prepared as directed under Ferri Peroxydum Hydratum. Collect and preserve the precipitate as the last. M. BOUCHARDAT prefers it to the proto-sulphuret as an antidote for sublimate, white arsenic, and the salts of lead and copper.

FERRI TARTARIZATUM. E. and D. See Ferri Potassio-tartras.

FLORES AURANTII (orange flowers), are preserved by mixing them with half their weight of salt.

FOLIA SENNÆ SPIRITU EXTRACTA. PRUS. PH. Macerate senna with 4 parts of rectified spirit for 2 days, then express and dry it. [Supposed to render it milder.]

FOTUS DULCAMARÆ. See Decoctum Dulcamaræ.

GARGARISMA CALCIS CHLORINATÆ. Chloride of lime ʒij, water Oj; triturate, filter, and add clarified honey ℥j.

GARGARISMA CHLORINII. MID. H. Chlorine water f℥ij, water f℥x. F. H. Chlorine water ℥ss, water ℥iv, syrup ℥ss, gum tragacanth gr. x.

GARGARISMA MANGANESII ACETATIS. Acetate of manganese ʒj, water f℥vij, clarified honey ℥j. [The chloride and the sulphate of manganese are also used, about ʒss or ℈ij to ℥vj of barley water, &c.]

GARGARISMA QUERCI. As Decoctum Querci.

GARGARISMA RESTRINGENS. CH. CROSS H. Alum ʒij, honey ʒij, water Oj.

GARGARISMA SIMPLEX. See Gargarisma.

GARGARISMA SINAPIS. M. FLEURY. Black mustard-seed, bruised, ʒiv, salt ℈iv, vinegar ℈viij, warm water f℥vij. Digest, and filter.

GARGARISMA SODÆ BORATIS. See Gargarisma Boracis.

GLANDES QUERCUS TOSTÆ. PRUSS. PH. Acorns, freed from their coating, and roasted in the same manner as coffee, and crushed. [Mixed with coffee, as a *tonic.*]

GUTTÆ SULPHURIS CARBURETI, LAMPADIUS. Bisulphuret of carbon fʒij, ether f℥j. A few drops on sugar. WUTZER. Bisulphuret of carbon ʒj, alcohol ʒij. From 5 to 10 or 15 drops, 3 times a day, *for rheumatism.*

HAUSTUS AMMONIÆ SESQUICARBONATIS. GUY'S H. Sesquicarbonate of ammonia ℈j, water f℥j, lemon-juice f℥ss. To be given effervescing.

HAUSTUS IPECACUANHÆ CUM ANTIMONIO. GUY'S H. Ipecac. wine fʒvj, antimonial wine fʒij. Mix.

HAUSTUS PYROXYLICUS. Pyroxylic spirit ♏v, comp. tincture of cardamoms fʒj, water fʒx.

HEPAR SULPHURIS. D. See Potassii Sulphuretum.

HEPAR ANTIMONII. Mix equal parts of black sulphuret of antimony and nitre, deflagrate them in a crucible, and pour out the fused mass.

HYDRARGYRI BICHLORIDUM CUM ALBUMINE. Mix ʒiv of corrosive sublimate with the whites of 6 eggs, very perfectly, and dry on plates in a stove.

HYDRARGYRI BROMIDUM. When a solution of bromide of potassium is added to a solution of proto-nitrate of mercury, an insoluble white precipitate falls, which is a bromide, or subbromide of mercury. Dose, one grain twice a day. By the direct action of bromine on mercury or its peroxide, a soluble salt is obtained, the dose of which is from 1-16th to 1-4th of a grain.

HYDRARGYRI CHLORO-IODIDUM. M. CAVENTOU. Dissolve bichloride of mercury in alcohol, and add an equal weight of biniodide of mercury; then carefully evaporate the mixed solutions to dryness. It is said to be more active than either of its constituents.

HYDRARGYRI PERNITRATIS LIQUOR. D. In f℥iss of pure nitric acid, diluted with f℥iss of distilled water, dissolve, by heat, ℥ij of pure mercury, and evaporate the solution to f℥iiss. [The same as Hydrargyri Deuto-nitras Liquidus.]

HYDRARGYRI ET AMMONIÆ NITRAS. WARD. Nitric acid ℥xvj, add gradually sesquicarbonate of ammonia, ℥viij; afterwards digest in a sand-bath with ℥iv of quicksilver, and when that quantity is dissolved, add more quicksilver by small quantities till the fluid ceases to act on it. Then evaporate the solution, and crystallize by refrigeration.

HYDRARGYRI SULPHAS. [Persulphas, 1826.] D. Place 10 ounces of quicksilver in a porcelain capsule with f℥vj of oil of vitriol, and apply heat until nothing remains but a white dry crystalline salt.

Hydrargyrum Purum. D. Having introduced 3 pounds (av.) of quicksilver into a small glass retort, over the body of which a hood of sheet iron is suspended, let the heat of a gas lamp be applied until two-thirds of the metal have distilled over. Boil this with f℥ss of pure muriatic acid, and f℥ij of distilled water; let it be washed entirely from acid, and dried by heat. P. directs it to be distilled from an iron or earthen retort, to which is fixed a tube of moistened linen, dipping into water: the metal to be dried, and passed through chamois leather. [Quicksilver may also be purified by heating it to 104° F., agitating it with a little strong solution of nitrate of mercury, and straining.]

Hydrargyrum et Stibium Sulphurata. See Æthiops Antimonialis.

Hydrogenium Carburetum. The mixed carburetted hydrogen gas, in the form of coal gas, is sometimes employed as a palliative in consumption. Dr. R. Clanny recommends it to be passed through water, then agitated with fresh precipitated carbonate of lead, and mixed in the gasometer with an equal quantity of common air. 12 cubic inches of the mixed gas to be inspired 3 or 4 times a day, and the quantity gradually increased to 20 C. I. [For *Sulphuretted* Hydrogen, see Acidum Hydrosulphuricum.]

Hydrolata. Distilled waters. See Aquæ Distillatæ.

Hyoscyamina. From henbane, as Lobelina. Dose not ascertained.

Ilicina. Boil a clear decoction of holly with animal charcoal stirring it constantly; let it settle, collect the deposited charcoal, wash it with cold water, dry it, and treat it with boiling alcohol; let the filtered liquid be evaporated to dryness. *Febrifuge.* Dose, gr. vi—xxiv?

Infusum Adianti. Canadian maidenhair ℥ss, boiling water Oij. Infuse till cold. Pectoral. Ad libitum.

Infusum Anthemidis et Aurantii. Dr. Percival. Chamomile flowers ℥j, dried orange-peel ℥ss, cold water ℔iij. Macerate for 24 hours.

Infusum Asclepiadis. Bark of the root of Ascl. Syriaca (common silk-weed) ℥j, boiling water Oj. Dose ℥j—℥iss? *In cough and dyspnœa.*

Infusum Carnis Bubulæ. *Beef Tea.* Professor Liebig. Let

℔j of beef, free from fat, be minced very small, as for sausage-meat; mix it with an equal weight of cold water, and heat it slowly to boiling; let it boil for a minute or two, and strain it through a cloth. It may be colored with roasted onion or burnt sugar, and salted to the taste. See also, Jusculum cum Carne Bovis.

INFUSUM CARTHAMI. Safflower ʒij, boiling water f℥xvj; infuse for an hour. By wineglassfuls, as a *diaphoretic.*

INFUSUM CARUI. Dr. WOOD. Bruised caraways ʒij, boiling water f℥xvj. A wineglassful, in *flatulence.*

INFUSUM CATARIÆ. Dry catmint ℥ij, boiling water Oj.

INFUSUM CINCHONÆ. L. Bruised yellow cinchona ℥j, boiling distilled water Oj; macerate for 2 hours in a covered vessel, and strain. E. directs under this name ℥j of any species of cinchona, according to prescription, in coarse powder, to infuse in Oj of boiling water for 4 hours. D. Coarsely powdered crown or pale bark ℥j, boiling water Oss; infuse 1 hour, and filter.

INFUSUM CINCHONÆ PALLIDÆ. L. With pale cinchona, as Inf. Cinchonæ. Dose, of either infusion, f℥j to f℥iij.

INFUSUM CINCHONÆ SPISSATUM. L. Macerate ℔iij of coarsely pulverized yellow bark in Ovj of [cold] distilled water, as directed for Extract of Bark, and strain. Evaporate the mixed infusions to one-fourth, and set aside for the dregs to subside. Pour off the clear liquor, and strain the remainder. Then mix, and again evaporate till the specific gravity becomes 1·200. To this, when cold, gently drop in rectified spirit in the proportion of fʒiij to each fʒj of liquid. Lastly, set aside for 20 days, that the dregs may entirely subside. [fʒj is equivalent to f℥j of bark, or Oj of the infusion.]

INFUSUM CINCHONÆ PALLIDÆ SPISSATUM. L. In the same manner, from pale bark.

INFUSUM COPALCHI. Dr. STARK. Bruised bark of copalkecroton ℥ss, boiling water Oj; infuse for 2 hours, and strain. Dose, f℥ss 3 times a day. A warm bitter.

INFUSUM CONTRAYERVÆ. Dr. PEREIRA. Powdered contrayerva ʒiv, boiling water f℥vj. Dose, f℥j to f℥ij.

INFUSUM COTULÆ. From dried flowers of Anthemis cotula, as Inf. Anthemidis.

INFUSUM DRACONTII. Skunk-cabbage-root ℥j, boiling water Oss.

INFUSUM EUPATORII CANNABINI, may be made as Infusum Eupatorii.

INFUSUM FRASERÆ. American colombo ℥j, boiling water f℥xvj. Dose, ℥j to ℥ij.

INFUSUM FULIGINIS ALKALINUM. Wood-soot O¼, hickory ashes Oj, boiling water Oiv; infuse 24 hours, and decant. A popular American remedy for *dyspepsia with acidity;* f℥iss 3 times a day.

INFUSUM GUACO. SIMMONDS. Bruised leaves and stems of guaco (Mikania Guaco) ℥j, boiling water Oj.

INFUSUM MARRUBII. Dried horehound [ʒiv, Dr. PEREIRA; ℥j, Dr. ROYLE], boiling water Oj. Dose ℥j to ℥ij.

INFUSUM PARIETARIÆ. RATIER. Dry pellitory of the wall ℥j, boiling water Oiss: infuse half an hour, and strain. By wineglassfuls, in *calculous disorders, dropsies,* &c.

INFUSUM POLYGALÆ. D. Bruised polygala root (Senega) ℥ss, boiling water f℥ix. Digest 1 hour, and strain.

INFUSUM SALICIS. Dr. ROYLE. Bark of the more bitter and astringent kinds of willow ℥j, boiling water Oj. A wineglassful every 2 or 3 hours.

INFUSUM SAPONARIÆ. *Tisane de Saponaire.* P. Soapwort-root ℥j, liquorice-root ℥ij, boiling water f℥xxxvj; macerate for 4 hours.

INFUSUM SARZÆ ACIDUM. Dr. HANCOCK. Sarsaparilla ʒx, boiling water Oj, muriatic acid ♏xxx to ♏xl. Infuse in a glass vessel for some hours, and strain. Dr. H. says the efficacy of the infusion is greatly increased by the acid.

INFUSUM SARSAPARILLÆ COMPOSITUM. D. 1826. Sarsap. ℥j [cold], lime water f℥xvj; macerate in a closed vessel for 12 hours, and strain. Dr. O'BEIRNE prescribes ℥ij of sarsaparilla, ʒij of liquorice root, to Oj of lime water; to macerate 24 hours. Dose, f℥iv to f℥vj, twice a day.

INFUSUM SARZÆ FRIGIDUM. GUY'S H. Sarsa ℥ij, lime water Oij: rub the sliced sarsaparilla with the lime water, in a marble mortar with a wooden pestle, for ¼ of an hour; then macerate, with occasional stirring, for 6 hours. Dose f℥ij to f℥iv.

INFUSUM SENNÆ. E. Infus. Sennæ Compositum, L. & D.

	L.		D.		E.	
Senna, . . .	ʒxv	..	ʒiv	..	ʒxij	Infuse for
Ginger, . . .	℈iv	..	ʒss	..	℈iv	one hour
Boiling water, .	Oj	..	Oss	..	Oj	and strain.

Dose, f℥ij to f℥iv.

INFUSUM SENNÆ CUM COFFEA. Mix infusion of senna with an equal quantity of infusion of roasted coffee. *For children.*

INFUSUM VETIVERIÆ. Roots of andropogon muriaticum (vetiver) ℥j, boiling water Oss; infuse till cold. Dose, ℥ss. [A weak infusion, ʒj, or ʒij to Oj of water, is used *ad libitum, in slight fevers.*]

IODINIUM PURUM. D. Place iodine in a deep circular porcelain capsule, and having covered this accurately with a glass matrass filled with cold water, apply a water heat to the capsule for 20 minutes, then, withdrawing the heat, allow it to cool. Should the sublimate attached to the bottom of the matrass include acicular prisms of a white color and pungent odor, let it be scraped off with a glass rod, and rejected. The matrass being returned, apply a gentle and steady heat, so as to sublime the entire of the iodine. Separate it from the bottom of the matrass, and immediately enclose it in a bottle furnished with an accurately ground stopper.

IODINII CHLORIDUM. SOUBEIRAN. Diffuse iodine in water, and pass into it a current of chlorine gas: a liquid of a deep red color is obtained, the irritating vapor of which has been tried in some affections of the eyes by Dr. TURNBULL.

IODINII LIQUOR COMPOSITUS. E. See Liquor Iodinei C.

LACTUCINA. *Lactucine.* LENOUR. Exhaust lactucarium with boiling alcohol. Redissolve what is deposited on cooling in sufficient hot alcohol, digest with animal charcoal, filter while hot, and let it cool.

LICHEN ISLANDICUS PRÆPARATUS. *Iceland moss deprived of its bitterness.* BERZELIUS. Macerate ℔ij of Iceland moss in ℔xxxvj of water containing ℥ij of pearlash, for 24 hours. Wash the moss thoroughly without pressure. M. ROBINET steeps the moss in cold water, renewed every 6 hours, for 3 days. M. COLDEFY heats the water to 140° F., strains, and repeats this 2 or 3 times.

LIMONADUM MAGNESIÆ AERATUM. DALLIER. Pure citrate of

magnesia ℥j, heavy carbonate of magnesia ʒiiss, citric acid in coarse powder ʒiv, refined sugar (powdered, and aromatized with lemon) ʒxj. Mix; for a pint of water.

LINIMENTUM ALLII. Juice of garlic, mixed with olive oil. *Used in infantile convulsions.*

LINIMENTUM ANTISPASMODICUM. HUFELAND. Oil of cajeput ℈j, oil of mint ℈j, compound camphor liniment ℥j, laudanum ʒj. Mix.

LINIMENTUM CALCIS CHLORINATÆ. SCHOENLEIN. Chloride of lime ℥j, soap ℥ij, water q. s. *For Itch.*

LINIMENTUM CAMPHORÆ ACETICUM. BRANDE. Tincture of camphor f℥iij, acetic acid ℥j. Mix.

LINIMENTUM CHLOROFORMI. WAHU. Chloroform ʒj, rectified spirit ʒij; dissolve, add ʒvj of oil of almonds, and agitate strongly.

LINIMENTUM COLCHICI. EAR INFIRMARY. Soap liniment f℥j, wine of colchicum seed f℥ss. Mix.

LINIMENTUM COLCHICI CUM CAMPHORA. DR. LAYCOCK. Tincture of colchicum, and comp. tincture of camphor, in equal quantities.

LINIMENTUM COLOCYNTHIDIS. HEIM. Tincture of colocynth ℥ss, castor oil ℥iss. A teaspoonful to be rubbed over the belly night and morning; as a purgative, or to disperse swollen glands.

LINIMENTUM GLYCERINII. MR. STARTIN. Soap liniment ℥iij, pure glycerine ℥j, extract of belladonna ʒj. Mix. *For gouty, rheumatic, and neuralgic pains; bruises, sprains,* &c. A little veratrine is sometimes added.

LINIMENTUM GLYCERINÆ [GUMMOSUM.] Powdered tragacanth ʒij to ℥ss, lime water ℥viij, pure glycerine ℥j, rose water ℥iij. *For superficial burns, excoriations, chaps of lips or nipples,* &c.

LINIMENTUM HYDRARGYRI CUM IODINEO. CUT. H. Iodine ℥ss, glycerine ℥ij, olive oil ℥iiiss, stronger mercurial ointment ℥ij. Dissolve, and mix.

LINIMENTUM HYDRARGYRI NITRICO-OXYDI. CUT. H. Castor oil ℥iv, lard ℥iv, levigated nitric oxide of mercury ʒij, oil of bitter almonds ʒss. Mix.

LINIMENTUM IODINII CUM OPIO. CUT. H. Equal parts comp. tincture of iodine and tincture of opium.

LINIMENTUM OLEI TEREBINTHINÆ. See Linimentum Terebinthinatum. GUY'S H.

LINIMENTUM PLUMBI ET ALBUMINIS. SCHWARTZE. Fresh linseed oil ℥viij, whites of 6 eggs, liquid diacetate of lead ℥j.

LINIMENTUM ZINGIBERIS. Dr. A. TURNBULL. Prepare a strong essence of ginger, by percolation, or by digestion and expression, with two parts of rectified spirit to one of ginger; decolorize it with animal charcoal, and filter. To be rubbed for 5 or 10 minutes over the whole forehead, as a remedy for *short-sightedness.* [Some ointments have also been termed Liniments. See UNGUENTA.]

LINTEUM. *Lint. Charpie.* It is made from linen rags carefully cleaned, and scraped with a knife, by means of a suitable apparatus. There are also several kinds of lint directly manufactured from linen or cotton.

LINTEUM NIGRUM. Mr. HIGGINBOTTOM. Dissolve ʒij of nitrate of silver in f℥iv of distilled water; saturate ℥j of fine lint with the solution, and expose it in a flat vessel to dry. Used in the treatment of old ulcers. [FRICKE'S LINTEUM INFERNALE is made with a weaker solution, gr. x to f℥j.]

LIQUOR ACIDI ARSENIOSI HYDROCHLORICUS. See Liquor Arsenici Chloridi.

LIQUOR ACONITINÆ. Dr. F. W. HEADLAND. (See p. 21.) Dissolve aconitine, gr. j, in rectified spirit, ʒj; add distilled water ʒix. (Each fluid drachm contains $\frac{1}{10}$th of a grain, and each drop $\frac{1}{600}$.) Dose, internally, ♏v.—♏xij.

LIQUOR ANIXII. Spirit of hartshorn saturated with sulphuric acid. Dose, 60 drops.

LIQUOR AMMONIÆ CITRATIS. L. Citric acid ℥iij, distilled water Oj; dissolve, and add ℥iiss of sesquicarbonate of ammonia, or q. s. to neutralize it. Dose, fʒiiss to fʒiv.

LIQUOR AMMONIÆ SUCCINATUS. See Liquor Cornu C. Succinatus.

LIQUOR AMMONIÆ TARTRATIS. May be made with ℥iij of tartaric acid, Oj of water, and ℥ii¼ or q. s. of sesquicarbonate of ammonia. [For the empyreumatic form, see Liq. Cornu Cervi Tartarisatus.]

LIQUOR ANTIMONII TARTARIZATI. D. Tartarized antimony 54 grains, distilled water Oj, dissolve, filter, and add f℥vij of rectified spirit. Dose, as Vinum Antimonii Potassio-tartratis.

LIQUOR ANTIMONII TERCHLORIDI. D. On 1℔ av. of prepared sulphuret of antimony pour Oiv of com. muriatic acid, and constantly stirring, beneath a flue with a good draught, apply a gentle heat, which must be gradually augmented as the development of gas begins to slacken, and finally kept at a boiling temperature for 15 minutes. Strain through calico, returning what passes first; and transfer the clear liquid into another capsule, and boil it down to Oij. The sp. gr. should be 1·470.

LIQUOR ANTINEPHRITICUS. ADAMS. Poppy heads ℥vj, water Oiss; boil to ℥viij, strain with pressure, and add ℥j of nitre. Dose, ʒij, night and morning, in warm linseed tea. *In painful affections of the urinary organs.*

LIQUOR ANTIPODAGRICUS. BEGUIN. Mix one part of fuming liquor of Boyle with three of spirit of wine. Dose, 30 or 40 drops. As *sudorific in gout;* also applied externally with camphor.

LIQUOR ARSENIATIS AMMONIÆ. H. OF ST. LOUIS. Arseniate of ammonia gr. iv, distilled water f℥iv, spirit of angelica fʒij. Dose, ♏xij to xxx. [There are other formulæ for this solution, differing in strength from the above. Dr. NELIGAN gives as BIETT'S—Arseniate of ammonia gr. iss, distilled water f℥iij, spirit of angelica fʒvj. Dose, fʒj to fʒiij. BOUCHARDAT says, gr. vj to ℥viij of distilled water. Dose, from 12 drops to ʒj.]

LIQUOR ARSENIATIS SODÆ. PEARSON'S Arsenical Solution. Arseniate of soda gr. iv, distilled water f℥iv. Dose, from ♏xij to ♏xxx in the day.

LIQUOR ARSENICI CHLORIDI. L. Bruised arsenious acid ʒss, hydrochloric acid fʒiss, distilled water f℥j; boil until dissolved; then add so much distilled water that the whole shall measure exactly f℥xx. [This was previously in use under the name of DE VALANGIN'S *Mineral Solvent.* Dr. Farr gives 3 drops 3 times a day, increasing the dose 1 drop daily till 10 drops are taken for each dose.]

LIQUOR ARSENICI ET IODINII. Dr. DUNGLISON. Compound solution of iodine (Liquor Iodinii Comp. U. S.) ℥j, solution of arsenite of potash ℥iv. Mix. Dose, 5 drops. [It loses its color.]

LIQUOR CALCII CHLORIDI. L. *Calcis Muriatis Solutio,* E. Chloride of calcium (dry muriate of lime) ℥iv, [℥iij, D.]

[crystals ℥viij, E.], distilled water f℥xij. Mix. Dose, from ♏xv to fʒj.

Liquor Calcis Muriatis. L. 1824. See Liquor Calcii Chloridi.

Liquor Chiraytæ. Treat ℥iv of bruised chirayta as directed for Liq. Calumbæ. The water may be either cold or newmilk-warm: 1 part to 7 of water makes the Infusion.

Liquor Cinchonæ. See Infusum Cinchonæ Spissatum.

Liquor Cornu Cervi. See Liquor Volatilis Cornu Cervi.

Liquor Cornu Cervi Succinatus. P. Neutralize true spirit of hartshorn (or a solution of ℥j of salt of hartshorn in ʒviij of water) with acid of amber.

Liquor Cornu Cervi Tartarizatus. As the last, substituting tartaric for succinic acid.

Liquor Creasoti. Reichenbach. Creasote ʒij, rectified spirit ʒiv, warm distilled water ℔iss.

Liquor Ergotæ. See Essentia Secalis Cornuti.

Liquor Ferri Acetatis. See Ferri Acetas, D. The Prus. Ph. directs the oxide precipitated from ℥vj of liquor ferri sesquichloridi by ammonia, to be washed, pressed, and dissolved in ℥vij of strong acetic acid.

Liquor Ferri Chlorati [Chloridi]. Prus. Ph. Put into a bottle sufficiently large ℥ij of iron wire, and add ℥x of hydrochloric acid (sp. gr. 1·12), and ℥v of distilled water. Set aside in a warm place for 24 hours, shaking occasionally; then filter rapidly, and add 10 drops of hydrochloric acid, and keep it in well-stopped 2-ounce bottles. It contains 10·8 per cent. of iron.

Liquor Ferri Sesquichlorati [Sesquichloridi]. Prus. Ph. Heat ℥xij of the last solution with ℥iij of hydrochloric acid, in a porcelain vessel, gradually adding ℥iiiss of nitric acid (sp. gr. 1·20), or so much that the solution shall not yield a green or blue color in a solution of red prussiate of potash. Evaporate with a gentle heat, so that it may be solid when cold; dissolve in ℥vj of distilled water, adding as much hydrochloric acid as is required to produce a clear solution with the aid of heat. Evaporate to ℥vj, and add ℥iss of distilled water or q. s. to make the sp. gr. 1·535 to 1·540.

LIQUOR FERRI IODIDI. U. S. Mix ℥ij of iodine with f℥v of water, and add ℥j of iron filings; stir frequently, and heat the mixture gently till it assumes a greenish color; then filter into a glass bottle containing ℥xij of powdered sugar; and after it has passed, pour distilled water on the filter, until the filtered liquor, including the sugar, measures f℥xx. Lastly, shake the bottle till the sugar is dissolved. It contains about 58 grains of iodide of iron in f℥j. [CUT. H. directs, iron wire ℥iv, iodine ℥iiss, water Oiij. Dose, ♏xv to ʒj.] See also Solutio Ferri Iodidi, and Syrupus Ferri Iodidi. E.

LIQUOR HYDRARGYRI BICHLORIDI. L. Bichloride of mercury ℈ss, hydrochlorate of ammonia ℈ss, distilled water Oj; dissolve. It contains gr. j of sublimate in f℥ij, or 876 grains. Dose, fʒss to fʒij. [P. (*Liqueur de Van Swieten*) directs 1 grain of the bichloride, 100 of rectified spirit, and 900 of distilled water. PRUS. PH. is *twice* the strength of L.]

LIQUOR HYDRARGYRI NITRICI [PROTO-NITRATIS]. PRUS. PH. Protonitrate of mercury ℥j, distilled water ℥viij, nitric acid (sp. gr. 1·2) ℈iiiss; filter, adding water, if necessary, to make its density 1·100. Dose, 1 to 5 drops.

LIQUOR INDIGO SULPHATIS. Digest 1 part of powdered indigo in 10 of sulphuric acid; when dissolved, dilute it with water. As a *Test.*

LIQUOR MAGNESIÆ TARTRATIS. M. AIRAT. Tartaric acid ℥xv¼, distilled water Oxx, fresh calcined magnesia (diffused in ℥xvj of distilled water) ℥iij ʒj; mix. Dose, as a purgative, f℥xv.

LIQUOR MORPHIÆ MURIATIS. D. See Liquor Morphiæ Hydrochloratis.

LIQUOR NITRI CAMPHORATUS. BAUME. Nitre ʒiv, water ℥iv; dissolve, and add ℈ij of spirit of camphor. Agitate and filter. Dose, 6 to 24 drops.

LIQUOR OPII MURIATICUS. Dr. NICHOL'S *Muriate of Opium.* Powdered Turkey opium ℥j, distilled water f℥xx, muriatic acid fʒj. Mix, shake it frequently every day for a fortnight, then strain, and filter. Dose, from 20 to 40 drops. Dr. N. considers it preferable to every other preparation of opium. [We have taken the liberty of slightly altering the names of this and some kindred compounds, to prevent mistake, and to promote uniformity of nomenclature among analogous preparations.]

LIQUOR PYROTARTARICUS RECTIFICATUS. SAX. PH. Half fill an iron or earthen retort with cream of tartar, and distil with a gradually increased heat, into a large receiver furnished with a safety tube. Redistil the liquid. Dose, 10 to 20 drops, repeated.

LIQUOR SENNÆ AROMATICUS. Dr. TWEEDIE. Exhaust 15℔s (av.) of Tinnevelli senna with 4½ or 5 gallons of water, by displacement, or by maceration and expression. Evaporate the liquor to 10℔s. (av.) Concentrate 6℔s (av.) of treacle over a water-bath until a little of it becomes nearly dry on cooling; dissolve this in the strained liquor. When cold, add Oiss of tincture of ginger, and water, if necessary, to make up Oxij.

LIQUOR SODÆ. L. (Liquor Sodæ Causticæ, D.) *Soap Lees.* L. directs it to be prepared in the same manner as Liquor Potassæ, from f℥xxxj of crystallized carbonate of soda, ℥ix of quick lime, and Cj of boiling distilled water. Sp. gr. 1·061, contains 4 per cent. of soda. D. directs it to be made from 2℔s. (av.) of carb. of soda, 10 ounces of lime, and Cj f℥vij of distilled water; proceeding as directed for Liquor Potassæ. Sp. gr. 1·056. [P. directs it to be made by dissolving pure soda in water to form a solution of 1·334 density; containing about 31 per cent. of soda. PRUS. PH. prescribes ℔iv carb. soda, ℔xx of water, and ℔j of lime. It is of nearly the same strength as the L. & D.] It should be kept in well-stopped green-glass bottles.

LIQUOR SODÆ CARBONATIS. D. Cr. carbonate of soda ℥iss, distilled water Oj: dissolve and filter. Sp. gr. 1·026.

LIQUORES VINOSI. Dr. B. LANE'S *Medicated Wines.* Permanent preparations of aloes, senna, calumba, gentian, rhubarb, and other vegetable drugs may be made by preparing a strong infusion (of double or quadruple strength) of the substance, adding to it 60 ounces of white sugar for 7 pints of the infusion, and sufficient yeast to produce fermentation. Let them ferment in casks or jars, at first open, and afterwards lightly closed, at a temperature of about 65°, till the action subsides; then draw off the clear liquid into fresh vessels, and keep them closed till it is fit for bottling.

LOBELINA. Mr. BASTICK. Macerate ℔ij of lobelia inflata for 48 hours in Cj of alcohol mixed with ℥iij of sulphuric acid. Filter the solution, and add powdered quick lime till it has an alkaline reaction. Again filter, and saturate the filtrate with sulphuric acid in slight excess, filter, and evaporate to one fourth. Add a little water to the residue, and evaporate all the remaining alcohol. Filter, saturate the filtrate with solution of carbonate of potash, and agitate the liquid with successive portions of æther till it no longer dissolves anything. By evaporating the æthereal solution, lobelina remains. It may be rendered colorless, by dissolving in alcohol and agitating with animal charcoal. Dose, not ascertained.

LOTIO ACIDI NITRICI. CUT. H. Dilute nitric acid f℈v, tincture of myrrh f℈ss, water Oj. To be diluted with 1, 2, or 3 parts of water.

LOTIO ACONITINÆ. Dr. F. W. HEADLAND. To liquor aconitinæ, ℈x, add glycerine ℈ij. (℈ss at a time to be rubbed on to the face, &c., in *neuralgia.*)

LOTIO AMMONIÆ MURIATIS CUM ARNICA. CARUS. Sal ammoniac ℈j to ℈ij, rue water f℥ix, vinegar of rue ℥iv, tincture of arnica ℈j to ℈ij.

LOTIO ANTIMONII TARTARIZATI. Dr. CLOC. Dissolve gr. x of emetic tartar in ℔j of water. Linen cloths wet with the lotion to be applied, and frequently changed.

LOTIO BELLADONNÆ COMPOSITUM. CUT. H. Extract of belladonna ℥ss, hydrocyanic acid ℈ij, glycerine ℥j, water f℥xviij; mix. ℥j to be mixed with ℥j to ℥iij of water.

LOTIO BISMUTHI NITRATIS. CUT. H. Trisnitrate of bismuth ℥iss, bichloride of mercury ℈vss, spirit of camphor ℈ij, water Cj; mix. To be diluted with from 1 to 3 parts of water.

LOTIO BORACIS CUM CRETA. Dr. JOHNSON'S *Lotion for Sore Nipples.* Borax ℈ij, precipitated chalk ℥j, rose water ℥iij, spirit of wine ℥iij.

LOTIO GALLÆ. St. B. H. Bruised nutgall ℈ij, boiling water Oj. Infuse, and strain. MID. H. ℈iij to f℥xij.

LOTIO GLYCERINÆ CUM CANTHARIDE. Mr. STARTIN. Aromatic spirit of ammonia ℥j, glycerine ℈iv, tincture of cantharides ℈j—ij, rosemary water f℥xiv. Once or twice a day to the hair, with a wet hair-brush.

LOTIO GLYCERINÆ CUM ACIDO NITRICO. Mr. STARTIN. Dilute nitric acid ℈ss to ℈j, trisnitrate of bismuth ℈ss, tincture of digitalis ℈j, glycerine ℈iv, rose water f℥viiiss. To allay itching, *in prurigo,* &c.

LOTIO HYDRARGYRI CHLORIDI CUM CALCE. See Lotio Hydrargyri Cinerea.

LOTIO HYDROCYANICA ALKALINA. Dr. A. T. THOMSON, *in milk scall.* Bicarbonate of soda ʒij, milk ℥viij, hydrocyanic acid fʒss.

LOTIO IODO-SULPHURATA. DAUVERGNE. Dissolve ʒvj of iodide of potassium in ℥iij of water, and add ʒiij of iodine. Dissolve also ℥iv of sulphuret of potassium in ℥viij of water. Mix a teaspoonful of the former solution with a tablespoonful of the latter, and put it into a washhand-basin of warm or cold water. *In some skin diseases.*

LOTIO OPII CUM ALUMINE. CUT. H. Tincture of opium ℥j, alum ℔ij, tincture of galls ℥iij, water Cj. Mix. f℥j to ℥j or ℥iij of water.

LOTIO POTASSII IODIDI. Dr. O. WARD uses ʒj iodide of potassium in from 8 to 16 ounces of water for the cure of *itch.*

LOTIO POTASSÆ SULPHURETI. St. B. H. Sulphuret of potash ʒij, water Oj.

LOTIO RUBRA. CUT. H. Bichloride of mercury gr. xviij, bisulphuret of mercury gr. ix, creasote ♏vj, water f℥viij. f℥j to f℥j—iij of water.

LOTIO RUBRA COMPOSITA. CUT. H. Equal measures of lotio rubra, lotio nigra, and water. f℥j to f℥j—iij of water.

LOTIO STAPHISAGRIÆ. Powdered stavesacre seeds ʒiv, water Oiss. Boil.

LOTIO SULPHURIS. CUT. H. Precipitated sulphur ℥x, spirit of camphor ℥ss, glycerine ℥iv, vermilion ʒij, water Cj. Mix. f℥j to f℥j—iij of water.

LOTIO SULPHUREA COMPOSITA. CUT. H. Powdered white hellebore ℥iss, boiling water Cj. Macerate for a night, strain, and add ʒij of bichloride of mercury, ʒij of white precipitate, and ℥vj of diluted sulphurous acid. [No form is given for the latter ingredient.] f℥j to be mixed with f℥j—iij of water.

LOTIO SULPHUREA DEPILATORIA. CUT. H. Fresh lime ℔j, water Cj, hydrosulphuric acid q. s. [M. BOUDET recommends, as the best depilatory, crystallized hydrosulphate of soda 3 parts, powdered quicklime 10 parts, starch 10 parts; to be mixed with water at the time of using. To be scraped off in a minute or two.]

LOTIO SULPHURETI SODÆ. Dr. BARLOW. *For Tinea*, &c. Sulphuret of soda ʒij, white soap ʒiiss, rectified spirit ʒij, lime water f℥vij.

LOTIO ZINCI IODIDI. Dr. ROSS. Boil from ʒj to ʒij of iodine with half its weight of zinc, in f℥viij of water, until the liquid is colorless, and filter. Applied, by means of a sponge, to *Enlarged Tonsils.*

MAGNESIÆ CITRAS. Dissolve citric acid in water, and add to the hot solution carbonate of magnesia till it ceases to be acted on; filter the solution while hot, and set aside to crystallize, concentrating it by evaporation, if necessary. Laxative, rather milder than the sulphate. This salt is apt to take the form of an insoluble hydrate. DORVAULT says the following method yields a neutral salt, which forms a permanent solution with 8 or 10 times its weight of water. Fuse 100 parts of citric acid in its water of crystallization by heating it in a water-bath, and incorporate with it 29 parts of calcined magnesia. The pasty product soon hardens, when it should be reduced to powder, and preserved for use. Or 64 parts of common carbonate of magnesia may be substituted for the calcined. [Others recommend the dry ingredients to be kept mixed, and a portion of it mixed with water when a solution of the salt is required. Pulverize 14 parts of citric acid, dry it carefully, and gradually add 10 parts of dry carbonate of magnesia. When required for use, add it gradually to the water previously placed in a mortar. M. THEVENOT directs 3 parts of dry citric acid in powder to be mixed with 1 of calcined magnesia; this is slightly acid. ROGE'S purgative consists of calcined magnesia 8 parts, carbonate of magnesia 4, dry citric acid 26, sugar (aromatized with lemon) 50 parts. See Liquor Magnesiæ Citratis.]

MAGNESIÆ BORO-CITRAS. CADET. Dissolve 260 grains of citric acid in Oiiiss water; add this gradually to 113 grains of boracic acid, and 80 grains of calcined magnesia in a porcelain vessel, so as to form a paste; then add the rest of the solution, boil to a paste, and dry it carefully.

MAGNESIÆ FERRO-SULPHAS. The salt sold under this name is sulphate of magnesia, containing 5 per cent. of sulphate of iron.

MAGNESIÆ, FERRI, ET QUINÆ SULPHAS. The article thus named appears to be made by adding a little sulphate of quinine to the preceding.

MAGNESIÆ TARTRAS. PEREIRA. Saturate a solution of tartaric acid with carbonate of magnesia, and evaporate to dryness. Dose, ℈j to ℈iij, in chronic maladies of the spleen. [RADMACHER.]

MAGNESIÆ POTASSIO-TARTRAS. MAILLIER. Boil 30 parts of cream of tartar, 8½ (or q. s.) of carbonate of magnesia, in 700 of water, and set aside to crystallize.

MAGNESIÆ ET POTASSÆ BORO-TARTRAS. M. GAROT. Borotartrate of potash 100 parts, water 600, carbonate of magnesia 24; boil, filter, evaporate to a paste, and dry at a gentle heat. It is taken in the following form: the above paste ℥j, citric acid ʒss, syrup of lemon peel ℥ij, water Oss.

MALORUM SUCCUS. *Verjuice.* Bruise wild apples (crabs), and express the juice.

MANGANESII ACETAS. Dissolve the carbonate of manganese in strong acetic acid, and evaporate, that crystals may form. Dose, 5 to 10 grains.

MANGANESII CHLORIDUM *vel* MURIAS. Saturate muriatic acid with carbonate of manganese, and evaporate to dryness by a gentle heat. Preserve it in closely-stopped bottles. Dose, 3 to 10 grains.

MANGANESII IODIDUM. Digest recently precipitated carbonate of manganese with fresh hydriodic acid, filtering and evaporating, the access of air being prevented. See Pilulæ Manganesii Iodidi, and Syr. M. I., for the best method of exhibiting it.

MANGANESII MALAS. From the fresh carbonate and malic acid, as Mang. acetas. Dose, 2 to 6 grains.

MANGANESII OXYDUM HYDRATUM. It may be precipitated from the sulphate by caustic potash or ammonia, and the precipitate well washed. It requires to be used while fresh, mixed with syrup, or an oily emulsion.

MANGANESII PHOSPHAS. Into a solution of sulphate of manganese drop a solution of phosphate of soda, collect, wash, and dry the precipitate, and keep it in well-closed bottles.

MANGANESII TARTRAS. Saturate a solution of tartaric acid with fresh carbonate of manganese, and evaporate. See Syrupus Mang. Tartratis. [These compounds of manganese are employed by M. HANNON, in *Anæmia*, *Cachectic diseases*, &c.

The insoluble preparations, as the carbonate, phosphate, and oxide, should be first used; then the soluble salts. The use of this remedy does not require to be persevered in so long as that of iron.]

MARRUBINA. MARRUBINE. A vegetable principle from white horehound, substituted for quinine.

MASTICATORIA. *Masticatories.* See Pilæ Masticatoriæ.

MEL FILICIS. DUNGLISON. Æthereal extract of fern ʒss, honey of roses ℥ss. Mix. Half at bed-time, the rest in the morning. *For Tapeworm.*

MISTURA ACACIÆ. L. Mucilago, E.; Muc. Acaciæ, D. and U. S. *Mucilage.* Gum arabic ℥x (E. ℥ix), water Oj. L. directs the powdered gum to be dissolved in boiling water. E. directs the gum to be dissolved in cold water (which is better), and strained through linen. D. directs 4 ounces of gum to be dissolved in 6 ounces of water, and strained through flannel. U. S. Powdered gum ℥iv, boiling water f℥viij. Dr. CHRISTISON recommends the gum to be tied in linen.

MISTURA ACIDA. See Julepum Acidum.

MISTURA AMMONIÆ PHOSPHATIS. CUT. H. Phosphate of ammonia ℥j, sesquicarbonate of soda ʒiv, compound tincture of lavender ʒss, water Oj: mix, and dissolve. Dose, ʒij—iv, in water.

MISTURA AMYGDALÆ AMARÆ. GUY'S H. directs it to be made as Mist. Amygdalæ, substituting bitter almonds for sweet. D. 1826 [Mist. Amygdalæ]. Sweet almonds, blanched, ℥iss; bitter almonds, blanched, ℈ij; white sugar ℥ss, water Oij. [BERAL directs sweet almonds ʒvj, bitter ʒij, water f℥xvj.]

MISTURA ANISATA. GLAS. H. Refined sugar ʒiij, mucilage ʒj, oil of aniseed ʒiss; rub together, and add gradually f℥vj of cinnamon water. Dose, f℥j.

MISTURA ANTIMONII POTASSIO-TARTRATIS. CUT. H. Potassio-tartrate of antimony ℈ss, tincture of digitalis ℥j, nitre ℥ss, comp. tragacanth powder ℥ss, water Oij. Mix. Dose, ʒij—iv.

MISTURA ARGENTI NITRATIS. TROUSSEAU. Nitrate of silver gr. j, distilled water f℥vss, syrup ℥ss. Dose, ℥j daily, *in hooping cough.*

MISTURA BENZOATA. Dr. G. BIRD. Benzoic acid ℈ij, carbonate

of soda ʒiss, phosphate of soda ʒiij, boiling water ℥iv; dissolve, and add cinnamon-water f℥viiss, tincture of henbane fʒiv. Dose, fʒj 3 times a day.

MISTURA BIBERINÆ. Dr. PEREIRA. Subsulphate of biberine ʒss, diluted sulphuric acid ♏xxv, syrup f℥j, tincture of orange-peel f℥j, water f℥iv. A tablespoonful three times a day. [GL. H. Sulphate of beberine ʒj, aromatic sulphuric acid ʒij, water ℥viij.]

MISTURA BISULPHURETI CARBONIS. CLARUS. Bisulphuret of carbon ℈j, sugar ʒij, milk ℥vj. Dose, ℥ss 4 times a day.

MISTURA CAFFEINÆ. VANDEN-CORPUT. Caffein gr. vij, distilled water f℥iij, hydrochloric acid 2 drops, syrup of orange-flower water ℥ss. Mix. Dose, a tablespoonful.

MISTURA CAFFEINÆ CITRATIS. *Potion contremigraine.* Syrup of citrate of caffein ℥j, water (or any agreeable diluent) ℥v. A tablespoonful frequently.

MISTURA CEREVISIÆ. See Mistura Fermenti.

MISTURA CHLOROFORMI. WAHER. Put into a bottle 30 or 40 drops of rectified spirit, add 15 to 20 drops of chloroform, close the bottle and shake strongly; then add ℥j of syrup, and ℥iij of water.

MISTURA CINCHONÆ OPIATA. Dr. WOOD. Red cinchona ℥ss, confection of opium ʒj, lemon juice ʒij, Port wine f℥iv. A third part every 3 hours; *in intermittents.*

MISTURA EMETO-CATHARTICA. GLAS. H. Tartarized antimony gr. ij, sulphate of magnesia ℥ij, water ℔ij. Dose, f℥ij every 2 hours.

MISTURA FEBRIFUGA CLUTTONI. CLUTTON'S Febrifuge tincture f℥ss, water f℥vij, syrup (simple, or of red poppies, &c.) fʒiv. Dose, f℥ss.

MISTURA FERMENTI CAMPHORATA. Dr. JONES LAMPREY. Yeast ℥x, camphor ʒss, spirit of nitric æther fʒiv. Dose, f℥j every 2 or 3 hours, *in petechial typhus.*

MISTURA FERRI ARSENICALIS. CUT. H. Arsenious acid ʒss, hydrochloric acid ʒj, tincture of sesquichloride of iron ℥vj, water Oviij. Dose, fʒj to ij in water; fʒj contains gr. $\frac{1}{40}$ of arsenious acid.

MISTURA FERRI IODIDI. GLAS. H. Syrup of iodide of iron ʒij, syrup of ginger ℥j, water ℥v. Mix. Dose, ℥ss three times a day.

MISTURA GLYCYRRHIZÆ COMPOSITA. U. S. Liquorice powder [Extract], gum arabic, sugar, each ʒiv, camphorated tincture of opium f℥ij, antimonial wine f℥j, spirit of nitric ether f℥ss, water f℥xij. Rub the liquorice, gum, and sugar, with the water gradually poured upon them, then add the other ingredients, and mix. [A modification of Mistura Fusca.]

MISTURA MAGNESIÆ SULPHATIS CUM ANTIMONIO. CH. Sulphate of magnesia ℥iv, tartarized antimony gr. ij, water Oj.

MISTURA MAGNESIÆ SULPHATIS CUM COFFÆA. M. COMBES. Sulphate of magnesia ℥j, ground roasted coffee ℥½, water Oj; boil for 2 minutes, remove from the fire, let it infuse for a few minutes, strain, and sweeten. By glassfuls, till it operates.

MISTURA OLEOSO-BALSAMICA. PRUS. PH. Essential oils of lavender, cloves, cinnamon, thyme, lemon, nutmeg, neroli, of each ℈j, Peruvian balsam ʒj, highly rectified spirit ℥x. Digest, and filter.

MISTURA PYROTARTARICA. SAX. PH. Compound spirit of angelica ℥vj, rectified pyrotartaric liquor (Liq. Pyrotartaricus rect.) ℥iv, sulphuric acid ℥ss (by weight). Mix. Has been recommended in *cholera*. Dose, 20 drops.

MISTURA QUINÆ CUM OPIO. CUT. H. Disulphate of quinine ʒvss, dilute sulphuric acid ℥iiss, tincture of opium ℥iiss, oil of caraway 20 drops, water Cj. Dose, ʒij—iv in water.

MISTURA SULPHURICA ACIDA. HALLER'S ELIXIR. PRUS. PH. To ℥iij of rectified spirit add gradually ℥j of pure sulphuric acid. Dose, 5 to 20 drops, diluted.

MISTURA VULNERARIA ACIDA. PRUS. PH. (*Aqua Vulneraria Thedeni.*) Vinegar ℔iij, proof spirit ℔iss, diluted sulphuric acid (1 part acid to 5 water) ℥vj, clarified honey ℔j. *For outward use.*

MORPHIÆ ACETATIS LIQUOR. See Liq. Morphiæ Acetatis.

MORPHIÆ ET CODEIÆ HYDROCHLORAS. GREGORY'S salt of opium. This is obtained in making the hydrochlorate of morphia, unless the morphia is precipitated by ammonia.

MORPHIÆ MURIATIS LIQUOR. D. *Solutio*, E. Muriate of morphia ʒiss, rectified spirit f℥v, distilled water f℥xv. See Liquor Morphiæ Hydrochloratis.

MORPHIÆ HYDRIODAS CUM IODINIO. BOUCHARDAT'S *Iodure d'iodhydrate de morphine.* Mix an acid solution of sulphate of morphia with an ioduretted solution of iodide of potassium, keeping the liquid at the temperature of 140° for an hour. Pour off the liquid, wash the scales, and dry them. Dose, gr. ¾ at bedtime.

MORPHIÆ ET ZINCI HYDRIODAS CUM IODINIO. BOUCHARDAT. Boil ℈j of ioduretted hydriodate of morphia with f℥ij of water and ℈x of zinc. After some days' action, filter the boiling liquid, which deposits the salt. [gr. iss in 8 pills, with marsh-mallow root and syrup; 1 or 2 daily, in *gastralgia*, &c.]

MUCILAGO HORDEI. D. Ground pearl barley ℥ss, water f℥xvj: triturate the barley with the water gradually added, and boil for a few minutes.

MUCILAGO OLEOSA. MIALHE. Powdered gum arabic ℥vj, white sugar ℥iij, almond oil ℥iij, water ℥viij. Mix. As a vehicle for medicines, an excipient for pills, &c.

NARCOTINÆ MURIAS. Exhaust opium by alcohol, add to the liquid sufficient ammonia to render it turbid; distil off ¾ of the spirit, and let the remaining fluid cool. Wash the crystalline mass with water, then dissolve it in water acidulated with muriatic acid (Oj of water, and ʒss of acid for each ℔j of opium); filter and evaporate to dryness. Dose, as an antiperiodic, 3 grains in the intermissions: in larger doses it is powerfully sudorific and calmative, as well as antiperiodic. [Dr. STEWART.]

NICOTIA. M. ORFILA. The vapor of tobacco is passed into cold water acidulated with sulphuric acid. An excess of an alkali is then added, and the nicotia set free is volatilized by heat. (An oily, colorless, strongly alkaline fluid, sp. gr. 1·048, boiling at 77° F. Very poisonous.)

OLEUM ALLII. A volatile oil (sulphuret of allyle) is obtained from garlic by distillation, which is a powerful irritant. A stimulating infused oil, is used externally in palsy and rheumatism.

OLEUM ALOETICUM. Distilled from socotrine aloes, as Ol. succini; externally, as a vermifuge.

OLEUM ANDÆ. Obtained by expression from the seeds of Anda Gomesii. *Purgative.* Dose, 20 to 30 drops in sugar. Dr. NORRIS prescribed 50 drops, but Dr. URE found 20 usually sufficient.

OLEUM ANISI. From Aniseeds. Dose, 2 to 8 drops.

Oleum Cadinum. *Huile de cade.* An empyreumatic oil obtained by dry distillation of the wood of the juniperus oxycedrus. But oil of tar is often substituted for it. Dose, a few drops in skin diseases, but chiefly externally.

Oleum Calami. By distillation from the rhizomes of acorus calamus.

Oleum Camphoræ Nitricum. Fee. Pulverized camphor 208 grains, nitric acid ℥j, dissolve without heat, and decant the oil.

Oleum Capsici. Dr. Turnbull. Heat in a water-bath ℥iv of cayenne pepper with Oj olive oil for 6 hours, and strain. Externally as a rubefacient in *cholera*, &c.

Oleum Iodatum. Marschal's *Iodized Oil.* Oil of almonds 15 parts, iodine 1 part. Triturate, and digest till dissolved.

Oleum Jatrophæ. Expressed from the seeds of jatropha curcas, or physic nuts; as Oleum Crotonis.

Oleum Juglandis. Expressed from walnuts, as Oleum Amygdalæ.

Oleum Lumbricorum. E. 1744. Washed earthworms ℔ss, olive oil Oiss, white wine Oss. Boil gently till the wine is consumed, and press, and strain.

Oleum Macidis. What is commonly termed *oil of mace* is expressed from nutmegs; but a volatile oil is obtained from mace by distillation.

Oleum Mudaris. Digest 10 grains of mudar bark in f℥j of olive oil, and strain. Applied with a camel-hair pencil to *cutaneous ulcers.*

Oleum Ophioglossi. From adder's tongue, as Ol. Belladonnæ.

Oleum Origani. From marjoram, by distillation. But the red oil sold under this name is obtained from common thyme (thymus vulgaris).

Oleum Pyrethri. Digest pellitory root in twice its weight of olive oil, and strain. Used in frictions as a rubefacient.

Oleum Succini. U. S. Half fill a glass retort with powdered amber mixed with an equal weight of sand, and distil by sand-bath, with a gradually increasing heat; then separate the oil from the acid liquor and concrete acid.

OLEUM TABACI [EMPYREUMATICUM]. U. S. Put ℔j of tobacco, in coarse powder, into a retort of green glass, connected with a refrigeratory, with a tube for the escape of incondensible products; then heat the retort by sand-bath gradually to dull redness, and keep it so until empyreumatic oil ceases to pass over; separate the oily liquid from the watery portion, and keep it for use. *Poisonous.*

OLEUM TANACETI. By distillation from the fresh tansy.

OLEUM TEREBINTHINÆ SULPHURATUM. Sulphurated linseed oil 1 part, oil of turpentine 3 parts.

OLEUM THYMI. The oil of common thyme is sold in the shops as Oleum Origani.

OLIVINA. *Olivine.* LANDERER. Treat olive-leaves with acidulated water, concentrate, precipitate with ammonia, redissolve the washed precipitate in a diluted acid, purify with animal charcoal, filter, and reprecipitate with ammonia.

OPII MURIAS. See Liquor Opii Muriaticus.

OXYGENIUM. P. *Oxygen Gas.* Heat chlorate of potash in a small retort or flask of green glass, as long as gas is disengaged, and collect the gas in a proper apparatus. [The process is much expedited by mixing the chlorate with an eighth part (in bulk) of black oxide of manganese.]

OXYMEL SCILLÆ COMPOSITUM. MANCH. H. Oxymel of squills f℥j, spirit of nitric ether ℥ss, tincture of tobacco f℥ss.

PASTA GUTTÆ PERCHÆ STYPTICA. Mr. BEARDSLEY. Gutta percha ℥j, Stockholm tar ℥iss or ℥ij, creasote ʒj, shell-lac ℥j, or q. s. to render it sufficiently hard. To be boiled together, with constant stirring, till it forms a homogeneous mass. For *alveolar hæmorrhage*, and as a stopping for teeth in toothache. To be softened by moulding with the fingers.

PESSI. The following *Medicated Pessaries* are used by Dr. SIMPSON:—

Pessus Aluminis. Alum, catechu, wax, each ʒj, lard ʒvss.

Pessus Belladonnæ. Extract of belladonna ℈ss, wax gr. xxiiss, lard, ʒiss; in each pessary.

Pessus Hydrargyri. Strong mercurial ointment ʒss, wax ʒss, lard ʒj. Mix.

Pessus Plumbi. Acetate of lead gr. viiss, white wax gr. xxiiss, lard ʒiss.

Pessus Plumbi Iodidi. Iodide of lead gr. v, wax gr. xxv, lard ʒiss.

Pessus Tannini. Tannin ℈ss, wax gr. xxv, lard ʒiss.

Pessus Zinci. Oxide of zinc gr. xv, white wax gr. xxiiss, lard ʒiss.

PHILLYRINÆ SULPHAS. M. JACHELLI. From the leaves and twigs of Phillyrea latifolia, nearly as for Quinæ sulphas [D.], for which it is said to be a substitute. Dose, gr. xij—xv.

PHOSPHORUS RUBER. *Red, or Amorphous Phosphorus.* This is an allotropic modification of phosphorus, produced under certain conditions. It is less inflammable, less soluble, and less active than the common phosphorus. It is produced when phosphorus is exposed in closed glass tubes to the action of a continued heat.

PILULÆ ACIDI CARBONICI. Mr. MORSON. Mix ʒss of bicarbonate of soda, add gr. xxv of tartaric acid, coarsely powdered, with the smallest possible quantity of syrup and mucilage to form a mass. Divide into 12 pills.

PILULÆ ALÖES ET HYDRARGYRI. GL. H. *Abernethy's Pills.* Mercurial pill, aloetic pill, of each ʒss, syrup q. s. Mix, and divide into 12 pills.

PILULA ALOES CUM SAPONE. L. Powdered extract of Barbadoes aloes, soft soap, extract of liquorice, of each equal parts, treacle q. s. [Probably intended as a substitute for Pilulæ Aloes Dilutæ.] Dose, gr. v—xv.

PILULÆ ANTICHOLERICÆ ARABICÆ. Assafœtida, asclepias gigantea, and opium, of each gr. iss, in each pill. One every ½ or ¾ hour, broken down in a spoonful of brandy and water, till the symptoms yield. After vomiting and purging have ceased, if prostration and spasms are urgent, give ½ or ¼ doses. Black pepper is substituted for asclepias in this country.

PILULÆ ANTIMONII COMP. St. B. H. Tartarized antimony gr. j, guaiacum ʒss, pill of aloes and myrrh ʒss, treacle q. s.; make 16 pills.

PILULÆ ARGENTI CHLORIDI. MIALHE. Nitrate of silver gr. xv, chloride of sodium ʒj, starch gr. xlv, gum gr. xv, water q. s. Divide into 100 pills. MIALHE affirms that the fresh precipitated chloride is partially soluble in chloride of sodium.

PILULÆ ATROPIÆ. BOUCHARDAT. Atropine gr. j; powdered althæa root, and honey, q. s. to make 50 pills. Dose, to commence with 1 to 2 pills.

PILULÆ BELLADONNÆ CUM CAMPHORA. Dr. DEBREYNE'S *Pills for Hysterical Complaints.* Camphor ʒiij, assafœtida ʒiij, extract of belladonna ʒj, extract of opium gr. xv, syrup of gum q. s. In 120 pills; 1 pill the first day, 2 the second, and so on till 6 are taken in 24 hours.

PILULA COLOCYNTHIDIS COMPOSITA. L. (In the place of Extractum Coloc. Comp.) Extract of colocynth ʒj, p. extract of aloes ʒvj, p. scammony ʒij, p. cardamom ʒss, soft soap ʒiss. Mix the powders, add the rest, and beat altogether into a mass. Dose, gr. iv to xij.

PILULÆ COLOCYNTHIDIS. E. [PIL. COL. COMPOSITÆ, D.]

	E.	D.
Aloes (Socot. or E. Ind.; hepat. D.), ...	8 parts.	℥ij
Colocynth pulp, in powder, ...	4 parts.	℥j
Scammony, in fine powder, ...	8 parts.	℥j
Castile soap, in powder, ...	—	ʒj
Sulphate of potash, ...	1 part.	
Oil of cloves, ...	1 part.	fʒj
Rectified spirit, ...	q. s.	
Treacle, ...	—	ʒx

Mix, and form a mass. (Divide into 5-grain pills, E.)

PILULÆ DIAPHORETICÆ. See Pil. Antimonii Comp., and Pil. Anodynæ Mercuriales.

PILULÆ DIGITALINÆ COMPOSITÆ. FALKEN. Digitaline gr. ¾, squill gr. 75, pure scammony gr. 75. Mix by long trituration, and form a mass with syrup of gum. Divide into 100 pills; and silver them. Give 2 pills, then 4, and afterwards 6 daily, *in dropsy, with disordered circulation.*

PILULA FERRI SUPERPHOSPHATIS. The compound (Ferri Biphosphas) made into pills alone or with liquorice powder. Dose, gr. j—ij.

PILULÆ FERRI SULPHURETI. BIETT. Sulphuret of iron ʒss, althæa powder gr. xv, syrup q. s.; in 20 pills; 1 to 4 daily, in *scrofulous eruptions.*

PILULÆ GENTIANÆ CUM FERRO. GUY'S H. Extract of gentian ʒj, sulphate of iron ℈j. Mix, and divide into 20 pills—one 3 times a day.

Pilulæ Hydrargyri Bichloridi cum Albumine. Albuminated bichloride of mercury gr. lxxv, powdered althæa gr. lxxv, syrup of gum q. s. Make 100 pills. 1 daily.

Pilulæ Iodoformi. Dr. Glover. Iodoform ʒj, bread-crumb and mucilage q. s. Divide into 30 pills. Bouchardat. Iodoform ℥ss, extract of wormwood q. s.; mix, and divide into 36 pills. One 3 times a day, *in scrofulous affections*, &c.

Pilula Ipecacuanhæ cum Scilla. L. (Pilulæ Ipecacuanhæ Compositæ. L. 1836.) Compound ipecacuanha powder ʒiij, fresh dried squill ʒj, ammoniacum ʒj, treacle q. s. Beat all together. Dose, gr. v to x.

Pilulæ Juglandis. M. Negrier. Extract of walnut leaves ʒj, powdered walnut leaves q. s. to form a mass, to be divided into 20 pills. 2 or 3 in the day.

Pilulæ Manganesii Carbonatis. M. Hannon. Dissolve separately ℥xvij of crys. sulphate of manganese, and f℥xix of carbonate of soda in water q. s. Mix the solutions, and add to every ℥xvij of the liquid, ℥j of syrup, and allow the precipitate to subside in a well-closed bottle. Pour off the supernatant liquid, wash the precipitate with sugared water, express, mix it with ℥x of honey, and evaporate rapidly to a pill-consistence. Dose, from 4 to 10 four-grain pills daily; *in anæmia, chlorosis*, &c.

Pilulæ Manganesii Iodidi. M. Hannon. Iodide of potassium ℥j, dried sulphate of manganese ℥j; mix with honey q. s. to form a pill-mass; divide into 4-grain pills. Dose, from one pill daily, gradually increased.

Pilulæ Manganesii Malatis. M. Hannon. Malate of manganese gr. xv, powdered cinchona gr. xv, honey q. s.; for 20 pills; 3 to 5 or 6 daily.

Pilulæ Manganesii Muriatis. Niemann. Muriate of manganese ℈ij, gum arabic ℈ij, liquorice ℈j. Mix.

Pilulæ Manganesii Tartratis. As Pil. Mang. Malatis.

Pilulæ Manganesii et Ferri Sulphatis. M. Hannon. Sulphate of iron ℥xiij, sulphate of manganese ℥iiiss, carbonate of soda ℥xviiss, honey ℥x, syrup q. s. to make a mass, to be divided into 4-grain pills. Dose, from 2 to 10 pills daily.

Pilulæ Rhei et Zingiberis. Rhubarb ʒiiss, ginger ʒiss, syrup q. s. In 5-grain pills.

PILULÆ SMUCKERI. Galbanum ʒj, sagapenum ʒj, soap ʒj, rhubarb ʒiss, tartar emetic gr. xvj, liquorice juice ʒj. Mix.

PILULÆ SODÆ ARSENIATIS. ER. WILSON. Arseniate of soda gr. ij; dissolve in distilled water q. s., and add p. guaiacum ʒss, oxysulphuret of antimony ℈j, mucilage q. s. Mix carefully, and divide into 24 pills. Dose, 1 pill.

PIX BURGUNDICA PRÆPARATA. Burgundy pitch, strained as Ammoniacum Præparatum.

PLUMBI SUBACETATIS LIQUOR COMPOSITUS. D. See Liquor Plumbi Diacetatis Dilutus.

POPULINA. Boil the bark of the root of populus tremula in water, evaporate with a gentle heat, and set aside to crystallize. Purify by solution in alcohol, and digestion with animal charcoal; filter and crystallize.

POTASSÆ AQUA. E. See Liquor Potassæ.

POTASSÆ CHROMAS FLAVA. The commercial yellow chromate of potash, manufactured on the large scale by heating chromate of iron with pearlash and nitre, may be purified by recrystallization. Dose, as an emetic, gr. ij—iv to adults; to children, gr. j—iss; as an alterative and expectorant, gr. ⅛ to ½. *Externally*, ʒss to ʒiss dissolved in f℥j of water, to destroy fungus; a weaker solution, ʒj to f℥xxxij, as an antiseptic, to living and dead parts. [Dr. PEREIRA.]

POTASSÆ FERRO-PRUSSIAS. See Potassii Ferro-cyanidum.

POTASSÆ ET UREÆ FERRO-CYANIDUM. M. BAUP has not made known his method of preparing this compound, which he states to be efficacious in intermittent fevers. But it contains from 72·2 to 77·8 per cent. of ferro-cyanide of potassium, 10·2 to 13·1 of urea, and 12·2 to 9·6 of water. It is mixed with honey, and divided into 3-grain pills, of which 10, 15, or 20 are given daily.

POTASSÆ HYPOCHLORIS. See Liquor Potassæ Chlorinatæ.

POTASSÆ IODAS. Fuse iodide of potassium in a capacious crucible, and gradually add to the fused salt, after removing it from the fire, 1½ part of chlorate of potash. Wash the mass with warm water, which leaves the iodate undissolved.

POTASSÆ NITRAS PURUM. D. Dissolve 4 pounds (av.) of commercial nitre in Oij of boiling water; let the heat be withdrawn, and the solution stirred constantly as it cools, that the salt may be obtained in very minute crystals. Wash these with cold distilled water till that which trickles through ceases to give a precipitate in sol. of nitrate of silver. Dry it in an oven. Dose, gr. v to ℈ij.

POTASSII IODIDI LIQUOR COMPOSITUS. D. See Liquor, &c.

POTASSII SULPHURETUM. E. & U. S. Sulphur ℥j, carbonate of potash ℥iv [℥ij, U. S.]; triturate them well together, and heat them in a covered crucible till they form a uniform fused mass, which, when cold, is to be broken into fragments, and kept in well-closed vessels. L. 1836, directed the same proportions. D. (Hepar Sulphuris) directs ℥iv of sublimed sulphur to ℥vij of carbonate of potash. Dose, gr. iij—x.

PTISANA MEZEREI. Mezereon bark ʒij, water Oiiss; boil to Oi¾, and strain.

PTISANA ORYZÆ. P. *Rice Water.* Infuse ʒiij of liquorice root in Oij of a decoction of ʒv of washed rice.

PRUNUM PRÆPARATUM. L. See Pulpa Prunorum.

PULVINA LUPULI. A pillow containing dried hops: used to allay restlessness.

PULVIS AEROPHORUS. PRUS. PH. Bicarbonate of soda ʒiv, tartaric acid ʒiij, refined sugar ʒvij. Reduce them separately to powder, dry well, and mix. Keep them in a close vessel.

PULVIS AEROPHORUS LAXANS. PRUS. PH. (*English Seidlitz Powders.*) Rochelle salts ʒij, bicarbonate of soda ℈ij; mix. In a separate paper give ʒss of tartaric acid (all in powder).

PULVIS ANTIARTHRITICUS. *Duke of Portland's Powder.* Round birthwort, gentian, tops of lesser centaury, tops of ground pine, and germander, of each equal parts. Dose, ʒj.

PULVIS CALAMINÆ [CUM AMYLO]. CUT. H. True calamine powder ℥j, starch ℥j. Mix.

PULVIS CALCIS PHOSPHATIS SACCHARATUS. Precipitated phosphate of lime gr. xv, white sugar gr. lxxxv; triturate, and divide into 20 packets. 2 or more daily, according to age of child. *In rickets,* &c.

PULVIS CAPUCINORUM. NIEMANN. Cevadilla, stavesacre, parsley-seed, and snuff, of each equal parts; mix. *To destroy vermin in the head;* but requires caution.

PULVIS CASTILLONI. Castillon's Powder. Sago, salep, tragacanth, each ʒj, prepared oyster shells ℈j, cochineal q. s. to color it. Boil ʒj in Oj of milk, as diet, *in chronic diarrhœa.*

PULVIS CATECHU COMPOSITUS. D. Catechu, kino, of each ℥ij; cinnamon, nutmeg, of each ℥ss. Reduce to a powder, pass through a fine sieve, and keep it in well-stopped bottles.

PULVERES EFFERVESCENTES CITRATI. D. Citric acid ʒix; divide into 18 powders. Bicarbonate of soda ʒxj (or bicarbonate of potash ʒxiij); divide into 18 parts. The acid and alkaline powders should be kept in papers of different colors.

PULVERES EFFERVESCENTES TARTARIZATI. D. Tartaric acid ʒx; reduce to powder, and divide into 18 parts. Bicarbonate of soda ʒxj (or of potash ʒxiij); divide into 18 parts. Keep the acid and alkaline powders in papers of different colors.

PULVIS GLYCYRRHIZÆ COMPOSITUS. PRUS. PH. Senna ℥vj, liquorice-root ℥vj, fennel seed ℥iij, sulphur ℥iij, refined sugar ℥xviij. Mix the powders.

PULVIS GUMMOSUS. Gum arabic ℥iij, liquorice ℥j, refined sugar ℥ij. Mix.

PULVIS MAGNESIÆ CUM RHEO. PRUS. PH. Carbonate of magnesia ℥j, oleo-saccharum of fennel ʒiv, rhubarb ʒij, orris ℥iss. Mix.

PULVIS POTASSÆ SULPHATIS CUM RHEO. Dr. A. T. THOMSON. Sulphate of potash gr. x, rhubarb gr. iij, calumbo gr. vj. Two or three times a day in *mesenteric disease.*

PULVIS QUINÆ SULPHATIS ET TABACI. HUG. Disulphate of quinine gr. xij, snuff ℥j, *for nervous headaches.*

PULVIS SALICIS COMPOSITUS. HUFELAND'S *Quinquine factice.* Willow bark, chestnut bark, gentian, calamus, herb bennet, of each equal parts. Pulverize and mix.

PULVIS STRYCHNIÆ CUM SACCHARO. GL. H. Strychnia gr. j, refined sugar ℈j. Mix, and divide into 8 powders.

PULVIS VERMIFUGUS. P. Corsican worm-moss ℥j, worm-seed ℥j, rhubarb ℥ss; mix. E. H. Scammony ʒj, calomel ʒj, rhubarb ʒiij. (The doses of the above are not given.) BAUME. Quicksilver ʒiij, Æthiop's mineral ʒij, white sugar ʒviij; triturate till the mercury disappears. Dose, gr. v to ℈j, twice a day. P. 1818. Æthiop's mineral ʒj, scammony ʒj; mix. SWEDIAUR. Tin filings ʒij, sulphate of iron gr. v; mix, for 6 doses. One every two hours. GERM. H. Male fern gr. xxiv, gamboge gr. ij.

QUINÆ ARSENIS. *Arsenite of Quinine.* M. SOUBEIRAN. Dissolve 500 grains of disulphate of quinine in distilled water with a few drops of diluted sulphuric acid; precipitate by ammonia, wash the precipitated quina, press it, and dissolve it in f℥viij of rectified spirit; then add 72 grains of arsenious acid, heat them together, and filter. The arsenite crystallizes on cooling.

QUINÆ DIARSENIS. Mr. KINGDON. Boil 64 grains of arsenious acid with 32 grains of carbonate of potash in f℥iv of distilled water for half an hour, and add water to make up f℥iv. To fʒv of this solution add ℈ij of disulphate of quinine previously dissolved in boiling water. Collect the precipitate on a filter, wash it, and leave it to dry. Dose, gr. ⅓ twice a day, in pills with bread.

QUINÆ DISULPHAS. See after Quinæ Sulphas.

QUINÆ MURIAS. *Muriate, or Hydrochlorate of Quinine.* D. Dissolve 123 grains of chloride of barium in f℥ij of distilled water, and 437½ grains of sulphate of quinine in Oiss of boiling water. Mix, evaporate to half, filter, and again evaporate, by steam or water heat, until crystalline spiculæ appear. Let it cool, and dry the crystals on blotting paper. Concentrate the liquid for an additional product. It may also be made by saturating dilute muriatic acid with quinine. PRUS. PH. (Chinium Hydrochloratum.) Dissolve ʒv of chlorate of barium in ℔j of boiling water, and gradually add ℥ij of sulphate of quinine. Boil for a few minutes, and filter whilst hot; dry the crystals which form. P. directs 100 parts of sulphate of quinine to 30 of cr. chloride of barium.

QUINOIDINA. (*Chinioideum.* PRUS. PH.) This is obtained from the mother liquors of sulphate of quinine manufactories, by precipitation with a carbonated alkali. It is purified by dissolving it in diluted sulphuric acid, passing sulphuretted hydrogen through the solution, filtering, boiling, and precipitating by carbonate of soda, washing the precipitate, drying it, and reducing it to powder.

RESINA IRIDIS. Lixiviate powdered orris root with ether, and let the clear tincture evaporate spontaneously. Chiefly used as a perfume.

Rheina. The crystalline bitter and purgative principle of rhubarb. It may be obtained from the infusion of rhubarb, in the same manner as digitaline (q. v.) from foxglove, by Labourdais' process. Dose, gr. j—ij. Some state that it is a simple tonic.

Rubinus Antimonii. Fuse together 5 parts of black sulphuret of antimony with 1 of carbonate of potash, and preserve the lower layer of the fused mass for use.

Sapo Hydrargyri Bichloridi. Sir H. Marsh. Beat ℥ij of white Windsor soap in a marble mortar till perfectly smooth; add ℈j of corrosive sublimate previously triturated with fʒj of rectified spirit, and beat the whole into a uniform paste, adding six drops of otto of rose. In some chronic forms of *cutaneous disease.*

Sapo Hydrargyri Precipitati Albi. Sir H. Marsh. Beat ℥ij of white Windsor soap in a marble mortar, add fʒj of rectified spirit, ʒij of white precipitate, and 10 drops of otto. Beat the whole to a uniform paste.

Sapo Hydrargyri Precipitati Rubri. Sir H. Marsh. White Windsor soap ℥ij, rectified spirit fʒj, powdered red precipitate ʒj, otto 6 drops. Proceed as in the last.

Sarsaparillina. See Smilacina.

Senegina. *Senegin*, or *Polygalic Acid.* Exhaust senega root with rectified spirit, evaporate the clear tincture to the consistence of treacle, agitate it with ether, and let the mixture stand at rest to deposit crystals. Acrid, poisonous.

Sodæ Aqua Effervescens. See Aqua Sodæ Effervescens.

Sodæ Carbonatis Liquor. D. See Liquor Sodæ Carbonatis.

Sodæ Bicarbonas. (*Sesquicarbonas.* L. 1836.) L. gives no process, but directs that it should yield no precipitate with bichloride of platinum or sulphate of magnesia, unless heat is applied. What is thrown down by chloride of barium should dissolve in hydrochloric acid. 100 grains gives off 51·7 grains of carbonic acid when added to dil. sulphuric acid.

E. directs carbonic acid to be passed, by a tube reaching to the bottom, into a vessel containing a mixture of one part of crystallized and two of dried carbonate of soda; and the salt, when it ceases to absorb gas, to be dried in the air, or at a temperature not above 120°. To procure the carbonic acid gas, fill with fragments of marble a glass jar, open at the bottom and tubulated at top; close the bottom so as to keep in the marble, without preventing the free passage of a fluid; and having connected the tubulature by a bent tube and corks with an empty bottle, and this with the vessel containing the soda, immerse the jar in diluted muriatic acid, contained in any convenient vessel. When the whole apparatus is filled with gas, secure the last cork tightly, and let the action go on till morning, or till the gas is no longer absorbed by the salt. Remove the damp salt which is formed, and dry it in the air, or at a temperature not above 120°.

D. directs the carbonic acid (from 16 oz. or q. s. of chalk, Oiss of muriatic acid, and Oiij of water) to be passed into a solution of 2℔ av. of cr. carbonate of soda in Oij of distilled water, as directed for bicarbonate of potash.

U. S. directs pieces of crystallized carbonate of soda to be spread on a pierced partition near the bottom of a wooden box with a close cover: and carbonic acid passed into the box beneath the partition, until the carbonate of soda is fully saturated. Dose, gr. x to ʒj.

Sodæ Sulphas Exsiccata. *Effloresced Glauber Salt.* Expose the crystals to a warm dry air till they fall into powder. They lose half their weight; the dose is reduced in the same proportion.

Sodæ Bisulphis. Dissolve crys. carbonate of soda in twice its weight of water, and pass sulphurous acid in excess through the solution. Set aside to crystallize. Dose, ʒss to ʒj. Its solution is used to preserve *subjects.* The *neutral sulphite* is obtained by saturating the bisulphate with carbonate of soda.

Soda Tartarizata. L. 1809. See Sodæ Potassio-tartras.

Sodæ Tartras. To a solution of tartaric acid, add carbonate or bicarbonate of soda q. s. to neutralize it; evaporate, and set aside to crystallize. Dose, as a purgative, ʒij—iv; as a diuretic and antilithic ℈j to ʒj largely diluted. It is more frequently taken in the form of *Soda Powders.*

Sodæ Valerianas. D. Dilute ℥viss of oil of vitriol with Oss of water; dissolve ℥ix of powdered bichromate of potash with the aid of heat in Oiiiss of water. When both solutions are cooled put them in a matrass, and having added f℥iv of fusel oil (Alcohol Amylicum) shake together repeatedly till the temperature, which first rises to 150°, has fallen to 80° or 90°. A condenser being connected, apply heat so as to distil over about Oiv of liquid. Saturate this exactly with Oj or q. s. of solution of caustic soda, separate from the oil, which floats on the surface, and evaporate till the residual salt is partially liquefied. The heat should now be withdrawn, and when the salt has concreted, while still warm, it is to be divided into fragments, and preserved in well-stopped bottles. [Chiefly used for obtaining the other valerianates.]

SOLUTIO APERIENS. Prof. METTAUER. Socotrine aloes ℥iiss, bicarbonate of soda ℥vj, water Oiv, compound spirit of lavender f℥ij. Digest for 14 days and decant. Dose, f℥j or more half an hour after dinner and supper.

SOLUTIO ARGENTI NITRATIS CONCENTRATA. Mr. HIGGINBOTTOM. Dissolve ℈iv of nitrate of silver in fʒiv of distilled water. To be applied by a small sponge (1 inch by $\frac{1}{3}$) on a silver probe. [Instead of solid caustic in Erysipelas, &c.]

SOLUTIO ARSENIATIS AMMONIÆ and SOLUTIO ARSENIATIS SODÆ. See Liquor Arseniatis Ammoniæ, &c.

SOLUTIO ARSENICALIS ACIDA. CUT. H. Arsenious acid ʒiiss, hydrochloric acid ℥ss, water f℥xxxiiss. Boil till the arsenic is dissolved, and add ʒj of syrup of saffron. Make it up f℥xxxiv. Dose, ♏iij to ♏vj.

SOLUTIO ARSENICALIS ALKALINA. CUT. H. Arsenious acid ʒiiss, solution of potash ℥j, water f℥xxxij. Boil till dissolved, then add ℥j of comp. tincture of lavender, and water to make up ℥xxxiv. Dose, ♏iij to ♏vj.

SOLUTIO AURI AMMONIO-CHLORIDI. FURNARI. Ammonio-chloride of gold gr. x, distilled water and rectified spirit, each ℥xiiss. Dose, a teaspoonful morning and evening, in sugared water; *against dysmenorrhœa* and *amenorrhœa.*

SOLUTIO BARYTÆ MURIATIS. E. Muriate of baryta (chloride of barium) ʒj, distilled water f℥j : dissolve.

SOLUTIO CAMPHORÆ E CHLOROFORMO. Messrs. T. & H. SMITH. Camphor ʒiij, chloroform fʒj. Dissolve. [For exhibiting camphor, with yolk of egg in emulsions.]

SOLUTIO CANTHARIDIS ÆTHERIALIS. Mr. TOYNBEE. Æther 3 parts, cantharides 1 part: exhaust by percolation.

SOLUTIO CHLOROFORMI. BOUCHARDAT. Chloroform ℥j, rectified spirit ℥j, water ℥x. Used chiefly as a lotion to allay itching.

SOLUTIO FERRI ALUMINOSA. SWEDIAUR. Calcined sulphate of iron ℈x, alum ℈v, water q. s. to dissolve them, sulphuric acid 15 drops. Dose, 10 to 15 drops. [Once a celebrated nostrum in Germany, under the name of *Tinctura Nervosa.*]

SOLUTIO FERRI BROMIDI. MOHR. Mix 1 part of iron filings with 3 of water in a stopped vial, add 1 part of bromine, and shake till the solution has assumed a greenish hue. It must be kept on the iron, and decanted or filtered when wanted for use.

SOLUTIO FERRI ET QUINÆ PHOSPHATIS. Dr. CATTELL states that it contains phosphoric acid, quina, and oxide of iron; but he has not given the quantities or process.

SOLUTIO HYDRARGYRI COMPOSITA. CUT. H. Corrosive sublimate ʒvj, arsenious acid ʒiiss, hydrochloric acid ℥j, boiling water f℥xxxij; boil, and make up ℥xxxiv. Dose, ♏iij to x.

SOLUTIO HYDRARGYRI BICHLORIDI. MIALHE. Bichloride of mercury 1 part, muriate of ammonia 2 parts, chloride of sodium 2 parts, distilled water 1000 parts. Dissolve. Dose, fʒj 3 or 4 times a day.

SPIRITUS. *Spirits.* Under this head are placed distilled spirits, simple and compound; with a few alcoholic solutions, and æthereal spirits. In preparing the distilled spirits, the seeds, &c., are to be bruised; the E. P. and other Ph. direct previous maceration for two or more days. D. now substitutes for most of the distilled spirits, solutions of 1 part of essential oil in 9 of rectified spirit. See ESSENTIA. [The spirit which forms the basis of these compounds is not prepared by pharmacists, but is a separate branch of manufacture. The Colleges, however, have indicated, by their densities, the strength of the spirits to be employed. The following table shows the specific gravity of the spirits used in the following compounds:]

Alcohol, D.,	·795
——— E.,	·796
Alcool Absolu. Paris Codex,	·796
Alcool at 40° P. C.,	·810
Spiritus Vini Alcoholisatus. PRUS. PH.,	·810 to ·813
Spiritus Fortior, D.,	·818
Spiritus Rectificatissimus. HANN. PH.,	·822
——— PRUS. PH.,	·833 to ·835
Spiritus Rectificatus. L. and E.,	·838
——— D.,	·840
Spiritus Vini. PRUS. PH.,	·840 to ·845
Alcohol du Commerce, 33°. P.,	·863

Spiritus Vini Rectificatus. Prus. Ph.,	·897 to ·900
——— Tenuior. L. and D.,	·920
——————— E.,	·912
Alcohol faible. P.,	·923
Spiritus Tenuior. L. 1824,	·930

Spiritus Ætheris Aromaticus. L. 1824. *Elixir Vitrioli dulce.* Cinnamon ʒiij, cardamom ʒiss, long pepper ʒj, ginger ʒj, spirit of s. æther f℥xvj. Macerate 14 days in a stopped bottle, and strain. Dose, fʒss to fʒj.

Spiritus Æthereus Nitrosus. D. Put f℥vj of rectified spirit in a quart matrass, and connect this with a Liebig's condenser, whose further extremity is fitted loosely by a collar of tow into a thin 8-ounce phial. Add f℥j of water to f℥iij of pure nitric acid, and having introduced half the mixture into the matrass through a siphon safety-tube, close the mouth of this tube with a cork, and apply for a few moments a gentle heat, so as to cause a commencement of ebullition. When the action produced has relaxed, introduce gradually the rest of the acid, so as to restore it. The action having ceased, agitate the distilled product with half its bulk of solution of ammonia, allow the mixture to rest for a few minutes, and having separated the supernatant ethereal liquid, mix f℥iv of it with Oij f℥ij of rectified spirit, and preserve it in small strong and accurately stopped bottles. The condenser should be fed with ice-cold water, and the phial surrounded by a mixture of 1 part of salt and 2 of pounded ice; or with a mixture of 8 parts sulphate of soda in small crystals, and 5 of muriatic acid. [The following process, founded on that of Liebig, is recommended by Mr. James Grant, in the *Pharmaceutical Journal.* Mix ʒij of powdered starch with fʒj of rectified spirit in a glass flask; to these add fʒj of nitric acid (sp. gr. 1·36), apply a gentle heat if necessary, until slight effervescence takes place, and pass the disengaged nitrous æther first into a washing bottle, then into f℥ix of rectified spirit. It is desirable to ascertain whether the product be free from prussic acid, with which Liebig's nitrous æther is said to be contaminated. See page 23.]

Spiritus Æthereus Oleosus. D. Mix Oiss of oil of vitriol with Oj of rectified spirit, in a glass matrass; connect this with a Liebig's condenser, apply heat, and distil till a black froth begins to rise. Separate the uppermost stratum of the distilled liquid, and having exposed it to the air for 24 hours, let the oil be transferred to a moist paper filter, and washed with a little cold water. Dissolve it in Oss of rectified spirit, mixed with f℥v of sulphuric æther. [This is almost identical with Spiritus Ætheris Compositus.]

Spiritus Calami. P. Calamus root ℔j, sp. of wine (·863) ℔viij; macerate 4 days, and distil nearly to dryness.

Spiritus Colchici Ammoniatus. *Tinct. Colchici Composita.*

Spiritus Cœruleus. Han. Ph. Wormwood, scordium, savin, lavender-flowers, of each ℥iiss; proof spirit Ov; distil Oiiss, and add ʒvj of verdigris, water of ammonia ℥ix. *For outward use.*

Spiritus Dilutior. E. See Spiritus Tenuior.

Spiritus Febrifugus Cluttoni. See Spiritus Ætheris Muriatici. The original form is—Oil of sulphur by the bell, oil of vitriol, and sea salt, of each ℥j, spirit of wine ℥vj. Let them digest for a month, then distil to dryness.

Spiritus Ferri Chlorati Æthereus. Prus. Ph. See Tinct. Ferri Chloridi Ætherea.

Spiritus Formicarum. Prus. Ph. Ants (fresh collected and clean) ℔ij, spirit of wine (at ·900) ℔iv, water q. s. Distil ℔iv. Dose, 20 to 60 drops; also *used outwardly.*

Spiritus Fortior. D. Carbonate of potash (heated to low redness and reduced to powder in a warm mortar) ℥viij, rectified spirit Oiv; let them be shaken in a bottle occasionally for four hours, at about 100° F. After settling for 20 minutes, separate the upper layer (about 74 fl. ounces) by a syphon, and distil it with a Liebig's condenser, and chloride of zinc bath, until the product amounts to 72 fl. ounces (sp. gr. ·818).

Spiritus Pyroxylicus. *Wood Spirit.* When the acid liquor obtained by the dry distillation of wood (beech or birch), after separating the tar, is distilled, the first portions which come over are chiefly wood spirit, which is rectified by one or more distillations. It is further purified by redistilling it over lime. D. states its sp. gr. to be ·846, but it may be obtained as low as ·813. The purest kinds of pyroxylic spirit constitute Dr. Hastings's *Medicinal Naphtha.* Dose, ♏xij—xv, 3 times a day, increased as the patient can bear it. *In consumption.*

Spiritus Spilanthi. Beral. Bruised Para cress (Spilanthes oleracea) in flower 1 part, spirit of ·863 sp. gr. 2 parts; macerate 2 or 3 days, and distil 2 parts.

SPIRITUS VANILLÆ. NIEMANN. Bruised vanilla 1 part, rectified spirit 12 parts, water 12; distil 12 parts.

STANNI PROTOCHLORIDUM. It is obtained, in solution, by digesting granulated tin in strong muriatic acid, as long as hydrogen gas is given off. [Used as a Test.]

STIBIUM SULPHURATUM, &c. See Antimonii Sulphuretum, &c.

STRYCHNIÆ MURIAS. D. On ℥j of strychnia pour f℥j, or q. s., of dilute muriatic acid, and adding f℥iiss of distilled water, apply heat till a perfect solution is obtained. Let this cool, and let the crystals be dried on bibulous paper. By evaporating the residual liquid to ⅓ of its bulk, and allowing it to cool, an additional quantity of the salt will be obtained.

STYRAX PRÆPARATA. L. (S. Colata.) Dissolve ℔j of storax (liquid) in Oiv of rectified spirit, strain through linen, distil off most of the spirit, and evaporate what remains by water-bath to a due consistence. [Styrax Purificata, D. 1806, was made by softening storax in tepid water, and expressing it between warm iron plates.]

SUCCUS ACONITI. See Succi Alcoholati. It is less active than the tincture of the dried root.

SUCCUS BELLADONNÆ [Alcoholatus]. Mr. BENTLEY. See Succi Alcoholati. Dose, from ♏xx.

SUCCUS CONII. [BENTLEY.] As the other Succi Alcoholati. Dose, from ♏xx.

SULPHUR FUSCUM. This is sulphur in an amorphous state, obtained by melting sulphur, increasing the heat till it becomes brown and viscid, and continuing it at that temperature for half an hour. It may be made into pills by softening it with hot water. Three to four 2-grain pills daily.

SULPHURIS HEPAR. See Potassii Sulphuretum.

SULPHURETUM ANTIMONII. See Antimonii Sulphuretum. [For the sulphurets, see their respective bases.]

SUPPOSITORIUM SODÆ SULPHATIS. PHŒBUS. Dried sulphate of soda ʒij, powdered soap ʒiv, honey q. s. For 4 suppositories. To be smeared over with oil when applied.

SYRUPUS ACACIÆ. U. S. Gum arabic ℥ij, sugar ℥xv, water f℥viij. Dissolve the gum in the water without heat, then the sugar with a gentle heat, and strain.

Syrupus Anticatarrhalis. M. Mouchon. To 3000 parts of boiling water add 250 parts of red poppy petals; infuse, strain with pressure, filter, mix it with 8000 parts of simple syrup previously reduced by boiling to 7500, and add a filtered solution of 30 parts of extract of henbane in 500 parts of orange-flower water.

Syrupus Atropiæ. Bouchardat. Atropine gr. iss, water (acidulated with a few drops of muriatic acid) ʒiiss, syrup f℥xxv. Dose, fʒiv, equivalent to gr. $\frac{1}{34}$.

Syrupus Caffeæ. Concentrated infusion of fresh-roasted coffee ℥iv, refined sugar ℥viij; dissolved in a closed vessel by a gentle heat.

Syrupus Caffeinæ Citratis. Hannon. Citrate of caffein ℈j, syrup ℥j. See Mistura Caffeinæ Citratis.

Syrupus Cannabinæ. Bouchardat. Tincture of cannabine (1 part of the resin to 10 of r. spirit) 1 part, simple syrup 100 parts. By spoonfuls.

Syrupus Castorei Compositus. M. Lebrou. Valerian water ℥v, cherry-laurel water ℥iiss, castor (dissolved in spirit q. s.) ʒiij, white sugar ℥xv. *In spasmodic asthma*, &c.

Syrupus Chimaphilæ. Mr. Procter. Macerate ℥iv of bruised leaves of umbellate winter-green in f℥viij of water for 36 hours, then subject it to percolation till f℥xvj of liquid have passed; reduce to half, and dissolve in it ℥xij of sugar. Dose, ℥ss to ℥j.

Syrupus Codeiæ. Codeia ℈j, water fʒiv, sugar ℥viij. Dose, a tea-spoonful, in *hooping-cough*.

Syrupus Croci [Vinosus]. P. Saffron ℥j, Malaga wine ℥xvj; macerate, strain, and add sugar ℥xxiv.

Syrupus Ferri Acetatis. Mr. Roper. Dissolve ℔ij of white sugar in Oss of water by water-bath, and add f℥xj of solution of acetate of iron. [Mr. Roper's acetate of iron is thus made: Dissolve ʒj of iron wire in fʒiv of muriatic acid diluted with fʒiv of water; add Oiv of water, and precipitate with f℥v of liquid potassæ: set aside for 24 hours, draw off the supernatant liquid with a syphon; fill again with water, and repeat the process a third time. Collect the precipitate on a linen filter, dissolve it in f℥ij of strong acetic acid, add water to make up f℥x, set aside for 24 hours, and filter. To make the ammonio-acetate add to Oj of the filtered liquor f℥ss of strong liquor ammoniæ. But for the syrup it is used without the ammonia.]

Syrupus Ferri et Potassii Iodidi. Dissolve ℥j of iodide of potassium in f℥vj of hot water, add f℥xij¼ of syrupus ferri iodidi, L., and sufficient simple syrup to make up Oiss. [There is no authorized formula; this contains gr. ij of each salt in f℥j.]

Syrupus Ferri Potassio-tartratis. M. Mialhe. Dissolve ℨiv of potassio-tartrate of iron in fℨiv of cinnamon water, and mix the solution with ℥xvj of simple syrup. A teaspoonful contains about 2 grains of the salt.

Syrupus Ferri Sesquinitratis. Mr. Duhamil. Clean iron wire ℨvj, nitric acid f℥iss, water f℥viij: let the mixture stand for 12 hours, or till all action has ceased, stirring it occasionally. Filter the solution, and dissolve in it ℥xiv of white sugar. Dose, 16 drops.

Syrupus Ferri Superphosphatis. Mr. Greenish. Superphosphate of iron (see Ferri Biphosphas) ℈ij, simple syrup fℨviij. Dose, ♏xij—xxiv.

Syrupus Iodinii cum Acido Tannico. Puche. Iodide of potassium ℨv, iodine gr. xv, tannin ℨss, syrup of orange-peel ℥xiv.

Syrupus Manganesii Malatis. M. Hannon. Malate of manganese ℥j, simple syrup ℥xvj, spirit of lemon-peel ℨij. Dose, ℨss to ℨj.

Syrupus Manganesii Phosphatis. M. Hannon. Phosphate of manganese ℨss, syrup of Tolu ℥iij ℨiij, syrup of cinchona ℥v, spirit of lemon-peel ℨiss, powdered tragacanth ℈ss. Mix quickly, and preserve in a well-stopped bottle.

Syrupus Manganesii Tartratis. It is made with tartrate of manganese, as Syr. Manganesii Malatis.

Syrupus Marrubii. P. Dried horehound ℥j, horehound water ℈ij: digest in a water-bath for two hours, strain, and add sugar ℔iv.

Syrupus Mezerei. Cazenave. Alcoholic extract of mezereum gr. j, simple syrup ℥x.

Syrupus Mori. L. Strained juice of mulberries Oj, sugar ℔iiss; dissolve with a gentle heat, set aside for 24 hours, remove the scum, and pour off the clear syrup from the dregs.

Lastly, add f℥iiss of rectified spirit. [SOUBEIRAN directs the mulberries to be crushed with the hand, and left to ferment for 2 or 3 days, not allowing it to proceed so far as to injure the color of the juice.]

SYRUPUS PHELLANDRII. MIALHE. Infuse ℥j of the seeds of phellandrium aquaticum in ℥iij of boiling water; when cold, strain, and add to the filtered infusion ℥x of simple syrup previously reduced by evaporation to ℥vij. Dose, ʒj—iv. *In bronchitis*, &c.

SYRUPUS QUINÆ IODIDI. Mr. DAVENPORT'S contains gr. j in each fʒj [perhaps held in solution by hydriodic acid?].

SYRUPUS QUINÆ SULPHO-TARTRATIS. Sulpho-tartrate of quinine 1 part, water 3, hot syrup 20 parts.

SYRUPUS QUINÆ LACTATIS. BOUCHARDAT. Lactate of quinine gr. xv, water ℥j; dissolve and add ℥ij of syrup. By teaspoonfuls, *in intermittents of children*.

SYRUPUS RHEI AROMATICUS. U. S. *Spiced Syrup of Rhubarb.* Rhubarb ℥iiss, cloves ℥ss, cinnamon ℥ss, nutmeg ʒij, proof spirit f℥xxxij; macerate for 14 days, strain, evaporate by water-bath to f℥xvj, filter while hot, and mix with Oiv f℥xvj of syrup previously heated. It may also be prepared by percolation. Dose, for *infantile bowel complaints*, fʒj.

SYRUPUS RIBIUM (*Syrup of Currants*); SYRUPUS RUBI IDÆI (*Raspberries*); SYR. RUBI FRUTICOSI (*Blackberries*); &c. As Syrupus Mori [P.], or Syrupus Limonis.

SYRUPUS SALICARIÆ. Infuse ℥iij of flowering tops of willow-herb in boiling water q. s. to obtain ℥v of infusion; add this to ℥xx of syrup previously evaporated to ℥xv.

SYRUPUS SENEGÆ. U. S. Bruised seneka root ℥iv, water f℥xvj; boil to f℥viij, strain, and add sugar ℔j; make a syrup. Or—take of senega in coarse powder ℥iv, water f℥iv; let them stand 12 hours; then put it in a displacement apparatus, and gradually pour water upon it until the liquid passes nearly tasteless. Evaporate it to f℥viij, and make a syrup with f℥xv of sugar. U. S., 1851, substitutes for the water a mixture of f℥viij of spirit, and f℥xxiv of water.

SYRUPUS SPIGELIÆ ET SENNÆ CONCENTRATUS. See Extractum Spigeliæ et Sennæ Fluidum, U. S.

SYRUPUS SYMPHYTI. E. 1744. Mr. BOYLE'S Syrup. Fresh

comfrey root ℔ss, plantain leaves ℔ss; bruise, express the juice, boil to half, and make a syrup with an equal weight of sugar.

SYRUPUS VALERIANÆ. P. Bruise ℔j of valerian root, and put it into a still with ℔viij of water. In 12 hours distil off ℔iss; strain and filter what remains, mix the liquor with ℔viij of simple syrup, evaporate to ℔viss, and add the distilled water.

TAFFETAS ANGLICUM. *Court Plaster.* See Emplastrum Ichthyocollæ.

TAFFETAS VESICANS. OETTINGER. Stretch taffeta on a frame, and brush it over twice with a solution of isinglass; when quite dry brush it over twice, at short intervals and in the same direction, with the following solution, repeating the application a third and fourth time, at intervals of 24 hours. Cantharidal æther, sulphuric æther, of each ℥x; boiled turpentine and black resin, of each ℥iiss; mix and dissolve. It is recommended to apply over it, some days after the last coating of the cantharidal solution, a solution of isinglass of a gelatinous consistence. This is to be wiped off before applying it to the skin, with a wet rag. [The same method answers for *paper*, which should be laid on a smooth plank.]

TAMARINDUS PRÆPARATUS. L. Tamarinds ℔j, water q. s. to cover them: macerate with a gentle heat for four hours, then finish as directed for Prunes. [See Pulpa Prunorum.]

TEREBINTHINA COLATA. Common raw turpentine, melted in a still, and strained while warm.

TEREBINTHINA COCTA. P. Put Venice (larch) turpentine in a basin with water, and boil, until a portion thrown into cold water assumes a pilular consistence. When required to form it into pills, soften it by warm water, and roll the pills in powdered starch. PRUS. PH. describes Ter. Cocta as the resin left in distilling oil of turpentine.

THERIACA ANDROMACHI. L. 1746. *Venice Treacle.* It consists of 61 ingredients, and contains 1 grain of opium in 75. The Theriaca of P. consists of 72 ingredients, and contains gr. j of opium in 72. For these polypharmic electuaries (which are rarely prescribed in this country, and probably never made according to the authorized formulæ) may be substituted the following:

THERIACA EDINENIS. E. 1744. Serpentary, valerian, contrayerva, each ℥iv; aromatic powder ℥iij, guaiacum resin ℥ij, castor ℥ij, nutmeg ℥ij, saffron ℥j, opium ℥j, clarified honey ℥lxxv. Dissolve the opium in a little wine, and mix it with the other dry ingredients in powder, and the honey. It contains 1 gr. of opium in 100. Most of the foreign formulæ for Theriaca contain sulphate of iron.

THRIDACIUM. *Thridace.* This name is applied both to Lettuce Opium (Lactucarium), and to the extract of the stalks (Extr. Latucæ Concentratum).

TINCTURA ABELMOSCHI SEMINUM. Dr. R. REECE. Musk seed ℥ij, proof spirit f℥xvj. Digest seven days, and strain. Dose, fℨj.

TINCTURA ACAROIDIS. Botany-bay resin ℥j, rectified spirit ℥viij.

TINCTURA ACONITI. L. (Tinct. Aconiti *Radicis*, D., and U. S.) L. Coarsely powdered aconite root ℥xv, rectified spirit Oij. Macerate for 7 days, express, and filter. [This is nearly as strong as Dr. TURNBULL'S *Tinc. Aconiti Concentrata.* Dose, ♏v to ix, but chiefly for outward use.] D. Dried aconite root cut small 10 oz., rectified spirit Oj; macerate for 14 days, express, and filter. [This is stronger than the last. Dose, ♏iv to viij, with caution. The following are also in use: U. S. Bruised aconite root ℔j, rectified spirit f℥xxxij. Macerate for 14 days, express strongly, and filter. Dose, as L. Dr. FLEMING. Macerate ℥xvj of the powdered root with f℥xvj of rectified spirit for 4 days; strain, and treat the aconite by percolation with more spirit, until the tincture obtained amounts to f℥xxiv. As an *anodyne, aneuralgic, and calmative,* Dr. F. gives ♏iij 3 times a day, increasing the dose one minim daily, if required. As an *antiphlogistic* he gives ♏v, repeated in 4 hours, and afterwards half the dose, if required. Its effects must be carefully watched. Dr. TURNBULL'S *Tinc. Radicis Aconiti Concentrata* is made by digesting the powdered root with twice its weight of rectified spirit, for 7 days. *For outward use.* Dr. PEREIRA directs ℔j of the root to Oiss of spirit, which is nearly identical with Dr. Turnbull's. Dose as L. above. Dr. TURNBULL has also described a weaker tincture—℥j of the powdered root to f℥vj of rect. spirit. Dose, from 10 drops.]

TINCTURA AROMATICA ACIDA. PRUS. PH. Nearly as Acidum Sulphuricum Aromaticum, E.; but with only ℥j of acid.

Tinctura Aurantiorum Immaturorum. Unripe orange-berries ℥iv, proof spirit Oj.

Tinctura Atropiæ. Mr. W. Cooper. Dissolve gr. j of atropine in fʒj of rectified spirit, and add fʒvij of distilled water. Dose, from ♏xv. One drop applied to the eye, morning and night, to keep up dilatation of the pupil. Bouchardat directs one grain of atropia to 100 of spirit. Dose, from 1 to 5 drops.

Tinctura Extracti Belladonnæ. Mr. Blackett. Extract of belladonna ʒx, proof spirit ℔j. Dose, ♏ij—iij.

Tinctura Chinæ Corticis. See Tinctura Cinchonæ.

Tinctura Chirettæ. D. Chiretta herb ℥v, proof spirit Oij; macerate for 14 days, strain, express, and filter.

Tinctura Cocci Cacti. D. Cochineal in fine powder ℥ij, proof spirit Oj. Macerate for 14 days, strain, express, and filter. [Probably intended chiefly as a coloring tincture; but it is also prescribed as an *antispasmodic and sedative.* Dose, fʒss—ij.]

Tinctura Colchici e Radice. P. Macerate 1 part of the dried cormi in 4 parts by weight of proof spirit.

Tinctura Cynaræ. Fresh artichoke leaves, bruised, ℔ij, rectified spirit ℔j; digest for 7 days, express, and filter.

Tinctura Colocynthidis. Prus. Ph. Dahlberb's *Tincture.* Colocynth pulp (cut small and free from seeds) ℥j, aniseed ʒj, proof spirit ℔j. Digest for 8 days, express, and filter. Dose, 6 to 20 drops.

Tinctura Copalchi Corticis. Bruised copalche bark ℥j, proof spirit Oj. 1 to 2 teaspoonfuls 2 or 3 times a day.

Tinctura Coptis. Dr. Wood. Gold-thread root ℥j, proof spirit f℥xvj. Dose, ʒj. *Tonic.*

Tinctura Elaterinæ. Morries. Elaterine gr. j, nitric acid 4 drops, rectified spirit, f℥j. Dose, fʒss.

Tinctura Erigeronis. Dried Canada flea-bane (Erigeron Canadense) ℥iv, proof spirit Oj. Macerate, express, and filter.

Tinctura Ferri Potassio-Acetatis. Mr. Donovan. Mix in a matrass ℥ij of precipitated carbonate (sesquioxide) of iron, and f℥xvj of acetic acid; when the effervescence is over, boil the mixture till reduced to f℥xij, and when cold filter. Expose the solution in a shallow dish for 3 days, pour it into a glass vessel large enough to hold 3 or 4 volumes of liquid; to this gradually add ʒxv of carbonate of potash, and when the effervescence is over, f℥xxiv of rectified spirit, and filter.

TINCTURA FERRI AMMONIO-CHLORIDI. L. *Tinc. Ferri Ammoniati.* Ammonio-chloride of iron ℥viij, proof spirit and distilled water, of each Oj. We have ventured here to correct an obvious error. The College, in adding Oj of water to the previous tincture, has neglected to increase the quantity of ammonio-chloride. That the tincture was intended to be of the same strength as before is plain from the note—that "f℥j yields, potash being added, 5·8 grains of sesquioxide of iron." It is therefore evident that ℥viij of the ammonio-chloride were intended, though ℥iv only are ordered. Dose, ♏xxx to fʒij.

TINCTURA FERRI CYDONIATI. As Tinct. Ferri Pomati, substituting quince juice for apple juice in preparing the extract.

TINCTURA FERRI POMATI. PRUS. PH. *Tinc. Ferri Malatis.* Extract of malate of iron (Ext. Ferri Pomati) ℥ij, spirituous cinnamon water ℥xij. Dissolve and filter. Dose, ♏xv to xxx.

TINCTURA GALLÆ COMPOSITA. GIBERT. Bruised galls ℥iv, water ℥viij, rect. spirit ℥viij, Cologne water ʒij.

TINCTURA GEI COMPOSITA. Avens root ℥iss, angelica root ℥j, tormentil root ℥j (all bruised), stoned raisins ℥ij, French brandy Oij. Macerate for a month in a warm place, and filter. Dose, f℥ss.

TINCTURA GUTTÆ PERCHÆ. Gutta percha in small pieces ℥j, chloroform ʒvj, digest till dissolved, and strain through muslin. Externally, *in some scaly diseases.*

TINCTURA HIBISCI ABELMOSCHI. Dr. REECE. Musk seed ℥ij, proof spirit f℥xvj. Digest 7 days. Dose, fʒj.

TINCTURA MATICO. D. Matico leaves in coarse powder ℥viij, proof spirit Oij. Macerate for 14 days, express, and filter. [Dr. JEFFREYS directs ℥vj to Oij.] Dose, fʒss to ʒij. *Styptic and astringent in hemorrhage.*

TINCTURA NICOTIANÆ. PRUS. PH. Fresh leaves of tobacco ℔j, rectified spirit ℔j: bruise the leaves in an earthen mortar, and digest with the spirit for four days; express, and filter. Dose, not more than 30 drops. [For another form, see Tinctura Tabaci.]

TINCTURA OPII AROMATICA. *Alcoolé d'opium cinnamomé.* GUIBOURT. Extract of opium 2 parts, rectified spirit 11 parts, cinnamon water 11 parts; dissolve, and filter.

TINCTURA OPII ECCARDI. ECCARD'S, or BAMBERG'S *Thebaic Tincture.* Opium ℥ij, cloves ʒj, cinnamon water f℥viij, rectified spirit ℥iv. Digest in a warm room for six days, and strain.

TINCTURA OPII FŒTIDA. *Elixir Fétida.* FULDA PH. Castor ℥iv, assafœtida ℥ij, salt of hartshorn ʒj, dry opium ʒiv, rectified spirit (sp. gr. 850) ℥xxxij (about Oij). Dose, ♏xv to ʒj.

TINCTURA PIPERIS. Black pepper ʒj, rectified spirit ℥vj.

TINCTURA QUINÆ COMPOSITA. L. Disulphate of quina ℈xvj, tincture of orange peel Oij. Digest for 7 days, or till dissolved, and filter. [The whole of the sulphate will scarcely dissolve, at least without the assistance of heat. fʒj should contain gr. j of the sulphate.]

TINCTURA QUINÆ HYDROCYANOFERRATIS. Mr. DONOVAN. Ferroprussiate of quinine gr. xxxij, rectified spirit f℥j. Dose, fʒj.

TINCTURA SEMINIS COLCHICI. See Tinct. Colchici.

TINCTURA SENNÆ AROMATICA. See Tinctura Rhei et Sennæ.

TINCTURA SPILANTHI. Bruise the flowering herb (*Para cress*), and macerate it for some days with an equal weight of rectified spirit; then express, and filter. *Sialagogue.*

TINCTURA SUMBULI. There is no authorized formula. Dr. H. LANE directs ℥v of the bruised root to be macerated for 7 days with Oij of proof spirit. *Stimulant.* Dose, ♏x to fʒss? [2 parts of this with 1 of the next form the Compound Tincture.]

TINCTURA SUMBULI ETHEREA. As the last, substituting spirit of sulphuric ether for rectified spirit. Dose, ♏x—xx.

TINCTURA VETIVERIÆ. Vittie-vayr (roots of Andropogon muricatum) ℥j, proof spirit Oss. Dose, a teaspoonful; *stimulant and sudorific.*

TINCTURA WARBURGII. WARBURGH'S *Fever Drops.* A secret remedy, said to be exactly imitated by the following: Aloes, zedoary, each ℈ij, camphor, angelica root, each gr. ij, saffron gr. iij, proof spirit ℥iij. Put the tincture into 5 drachm bottles, adding to each gr. vj of sulphate of quinine.

TINCTURA ZEDOARIÆ COMPOSITA. (WEDEL'S *Essentia Carminativa.*) Zedoary ℥iv, calamus, galangal, each ℥ij, chamomile, aniseed, caraway seed, each ℥j, bay-berries, and cloves, each ʒvj, orange-peel, and mace, each ʒiv, peppermint water, and rectified spirit, each ʒxxiv. In 6 days strain, and add muriatic ether ℥iv.

TROCHISCI AGARICI. L. 1720. White agaric ℥iij, ginger ʒij, mucilage of tragacanth q. s. [This was intended to render the agaric milder.]

TROCHISCI ALHANDAL. See Colocynthis preparata.

TROCHISCI ALUMINIS. Dr. T. THOMPSON. Alum ʒij, catechu ʒiij, p. acacia, white sugar, each ʒiij, p. tragacanth ʒiss, rose water q. s. To form a mass for 60 lozenges. *In hæmoptysis, relaxed sore throat,* &c.

TROCHISCI CAFFEINÆ. Citrate of caffein ʒj, sugar ℥j, mucilage of tragacanth q. s. Mix, and divide into 60 lozenges.

TROCHISCI EXTRACTI CINCHONÆ. Dry extract of bark ʒx, sugar ℥xj, powdered cinnamon ʒj, mucilage of tragacanth q. s.; in 10-grain lozenges.

TROCHISCI FERRI ET MAGNESIÆ CITRATIS. *Van den Corput.* Citrate of iron and magnesia 5 parts, sugar 40, saccharide of vanilla (saccharum vanillæ) 2, mucilage of tragacanth 5. Mix, and divide into tablets of 16 grains each.

TROCHISCI MAGNESIÆ CITRATIS. M. MARCHAND. Soluble citrate of magnesia ʒxiiss, sugar (aromatized with a little oil of orange-peel) ʒxiiss, mucilage of tragacanth q. s. Divide into 100 tablets.

TROCHISCI PYRETHRI. Tincture of pellitory ℥j, sugar ℥viij; mix, dry, and form into lozenges with mucilage of tragacanth.

TROCHISCI SCAMMONII. BOURIERES. Resin of scammony ʒiv, calomel ʒiv, sugar ℥vj, tragacanth ʒss, tincture of vanilla f℈ij. In 300 lozenges. One or two for a child; 2 to 4 for an adult.

UNGUENTUM ACONITINÆ. Dr. F. W. HEADLAND. Mix thoroughly aconitine, gr. ij, and ceratum cetacei, ℥j. (To be rubbed on the face, in small portions at a time, in neuralgic affections.)

UNGUENTUM ACONITINÆ FORTIUS. Dr. F. W. HEADLAND. Mix thoroughly aconitine, gr. iv, with ceratum cetacei, ℥j. (To produce a rapid and powerful effect.) The above proportions must be followed when the alkaloid is pure. For two grains here ordered, Dr. Fleming used sixteen, while Dr. Turnbull and Mr. Phillips recommended eight. The high price at which the pure aconitine has been hitherto sold, 3s. to 3s. 6d. a grain, has prevented this valuable remedy from being so extensively employed as it deserves. But we have been assured by Dr. Headland, that by following his formula, the alkaloid may be obtained at a cost not exceeding *sixpence* the grain.

UNGUENTUM HYDRARGYRI HYDROCHLORATIS. CUT. H. Levigated sal ammoniac ℥ij, mercurial ointment ℥vj, oil of bitter almonds ʒj. Mix.

UNGUENTUM ANTHEMIDIS. M. BAZIN. Freshly powdered chamomile flowers, olive oil, and lard, in equal quantities. For the cure of *itch.*

UNGUENTUM ANTIMONIALE CAMPHORATUM. Dr. FABURE'S *Ointment for chronic affections of the liver.* Muriate of ammonia ʒj, tartarized antimony ʒss, camphor gr. xxv, musk gr. x, lard ℥j.

UNGUENTUM ANTI-HERPETICUM. CHEVALLIER. Chloride of lime ʒiij, subsulphate of mercury ʒij, oil of almonds ʒvj, lard ℥ij. ALIBERT. Red sulphuret of quicksilver ʒiss, camphor ʒss, cerate ℥ij.

UNGUENTUM ANTIPERIODICUM. Lard ℥iij, sulphate of quinine ʒj, subcarbonate of iron ℈ss, opium gr. iij. To be rubbed on the skin previously washed with soap.

UNGUENTUM CADMII. RADIUS. Sulphate of cadmium gr. j to ij, lard ʒj. *For removing specks from the cornea.*

UNGUENTUM CAFFEINÆ. Citrate of caffeine gr. viij, lard ʒj. Mix.

UNGUENTUM CALCIS CHLORIDI CUM BORACE. Chloride of lime ʒj, borax ʒj, lard ℥j. *For chilblains.*

UNGUENTUM CAPSICI. Dr. TURNBULL. Evaporate concentrated tincture of capsicum to the consistence of a jelly, and mix ʒiij of the extract with ʒvj of lard. For external use, as a stimulant. Dr. T. states that it is of importance that the capsicum be free from salt, otherwise it will vesicate.

UNGUENTUM CHLOROFORMI. M. BOUIS. Chloroform 60 drops,

lard ℥j; mix, and keep it in a wide-mouthed stopped bottle. *In neuralgia.*

UNGUENTUM EXSICCANS. HAN. PH. Wax ʒiss, olive oil ℥j; melt, and add prepared bole ʒj, oxide of zinc ʒss.

UNGUENTUM FERRI OXYDI NIGRI. BREFELD. Beef suet ℥xvj, lard ℥xvj, black oxide of iron ℥ij; heat them together in an iron vessel, constantly stirring them with an iron rod till the mixture becomes black; let the sediment subside, pour off the liquid ointment, and add to it Venice turpentine ℥ij, oil of bergamot ʒj, bole (rubbed with a little olive oil) ℥j; mix thoroughly. (A modification of WAHLER'S *Ointment for Chilblains.*)

UNGUENTUM GALLÆ. D. Galls in very fine powder ʒj; ointment of white wax ʒvij; rub together until a uniform mixture is obtained.

UNGUENTUM HEDERÆ. Bruise fresh ivy leaves and boil them with 2 or 3 times their weight of lard until the leaves become crisp; then strain and press. A stimulating application to *indolent ulcers* and to *corns.*

UNGUENTUM HYDRARGYRI. L. E. & D. (*Ung. Hydrargyri Fortius,* L. 1836.) E. Mercury ℔ij, lard ℥xxiij, suet ℥j. L. The same, but half the quantity. Rub the mercury with the suet and a little of the lard until the globules disappear; then add the rest of the lard, and mix. D. directs ℔j each of pure mercury and prepared lard. [This ointment is not well prepared so long as metallic globules may be seen in it with a magnifier of 4 powers. E.] D. & P. omit the suet. [The extinction of the quicksilver may be greatly facilitated by triturating it with a portion of *old* mercurial ointment, as recommended by Mr. HIGGINBOTTOM of Northampton, in 1814, and as adopted in the last edition of the Prussian Pharmacopœia; or otherwise by employing lard which has been long exposed in a finely divided state to the action of the air. See Adeps oxygenatus. Several other modes of abridging the time and labor required in accomplishing this object have been proposed; but none of them are more effectual, or freer from objection, than these.]

UNGUENTUM HYDRARGYRI CUM AMYLO. M. BRIQUET. Mercurial ointment ℥j, powdered starch ʒij. Mix. To prevent pitting in small-pox; smeared over the face night and morning.

UNGUENTUM HYDRARGYRI CUM BELLADONNA. MANCH. H.

Strong mercurial ointment ℥j, liquid ammonia ʒvj, extract of belladonna ʒiv. Mix.

Unguentum Hydrargyri Iodidi Rubri. D. Red iodide of mercury ʒj, ointment of white wax ʒvij. Mix by trituration.

Unguentum Iodinii. U. S. Iodine ℈j, rectified spirit ♏xx; rub together, and add ℥j of lard. [Guy's H. Iodine gr. xv, lard ℥j. For E. see Unguentum Iodinii Compositum.]

Unguentum Iodoformi. Dr. Glover. Iodoform ʒss, to ʒj, simple cerate ʒviij. Mix.

Unguentum Juglandis. Negrier. Extract of walnut leaves ʒiij, lard ʒiv, oil of bergamot 1 drop. Mix.

Unguentum Lycopodii. Lycopodium ʒj, lard ℥j. *In excoriations.*

Unguentum Maturans. Canquoin. Acetate infusion of mezereon, treacle, olive oil, each ℥iss, ox-gall ʒij, evaporate to the consistence of honey, and add of basilicon and emplastrum fuscum, each ℥iss, calomel ʒj. *For indolent ulcers,* &c.

Unguentum Picis. L. (*Ung. Picis Nigræ,* 1836.) *Black Basilicon.* Black pitch, wax, resin, of each ℥xj, olive oil Oj; melt together, and strain through linen.

Unguentum Precipitati Albi. E. White precipitate ʒij, lard ℥iij. Melt the lard, add the precipitate, and stir till cold.

Unguentum Propolis. Strained propolis ʒj, olive oil ʒiss. Melt together. *In hæmorrhoidal disorders.*

Unguentum Quinæ Sulphatis. Antonini. Sulphate of quinine ʒj, alcohol ʒij, sulphuric acid 10 drops, lard ℥ss. To be rubbed on the groin, *in intermittents.*

Unguentum Resinæ. D. Resin in coarse powder ℔ss, yellow wax ℥iv, prepared lard ℔j. Melt together, strain through flannel, and stir until it concretes.

Unguentum Stimulans. E. Wilson. Powdered cantharides ℥iij, lard ℥xij; macerate with a moderate heat for 24 hours, and filter through paper. To dilute it, use pomatum.

Unguentum Sulphuris cum Pice. Guy's H. Sulphur ointment ℥ij, tar f℥ij. Mix.

Unguentum Acidi Tannici Compositum. Cut. H. Tannin ℥ss, Æthiop's mineral ℥ss, zinc ointment ℥viij, compound lead ointment ℥viij. Mix.

Urea. Evaporate urine to the consistence of a syrup; when cold add nitric acid until a crystallized mass is obtained, wash this repeatedly with cold water, and press it between blotting paper. Neutralize by a solution of carbonate of potash in 3 parts of water, and evaporate to dryness. Treat the residue with alcohol, and concentrate, that the urea may crystallize. *Diuretic.* Dose, ℈ss to ʒj. See Urea Factitia.

VEGETABILIA PRÆPARATA. L. The purified gum-resins and the pulps of fruit are noticed elsewhere. See Ammoniacum Præparatum, Cassia Præparata, Pulpæ, &c. [Under Ammoniacum Præparatum, page 448, we have omitted to state that the mixture should be *constantly stirred.* Mr. BRANDE recommends reducing the gum-resins to powder in cold weather, and passing the product through a sieve. M. GOBLEY heats them in a tinned copper vessel, with 3-8ths their weight of proof spirit, stirring with a wooden spatula, and strains through a linen cloth.]

VINUM CAMPHORATUM. PRUS. PH. Camphor, and gum acacia, in powder, each ʒij; mix accurately, and gradually add ℔j of white wine.

VINUM CASCARILLÆ. M. BERNARDEAU. Cascarilla ℥j, Malaga wine Oj. Dose, f℥j twice a day, *in consumption.*

VINUM CATECHU. SOUBEIRAN. Tincture of catechu 1 part, red wine 12. Mix, and after a few days filter.

VINUM CENTAURII COMPOSITUM. HOFFMANN'S *Elixir Viscerale.* Centaury, orange peel, extract of blessed thistle, gentian, myrrh, cascarilla, each ʒj, sherry Oij.

VINUM CINNAMOMI. BERAL. Cinnamom ℥j, Alicant wine ℥xvj. Macerate and filter. Sugar is sometimes added.

VINUM EUPATORII. GESNER. Hemp agrimony ℥j, white wine Oj; digest and strain.

VINUM OLIVÆ. LOUIS. Fresh olive leaves ℥ij, white wine ℥xxxij. Half a glass twice a day.

VINUM STIBIATUM. See Vinum Antimonii Potassio-tartratis.

ZINCI CHLORIDI LIQUOR. D. Sheet zinc ℔j, muriatic acid Oiiss, water Oiiss; heat in a porcelain capsule until the metal is dissolved; filter through calico, and having added f℥j of solution of chlorinated lime, boil down to Oj. When the solution has cooled, place it in a bottle with ℥j of prepared chalk; and having added sufficient distilled water to make up Oij, shake the mixture occasionally for 24 hours. Finally filter, and preserve the product in a well-stopped bottle. Sp. gr. 1593.

ZINCI ET AMMONIÆ IODIDUM. BOUCHARDAT. Pour a clear solution of iodide of zinc into liquid ammonia, dissolve the precipitated salt in boiling ammonia, and let it crystallize by cooling. Dose, gr. ¼ with the same quantity of extract of belladonna, gradually increased to gr. ij, twice a day. *In chorea, epilepsy*, &c.

ZINCI OXYDUM HYDRATUM. The *hydrated* oxide is obtained by precipitating a solution of pure sulphate of zinc by solution of potash, avoiding excess.

ZINCI TANNAS. Saturate a solution of tannic acid with hydrated oxide of zinc, fresh precipitated and still moist; filter the solution, and evaporate to dryness. *Astringent;* chiefly used in *injections.*

TESTS.

The Pharmacopœias direct the following Tests to be used in ascertaining the purity of medicines. The formulæ have already been given.

AMMONIÆ OXALAS, E.; ACIDUM HYDROSULPHURICUM *recens præparatum*, L. (see Acidum Sulphydricum); Liquor Argenti Nitratis, L.; Solutio Argenti Nitratis, E.; Solutio Argenti Ammoniati, E.; LIQUOR BARII CHLORIDI, L.; BARYTÆ NITRAS, E.; SOLUTIO BARYTÆ NITRATIS, E.; SOLUTIO SODÆ PHOSPHATIS, E.; LIQUOR CHLORINII *recens præparatus*, L. (see Chlorinii Liquor); LACMUS (see Charta Exploratoria); PLATINI BICHLORIDUM, L.; POTASSII ET HYDRARGYRI IODO-CYANIDUM, L. (see Hydrargyri et Potassii Iodo-cyanidum); LIQUOR INDIGO SULPHATIS, L.; STANNI PROTOCHLORIDUM, L.

PREPARATIONS AND COMPOUNDS OF THE MORE IMPORTANT ARTICLES OF MATERIA MEDICA, CONTAINED IN THE FORMULARY.

Abbreviations:—Ac., Acidum; Aq., Aqua; Barb., Barbadensis; Co., Compositus; Conf., Confectio; Dec., Decoctum; Dil., Dilutum; Emb., Embrocatio; Emp., Emplastrum; Ess., Essentia; Garg., Gargarisma; Gt., Guttæ; Inf., Infusum; Inj., Injectio; Lin., Linimentum; Mist., Mistura; Ol., Oleum; Pil., Pilula, or Pilulæ; Pulv. Pulvis; Sp., Spiritus; Syr., Syrupus; Tinct., Tinctura; Troch., Trochisci; Ung., Unguentum; Vin. Vinum.

ACACIA. *Gummi Acaciæ,* E. *Gum Arabic.* Mucilago, Mist. acaciæ; Emulsio acaciæ; Mist. Arabici, oleosa; Pasta althææ, jujubæ, pectoralis, &c.

ACETUM. *Vinegar.* Acetum distillatum: Syr. aceti; Oxymel; Acetum capsici, colchici (E.), digitalis, lavandulæ, opii (E.,) rubi idæi, rutæ, scillæ (E.), sinapis, &c.

ACIDUM ACETICUM. *Acetic acid.* Acidum aceticum (L. E. & D.); Ac. acet. glaciale (D.), forte (D.), dilutum (L. & D.); Ac. pyroligneum (E.); Acetum aromaticum (P.), antisepticum; Ac. acet. camphoratum; Mist. aceti; Oxymel; Acet. cantharidis, colchici, opii (D.), scillæ (L. & D.)

ACIDUM HYDROCHLORICUM, L. [Muriaticum, E. & D.] *Muriatic or hydrochloric acid.* Acidum hydrochloricum [muriaticum, E. & D.], purum, dilutum; Collutorium, Garg., Julepum; Linimentum muriaticum.

ACIDUM NITRICUM. *Nitric acid.* Ac. nitricum alcoholisatum, purum, fumans, dilutum; Ac. nitro-muriaticum; Causticum nitricum; Haust., Lotio, Julepum acidi nitrici.

ACIDUM SULPHURICUM. *Sulphuric acid.* Acid. sulphuricum purum, dilutum, aromaticum; Elixir acidum Halleri; Causticum sulphuricum; Ung. acidi sulphurici.

ACONITUM. *Leaves (E.), leaves and root (L. & D.) of monkshood (Aconitum Napellus).* Ext., Ext. alcoholicum, ammoniatum, siccum; Pil. aconiti; Tinct. aconiti foliorum, U. S. & P.; Tinct. aconiti [radicis], L., E., D., U. S., Fleming's, Turnbull's; Tinct. ac. ætherea; Ung. aconiti ammoniatum. Aconitina; Liquor aconitinæ; Lotio, et Embr. aconitinæ; Ung. aconitinæ.

ÆTHEREA. *Ethers.* Æther [sulphuricus], lotus; Sp. ætheris co., aromaticus; Sp. æthereus oleosus; Aq. ætheris; Syr. ætheris; Æther aceticus; Sp. Ætheris acetici; Æther chloricus; Chloroformyl; Æther muriaticus; Sp. ætheris muriatici; Sp. febrifugus Cluttoni; Æther nitricus; Sp. ætheris nitrici; Æther cantharidale, ioduretus, phosphoratus; Collodium; Tinct. æthereæ (various).

ALOES. *Aloes.* (Hepatic, Barbadoes, Socotrine, and Indian.) Aloes colata; Aloina; Collyrium Aloeticum; Dec. aloes co., concentratum; Enema aloes; Extr. aloes, Barb.; Ext. rhei co.; Ext. coloc. co.; Inf. aloes; Pil. aloes, comp., et assafœtidæ, dilutæ, et Ferri, et Hydrargyri, cum mastiche, cum rheo, cum myrrhâ, cum sapone, rosatæ, et zingiberis, et terebinthinæ; Pil. Anderson, coloc. co., cambogiæ co., rhei co., sagapeni co., Pulvis aloes co., cum canellâ, cum ferro; Pulv. Anthemidis cum aloe; Solutio Aperiens; Suppositorium anthelminticum; Tinct. aloes, comp. alkalina, ætherea; Tinct. Benzoes co., Myrrhæ et Aloes, Rhei et Aloes; Ung. Aloes; Vin. Aloes, alkalinum.

ALUMEN. *Alum.* Alumen ustum; Garg., Lotio, Inj. Cataplasma, Conf. aluminis; Fotus astringens; Liq. aluminis co.; Pulv. alum co., Pulv. alum cum capsico; Pulv. cubebæ cum alumine; Pulv. aluminis gummosus, saccharatus, opiatus; Pulv. stypticus; Serum aluminis, Ung. aluminis.

AMMONIA. Ammoniæ arsenias, benzoas, bicarbonas, sesquicarbonas, citras, hydriodas, hydrochloras [murias], hydrosulphuretum, nitras, nitro-sulphas, oxalas, phosphas, sulphas, succinas, tartras; Ceratum Ammoniacale; Liq. Ammoniæ, fortior, sesquicarbonatis, acetatis, citratis, tartratis; Empl. ammoniæ; Haust., Inj., Lin. ammoniæ; Mist. ammoniæ acetatis, sesquicarbonatis, muriatis, oleosa, phosphatis; Sp. ammoniæ, aromaticus, comp., fœtidus; Ung. ammoniæ carb., hydriodatis.

ANTIMONIUM. *Antimony.* Antimonii chloridum, terchloridum liquor, cinis, crocus, oxydum, oxychloridum, oxysulphuretum, sulphuretum ppm., tersulphuretum [sesquisulphuretum], sulph. aureum, sulph. precipitatum, potassio-tartras [tartarizatum, E. & D.], regulus, rubinus, tannas; Antimonium calcinatum, vitrifactum; Ant. et sodii sulphuretum; Kermes minerale; Ant. vitrum ceratum; Liq. ant. tartar.; Vin. ant. potassio-tartratis; Emp. antimo. potassio-tart., cum saccharo, cum acido sulph., camphoratum.

ARGENTUM. *Silver.* Argenti ammonio-chloridum, chloridum, cyanidum, iodidum, nitras, oxydum, pulvis; Collyrium, Enema, Inj., Liquor, Lotio, Mist., Pil., Sol., Ung., Argenti nitratis; Liq. arg. acetatis; Pil. arg. iodidi, ammonio-chloridi, chloridi; Pulv. arg. co.; Sol. arg. ammoniati; Ung. arg. oxidi.

ARSENICUM. *Arsenic.* Arsenicum purum; Acid. arseniosum purum; Arsenicum album ppm., sublimatum; Ac. arsenicum, Ammoniæ arsenias, Ars. iodidum; ars. antimoniatum; Liq. pot. arsenitis; Liq. arsen. ammoniæ; Liq. ars. chloridi; Liq. arsenici et iodinii; Liq. ars. periodidi; Pot. arsenias; Sodæ arsenias; Pulv. arsenicalis; Quinæ arsenias; Sol. arsenicalis acida et alkalina; Ung. arsenici, cum sulphure, iodidi, &c.

ASSAFŒTIDA. Empl., Enema, Haust., Mist., Pil., Tinct. assafœtidæ; Assafœtidæ ppa.; Pil. Galbani co.: Sp. ammoniæ fœtidus.

AURUM. *Gold.* Auri pulvis, chloridum, cyanidum, iodidum, oxydum; Auri et sodii chloridum; Aurum stanno paratum; Pil auri co., auri et sodæ muriatis; Pulv. auri co., auri et ferri; Syr. auri; Troch. auri cyanidi; Ung. auri.

BARIUM, and BARYTA. *Barium, and its oxide Barytes.* Barii bromidum, chloridum, iodidum, sulphuretum; Barytæ carbonas, nitras, murias; Liq. barii chloridi; Pil. barii chlor.; Sol. barytæ muriatis; nitratis; Ung. barii iodidi.

BELLADONNA. *Leaves* (fresh and dried, L. &. E.) *and root of* Atropa Belladonna; *deadly nightshade.* Cataplasma, Cerat., Empl., Enema, Inf., Ext., Ext. alcoholicum, Ext. baccarum, Ext. siccum, Lin., Lin. co., Lotio, Lot. co.; Oleum, Pil., Pessus, Pulv. saccharatus, Solutio, Syr.

Tinct., Tinct. ætherea, Ung. Belladonnæ; Ung. bellad. antimoniatum. Atropia; Atropiæ sulph., Collyr. atropiæ, Sol. atropiæ.

BENZOINUM. *Benzoin.* Acidum Benzoicum; Aq. Benzoata; Balneum benzoicum; Fumigatio balsamica; Mist. benzoata; Ol. benzoinum, Tinc. benzoini, comp., Pil. benzoes; Pulv. ac. benz. co. Benzoas ammoniæ, potassæ, sodæ; Pulv. benz. astringens.

CALX. *Lime; Oxide of Calcium.* Calx (viva); Calx e testis; Calcis hydras; Liq. calcis; Aq. calcis. co.; aq. calcis carb.; Calcii bromidum, chloridum, iodidum, sulphuretum; Calcis acetas, carbonas prec., lactas, murias, phosphas; Calx chlorinata; Liq. calcis chlorinatæ; Catapl., Garg., Lotio calcis chlorinatæ; Creta ppa., Cer. cretæ; Ung. plumbi co.; Mist. cretæ; pulv. pro mist. cretæ; Pulv. cretæ co., cum opio; Haust. calcis; Lin. calcis, camphoratum, opiatum; Lotio calcis spirituosa, cum ac hydrocy.; Liq. calcis chloridi, Pil. calcis chloridi; Pulv. calcis phosph. sacch.; Syr. calcis.

CAMPHORA. *Camphor.* Bolús, Cigarra, Enema, Essentia, Emulsio, Haustus, Liquor, Balneum Ceratum camphoræ; Emp. camphoratum; Mist. camphoræ, cum lacte, cum myrrhâ, cum sp. ætheris nitr. carbonica; Lin. camphoræ, comp., aceticum, æthereum, terebinthinatum; Lin. hydrargyri, Lin. saponis, anodynum, cajeputi, ammoniæ co., ammoniæ camphoratum; Lin. Hungaricum, terebinthinatum; Oleum camphoratum, ol. camph. nitricum; Pil. camphoræ; Pulv. camph. nitratus; Solutio camphoræ carbonica, e chloroformo, et myrrhæ; Sp. vel Tinct. camphoræ; Tinct. camph. co., Tinct. opii camph; Vin. camphoratum.

CATECHU. Catapl. astringens; Garg. astr.; Bolus, Ext., Inf., Conf., Elect., Pulvis co., Syr., Troch., Tinct catechu.

CHIRETTA. Inf., Dec., Liquor, Pil., Tinct., chirettæ.

CINCHONA. *Cinchona or Peruvian Bark: red, yellow, and pale.* Bolus febrifugus, ad quartanum; Catap. antisepticum; Cer. cinchonæ; Cerevisia cinch.; Conf. cinch.; Dec. cinchonæ [flavæ et pallidæ], acidulatum cum serpentariâ; Elect. cinch. co.; Ext. cinchonæ, siccum, resinosum, fluidum; Garg. cinchonæ; Haust. cinch.: Mist. cinch.; Inf. cinchonæ, spissatum; Inf. cinch. sine calore, cum aquâ calcis, cum magnesiâ; Pulv. alterativus (CLINE); Pulv. cinch. co., cum antim., cum myrrhâ, cum rheo, laxans; Syr. cinchonæ, concentratus, vinosus; Tinct. cinch., comp., ammoniata; Vin. cinchonæ, et valerianæ. [For Quinine and its preparations, see QUINA, below.] Cinchonia; Cinchoniæ disulphas; Syr., Tinct., Vin. cinchoniæ.

COLCHICUM. *Seeds and corms of meadow saffron.* Acetum colchici; Colchicina; Ext. colchici; Ext. col. aceticum; Haust. colch., Mist. colch., Lin. colchici; Oxymel colchici; Pil. colchici cum opio; Pil. coloc. cum colchico; Pulv. colchici co.; Succus colchici; Syr. Colchici; Tinct. colchici [sem.], e radice, florum extracti; Tinct. colch. co.; Vin. colchici; V. colch. sem.; Vin. colch. opiatum.

COLOCYNTHIS. *Colocynth pulp.* Col. præparata; Enema, Extr.; Ext. comp.; Decoctum, Oleum colocynthidis; Pil. coloc. co., simpliciores, et calomelanos, et crotonis, et colchici, ferrosæ, et hyoscyami, cum scammonio; Tinct. colocynthidis; Vin. colocynthidis.

CONIUM. *Hemlock.* Cataplasma, Conf. Empl., Ext., Ext. alcohol., Inf.,

Mist., Oleum, Pil., Pil. conii co., Pil. conii cum hydr.; Tinct. conii, ætherea; Ung. Conii. Conia, Sol. coniæ, Syr. coniæ.

Copaiba. *Balsam of Copaiva.* Bolus, Ceratum, Emulsio, Enema, Elect., Ext., Haustus, Injectio; Mist. copaibæ, benzoata, cum hemidesmo, vinosa; Ol. copaibæ; Pil. copaibæ; Sol. copaibæ alkalina; Syr. copaibæ.

Cubebæ. *Cubebs.* Bolus cubebæ; Elect. cubebæ et copaibæ; Emulsio cubebæ; Enema cubebæ; Ess. cubebæ; Ext. cubebæ, fluidum; Mist. cubebæ; Oleum cubebæ; Pulv. cubebæ cum alumine; Tinct. cubebæ.

Digitalis. *Foxglove.* Acet., Catapl., Ext., Fomentum, Inf., Lin., Pil. digitalis; Syr. digitalis; Tinct. digitalis; Vin. digitalis. Digitalina; Pil. digitalinæ.

Ferrum. *Iron.* Ferrum reductum (pulvis); Limatura ferri, ppta, lævigata; Ferri acetas, ammonio-chloridum, ammonio-citras, ammonio-tartras, arsenias, bromidum, carbonas, carb. cum saccharo, chloridum chlor. hydratum, perchloridum, citras, et potassæ citras, et sodæ citras, et quinæ citras, ferro-cyanuretum, iodidum, lactas, oxydum nigrum (magneticum), sesquioxydum, oxydum rubrum, peroxydum, perox. hydratum, pernitratis liquor, phosphas, oxyphosphas, biphosphas, potassio-tartras, bitartras cum potassæ sulphate, proto-tartras, rubigo, sulphas, s. granulatum, s. exsiccatum, persulphas, et aluminæ bisulphas, sulphuretum, proto-sulphuretum hydratum, pers. hydratum, sulpho-cyanidum, tannas, valerianas; Ferrugo [peroxydum hydratum]; Aq. chalybeata aerata; Balneum ferri; Bolus ferri; Conf. ferri subc., Elect. ejusdem; Emp. ferri; Enema ferri muriatis, ferri percyanidi, f. tartarizata; Guttæ emmenagogæ; Haust. ferri effervescens, aeratus, et magnesiæ; iodidi, protoxydi; Inj. ferri iodidi; Liq. ferri acetatis alkalini, chloridi, sesquichloridi, citratis, iodidi, p. tart.; Mist. ferri aromatica; Mist. ferri co., Mist. ferri arsenicalis, Mist. ferri cum aloe, ferri iodidi; Pil ferri cum absinthio; Pil. ferri ammoniati, ammonio-citratis, arseniatis, bromidi chloridi, compositæ, carbonatis, cum aloe, et conii, et copaibæ, fœtidæ, cum gentianâ, iodidi, lactatis, percyanidi, subphosphatis, superphosphatis, sulphatis, sulphureti, et quinæ iodidi, manganesii et ferri; Pulv. ferri comp., cum ipecac., ferro-carbonicus; Saccharum Martis; Solutio ferri aluminosa, am. tart, bromidi, iodidi, sesqui-iodidi, oxysulphatis, et quinæ phosphatis, sulphatis; Syrupus ferri, sulphatis, acetatis, albuminatis, protochloridi perchloridi, ferri et quinæ citratis, potassio-citratis, iodidi, iod. comp., iod. et ferri chloridi, ferri lactatis, potassio-tart., sesquicarb., subcarb., sulphatis, sulphureti, per-phosphatis, superphosphatis, tannatis; Tinctura ferri acetatis, f. a. ætherea, potassio-acetatis, ammonio-chloridi, aurantiaca, cydoniata, proto-iodidi, pomati, sesquichloridi, tartarizati; Trochisci ferri citratis, et magn. citratis, iodidi, lactatis; Ung. ferri arseniatis, iodidi, oxydi, phosphatis, prussiatis, sulphatis; Vinum ferri, acetatis, citratis, iodidi; Chocolata ferri.

Hydrargyrum. *Quicksilver.* Hydrargyri acetas, ammonio-chloridum, bicyanidum, bromidum, iodidum, biniodidum, chloro-iodidum, proto-nitras, deuto-nitras liquidus, pernitras liq., oxydum, nitrico-oxydum (oxydum rubrum, E.), subsulphas, sulphas, phosphas, potassio-iodo-cyanidum, potassio-iodidum, precipitatum nigrum, et quinæ chloridum, subsulphas flavus, sulphuretum cum sulphure, bisulphuretum, tartras, potassio-tartras; Hydrargyrum purum, cum cretâ, cum magnesiâ; Balneum Hydr. bichloridi; Causticum hydrargyri; Cer. mercuriale, hydr. compositum, hydr. nitratis; Collyrium hydr. chloridi, bichloridi; Fumigatio mercurialis; Gargarisma hydrar. bichloridi. Guttæ hyd. bichloridi, Inject. hyd. bichl.; Julepum hyd. bich.; Liq. hyd. bich.; Liq. hyd. bicyanidi, cyanidi iodidi potassii: Liq. hyd. protonitratis and deuto-nitratis; Linim. hydrargyri, cum iodinio, nitratis, nitrico-oxydi; Lotio hyd. acetatis; Pessus hydrargyri; Pil. hydrargyri; Pil. hyd. aloeticæ, camphoratæ, cum colocynthide, cum conio, et hyoscyami, cum rheo, cum scillâ, cum stearino, cum sapone; Pil. hydr. acetatis; Pil. hydr. chloridi, comp., cum opio, cum scillâ; Pil. hydr. bichloridi, cum aconito, albumine, conio, glutine, guaiaco; Pil. hydr. et quinæ chloridi; Pil. hyd. iodidi, deuto-iodidi, et pot. iodidi, protoxydi, phosphatis, Hahnemanni, proto-nitratis; Pulv. calomelanos arsenicalis; P. hydr. comp.; Sapo hydr., bichloridi, precipitati albi et rubri; Sol. hydr. co.; Sol. hyd. bichloridi, deuto-iodidi; Syr. hydrargyri; Troch. calomelanos; Ung. hydrargyri, hydr. mitius, cum amylo, cum belladonnâ, camphoratum, cum ammoniæ muriate, opiatum, cum pice, cum sodâ, ioduretum, ammonio-chloridi, chloridi cum sapone; Ung. calomelanos, hydr. bichloridi, chloro-iodidi, cyanidi, iodidi, biniodidi, proto-nitratis; Ung. hydr. nitratis, mitius, nitrico-oxydi, oxydi cinerei, subsulphatis, biphosphatis, sulphureti rubri.

Hyoscyamus. *Henbane.* Catap., Emp., Extr., Haustus, Oleum, Pil., Syr., Tinct. Hyoscyami.

Iodinium. *Iodine.* Æther ioduretus; Aquæ iodinii; Balneum, Catapl., Causticum, Empl., Collyr., Garg., Iodinii; Liq. iodinii co., Mist. iod. cum sarsa, &c.; Pil. iodinii; Solutiones iodinii (Lugol's); Sol. iod. cum conio; Tinct. iodinii; Tinct. iod. co.; Syr. iod.; Syr. iod. cum tannino; Arsenici, barii, calcii, ferri, hydrargyri, magnesii, potassii, sodii, sulphuris, zinci iodidum; Liq. arsenici periodidi; Liq. ferri iod.; Pil. ferri iodidi; Syr. ferri iodidi; Syr. ferri iod. et chloridi; Syr. ferri et quinæ iodidi; vin. ferri iodidi; Pil. hydr. iodidi et biniodidi; Ung. hydr. iod. et biniod.; Empl. potassii iodidi; Mist. pot. iodidi; Pil. pot. iod.; Sol. p. iod.; Pil. sulph. iod.; Ung. sulph. iod.; Syr. zinci iodidi; Iodoformum; Pil. iodoformi.

Ipecacuanha. Enema, Ext., Haust. ipec., &c.; Mist. ipec. alkalina; M. ipec. et sennæ, &c.; Pil. ipec. co.; Pil. ipec. cum Scillâ, &c.; Pulv. emeticus; Pulv. ipec. co.; P. ipec. cum nitro, rheo, &c.; Syr. Ipec.; Tinct. Ipec.; Tinct. ipec. anisata; Troch. ipec.; Troch. ipec. cum camphorâ, &c.; Troch. ipec. et scillæ; Troch. morphiæ, et ipec.; Vin. ipec.; Lin. ipecac.; Ung. ipecacuanhæ.

Jalapa. *Jalap root.* Ext. jalapæ; Ext. jal. alkalinum; Pil. jalapæ; Pil. jalap. co., alkalina, cum colocynth, &c.; Pulv. jalapæ co., aurantiacus, cum ipec., &c.; Panes purgantes; Saccharum jalapæ; Syr. jalapinus; Tinct. jalapæ; Tinct. jal. comfortans; Sapo jalapinus; jalapina; Resina jalapæ.

Lobelia Inflata. Acet.; Ext.; Syr.; Tinct.; Tinct. ætherea, Whitlaw's.

Magnesia. Magnesia [calcinata]; Mag. calc. ponderosa; Magn. carbonas; Magn. carb. ponderosa; Magn. citras, boro-citras, phosphas, sulphas, ferro-sulphas, tartras, potassio-tartras; Magn. et quinæ sulphas; Haust. magnesiæ; H. magn. effervescens, sulphatis, &c.; Haust. aperiens, niger; Mist. aperiens; M. magn. bicarbonatis, sulphatis, &c.; Liq.

magn. carb., aeratus sulph., &c.; Pulv. magn. tartaricus, cum rheo; Pulv. rhei co.; Sol. magn. sulph., &c.

MANGANESIUM. *Manganese.* Manganesii acetas, carbonas, chloridum, iodidum, malas, oxydum hydratum, phosphas, sulphas, tartras; Garg. manganesii acet., oxydi; Pil. magnesii carbonatis, iodidi, malatis, muriatis, phosphatis, tartratis, et ferri sulphatis; Syr. mangan. iodidi, malatis, phosphatis, tartratis.

MATICO. Decoctum; Infus.; Liquor, Tinctura.

MORPHIA. Morphiæ acetas, bimeconas, hydriodas; Morph. hydriod. cum iodinio, cum zinco; M. hydrochloras, nitras, sulphas, tartras; Enema morphiæ; Liq. morphiæ acetatis, citratis, muriatis (hydrochloratis), sulphatis; Sol. morphiæ bimeconatis, muriatis, &c.; Syr. morphiæ acetatis, muriatis, sulphatis.

NUX VOMICA, ET STRYCHNIA. Ext. nucis vomicæ; Ext. aquosum; Haust. Inf., Pil. n. v.; Pulv. n. v. co.; Lin. nucis v.; Tinct. nucis vomicæ; Strychnia; Strychniæ acetas, hydriodas, murias, nitras, phosphas, sulphas; Collyr. str. acetatis; Lin. strychniæ; Mist. strychniæ; Pil. strychniæ; Pulv. strychn. cum saccharo; Sol. strychn. acetatis; Tinct. Ung. strychniæ.

OPIUM. Acetum opii; Aqua, Cerat., Conf., Elect., Emp., Enema Opii; Ext. opii; Ext. opii absque narcotinâ; Ext. opii per ferment., torrefacti, vinosum; Liquor opii aceticus, citricus, muriaticus, tartaricus, sedativus, concentratus; Collyr. opiatum; Linctus opiatus; Lin. opii; Oleum opiatum; Pil. opii; Pil. calomel, et opii; Pil. opii comp.; Pil. saponis cum opio; Pulv. cretæ cum opio; P. ipec. comp.; Suppositorium opii; Syr. opii; Tinct. opii; Tinct. opii acetata, ammoniata, aromatica, camphorata, Eccardi, fœtida; Vin. opii; Vin. opii ferment.; Guttæ nigræ; Troch. opii; Troch. glyc. cum opio; Ung. opii; Ung. opiatum cum felle, cum succo gastrico. [For Morphia and its preparations, see Morphia, above.]

PAPAVER; *Poppy:* and P. RHŒAS. *Red Poppy.* Catapl. papaveris; Collyr., Decoct., Emulsio, Syrupus, Fotus, Troch. papaveris; Syr. rhæados; Syr. anticatarrhalis.

PHOSPHORUS. Æther phosphoratus; Lin. phosphoratum; Mist. phosphori; Ol. phosp.; Sol., Tinct. ætherea phosphori.; Ung. phosphoratum; Acidum phosphoricum.

PIPER. *Pepper.* (P. nigrum; *Black Pepper.* P. longum; *Long Pepper.*) Conf. piperis; Ext. piperis fluidum; Ol. piperis; Ung. pip. nigri, comp. Tinct. piperis, stomachica; Piperina. Pil. piperinæ, cum hydrargyro; Pulv. piperis; P. cretæ co.; P. pepticus.

PLUMBUM. *Lead.* Plumbi acetas, diacetas, carbonas, chloridum, cyanidum, iodidum, nitras, oxydum hydratum, oxyd. semivitreum, ox. rubrum, saccharas, tannas; Collyr. Emp., Inj.; Lin.; plumbi; Emp. varia; Lotio plumbi acet., acet., diac., opiata, chloridi; Liq. Plumbi diac., d. dilutus; Pil. plumbi opiatæ, iodidi; Ung. plumbi acetatis, carbonatis c. camphoratum, comp., chloridi, iodidi, tannatis, Ung. plumbi cum aq. lauro-cerasi, cum ac. hydrocyanico.

POTASSA. *Potash, oxide of Potassium.* Potassæ acetas, arsenias, antimonias, arsenitis liquor, benzoas, boras, boro-tartras, carbonas, bicarbonas, chloras, chromas, citras, hydras, hydrocyanas, iodas, nitras, nitras fusa, silicas, sulphas, bisulphas, c. cum sulphuro, tartras, ammonio tartras, bitartras; Potassii bromidum, chloridum, iodidum, sulphuretum; Liq. potassæ; Liq. Pot. Brandishii; Liq. pot. acetatis, arsenitis, carbonatis, chlorinatæ, citratis, effervescens; Elect. pot. nitratis; Haust. pot. acetatis, citratis; Liq. potassii iodidi, cyanidi, sulphureti; Mist. pot. cum calce, pot. supertartratis; Mist. pot. bromidi, cyanidi, iodidi; Pulv. pot. nitr. co.; P. pot. sulph. cum rheo; Ung. potassii cyanidi, iodidi, iod. opiatum, sulphureti.

QUINA. *Quinine.* Quina; quina amorpha, q. impura; Quina acetas, arsenias, diarsenias, arsenis, citras, ferro-prussias, iodidum, kinas, lactas, murias, nitras, phosphas, sulphas (disulphas), sulphas neutralis, tannas, tartras, sulpho-tartras, valerianas; Embroc., Empl. quinæ; Haust. quinæ acidus, cum zinco; Liq. quinæ sulphatis (amorphous); Mist. quinæ muriatis, tartarica, cum coffeâ, cum opio; Pil. quinæ sulphatis, comp. cum camphorâ; Pil. q. ferrocyanidi; Pulv. quinæ aeratus, q. cum antimonio, cum morphiâ, &c.; Sol. q. sulphatis, et ferri, q. citratis, &c.; Syr. q. citratis, sulpho-tartratis, iodidi, et ferri iodidi; Syr. q. cum coffeâ, dikinatis; Tinct. quinæ comp., acida, impuræ, hydroferrocyanidi; Troch. quinæ.

RHATANIA. (Krameria triandria.) *Rhatany root.* Ext. krameriæ; Inf. krameriæ; Pil. rhat. et rhei; Suppos. rhataniæ; Syr. krameriæ; Tinct. krameriæ; Tinct. rhat. aromatica.

RHEUM. *Rhubarb.* Extr. rhei; Ext. rhei fluidum; Liquor rhei; Mist. rhei; Mist. rhei co.; Pil. rhei; Pil. rhei co., cum opio, sodâ, &c.; Pulv. rhei co.; et hydrarg., opiatus, salinus, &c.; Tinct. rhei; Tinct. rhei co.. anisata, rhei et aloes, et gentianæ, et sennæ; Troch. rhei, Troch. r. aromatici; Rheum ustum. Rheina.

SARSA. *Sarsaparilla root.* Dec. sarsæ; Dec. sarsæ comp.; Dec. s. cum sennâ cum icthyocollâ; Ess., Ess. Co., Ext. sarsæ; Ext. sarsæ co., alcoholicum, fluidum; Inf. sarsæ, frigidum, acidum, alkalinum; Liquor; Syr. sarsæ; Syr. s. comp., ioduretus, cum extr. sarsæ; Tinct. sarsæ, s. co., Pulv. alterativus (CLINE'S); Vin. sarsap. co.

SCAMMONIUM. *Scammony.* Conf., Haustus, Mist., Emulsio purgans, Panes scammonii; Pil. scam. co.; Pil. coloc. co. &c.; Pulv. scammonii comp., cum aloe, c. calomelane, &c.; Pulv. basilicus; Tinct. sc.; Troch. scammonii.

SCILLA. *Squill bulb.* Acetum, Bolus, Extr., Mel. scillæ; Mist. scillæ co.; Oxymel scillæ; Oxym. scillæ co.; Pil. scillæ comp., cum ammoniaco, cum crotone, cum hydrarg., &c., Pil. ipec. cum scillâ; Pulv. s. co.: Syr. scillæ; Syr. scillæ co.; Troch. scillæ, cum ipecac.; Tinct. scillæ, alkalina, &c.; Vin scillæ comp., V. scilliticum amarum; Ung. scillæ; Dec. scillæ comp.; Emp. scillæ co.

SENNA. Conf., Elect., Inf. sennæ; Inf. sennæ comp., cum coffeâ, limoniatum, tartarisatum, cum tamarindo; Haust. sennæ, niger. &c.; Liquor sennæ; Liq. sennæ aromat.; Mist. aperiens, sennæ, &c.; Syr. sennæ, concentratus; Tinct. sennæ comp., aromatica; Tinct. rhei et sennæ; Vin. sennæ.

SODA. *Soda, or Oxide of Sodium.* Sodæ acetas, arsenias, benzoas, biboras, carbonas, c. exsiccata, bicarbonas, clorinata, hydrosulphas, hydrosulphis, murias, phosphas, sulphas, bisulphas, potassio-tartras, valerianas; Sodii chloridum, iodidum, sulphuretum; Balneum sodæ chlorinatæ, alkalinum; Catap. sodæ chl.; Enema sodæ chl.; Garg. sodæ chl.; Collyr. sodii chloridi; Liq. sodæ (causticæ), carbonatis, effervescens; Liq. sodæ tart. efferv.; Mist. sodæ sulphatis, sodii chloridii; Pil. sodæ cum sapone, cum hydrargyro; Pulv. sodæ comp., cum hydrargyro, muriatis co.; sulphatis co.; Sol. sodæ carb., s. phosphatis; Syr. sodæ hyposulphitis; Troch. sodæ bicarb., chlorinatæ, cum zingibere; Saponis; Ung. alkalinum.

SULPHUR. Bals. sulphuris; Conf. sulph. co.; Elect. sulph. comp.; Elect. hæmorrhoidale; Elect. anti-rheumaticum; Lin. sulphuris cum sapone; Lotio sulphuris, comp.; Sulphur fuscum, lotum, precipitatum, hypochloridum, iodidum; Pulv. s. co.; Troch. sulphuris; Ung. sulphuris s. comp., alkalinum, cum carbone, cum pice, cum zinco; Ung. sulphuris hypochloridi, iodidi.

TARAXACUM. *Dandelion.* Decoctum, Extr., Ext., Fluidum, Mellago, Cremor, Liquor, Succus taraxaci.

TEREBINTHINA. *Turpentine.* Balneum, Bals., Conf., Elect., Enema, terebinthinæ; Lin. tereb.; Lin. tereb. aceticum, ammoniatum, vitriolicum; Mist. tereb.; Mist. tereb. Venetæ; Ol. tereb. purificatum; Pil. tereb., tereb. cum rheo; Sapo terebinthinæ; Tereb. colata, cocta; Ung. tereb. ammoniatum.

VALERIANA. *Valerian root.* Aqua valerianæ; Elect. anti-epilepticum, vermifugum; Ext. valer.; Ext. val. fluidum; Inf., Syr., Tinct. valerianæ; Tinct. valer. co., ætherea; Vin. cinchonæ et. valer.; Acidum valerianicum; Bismuthi, ferri. quinæ, sodæ, zinci valerianas; Pil. valer. co.; Pil. zinci valerianatis.

ZINGIBER. *Ginger.* Cerevisia, Empl., Lin., Ess., Syr. Tinct., Troch. Zingiberis.

ZINCUM. *Zinc.* Zinci acetas, carbonas, chloridum, chloridi liquor, cyanidum, ferrocyanidum, iodidum, Z. et ammoniæ iodidum, lactas, oxydum, oxydum hydratum, sulphas, tannas, valerianas; Collyrium, Garg., Inj., Lotio, zinci sulphatis, &c.; Mist. zinci co.; Pil. zinci sulph., cum gentianâ, myrrhâ, &c.; Pulv. Zinci cyanidi co.; Pulv. z. sulph. co.; Sol. zinci acetatis; ætherea, alkalina, sulphatis; Syr. zinci iodidi; Troch. zinci; Ung. zinci oxydi, cum myrrhâ, cum opio, et lycopodii; Ung. zinci cyanidi, iodidi, sulphatis; Causticum zinci, antimoniale, comp., cum opio; Pessus zinci.

www.ingramcontent.com/pod-product-compliance
Lightning Source LLC
LaVergne TN
LVHW021313110826
845150LV00003B/561

* 9 7 8 1 4 2 5 5 5 8 4 7 5 *